# Trace Metals and Infectious Diseases

# Strüngmann Forum Reports

Julia Lupp, series editor

The Ernst Strüngmann Forum is made possible through
the generous support of the Ernst Strüngmann Foundation,
inaugurated by Dr. Andreas and Dr. Thomas Strüngmann.

This Forum was supported by funds from the
Deutsche Forschungsgemeinschaft
(German Science Foundation)

# Trace Metals and Infectious Diseases

*Edited by*

Jerome O. Nriagu and Eric P. Skaar

*Program Advisory Committee:*

Rodney R. Dietert, Julia Lupp, Jerome O. Nriagu, Lothar Rink, Anthony B. Schryvers, and Eric P. Skaar

The MIT Press

Cambridge, Massachusetts
London, England

© 2015 Massachusetts Institute of Technology and
the Frankfurt Institute for Advanced Studies

Series Editor: J. Lupp
Assistant Editor: M. Turner
Photographs: U. Dettmar
Lektorat: BerlinScienceWorks

MIT Press books may be purchased at special quantity discounts
for business or sales promotional use. For information, please email
special_sales@mitpress.mit.edu.

The book was set in TimesNewRoman and Arial.
Printed and bound in the United States of America.

Library of Congress Cataloging-in-Publication Data

Trace metals and infectious diseases / edited by Jerome O. Nriagu and Eric P.
Skaar.
pages    cm. — (Strüngmann Forum reports)
Includes bibliographical references and index.
ISBN 978-0-262-02919-3 (hardcover : alk. paper)
1. Trace elements—Toxicology. 2. Trace elements—Environmental
aspects. 3. Communicable diseases. I. Nriagu, Jerome O., editor II. Skaar,
Eric P. (Eric Patrick), editor.
TD196.T7T725   2015
614.4—dc23
                                                            2014039756

10 9 8 7 6 5 4 3 2 1

# Contents

# The Ernst Strüngmann Forum

Founded on the tenets of scientific independence and the inquisitive nature of the human mind, the Ernst Strüngmann Forum is dedicated to the continual expansion of knowledge. Through its innovative communication process, the Ernst Strüngmann Forum provides a creative environment within which experts scrutinize high-priority issues from multiple vantage points.

This process begins with the identification of themes. By nature, a theme constitutes a problem area that transcends classic disciplinary boundaries. It is of high-priority interest, requiring concentrated, multidisciplinary input to address the issues. Proposals are received from leading scientists active in their field and reviewed by an independent Scientific Advisory Board. Once approved, we convene a steering committee to refine the scientific parameters of the proposal and select participants. Approximately one year later, a central gathering, or Forum, is held to which circa forty experts are invited.

Preliminary discussion for this theme began in 2012. Impetus behind this theme was the growing concern that human beings may inadvertently be contributing to an epidemic of trace metal deficiency—one that affects billions of people worldwide and is especially prevalent in developing countries. From January 26–29, 2013, the Program Advisory Committee met to transform the approved proposal into a working scientific framework that would support the ensuing discussion. The collective expertise and international experience of the committee members— Rodney R. Dietert, Jerome O. Nriagu, Lothar Rink, Anthony B. Schryvers, and Eric P. Skaar—were instrumental in refining the issues for debate.

From January 19–24, 2014, the Forum was held in Frankfurt am Main. The activities and discourse that surround a Forum begin well beforehand and conclude with the publication of this volume. Throughout each stage, focused dialog is the means by which issues are examined anew. Often, this requires relinquishing long-established ideas and overcoming disciplinary idiosyncrasies that might otherwise bias or inhibit joint examination. When this is accomplished, synergism results from which new insights can emerge.

This volume conveys the ideas and input of a diverse group of experts, each of whom assumed an active role, and it is comprised of two types of contributions. The first set provides background information on key aspects of the overall theme. Originally written in advance of the Forum, these chapters have been extensively reviewed and revised to provide current understanding on these key topics. The second set (Chapters 7, 13, 17, and 20) summarizes the extensive group discussions that transpired. These chapters should not be viewed as consensus documents nor are they proceedings; their purpose is to transfer the essence of the multifaceted discussions, to expose areas where opinions diverge and open questions remain, and to highlight topics in need of future enquiry.

An endeavor of this kind creates its own unique dynamics and puts demands on everyone who participates. Invitees must embrace the process with a willingness to probe beyond that which is evident, and I wish to extend my gratitude to all. A special word of thanks goes to the Program Advisory Committee as well as to the authors and reviewers of the background papers. The work of the moderators of the individual working groups (Robert Perry, Robert Black, Ellen Silbergeld, and Joseph Caruso) is gratefully acknowledged. In addition, I am especially grateful to the rapporteurs (Jennifer Cavet, Dieter Rehder, Leigh Ackland, and Wolfgang Maret), who drafted the group reports during the Forum and brought them to their final form. Most importantly, I extend my sincere appreciation to Jerome Nriagu and Eric Skaar, chairpersons of this 16th ES Forum. Their commitment and steady guidance throughout the entire process ensured a most vibrant intellectual gathering.

A communication process of this nature relies on institutional stability and an environment that encourages free thought. The generous support of the Ernst Strüngmann Foundation, established by Dr. Andreas and Dr. Thomas Strüngmann in honor of their father, enables the Ernst Strüngmann Forum to conduct its work in the service of science. In addition, the following valuable partnerships are gratefully acknowledged: the Scientific Advisory Board, which ensures the scientific independence of the Forum; the German Science Foundation, for its supplemental financial support; and the Frankfurt Institute for Advanced Studies, which shares its vibrant intellectual setting with the Forum.

Long-held views are never easy to put aside. Yet, when this is achieved, when the edges of the unknown begin to appear and the resulting knowledge gaps are able to be identified, the act of formulating strategies to fill them becomes a most invigorating activity. It is our hope that this volume will convey a sense of this lively exercise and inspire further scientific enquiry into the linkages between trace metals and the pathogenesis of infectious disease.

Julia Lupp, Program Director Ernst Strüngmann Forum
Frankfurt Institute for Advanced Studies (FIAS)
Ruth-Moufang-Str. 1, 60438 Frankfurt am Main, Germany
http://esforum.de/

# List of Contributors

**Ackland, M. Leigh**   Deakin University, Burwood Campus, Burwood 3125, Australia

**Andisi, Vahid Fa**   Departments of Microbiology, Immunology and Infectious Diseases, University of Calgary, Calgary, Canada

**Arrieta, Angel L.**   Department of Microbiology and Immunology, Life Sciences Institute, University of British Columbia, Vancouver, BC V6T 1Z3, Canada

**Bachman, Michael A.**   Department of Pathology, University of Michigan, Ann Arbor, MI 48109, U.S.A.

**Becker, J. Sabine**   Central Institute for Engineering, Electronics and Analytics, Forschungszentrum Jülich, 52425 Jülich, Germany

**Black, Robert E.**   Department of International Health, John Hopkins University, Baltimore, MD 21205, U.S.A.

**Bornhorst, Julia**   Institut für Ernährungswissenschaft, Universität Potsdam, 14558 Nuthetal, OT Bergholz-Rehbrücke, Germany

**Brunke, Sascha**   Department of Microbial Pathogenicity Mechanisms, Hans Knöll Institute, 07745 Jena, Germany

**Caruso, Joseph A.**   Department of Chemistry, University of Cincinnati, Cincinnati, OH 45221-0172, U.S.A.

**Cavet, Jennifer S.**   Faculty of Life Sciences, University of Manchester, Manchester, M13 9PT, U.K.

**Chan, Anson C. K.**   Department of Microbiology and Immunology, Life Sciences Institute, University of British Columbia, Vancouver, BC V6T 1Z3, Canada

**Contag, Christopher H.**   Stanford University School of Medicine, Stanford, CA 94305-5427, U.S.A.

**Darwin, K. Heran**   Department of Microbiology, NYU Langone Medical Center, New York, NY 10016, U.S.A.

**Dedoussis, George V.**   Harokopio University, Kallithea-Athens, Greece

**Dietert, Rodney R.**   Department of Microbiology and Immunology, College of Veterinary Medicine, Cornell University, Ithaca, NY 14853, U.S.A.

**DiRita, Victor J.**   Department of Microbiology and Immunology, University of Michigan Medical School, Ann Arbor, MI 48109-5620, U.S.A.

**Fierke, Carol A.**   Department of Chemistry, University of Michigan, Ann Arbor, MI 48109-1055, U.S.A.

**García-Barrera, Tamara**   Department of Chemistry and Materials Science, and Research Center on Health and Environment (CYSMA), University of Huelva, 21071 Huelva, Spain

**Giedroc, David P.**   Department of Chemistry, Indiana University, Bloomington, IN 47405-7102, U.S.A.

**Hagedoorn, Peter-Leon**   Department of Biotechnology, Delft University of Technology, 2628 BC Delft, The Netherlands

**Imlay, James A.**   Department of Microbiology, University of Illinois, Urbana, IL 61801, U.S.A.

**Kobylarz, Marek J.**   Department of Microbiology and Immunology, Life Sciences Institute, University of British Columbia, Vancouver, BC V6T 1Z3, Canada

**Lemire, Joseph**   Department of Biological Science, University of Calgary, Calgary, AB T2N 1N4, Canada

**Liu, Wenwen**   Department of Chemical Engineering, Northeastern University, Boston, Massachusetts, U.S.A. 02115 and Department of Prosthodontics, School of Stomatology, Capital Medical University, Beijing 100050, P.R. China

**Loutet, Slade A.**   Department of Microbiology and Immunology, Life Sciences Institute, University of British Columbia, Vancouver, BC V6T 1Z3, Canada

**Maret, Wolfgang**   Diabetes and Nutritional Sciences, King's College London, London, SE1 9NH, U.K.

**Matusch, Andreas**   Institute for Neuroscience and Medicine, Forschungszentrum Jülich, 52425 Jülich, Germany

**Moraes, Trevor F.**   Department of Biochemistry, University of Toronto, Toronto, ON M5S 1AS, Canada

**Murphy, Michael E. P.**   Department of Microbiology and Immunology, University of British Columbia, Vancouver, BC V6T 1Z3, Canada

**Navarro, Maribel**   Directoria de Metrologia Aplicada á ciências da vida, Instituto Nacional de Metrologia, Normalização e Qualidade Industrial, Rio de Janeiro, Brasil

**Nriagu, Jerome O.**   Center for Human Growth and Development, School of Public Health, University of Michigan, Ann Arbor, MI 48109-2029, U.S.A.

**Oros-Peusquens, Ana-Maria**   Institute for Neuroscience and Medicine, Forschungszentrum Jülich, 52425 Jülich, Germany

**Pacyna, Elisabeth G.**   NILU – Norwegian Institute for Air Research, 2027 Kjeller, Norway

**Pacyna, Jozef M.**   NILU – Norwegian Institute for Air Research, 2027 Kjeller, Norway and The Gdansk University of Technology, Department of Chemistry, Gdansk, Poland

**Perry, Robert D.**   Department of Microbiology, Immunology and Molecular Genetics, University of Kentucky, Lexington, KY 40536-0298, U.S.A.

**Pettifor, John M.**   Developmental Pathways for Health Research Unit, University of the Witwatersrand, Faculty of Health Sciences, Johannesburg 2193, South Africa

**Pfaffen, Stephanie**   Department of Microbiology and Immunology, Life Sciences Institute, University of British Columbia, Vancouver, BC V6T 1Z3, Canada

**Rehder, Dieter**   Department of Chemistry, University of Hamburg, 20146 Hamburg, Germany

**Rink, Lothar**   Institute of Immunology, 52074 Aachen, Germany

**Schryvers, Anthony B.**   Department of Microbiology, Immunology and Infectious Diseases, Calgary, AB T2N 4N1, Canada

**Silbergeld, Ellen K.**   Bloomberg School of Public Health, John Hopkins University, Baltimore, MD 21205, U.S.A.

**Skaar, Eric P.**   Department of Pathology, Microbiology and Immunology, Vanderbilt University Medical Center, Nashville, TN 37232-2363, U.S.A.

**Soares, Miguel C. P.**   Instituto Gulbenkian de Ciencia, 2780-156 Oeiras, Portugal

**Sundseth, Kyrre**   NILU – Norwegian Institute for Air Research, 2027 Kjeller, Norway

**Thiele, Dennis J.**   Department of Pharmacology and Cancer Biology, Duke University School of Medicine, Durham, NC 27710, U.S.A.

**Thompson, Richard B.**   Department of Biochemistry and Molecular Biology, University of Maryland School of Medicine, Baltimore, MD 21212, U.S.A.

**Verstraete, Meghan M.**   Department of Microbiology and Immunology, Life Sciences Institute, University of British Columbia, Vancouver, BC V6T 1Z3, Canada

**Visbal, Gonzalo**   Directoria de Metrologia Aplicada á ciências da vida, Instituto Nacional de Metrologia, Normalização e Qualidade Industrial, Rio de Janeiro, Brazil

**Wang, Fudi**   Laboratory of Nutrition and Metabolism, Center for Nutrition and Health, Department of Nutrition, School of Public Health, School of Medicine, and Institute of Nutrition and Food Safety, Collaborative Innovation Center for Diagnosis and Treatment of Infectious Diseases, Zhejiang University, Hangzhou 310058, P. R. China

**Wang, Mian**   Department of Chemical Engineering, Northeastern University, Boston, Massachusetts 02115, U.S.A.

**Webster, Thomas J.**   Department of Chemical Engineering, Northeastern University, Boston, Massachusetts 02115, U.S.A. and Center of Excellence for Advanced Materials Research, King Abdulaziz University, Jeddah, Saudi Arabia

**Weiser, Jeffrey N.**   Departments of Microbiology and Pediatrics, University of Pennsylvania School of Medicine, Philadelphia, PA 19104-6076, U.S.A.

**Weiss, Günter**   Department of Internal Medicine VI, Infectious Diseases, Immunology, Rheumatology, and Pneumology, Medical University of Innsbruck, 6020 Innsbruck, Austria

**Wessels, Inga**   Food Science and Human Nutrition Department, University of Florida Gainesville, FL 32611-0370, U.S.A.

**Ye, Bin**   Department of Microbiology and Immunology, Life Sciences Institute, University of British Columbia, Vancouver, BC V6T 1Z3, Canada

**Zhang, Lihong**   Laboratory of Nutrition and Metabolism, Center for Nutrition and Health, Department of Nutrition, School of Public Health, School of Medicine, and Institute of Nutrition and Food Safety, Collaborative Innovation Center for Diagnosis and Treatment of Infectious Diseases, Zhejiang University, Hangzhou 310058, P.R. China

# 1

# Introduction

Jerome O. Nriagu and Eric P. Skaar

The presence of a safe and adequate supply of trace metals in the environment is an evolutionary pressure that has constrained host–microbe relationships. All life forms need trace metals for nutrition and proliferation, and all organisms have evolved mechanisms to harvest the required amount of trace metals from the available pool in their particular environmental niche. This applies especially to pathogens which colonize host tissues and cause disease, and which have evolved highly efficient nutrient retrieval strategies to counteract trace metal deprivation by the host. In response to metal deprivation, pathogens elaborate elegant strategies to liberate and acquire trace metals required for growth. Additionally, under stress from trace metal deficiency, the demand of the invading parasites for the host's pool of trace metals can increase pathogenesis and disease (Abu-Kwaik and Bumann 2013). It is conceivable that these host–pathogen relationships are increasingly affected by the recent modifications of the natural biogeochemical cycles of trace metals in ways that may be significantly altering the type and levels of metals in the human host. These human-induced changes in environmental accumulation of toxic metals and depletion of essential trace elements in soils, water, and the food chain tend to be most intense in countries that have the highest burden of infectious diseases (Graham et al. 2012). We thus have an ongoing experiment of concurrent exposure of human populations to emerging metals, high levels of toxic metals and/or suboptimal amounts of essential metals, along with pathogenic organisms responsible for endemic infections in many countries. The consequences of this growing mutualism (of coexposure to metals and pathogens) on the pathogenesis of infectious diseases have been largely neglected.

Infectious diseases themselves can increase human susceptibility to the adverse effects of metal exposure, likely moderated through the immunological system and by chronic inflammation induced by the infection (Winans et al. 2011). Patients with infectious diseases can thus be considered to be at higher risk for chronic diseases because of metal exposure. Conversely, exposure to metals may aggravate diseases caused by pathogenic infections or even initiate these diseases following exposure to certain microbes. The combined effects of exposure to metals and pathogens on the burden of disease in human populations remain unknown, but they are no doubt being modified by the increasing contamination of the environment with metals. The multiple inter-actions between pollutant metals, pathogens, and the environment are obviously complex and difficult to disentangle. However, in the current context of emerging metals, emerging infectious diseases, and rapid alterations of metal levels in our environment, understanding the consequences of such interactions is necessary to protect the public's health.

Many parts of the world (especially in the developing areas of Africa, Asia, and South America) that are endemic for the most common infectious diseases of our time—including malaria, HIV/AIDS, diarrhea, upper respiratory tract infections, and tuberculosis—also have high prevalence rates of trace metal deficiencies. Likewise, the highest emission rates for toxic trace metals into the environment are occurring in many countries with high incidence of infectious diseases. Coexposure to pathogens and suboptimal amounts of trace metals significantly impacts human health because trace metals command a central position at the host–pathogen interface due to the essential demand for metals that are required for many metabolic processes in all cells (Failla 2003). For microbes that reside within a niche inhabited by substantial microbial populations (such as the human gut or respiratory tract), they must compete with these other coexisting species to obtain the required amount of various trace metals. Compounding this issue is that invading microbes must also compete for these nutrients with their host. Mammals have evolved complex strategies aimed at restricting the supply of essential nutrient metals to pathogens, which represents an effective strategy of host defense sometimes termed "host tolerance" or "nutritional immunity." Note that we use the term "host tolerance" to define processes by which the host can minimize damage caused by the pathogen resulting in a homeostatic relationship between host and microbe, and this is not to be confused with "immune tolerance" which defines a state of unresponsiveness of the immune system to substances that have the potential to elicit an immune response. Notably, pathogens can evoke multiple strategies to acquire the essential element metals from their hosts to satisfy the requirement for metals in processes, including proliferation, virulence, and persistence (Failla 2003; Haase et al. 2008). The control over the homeostatic balance of essential trace metals is a critical battlefield during host–pathogen interactions which determines the course of an infectious disease in favor of either the mammalian host or the microbial invader.

A plethora of studies in recent years has revealed a complex control network of molecules involved in the competition between host cells and invading pathogens for essential trace elements. These studies have aimed at elaborating either the host's mechanisms of metal restriction or the counteracting metal acquisition strategies employed by pathogens (Inadera 2006; Jomova and Valko 2011). Recently, the concept of nutritional immunity has expanded to include host-imposed metal toxicity as a strategy to protect against microbial challenge. The most thoroughly studied of the competition for metals involves the acquisition of iron, although there is a growing appreciation of the contribution of manganese, zinc, and copper to the outcome of host–microbe interactions. Limiting iron availability can be an efficient strategy to restrict extracellular bacteria, and such a strategy is also detrimental for intracellular pathogens. Indeed, there is now strong evidence to suggest that host-mediated alteration of iron homeostasis has direct impacts on the proliferation of microbes. Recent studies have also shown a clear-cut correlation between bacterial infections and removal of zinc from the serum. More generally, zinc deficiency can reduce immune defense against infections, chronic inflammatory disease, and reduced cellular activation, whereas high zinc can hamper effective signal transduction leading to various negative consequences. Iron homeostasis is in part linked to copper homeostasis. Copper deficiency predisposes mammals to infectious diseases, to some extent as a consequence of a lack of neutrophils induced by inadequate copper availability or supply (see Rehder et al., this volume).

Traditional wisdom holds that host-defense mechanisms are primarily a function of the immune system and can be deployed to detect and eliminate invading parasites. This paradigm has recently been challenged by studies showing that the human host uses two strategies for dealing with an infection that are not mutually exclusive: the ability (a) to limit parasite burden (resistance) and (b) to limit the harm caused by a given burden of parasites (tolerance). From an ecological perspective, resistance protects the host at the expense of the parasite, whereas tolerance saves the host from harm without having any direct negative effects on the parasite (Ayres and Schneider 2012). This distinction is useful because it recognizes the important fact that hosts can sometimes be quite healthy, despite high parasite burdens, or conversely die with parasite loads which are tolerated by others; in fact, pathogen burden and health are not always well correlated (Schneider and Ayres 2008; Ayres and Schneider 2012; Medzhitov et al. 2012). Although these two components, together, determine how well a host is protected against the effects of infection, studies of human defense against microbes have focused to date primarily on resistance; the possibility of tolerance and its implications have been comparatively less well studied (Miller et al. 2006). The linkage of metabolic cycles of trace metals to tolerance mechanisms in the host is one of the more important recent discoveries in the field of trace metals research.

Although only a few metals are known to be biologically essential (iron, molybdenum, manganese, zinc, nickel, copper, vanadium, cobalt, and selenium), there is growing realization that almost every element in the periodic table (including arsenic, bismuth, boron, cadmium, chromium, cobalt, copper, germanium, gold, iron, silver, lead, mercury, nickel, manganese, molybdenum, platinum, palladium, rhodium, ruthenium, thallium, tin, titanium, vanadium, and zinc) can also moderate a host's immune response to pathogens. Many trace metals and metalloids have been reported in human and animal experiments to display antiviral, antifungal, antibacterial, and/or antiprotozoa properties, but the mechanisms for these effects are only beginning to be uncovered.

However, the role of these metals on the tolerance defense strategies is currently unknown.

A close look at the modes of death from infections shows surprisingly that death is often not attributable to a direct effect of the pathogen or of any toxin it produces but rather is the consequence of the systemic inflammatory response in the host (Baillie 2014). Our own immune system can be responsible for destroying us. Although this has been known for some time, efforts to find effective therapies that alter the host response to infection to promote survival have not been tremendously successful. This failure may be related, in part, to the inability to distinguish between failed resistance and failed tolerance in monitoring the outcome of treatment. When failed tolerance is the underlying factor, boosting immunity and reducing pathogen burden (using drugs) may be ineffective, whereas enhancing tolerance (e.g., with trace metal intervention) may have salutary effects. Drug interventions that target tolerance pathways may also be more desirable when immune defenses are either inefficient, compromised, or cause excessive immunopathology. Boosting tissue tolerance could be a particularly useful strategy in diseases such as malaria, tuberculosis, and HIV, where pathogen control through vaccination or antimicrobial drugs is currently suboptimal (Medzhitov et al. 2012). Conceptually, it is appealing to reduce the effect of an infection by moderating the host environment as opposed to poisoning the pathogen with a toxic metal. In this sense, metallic compounds hold some promise as potentially effective, adequate, affordable, and safe chemotherapies to boost host tolerance as well as resistance.

Unlike the essential metals, exposure to many toxic heavy metals found in the environment may trigger autoimmunity (overactive immune system) or result in immunotoxicity (Dietert 2009). The manifestation of autoimmune diseases includes production of autoantibodies, inflammation and cytokines in various target organs, and deposition of immune complexes in vascular sites (i.e., immunopathology). At high enough doses, exposure to metals can exert direct toxicity on the immune system through suppression of the system as a whole or by the disruption (suppression) of immunoregulatory systems, and hence result in exaggerated responses to infections (Failla 2003). In terms of the combined effect of coexposure to essential and toxic metals, it is conceivable for the antibiological activity of one metal to amplify the activity of a distinct metal, leading to increased resistance (or tolerance) against infections. A few *in vivo* and *in vitro* studies have reported reduced host vulnerability in response to coexposure to two or more trace metals. On the other hand, the antibiological activity for one metal can be incompatible with the activity of another metal, which then can lead to enhanced virulence or morbidity following an infection. Competition phenomena between zinc and several trace metals (such as cadmium, lead, calcium, iron, manganese, and copper) have been documented in zinc supplementation trials; however, results are inconsistent because of failure to consider the basal zinc status during the experiments. There are some parts of the world where communities with high prevalence of iron, zinc, or selenium deficiency are being exposed to high levels of toxic metals (especially lead, mercury, and arsenic). Populations in such areas are well suited for epidemiological studies aimed at understanding the underlying mechanisms of how trace metal interactions moderate the outcome of an infection.

## General Perspectives from the Forum's Discussions

Interest in processes at the nexus of host–microbe–metal interactions has risen recently as a result of advancements in the study of metallomics (metal-containing biomolecules), proteomics, and genomics. These emerging fields have given rise to new developments in powerful analytical methods and technology for studying the identity, distribution, quantity, trafficking, fate, and effects of trace metals in biological systems. Applications of these advanced techniques to the study of metabolic cycles are yielding results and have placed scientists at the threshold of major paradigm shifts in our understanding of the relationships between homeostatic mechanisms of trace metals and pathogenesis of infectious diseases. This emerging field was thus well suited for an Ernst Strüngmann Forum, which applies a unique multidisciplinary framework to assess current knowledge and identify gaps and research opportunities on cross-cutting issues. The fields present at this Forum were broad: chemistry, biology/biochemistry, toxicology, nutrition, immunology, microbiology, epidemiology, environmental and occupational health, as well as environmental and veterinary medicine. The majority of participants shared common interests in the roles of metals in biology, and they were tasked with using their knowledge to discuss and create reports on how the metabolic cycles of trace metals relate to the pathogenesis of disease during infection. To prepare for this discussion, invited background papers provided reviews of critical topics as a basis for the group discussions. The stimulating dialog that ensued covered a wide range of views, insights, and perspectives on current knowledge and raised important open questions that should be addressed by future research initiatives. Detailed summaries of the current state of knowledge and future areas for further research and development are presented in the group reports. The overviews below are our perceptions of some of the general areas of concern expressed at the Forum.

Cavet et al. (Chapter 7, this volume) focus on the microbial perspective during host–microbe interactions. Their discussions were directed at five key areas deemed to require greater understanding:

1. Metal availability in distinct environments, including within and outside microbial cells, with some emphasis on intracellular metal availability and how metal-requiring proteins acquire their correct metal cofactors.

2.  The different levels and sources of metals available to microbes in distinct niches within the host.
3.  The effect of the metal status of a pathogen, as derived from its prior environment, on its ability to establish an infection or the severity of disease.
4.  The interplay between metals and the microbiota.
5.  How metal restriction and metal oversupply can inhibit microbial growth or cause their death.

Specific issues that are explored in detail by Cavet et al. include the nature of the pool of exchangeable metal inside cells; whether metalloforms of an enzyme differ depending upon circumstance; control of metallation status by thermodynamics of binding sites; metabolic metal shuttling (metal ligands and proteins); the diversity of ecological niches for microbes in the vertebrate host; the sources and forms of metals in different niches; metal speciation in the intracellular environment; microbial strategies for obtaining metals from host and the effects of metal restriction; how an overabundance of intracellular metals impedes cell growth; and the effect of metal import and export systems on microbial growth and pathogenesis. They also cover some of the most intense and exciting areas of research on metals in the biology of microbes.

Rehder et al. (Chapter 13, this volume) provide a comprehensive overview of the role of metal ions in infectious diseases from the host perspective, focusing on iron, copper, zinc and, to a lesser extent, manganese and the metalloid selenium. Additionally, recommended dietary allowances (RDAs) are addressed, as well as metal-based drugs in the treatment of tropical diseases. The issues highlighted by Rehder et al. include the roles of manganese, iron, copper, zinc, and selenium in immune function; the interplay of iron distribution between microbes and host cells; the impact of iron on anti-immune effector functions; the role of zinc in host resistance/susceptibility and tolerance; therapeutic effects of zinc in infectious diseases of children; the specific case of selenium and susceptibility to viral and bacterial infections and to parasites; and a commentary on the RDAs and related intake levels. Their report includes a discussion of the role of the gasotransmitters carbon monoxide and nitric oxide in relation to their interference with bound and free metal ions. To cope with the increasing concern about the epidemic of tropical diseases (such as leishmaniasis, Chagas disease, and malaria), drugs are being developed that are based on coordination compounds of metals, including copper, iron, ruthenium, and gold. The efficacies and limitations of such drugs are described by Rehder et al. This report synthesizes the current state of knowledge regarding the contribution of metals to infectious disease from the host perspective and offers recommendations for areas of future research.

Ackland et al. (Chapter 17, this volume) provide insights into current knowledge and gaps in our understanding of the interplay between trace metals in the environment and infection. The contributions of metal deficiencies to the global burden of infectious diseases are substantial for zinc and iron but less defined for other metals. How emerging metals relate to emerging pathogens, and hence influence the disease burden, is identified as a matter that deserves further research. Despite considerable research taking place separately on trace metals and infectious pathogens, little is currently known about the interactions between these two key determinants of health, especially in the host microbiota, where direct coexposure occurs. A number of global trends have been identified that have the potential to upset the natural host–microbe–metal nexus, including climate change, Western-style food processing, increasing reliance on infant formula and consumption of fast foods, as well as the commercialization of products with metalliferous nanomaterials. From an ecological perspective, the two main processes by which the environment can directly impact host–pathogen interactions are (a) the changing pathogenicity of infectious agents combined with the emergence and spread of drug resistance, and (b) the changing of host resistance to the pathogen. The contributions of metals to the specific mechanisms involved in each process are essentially unknown.

Ackland et al. note that failure to ascertain the environmental contribution to infectious disease etiology stems largely from limitations in our ability to assess the environmental exposures, which have traditionally been measured using questionnaires and geographical mapping. The need for a new exposure paradigm that can integrate many external and internal exposures from different sources over the life course is emphasized. Exposomics or environment-wide association studies offers one such approach to gain insight into the environmental component essential to improving our understanding of the predictors, risk factors, and protective factors in complex interactions between trace metals, the environment, and infective microbes. An understanding of the effects of such an environmentally determined exposome on susceptibility to infectious disease would be an important step in developing appropriate intervention strategies in many parts of the world.

Our understanding of the biology of metals in the context of infectious disease is necessarily advanced (and limited) by the available analytical tools. The broad aims of Maret et al. (Chapter 20, this volume) were to provide an overview of analytical techniques available for investigating the interaction of metals/metalloids within both microbe and host, to specify needs for technological improvements, and to identify emerging applications and analytical questions. Measurement of metals in biological samples should encompass the total metal content, chemical speciation of metals, and additional information about distribution in biological space and time. Maret et al. stress the need to generate data that can be used to understand the metallome, or the functions of all parts of systems biology. In their report, they identify gaps and needs in technology, upcoming methodological issues, and analytical ways to study therapeutic and preventive interventions that will address the host–microbe interaction, with a focus on further goals and potential applications.

In this regard, Maret et al. discuss the adaptation of hyphenated techniques in proteomics research that require protein separation, mostly chromatographic and electrophoretic, in combination with molecular mass spectrometry (ICP-MS, ES-MS, MALDI-MS). In addition, the pool of nonprotein-bound metals, which is increasingly drawing attention because it is "metabolically active," can be addressed with fluorimetric techniques that have detection limits down to the septomolar range of concentrations or even reach single molecule or single cell resolution with super-resolution microscopy. An important issue for further research is the development of isotope tracer techniques, which can be used in experimental designs that span a wide range due to the large differences in size, reproductive speed, and experimental tractability of microbes and host animals. Microbes and cultured cells can be grown in media containing radioactive or stable isotope tracers, and the total inventory of metal species can theoretically be identified and quantified by radioactivity detection or by the isotopic shift, respectively. In higher animals, tracer techniques allow application of uptake measurements and metal species turnover, but lack or bias the information on the total inventory of metals. Currently, localization and speciation of total metals or the metallome in higher animals is pursued only *ex vivo* in tissue sections or extracts of cells, tissues, or body fluids because many of these techniques are destructive in nature.

Significant insight into trace metals and infections can be gained from further development and improvement in the transgenic constructs of metal sensors/reporter proteins from the cellular to the organismal level. Permanent or conditional knockouts (KO) of metal chaperones, transporters, chelators, or storage proteins elucidate the mechanism of metal-related host defense, but typically require the use of KO mice. Fusions of fluorescent or luminescent proteins with metal-chelating proteins may report free metal ion concentrations. Luminescent reporter proteins expressed under the control of promoters for genes of interest allow for studying the regulation of metalloproteins or effector proteins responsive to metals and can provide an indication of the metal environment experienced by a pathogen during infection. In addition, Maret et al. review *in silico* approaches to metalloprotein function to predict and calculate the dynamics of metallomes for organisms, starting from their genome sequences. Attention is drawn to existing or upcoming genome-wide expression studies utilizing real-time polymerase chain reaction for identifying genes encoding metalloproteins, which are up- or down-regulated in the host or microbe upon mutual contact or may mediate metal modulation of infectious disease.

In their report, Maret et al. include a general overview of existing analytical methods for trace metals; in particular, inductively coupled plasma mass spectrometry (ICP-MS), which has been established as the workhorse in non-radioactive metal speciation studies and, when coupled to a laser ablation (LA) instrument, enables imaging at the mesoscopic scale. ICP-MS provides the lowest detection limits and the best sensitivities, highest concentration dynamic range, broad multiplex capability, and robustness toward matrix effects. Identification of metalloproteins after chromatographic or electrophoretic separation uses metal detection by ICP-MS (or autoradiography) and for protein determination by tryptic digestion, followed by high-resolution tandem mass spectroscopy. The experimentally determined amino acid sequences of the peptides are then compared with those organized in protein databases, yielding acceptable or unacceptable probabilities of correct identifications. Unfortunately, protein databases lack many metalloproteins and contain numerous mis-assignments of metalloproteins, which is a major shortcoming in the field of metallomics.

In summary, through this Forum we collectively sought to expand understanding of the linkage(s) between metals and the pathogenesis of infectious diseases, and to address the underlying mechanisms that moderate the outcome of infection. The dialog that emerged from a tremendously diverse group of international experts attests to the very real needs that exist in science. This volume aims to transfer the Forum's results. It provides an integrated summary of our current knowledge, highlights the contentious issues, and suggests critical areas for further research. We hope that it will spur future work and discovery in the service of humankind to alleviate the burden of infectious disease throughout the world.

The outcome of the Forum depended very much on the efficiency, helpfulness, and general guidance of Julia Lupp and the entire staff of the Strüngmann Forum. Their unflinching support and professionalism were appreciated by all who attended the meeting. The Forum benefited greatly from the work of the Program Advisory Committee members—Rodney R. Dietert, Julia Lupp, Jerome O. Nriagu, Lothar Rink, Anthony B. Schryvers, and Eric P. Skaar— who met in Frankfurt from January 26–28, 2013 to develop the scientific program for the Forum. Success, however, belongs to the moderators, rapporteurs, and all participants. In closing, we wish to thank the authors of the invited background papers as well as the rapporteurs, who share credit for the quality of material in this book.

# Host–Microbe Interactions: The Microbe Perspective

# 2

# Is Metal Uptake Related to Ecological Niche in the Vertebrate Host?

Joseph Lemire, Trevor F. Moraes,
Vahid Fa Andisi, and Anthony B. Schryvers

## Abstract

There is a complex interplay between the vertebrate host and the microbes that inhabit its mucosal surfaces in their competition for essential metal ions. Mucosal surfaces in the host constitute an array of diverse ecological niches that vary substantially in the availability of metal ions from the external environment and from the host. The microbes that inhabit different mucosal surfaces vary in the degree to which they are uniquely adapted to, and are restricted to, the host mucosal environment. This chapter reviews current understanding of metal ion homeostasis in the host, the mechanisms of metal ion acquisition in microbes, and the degree to which the specific mucosal niche impacts the repertoire of metal ion acquisition mechanisms that the microbes possess.

## Introduction

Our aim in this chapter is to provide a synopsis of the mechanisms of essential metal ion acquisition in microbes that inhabit the vertebrate host, highlighting how different mucosal environments may influence the repertoire of acquisition systems that are present. An appreciation of the relative exposure of microbes to metal ions from the environment or derived from the host and their available metal ion acquisition systems is an essential foundation for understanding the impact of metals ions on infection.

## Metal Ion Homeostasis in Vertebrates

Metal ions are essential to biological systems, as they participate in discrete chemistries that are not possible by organic molecules alone. Iron (Fe), zinc

(Zn), copper (Cu), and manganese (Mn) are essential to both bacterial and mammalian cells alike. However, the human body also requires molybdenum (Mo), selenium (Se), chromium (Cr), cobalt (Co) and other metals for select biochemistries. While the homeostasis (acquisition, distribution, storage, and elimination) of iron has received a great deal of attention, the homeostasis of some of the other aforementioned metals has not been as well defined.

## The Functional Role of Essential Metal Ions:
## A Brief Glance at Metallobiochemistry

A comprehensive review of the functional role of metals in biological systems is well beyond the scope of this chapter. In the sections below, discussion focuses on some of the well-studied biological roles of essential metals.

*Redox-Active Metals: Iron, Copper, Molybdenum,*
*Cobalt, Manganese, and Chromium*

Current understanding of Fe and Cu homeostasis stems from their vital and diverse functions in cellular chemistry. Indeed, iron is an essential player in ATP production, cellular division, DNA repair, and antioxidant defense, and is a required moiety for distributing oxygen in the human body. The ability of iron to undergo redox chemistry (i.e., $Fe^{2+} \leftrightarrow Fe^{3+}$) makes it ideal for participating in electron donor/receiving reactions in the electron transport chain and other important redox reactions. Copper also lends itself to electron transfer in the electron transport chain, as a critical cofactor in cytochrome *c* oxidase. The ability of copper to be oxidized ($Cu^{2+}$) or reduced ($Cu^+$) gives it utility in antioxidant defense in the enzyme Cu/Zn-superoxide dismutase (Cu/Zn-SOD) (Turski and Thiele 2009). The necessity of redox-active metals in attenuating reactive oxygen species is also evidenced by some cells expressing an Fe-dependent SOD.

   The human body requires cobalt in its corrin form as cobalamin (vitamin B12). The importance of bacteria to human health is demonstrated by our reliance on them for the synthesis of cobalamin. The versatility of the cofactor cobalamin gives it utility in a range of essential cellular pathways: fatty acid and amino acid metabolism, DNA synthesis, and energy production. Within these pathways, cobalamin participates in small molecule transfer. Some classic examples of this are methyl group transfer (methyl transferases) and hydrogen atom handling (ribonucleotide reductases) (Banerjee and Ragsdale 2003).

   In their free ionic form, molybdenum and chromium are typically found as oxyanions in biological systems: $MoO_4^{2-}$, and $CrO_4^{2-}$, respectively. However, human cells have found ways to exploit them for biological functions. Cofactor manipulation of molybdenum allows for the shuttling of electrons between molybdenum's IV, V, and VI oxidation state (Schwarz et al. 2009). This gives enzymes such as xanthine oxidase the capacity to participate in two electron transfer reactions. Currently, the debate on $Cr^{3+}$ necessity to human health and nutrition is still ongoing. Vincent (2010) proposed that $Cr^{3+}$ is involved in glucose metabolism, through the interaction with various aspects of the insulin-signaling pathway. To date, however, there has been no apparent mechanism that explains this phenomenon in detail.

As a micronutrient, manganese finds one of its most important utilities in Mn-dependent SOD in the mitochondria, and is therefore essential for antioxidant defense. The proposed mechanism of action for manganese in SOD is the formation of a $Mn^{3+}$ intermediate that oxidizes superoxide (Sheng et al. 2012).

*Nonredox-Active Metals: Zinc and Selenium*

Though not redox active, $Zn^{2+}$ finds use as a catalytic, structural, and regulatory cofactor in the cell (Maret 2013). One of the best-studied catalytic functions of zinc is the activation of water in carbonic anhydrase. Water activation by zinc in carbonic anhydrase allows for the formation of bicarbonate ($HCO_3^-$) from carbon dioxide ($CO_2$), an essential function for maintaining the pH of the blood. Zinc is also required for maintaining the structure of the Zn-finger family of transcription factors. Additionally, zinc has also been demonstrated to participate in cell signaling as a secondary messenger, thus inducing the expression of certain genes (Yamasaki et al. 2007).

Selenium is required to biosynthesize the noncoded amino acid selenocysteine. One of the better-documented functions of selenocysteine is its importance in glutathione peroxidase, an enzyme that can detoxify hydrogen peroxide ($H_2O_2$). Other notable enzymes that require selenocysteine to operate are deiodinases (removal of iodine from thyroid hormones) and formate dehydrogenases (detoxification of formate in the liver) (Rayman 2000).

**Acquisition and Transport of Essential Metal Ions**

Iron plays a critical role in biological redox reactions but its innate insolubility and the potential for free iron to mediate the generation of toxic by-products in the presence of oxygen has prompted the development of complex systems for maintaining its solubility through ligating to various organic acids and proteins. Thus mammals have developed effective systems for handling iron and regulating the level of available iron (De Domenico et al. 2008). Although less studied, there are likely complex systems for handling other essential metals. One critical component of metal ion homeostasis is the mechanism for uptake by gut epithelial cells, and studies have revealed several pathways (Figure 2.1). However, due to the varying forms of metal ions in dietary sources and the complexities introduced by the interplay with the gut microbiota, it remains to be seen whether there are additional metal ion uptake pathways and to what extent they contribute under varying dietary conditions and microbiota compositions.

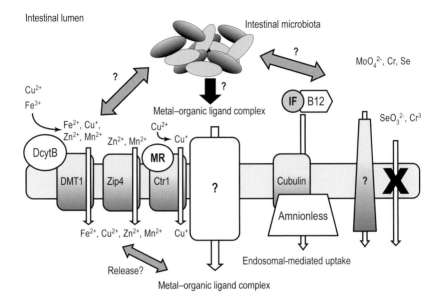

**Figure 2.1** Essential metal uptake into intestinal epithelium cells from the gut lumen. The divalent metals $Fe^{2+}$, $Cu^{2+}$, $Zn^{2+}$, and $Mn^{2+}$ can be transported by divalent metal transporter 1 (DMT1) (Vashchenko and MacGillivray 2013). $Fe^{3+}$ must be reduced to $Fe^{2+}$ by the duodenal cytochrome B (DcytB) prior to internalization by DMT1 (Kim et al. 2008; Lichten and Cousins 2009; Vashchenko and MacGillivray 2013). Zip4 and Ctr1 mediate the uptake of $Zn^{2+}$ or $Mn^{2+}$ and $Cu^+$, respectively (Kim et al. 2008; Lichten and Cousins 2009; Vashchenko and MacGillivray 2013). Reduction of $Cu^{2+}$ to $Cu^+$ by a metaloreductase, possibly DyctB, is required for import by Ctr1. Vitamin B12 (cobalamin) requires its own transporter complex—cubulin-amnionless—which internalizes a complex of B12 and intrinsic factor (IF) by an endosomal-dependent pathway (Kozyraki and Cases 2013). The exact transport mechanism of $MoO_4^{2-}$, Cr (III and VI), and Se remain a point of discovery and controversy (Lichten and Cousins 2009; Zeng et al. 2011; Mendel and Kruse 2012).

*Essential Metal Uptake by the Gut Epithelia*

The divalent metal transporter 1 (DMT1) is capable of transporting a number of the essential metal ions ($Fe^{3+}$, $Cu^{2+}$, and possibly $Zn^{2+}$ and $Mn^{2+}$) into the gut epithelial cell. This process, however, generally requires the activity of the duodenal cytochrome B (DcytB), which reduces dietary $Fe^{3+}$ to $Fe^{2+}$ or $Cu^{2+}$ to $Cu^+$ for transport by DMT1 into the intestinal epithelial cell (Vashchenko and MacGillivray 2013). Copper can also be transported by a high affinity Cu transporter, Ctr1, a process that also requires coupling to a metalloreductase (Kim et al. 2008). The Zip4 family of transporters on the apical surface of the intestinal epithelia specifically transports zinc, but may also transport manganese (Lichten and Cousins 2009).

Microorganisms also have strict requirements for iron, copper, zinc, and manganese and have mechanisms of acquisition that involve modifying the form of metal present in food sources. Current models for metal ion acquisition, however, do not generally account for how eukaryotic cells address the impact of the gut microbiota and compete for various forms of metal ions that may be present. The serendipitous discovery of siderocalin, a secreted protein that binds iron complexed to bacterial siderophores (Flo et al. 2004), provides an example of additional complexities in the competition between the microbiota and host in the competition for metal ions. An obvious question is whether there are additional surface proteins and systems in the gut epithelial that are devoted to acquisition of metal ion complexes that exist due to the presence of the gut microbiome.

Cobalamin (vitamin B12) is the form of cobalt that is transported by gut epithelial cells and there is a complex system for optimizing its utilization. Cobalamin is bound by the salivary gland-derived glycoprotein, haptocorrin (transcobalamin), in the upper gastrointestinal tract to protect the sensitive vitamin from acidic breakdown (Kozyraki and Cases 2013). Cobalamin is then passed from haptocorrin to the parietal cell-produced glycoprotein—intrinsic factor (IF)—in the duodenum following the degradation of haptocorrin. The cobalamin-IF complex is then transported from the lumen by an endosomal-dependent pathway into the enterocyte by the cubilin-amnionless complex (Kozyraki and Cases 2013).

The uptake of molybdenum, chromium, and selenium is poorly characterized. Molybdenum is likely absorbed as $MoO_4^{2-}$ by an active transport process, which may be impeded by the presence of competing anions such as sulphate (Mendel and Kruse 2012). Uptake of chromate through anion transporters is considered a source of toxic exposure. The entry of dietary Cr(III) into the human body may require coordination by an organic ligand (Lichten and Cousins 2009), and Se absorption is enhanced in its amino acid—selenocysteine and selenomethionine—form (Zeng et al. 2011).

*The Distribution of Essential Metals throughout the Body*

Bioaccessible dietary iron taken up by the enterocyte is transported to the basal membrane where it is loaded onto transferrin (Tf), a bi-lobed glycoprotein capable of binding two $Fe^{3+}$ with high affinity (Figure 2.2). Ferrous iron ($Fe^{2+}$) is exported from the enterocyte through ferroportin and converted to $Fe^{3+}$ by the ferroxidase hephaestin, for loading iron onto Tf (Vashchenko and MacGillivray 2013). Transferrin transports iron to cells that require iron for growth, particularly erythrocyte precursors which require iron for the oxygen transport protein hemoglobin. Iron is efficiently recycled in the body through (a) direct engulfment of senescent erythrocytes and other cells, (b) macrophages and hepatocytes, or (c) recapture of released hemoglobin or heme by the serum glycoproteins haptoglobin and hemopexin, and taken up by hepatocytes. The recycled iron from macrophages and hepatocytes is then loaded onto Tf through ferroportin and a ferroxidase, as in the enterocyte. The regulation of

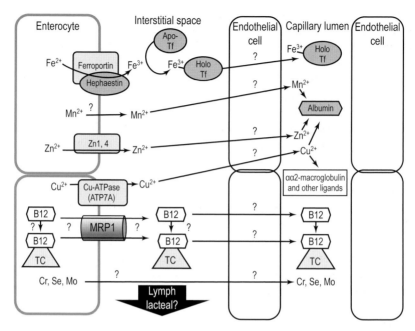

**Figure 2.2**   Essential metal transport from the enterocyte to the systemic circulation. Iron is transported from the enterocyte to the interstitial space via export through ferroportin and oxidation of $Fe^{2+}$ to $Fe^{3+}$ by hephaestin. This provides the form of iron that is bound by apo-transferrin (apo-Tf) (Vashchenko and MacGillivray 2013). $Zn^{2+}$ and $Cu^{2+}$ are both exported from the enterocyte by specific transporters: Znt1, 4 and ATP7A (Cu-ATPase), respectively (Kim et al. 2008; Lichten and Cousins 2009). Cobalamin (B12) is exported through MRP1, the multidrug protein, and binds to transcobalamin (TC) for distribution in the blood (Kozyraki and Cases 2013). As indicated by the numerous question marks, there is considerable uncertainty as to how the metal ions released from the basal membrane of the enterocyte are transported to the lumen of the blood vessels and bound to proteins thought to be responsible for their distribution throughout the body.

Fe homeostasis by hepcidin takes advantage of the critical role that ferroportin plays in export of iron from cells, and influences the stability of ferroportin (Zhang and Enns 2009).

Cobalamin is likely exported from the enterocyte through the multidrug resistance protein 1 (MRP1) transporter following release from the IF cubulin-amnionless complex via lysosomal acidification (Kozyraki and Cases 2013; Cole 2014). From the enterocyte, cobalamin is delivered through the systemic circulatory system by binding to transcobalamin (Kozyraki and Cases 2013). Further studies are required to establish whether cobalamin binds to transcobalamin before exiting the enterocyte, while in the interstitial space, or upon reaching systemic circulation.

Copper is exported from the enterocyte by a Cu-ATPase (ATP7A) (Kim et al. 2008) but the ligands that it binds for transport throughout the body are not firmly established, although albumin and $\alpha_2$-macroglobulin are likely candidates (Collins et al. 2010). It has also been suggested that the serum Fe oxidase, ceruloplasmin, may play an integral role in Cu transport through the systemic circulation, since 90% of serum copper is bound by ceruloplasmin. However studies in mice lacking ceruloplasmin demonstrated no apparent defect in Cu absorption or distribution (Kim et al. 2008).

Export of zinc from the enterocyte relies on the Zn transporters Znt1 and Znt4 (Lichten and Cousins 2009), whereas Mn export may rely on ferroportin (Madejczyk and Ballatori 2012). Albumin has been implicated as the molecule responsible for carrying both zinc and manganese in the blood (Michalke et al. 2007; Lu et al. 2008).

Although there is information on the pathways for exporting metal ions from the enterocyte, many questions remain: Where does the apo-Tf that binds the $Fe^{3+}$ at the basal membrane of the enterocyte originate (Figure 2.2)? Is apo-Tf produced locally by enterocytes or by leukocytes, or is it transported from the lumen of capillaries? Are the proteins involved in binding other metal ions also present at the basal surface of the enterocyte, and, if so, what is their origin? How is the Fe-loaded Tf transported to the lumen of blood vessels for distribution throughout the body? How are other metals ions, or metal ions complexed to proteins, transported into the lumen of the blood vessels? Are metal ions or metal ion complexes transported through the lymphatics along with cell fluids, just as chylomicrons are? Clearly, current gaps in our understanding of how metal ions enter the systemic circulation remain a field for future discovery in metal ion homeostasis (Figure 2.2).

## Mechanisms and Pathways for Metal Ion Acquisition in Microbes

### Sources of Metal Ions

The descriptions of metal ion homeostasis in the preceding section focused on the acquisition, distribution, and storage of metal ions within the body. As such, they provide insight on the forms of metal ions that would be available in the extracellular milieu during invasive infection (Hood and Skaar 2012) but do not necessarily provide information regarding what is available on mucosal surfaces.

Due to our understanding of Fe homeostasis, we have a good grasp of the sources of iron available to invading microbes within the mammalian host (Hood and Skaar 2012). The predominant form of extracellular iron within the body is in the form of Tf, which is normally partially saturated (~30%), resulting in rapid sequestration of any available $Fe^{3+}$ by Tf. The structurally related glycoprotein, lactoferrin (Lf), is normally at nearly 1,000-fold lower levels than that of Tf. However, since it is released from neutrophil granules at sites of infection and inflammation, the local concentrations can be substantial. The efficient recycling of hemoglobin and heme by haptoglobin and hemopexin not only limit the levels of free hemoglobin and heme, the levels of hemoglobin-haptoglobin and heme-hemopexin complexes are also kept very low, except under conditions of extensive hemolysis.

Although the study of homeostasis of other essential metal ions is less extensive than for iron, there are common features and considerations. The majority of the zinc, manganese, and copper in plasma is bound to albumin or other serum proteins, and calprotectin-releasing cells (e.g., neutrophils) can release calprotectin for Zn and Mn chelation (Hood and Skaar 2012). Just as there is some uncertainty of how metal ions from the diet are transported into serum (Figure 2.2), it is not readily apparent whether or how the components of serum involved in metal ion coordination are transported into the interstitial fluids, except when there is damage to blood vessels during infection or inflammation.

The production of Lf by glandular epithelial cells (Figure 2.3) has led to the general assumption that Lf would be more readily available on mucosal surfaces than Tf. This assumption has been shown, however, to be incorrect for the male genitourinary tract in humans (Anderson et al. 2003). Still, the levels of Lf increase upon gonococcal challenge, are likely due to the concomitant inflammatory response. It is important to consider that Lf is secreted in its apo form and does not in itself represent a means of delivering host iron to the mucosal surface. Lactoferrin will, however, readily complex any free $Fe^{3+}$ that is available. Similarly, the secretion of members of the S100 family of vertebrate proteins would result in chelation of other essential metal ions but would not provide a supply of host-derived metal ions (Hood and Skaar 2012). Aside from the process of bleeding, there currently are no well-described mechanisms by which host metal ion sources would be available on the mucosal surfaces where most microbes reside. Metal ions could certainly be transported to mucosal surfaces by the secretions from glandular cells, which are significant components on mucosal surfaces, but it may not be a well-controlled process. The prevalent forms of the metal ions on the mucosal surface are not well known.

When considering the availability of essential metal ions on various mucosal surfaces, one not only has to consider the degree to which external sources (food, dust particles) are available and the degree to which host sources may be available, but also the degree to which the microbes themselves influence the available sources. Many microbes produce and secrete small Fe-binding chelators, termed siderophores, which are capable of binding and sequestering iron in diverse environments. The selective capture by surface proteins enables the microbe to compete effectively for iron when the supply is limited. Comparable systems for the specific capture of copper, zinc, or manganese have not been identified, but the demonstration that some siderophores may have comparable affinities of iron, copper, and zinc (Brandel et al. 2012) suggests that under some conditions siderophores could provide a means for other essential metal ions to piggyback on siderophore-mediated systems. For

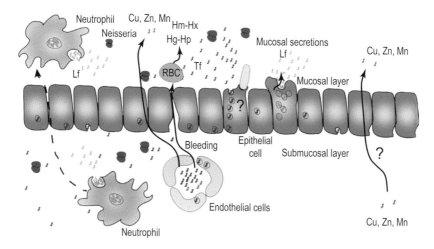

**Figure 2.3** Host-derived essential metal ion sources on mucosal surfaces. Potential routes for movement of host-derived metals to the mucosal surfaces consist of migration of host cells (neutrophil), bleeding, and mucosal secretions. The recent observation that *Helicobacter pylori* is capable of hijacking the Tf recycling system and bringing Tf-bound iron to the epithelial surface (Tan et al. 2011) begs the question of whether microbes on mucosal surfaces have a variety of undiscovered mechanisms for bringing essential metal ions to the mucosal surface. Not to be ignored is that some bacteria can be transcytozed across the epithelial cell layer and may reside in the submucosal space.

example, the Fe-binding catecholate siderophore yersiniabactin (Ybt) released by *Escherichia coli* also has the capacity to bind to copper. This Cu chelation capacity of Ybt contributes to higher Cu resistance in urinary tract infection isolates (Chaturvedi et al. 2012).

## Transport across the Cytoplasmic Membrane

Unlike the eukaryotic host, microbes (yeast, bacteria) do not transport complexes of metal ions with proteins into the cell. Thus the final stages of transport of metal ions across the cytoplasmic membrane are either with the free metal ion or as a metal ion complexed with small molecules. This process occurs irrespective of what the physiological source of metal ion is. The removal or capture of the metal ion from the host protein is a necessary prior step for protein-metal ion complexes, and the mechanisms vary considerably between Gram-negative and Gram-positive bacteria (Figures 2.4 and 2.5).

A common mechanism for the transport of essential metal ions across the cytoplasmic membrane is through the action of ATP-binding cassette (ABC) transporters (Rees et al. 2009). In addition to the cytoplasmic membrane complex, which consists of a cytoplasmic ATPase bound intimately to an inner membrane transporter, a specific binding protein component is normally

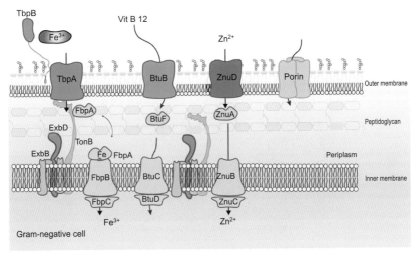

**Figure 2.4**  Metal ion transport in Gram-negative bacteria. In this figure, only trans-port systems in which transport across the inner membrane is mediated by an ABC transport system (FbpABC, ZnuABC, BtuFCD) have been included. These systems typically have a periplasmic binding protein (FbpA, ZnuA, BtuF) that delivers the metal ion or metal ion complex to an inner membrane complex consisting of an inner membrane transporter (FbpB, ZnuB, BtuC) and a cytoplasmic ATPase component (FbpC, ZnuC, BtuD). For completeness, a porin in the outer membrane (right-hand side) has been included, although it is an unlikely mode for transport of essential metal ions across the outer membrane. The ZnuD outer membrane transporter and the ZnuABC transport pathway represent the simplest system in which the outer membrane receptor binds Zn and transports it across the outer membrane. The BtuB outer membrane receptor and BtuFCD transport system for transporting vitamin B12 (cobalamin) is a representative for heme and siderophore receptors in that the metal ion complex is directly bound and transported into the cell. The most complex system represented by the TbpAB, FbpABC system involves removal of metal ion from the protein carrier at the cell surface and transport of the metal ion into the cell. This process may involve a lipoprotein component that facilitates the transport process by delivery of the metal-containing protein to the integral outer membrane receptor protein.

present as it not only confers specificity on the transport process but also is effective at capturing substrate for the transport process. In Gram-negative bacteria the binding protein is soluble and contained within the periplasmic space (Figure 2.4), whereas in Gram-positive bacteria the proteins are lipoproteins anchored to the cytoplasmic membrane (Figure 2.5).

A variety of ABC transport systems for essential metal ions have been identified and characterized in bacteria, including FbpABC for $Fe^{3+}$, ZnuABC for zinc, MntABC for manganese, and NosVFD for copper. Careful biochemical and physiological studies, however, may be needed to define the substrate preference of some transport systems clearly, particularly for the Mn transporters. The structural features of the periplasmic binding proteins and related lipoproteins that directly bind metal ions vary from the venus fly-trap structure of

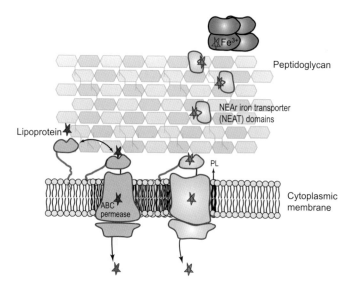

Gram-positive cell

**Figure 2.5**  Metal ion transport in Gram-positive bacteria. Metal ions or metal ion complexes (outlined as stars) can be captured directly by a tethered lipidated binding protein and transported across the inner membrane by the inner membrane permease-ATPase complex of the ABC transport system. A series of membrane-anchored proteins (proteins with near iron transporter, NEAT, domains) are required for the removal of heme from physiological heme sources such as hemoglobin or hemoglobin-haptoglobin complexes. After shuttling the heme between a series of NEAT domain proteins, the heme is transferred to the lipid-anchored binding protein and transported across the inner membrane by the ABC transporter complex.

the cluster 1 type (FbpA-Fe), which involves considerable domain movement upon metal ion binding, to the more rigid cluster 8/9 type (TroA-Zn) proteins (Krewulak and Vogel 2008). Thus, the processes of metal ion removal and transport into the cell may vary. ABC transporters are also responsible for the transport of iron-siderophore complexes, heme iron, and cobalamin (B12) into the cell. In addition, because the periplasmic binding proteins and lipoproteins all belong to the cluster 8 type, it is likely that the mechanism of removal and transport is similar to that proposed for the BtuFDC complex based on the atomic resolution structural information (Rees et al. 2009).

In addition to the ABC transporters illustrated in Figures 2.4 and 2.5, there are a variety of other essential metal ion transport systems in the cytoplasmic membrane, such as the FeoAB ($Fe^{2+}$), MntH (Mn), and ZupT (Zn) transporters, the latter being homologs of the eukaryotic NRAMP and ZIP transporter families. These transporters tend to have relatively broad substrate specificities *in vitro*, and determining whether their physiological role relates to a specific metal ion in the mammalian host can be elusive. Similarly it is unclear whether

ABC transport systems or these types of transporters play more important roles in different ecological niches or under different conditions.

## Transport across the Gram-Negative Outer Membrane

The Gram-negative outer membrane provides a semipermeable barrier containing substrate-specific porins and nonspecific porins that allow diffusion of small molecules of the appropriate size and charge characteristics to pass readily through their central channels along a concentration gradient (Figure 2.4). However, essential metal ions and metal ion complexes are generally in low concentrations in the external milieu; they move against a concentration gradient or are not suitable for passing through the standard porin proteins. Thus specific channels are required to facilitate the transport of metal ions and metal ion complexes across the outer membrane and serve to bind and capture the metal ion or metal ion complexes.

Most Gram-negative bacteria have outer membrane receptor complexes that mediate the transport of specific metal ions or metal ion complexes across the outer membrane belonging to the TonB-dependent class of outer membrane proteins. TonB-dependent receptors interact with the cytoplasmic membrane-anchored TonB complex that is required for providing energy for the transport across the outer membrane (Shultis et al. 2006). The simplest TonB-dependent systems are represented by ZnuD (a Zn-specific transporter), siderophore receptors, heme receptor proteins, and BtuB as they appear simply to bind the metal ion (Zn) or metal ion complex (iron-siderophore, heme, or cobalamin) and mediate its transport across the outer membrane in a TonB-dependent manner (Figure 2.4). The apparent independence of ZnuD-mediated Zn transport from TonB (Stork et al. 2010) is an interesting phenomenon, but whether it applies to acquisition of zinc from physiological sources in the host is still an open question. To some extent this is reminiscent of the inability to demonstrate a dependence for utilization of iron in Tf on the surface lipoprotein TbpB with TbpB-deficient strains until tested in the host (Baltes et al. 2002).

Additional complexities arise when metal ions or metal ion complexes are bound to proteins such as Tf, Lf, hemoglobin, hemoglobin-haptoglobin, or heme-hemopexin, and their removal is intrinsic to the overall transport process. The simplest are the single component receptors such as the TbpA2 receptor or heme/hemoglobin receptors (HmbR). The process for heme acquisition may be facilitated by production and secretion of protein hemophores to extract heme from hemoglobin and other heme sources, analogous to siderophores (Wandersman and Delepelaire 2004). The most complex are receptor transporter complexes consisting of a TonB-dependent integral membrane protein and a surface lipoprotein, which facilitates the efficiency of the transport process such as the TbpA-TbpB Tf receptors (Morgenthau et al. 2013) and the HpuA-HpuB hemoglobin-haptoglobin receptors (Rohde and Dyer 2004). The role of the accessory surface lipoprotein can be difficult to demonstrate, and the importance in the transport process may only become evident in the host (Baltes et al. 2002).

Structural studies with TonB-dependent transporters have led to insights into the process by which these proteins utilize energy transduced by the inner membrane TonB-Exb-ExbD complex (Figure 2.4) to mediate the transport of iron-siderophore complexes, nickel complexes, or vitamin B12 across the outer membrane (Noinaj et al. 2010). In addition, ongoing structural and functional studies are beginning to provide insights into how the surface receptor complexes are able to extract iron from Tf and mediate its transport across the outer membrane. Although there is some preliminary evidence, it is not well established whether the process of transport across the outer membrane is effectively coupled to the subsequent transport of ligand by the periplasm to the cytoplasm ABC transport system.

## Transport in Gram-Positive Bacteria

Although Gram-positive bacteria do not have to contend with the potential barrier that the Gram-negative outer membrane represents, they still have to deal with relatively low concentrations of essential metal ions that are frequently bound to host proteins. The high binding affinity of the lipoprotein component of ABC transporters may be sufficient for capturing some metal ions and metal ion complexes from the external milieu, but the competition with host proteins has required additional components for acquiring some metal ion or metal ion complexes (Figure 2.5). Thus production of siderophores provides one mechanism for acquiring iron from host Tf, and many bacteria produce lipoproteins capable of binding complexes of iron and siderophores produced by other bacteria (Beasley et al. 2011) (Figure 2.5). More complex systems involving a series of heme-binding proteins anchored to the cell wall are involved in acquiring heme iron from various physiological sources of heme. The cell wall-anchored proteins shuttle heme and deliver it to a lipid-anchored binding protein that transports heme iron into the cell through an ABC transport pathway (Tiedemann et al. 2012) (Figure 2.5).

## Metal Ion Acquisition on Mucosal Surfaces

### Metal Ion Acquisition in the Gastrointestinal Tract

Mucosal surfaces of the gastrointestinal tract represent a diverse set of ecological niches to which the colonizing microbes adapt, ranging from aerobic environments present in the oral cavity to the acidic environment of the stomach to the nearly anaerobic environment of the colon. The microbial communities that are established throughout the gastrointestinal tract are continuously exposed to microbes from the external environment, and this can impact the composition of the microbial flora and the development of disease.

Although the microbes may be well adapted to the local environment, many of the microbes in the lower gastrointestinal tract (stomach and intestine) are acquired through the fecal-oral route. Thus they must also adapt to survival outside of the human or vertebrate host. In addition, the microbes are exposed to varying food sources and may thus require diverse capabilities and strategies for metal ion acquisition. As a consequence, versatile mechanisms of metal ion acquisition, such as the siderophore-mediated Fe acquisition mechanism, are often found in pathogens and inhabitants of the gastrointestinal tract. The secretion of siderocalin (lipocalin2) by the host has been shown to limit proliferation of enteric pathogens that produce siderophores capable of being bound by siderocalin (Flo et al. 2004). The production of siderophores that are not bound by siderocalin is a strategy pathogens have used to overcome this growth limitation.

Although microbes colonizing the gastrointestinal tract are expected primarily to access food sources of metal ions, there are unique niches where access host Fe sources may be an advantage. For example, it has recently been demonstrated that *H. pylori* is able to modulate the Tf recycling pathway in host epithelial cells with CagA and VacA, resulting in transport of submucosal Tf to the epithelial surface (Tan et al. 2011). Clearly this is just one example of unique adaptations to specific niches within the diverse microbial surfaces of the gastrointestinal tract that are likely to be revealed with further study.

**Metal Ion Acquisition in the Respiratory and Genitourinary Tracts**

Unlike the gastrointestinal tract, where there is a large intake of material containing metal ions from the environment, the microbes that inhabit the mucosal surfaces of the genitourinary tract (particularly the male genitourinary tract) and upper respiratory tract—excluding the oral cavity and oropharynx—may rely primarily on host sources of metal ions (Figure 2.3). Since many of the microbes and pathogens that reside in this niche are acquired primarily from other hosts through the close contact and exchange of material from the host (e.g., respiratory droplets, direct exchange during sexual contact) they are highly adapted to the only niche they inhabit: the host's upper respiratory or genitourinary tract. This is reflected in a relatively small genome size, many host-specific interactions, and, commonly, natural transformation systems that facilitate antigenic variation of surface components.

Since metal ions on the upper respiratory and genitourinary tract mucosal surfaces may be primarily obtained from endogenous sources (Figure 2.3), it is perhaps not surprising that some bacteria which reside in this niche have developed mechanisms of acquiring metal ions directly from host proteins. Many of the host-specific receptors that bind to host Fe-containing complexes (Tf, Lf, hemoglobin-haptoglobin, heme-hemopexin) have only been found in bacteria that reside in the genitourinary and upper respiratory tracts (see Tf, Lf, Hg-Hp, Hm-Hx in Figure 2.3). It is also important to note that some bacteria are capable of attaching to host surface proteins to mediate transcytosis across epithelial cells, and thus may be able reside in the submucosal space (Sadarangani et al. 2011) where the host Fe-binding complexes would be readily available. This raises the question of whether the ability to use host proteins directly for Fe acquisition is restricted to bacteria that are capable of accessing a different niche. Genomic comparisons of pathogenic and commensal *Neisseria* species (Marri et al. 2010) suggest that some commensals have a different, and to some extent, mutually exclusive mechanism for Fe acquisition, which may be a reflection of different niches. Thus our current appreciation of the mechanisms of metal ion acquisition by bacteria which reside on the genitourinary and upper respiratory mucosal surfaces may be biased by the natural focus on disease-causing bacteria.

There has been a fairly extensive focus on the study of Fe acquisition mechanisms of the Gram-negative pathogenic bacteria which reside exclusively in the genitourinary and upper respiratory tracts that directly acquire iron from host proteins and do not produce siderophores. The lack of siderophore production is also observed in the important Gram-positive pathogen, *Streptococcus pneumoniae,* leading to an impression that reliance primarily on host-derived sources of metal ions by inhabitants of the genitourinary and upper respiratory tracts may lead to less reliance on siderophore-mediated mechanisms. This may reflect the inhabiting of a particular subniche or just a bias in the microbes being studied. A more important question regarding these mucosal surfaces is: What is the source of essential metal ions, and how do the inhabitants access them? The novel finding that *H. pylori* is capable of bringing Tf-Fe to the epithelial system by hijacking the recycling pathway begs the question of whether the inhabitants of the genitourinary and upper respiratory tracts have a diverse array of similar mechanisms for ensuring a sufficient supply of essential metal ions.

## Conclusions

It is readily apparent that there are many unanswered questions regarding metal ion homeostasis and the interplay between microorganisms that colonize and infect the vertebrate host. Many of the questions will be addressed through ongoing studies that are being pursued, but some questions may require new initiatives and collaborations. The following are a limited set of questions that we feel warrant attention:

- How do microbiota modulate the bioavailability of metal ions from dietary sources? What are the primary forms of metal ions that the enterocyte is exposed to as a consequence of microbiota actions?

- How are metal ions released from the enterocyte transported to the lumen of the blood vessels? What is the source of apo-Tf that accepts ferric ion from the enterocyte, and how does the resulting Fe-loaded Tf enter the lumen of the blood vessels?
- How are metal ions in serum delivered to the tissues? Are essential metal ions from the host a primary source for microbes that inhabit the upper respiratory and genitourinary tracts? If so, what are the primary mechanisms for delivery of metal ions onto the mucosal surfaces?

# 3

# Competition for Metals among Microbes and Their Host

Michael A. Bachman and Jeffrey N. Weiser

## Abstract

Both microorganisms and their eukaryotic hosts must acquire and compete for metal ions, often from scarce environmental sources, for their metabolism. Since metal ions can also be toxic, their cellular levels must be precisely regulated. The battle over these nutrients may affect the balance between microbe and host, impacting inflammatory responses and determining the outcome of this relationship during colonization and disease. This chapter examines aspects of the thrust and parry among bacteria residing in a host, and between bacteria and their host over metals.

## Introduction

Microbial metabolism requires the acquisition of numerous metals from environmental sources. Many microbes reside within a niche, such as the mammalian respiratory or urinary tracts, where these nutrients are available in extremely limited quantities. To be successful in such a niche where many species coexist, microbes must thus compete with one another to obtain required metals. Microbes that reside within a host face an additional challenge; namely, they must compete for these nutrients with their host, which may require the same metals for its metabolism. The most thoroughly studied of these biological battles over metals involves the acquisition of iron (Fe), although there is a growing appreciation over the struggle for manganese (Mn), zinc (Zn), and copper (Cu) among microbes and their hosts. Bacteria, for example, utilize iron for electron transport, amino acid synthesis, DNA synthesis, and protection from superoxide radicals. Under aerobic conditions, iron is primarily in the ferric [Fe (III)] oxidation state and readily forms insoluble complexes. Sequestration of scarce quantities of soluble iron is a prototypical protective response against invading bacteria, mediated by the Fe-binding proteins transferrin and lactoferrin and the storage protein ferritin. In contrast to Zn supplementation, which can be protective, nutritional supplementation with iron and Fe overload states is associated with an increased risk for certain bacterial infections. Additionally, in response to infection, the host increases production of hepcidin peptide hormone, which acts to block Fe uptake from the gut and the release of Fe stores, thereby restricting Fe levels in the bloodstream (Ganz 2009). To acquire iron within the host and counteract Fe binding by the host, bacteria must develop ways of scrounging iron directly from host sources or secrete siderophores that bind ferric iron with greater affinity. Growth limitation through the sequestration of essential elements or nutrients has been termed "nutritional immunity" and is now known to extend beyond Fe deprivation to other metals, including zinc and manganese (Hood and Skaar 2012).

## Cooperation and Competition among Bacteria for Metals

The scavenging of scarce amounts of ferric iron may provide an advantage to siderophore-expressers by depleting the availability of this limiting, required nutrient for competitors. Siderophore production may also be an altruistic or cooperative trait, where the cost of production for the individual is outweighed by the benefit to the group when other individuals can take up the siderophore-iron complex (Griffin et al. 2004). The fitness impact of siderophore-mediated cooperation on microbial ecology has been examined in detail using pyoverdin secreted by *Pseudomonas aeruginosa* (Buckling et al. 2007). These *in vitro* studies demonstrate that among closely related populations (kin selection), cooperative utilization of a close relative's siderophore is indeed favored. The *in vivo* relevance of these observations was subsequently shown in a wax moth larvae infection model, where a combination of pyoverdin-cooperating *P. aeruginosa* strains were more virulent compared to other combinations (Buckling et al. 2007).

In turn, microbes that are noncooperating cheats ("cheaters") avoid the energetic cost of siderophore production but are able to obtain iron by taking up siderophores made by their neighbors. Buckling et al. (2007) predict that cheats would be especially more fit under greater Fe-limiting conditions. *Neisseria gonorrhoeae*, for instance, produces no known siderophores but depends on host-derived, Fe-binding proteins, including transferrin and lactoferrin, for its iron (Strange et al. 2011). In addition, the gonococcus has been shown to acquire its iron from siderophores produced by other bacteria (termed "xenosiderophores"), such as the common catecholate class of siderophores. In this study, xenosiderophore-mediated growth was shown to be dependent on the *fbpABC* operon encoding the same ABC transport system that enables the gonococcus to transport iron into the cell from host Fe-binding sources. An additional strategy for microbes to conserve the energy required for Fe uptake is to cease production of siderophores when these are no longer needed. In fact, studies from the *P. aeruginosa* wax moth larvae infection model demonstrate that cheaters which no longer produce pyoverdin arise *de novo* under conditions where they have a selective advantage. The full extent of competitive and cooperative interactions involving Fe acquisition in extensive and heterogeneous microbial communities, such as within the mammalian gut, are likely to be complex and have yet to be fully explored.

Microbial competition for zinc *in vivo* has recently been demonstrated for the gut microbe *Campylobacter jejuni*. Expression of a high-affinity ABC transporter for Zn uptake was required for Campylobacter survival in chicken intestines in the presence of a normal microbiota, but not when chickens were reared under germ-free conditions with a more restricted microbiota. Differences in survival correlated with the presence of numerous Zn-binding proteins in the intestines of conventional chicks compared to the number in limited-microbiota chicks. This study concluded that the microbiota stimulates the production of host Zn-binding enzymes, which restrict the growth of bacteria that lack high-affinity Zn transporters (Gielda and DiRita 2012).

## Bacterial Infection Induces Metal Ion-Sequestering Components of Innate Immunity

Host–pathogen interactions often begin with colonization of mucosal surfaces. These relationships are highly specific, as certain microbial species are found only in particular microenvironments. We previously reported the use of transcriptional microarrays to screen host genes whose expression in the murine nasal mucosa was affected by colonization with the Gram-positive bacterium *Streptococcus pneumoniae* (Nelson et al. 2005). In this study, the most upregulated gene in response to colonization was lipocalin 2 (Lcn2, also known as siderocalin or neutrophil gelatinase-associated lipocalin, NGAL), whose expression was increased up to 65-fold during colonization as measured using qRT-PCR. Western analysis showed that Lcn2 was secreted into airway surface fluid in colonized animals. Immunohistochemical analysis localized Lcn2 expression primarily to Bowman's glands, which secrete Lcn2 into the nasal lumen where it bathes the colonized mucosa. Similar results were observed during colonization with the Gram-negative bacterium *Haemophilus influenzae*, suggesting that Lcn2 secretion is a general response to infection of the airways that may have a role in determining the establishment or maintenance of mucosal colonization (Nelson et al. 2005). Indeed, Lcn2 is induced by broad innate immune signals, including TLR4 stimulation and IL-1β (Chan et al. 2009).

Lcn2 contributes to antimicrobial defense by sequestration of a subset of microbial siderophores (Correnti and Strong 2012). Lcn2 specifically binds siderophores, such as the catecholate enterobactin (Ent), with an affinity similar to the *Escherichia coli* Ent receptor FepA; thus, it is able to compete with bacteria for Ent binding. Lcn2 is able to bind both ferric and aferric Ent, thereby depleting Ent from the microenvironment and inhibiting bacterial uptake of Ent-bound iron (Abergel et al. 2008). As a result, Lcn2 is bacteriostatic. Bacterial growth can be restored by the addition of excess iron or Ent. In a murine sepsis model, serum Lcn2 is protective against an *E. coli* strain that requires Ent to obtain iron (Flo et al. 2004). Accordingly, Lcn2-deficient mice (*Lcn2$^{-/-}$*), which are otherwise healthy, succumb more readily to invasive *E. coli* infection. Conversely, co-injection of *E. coli* and a siderophore to which Lcn2 cannot bind is sufficient to cause lethal infection in *Lcn2$^{+/+}$* mice.

As neither *S. pneumoniae* nor *H. influenzae* are known to produce or utilize siderophores, successful colonizers of the nasal passages appear to have evolved siderophore-independent mechanisms, such as the binding and utilization of host sources including heme, transferrin, and lactoferrin, to acquire essential iron and to evade the inhibitory effects of Lcn2. The Fe-sequestering effects of Lcn2 are likely an effective defense against Ent-dependent species in the mammalian respiratory tract. Indeed, high levels of Lcn2 correlate with increased survival of patients with Gram-negative bacterial pneumonia (Warszawska et al. 2013). In contrast, Lcn2 appears to be less of a determining factor in the composition of the gut flora where the Ent-expressing members of the Enterobacteriaceae family are abundant.

As is the case for ferric iron, the host also sequesters other metals required for microbial physiology during infection. To acquire zinc and manganese from the host reservoir, many bacterial species must express dedicated transport systems to compete for these metals. Virulence is often reduced when mutants of these Mn or Zn transporters are studied. Zinc is bound and sequestered from microbes when bound by albumin, 2-macroglobulin, and transferrin (Foote and Delves 1984; Moutafchiev et al. 1998). Additionally, the Zn status of the host affects immune functions (Knoell and Liu 2010; Nairz et al. 2010), and serum Zn levels are reduced upon infection or exposure to LPS, an effect that restricts availability of the metal to invasive microbes (Weinberg 1972; Liuzzi et al. 2005). Manganese is bound by apoferritin, lactoferrin, and transferrin (Macara et al. 1973; Lönnerdal et al. 1985; Davidsson et al. 1989; Critchfield and Keen 1992; Aschner and Gannon 1994; Moutafchiev et al. 1998). The extracellular protein calprotectin (a heterodimer of S100A8/ S100A9 or calgranulin A and B), a major product of neutrophils that migrate to sites of inflammation, binds manganese and possibly zinc (Kehl-Fie and Skaar 2010). Abscesses formed in response to *Staphylococcus aureus* infection are devoid of manganese. However, in mice lacking calprotectin, these are replete with manganese and have an increased bacterial burden, suggesting that calprotectin-mediated Mn chelation protects against disease (Corbin et al. 2008). It has also been postulated that other S100 proteins contribute to antimicrobial activity by restricting the bioavailability of other metals. At the other end of the spectrum, zinc may be toxic and levels elevated during inflammation. It has been proposed that zinc, like copper, accumulates in phagosomes and may contribute to host defense against intracellular pathogens (Botella et al. 2012). Within the phagocytic cell, NRAMP1 modulates microbial access to iron, manganese, and possibly zinc within vesicles. Thus, intracellular organisms must deal with cellular mechanisms that restrict survival through modulations of local metal concentrations. The scope of the battle with the host over levels of metals for microbial communities and interactions among the microflora *in vivo* has not yet been fully explored.

## The Battle between Microbes and Host over Metals Affects Inflammatory Responses

A number of cell culture studies have shown siderophore-dependent effects (Bierer and Nathan 1990; Coffman et al. 1990; Autenrieth et al. 1991, 1995; Britigan et al. 1994, 1997, 2000; Hileti et al. 1995; Tanji et al. 2001; Lee et al. 2005; Paauw et al. 2009). Many, but not all, of these effects are due to Fe sequestration, and together these reports indicate that both Fe deficiency and excess affects immune function. For example, in cultured human respiratory epithelial cells, treatment with aferric Ent produces a dose-dependent increase in proinflammatory signals, such as secretion of the chemokine IL-8, which promotes an influx of neutrophils (Nelson et al. 2007). Similar effects on pro-inflammatory signaling have been attributed to the microbial siderophore de-ferrioxamine, where the effect of Fe chelation was ascribed to the activation of p38 and extracellular signal-regulated kinase pathways (Choi et al. 2004). Furthermore, siderophores are potent activators of hypoxia inducible factor-1 (HIF-1), a global transcriptional regulator that enhances myeloid function and cytokine release (Peyssonnaux et al. 2005). However, the contribution of HIF-1 to siderophore-triggered inflammation during infection is unknown.

Through its interaction with Ent, Lcn2 can act as a signaling molecule. Two potential receptors for Lcn2 have been identified: megalin and 24p3R (Devireddy et al. 2005; Hvidberg et al. 2005). Megalin is expressed in kidney tubules and mediates uptake of siderophore-bound complexes with iron through endocytosis (Bao et al. 2010a). 24p3R is widely expressed in tissues, including the lung, as well as in lymphoid and myeloid cells. Although 24p3R has been shown to internalize Lcn2 alone or Lcn2 bound to a siderophore and to modulate Fe homeostasis and apoptosis, these findings are controversial (Correnti et al. 2012). In respiratory epithelial cells, Lcn2 is internalized and potentiates the cytokine release triggered by aferric Ent. In contrast, ferric Ent (Fe-Ent) does not elicit significant IL-8 release. Thus, aferric Ent may be a proinflammatory signal for respiratory epithelial cells, permitting detection of microbial communities that have disturbed local Fe homeostasis. Lcn2 expression by the host amplifies this signal. This may be a mechanism for the mucosa to respond to metabolic signals (i.e., the depletion of ferric iron) of expanding microbial communities (i.e., the expression of increasing amounts of siderophores).

Perhaps due to the actions of Lcn2, successful pathogens do not typically depend solely on Ent for iron and have evolved to use alternative siderophores that do not bind to Lcn2, allowing iron to be acquired even in its presence. An example in which the relative contribution of different Fe-scavenging systems has been studied *in vivo* is the Gram-negative member of the Enterobacteriaceae family, *Klebsiella pneumoniae*. *K. pneumoniae* is an opportunistic pathogen capable of colonizing multiple mucosal surfaces, including the nasopharynx, urinary tract, and large intestine of humans; it is also a common cause of bacterial pneumonia, urinary tract infection, and sepsis (Bachman et al. 2011). Isolates of *K. pneumoniae* invariably produce Ent, and a subset produces additional siderophores, including yersiniabactin (Ybt), aerobactin, and salmochelin. Salmochelin is glycosylated Ent (Gly-Ent) encoded by the *iroA* locus in some isolates of *K. pneumoniae, Salmonella enteric*, and *E. coli* (Fischbach et al. 2006). This cluster encodes the Ent glycosylase IroB that blocks Lcn2 binding, IroC for export, IroN for import, IroE for linearization, and IroD to degrade Gly-Ent and release iron. Transformation of *E. coli* with the *iroA* locus is sufficient to allow for lethal infection in $Lcn2^{+/+}$ mice. Conversely, disruption of either the *iroC* exporter or *iroB* glycoslyase attenuates virulence in a mouse model of systemic *Salmonella* infection (Crouch et al. 2008).

To study each potential effect of Lcn2, Lcn2-deficient mice and *K. pneumoniae* mutants predicted to be susceptible to Lcn2-mediated Fe sequestration (*iroA ybtS* mutant) or inflammation (*iroA* mutant) or to not interact with Lcn2 (*entB* mutant) were compared in a *K. pneumoniae* colonization model (Bachman et al. 2009). During murine nasal colonization, the *iroA ybtS* double mutant was inhibited: *iroA, entB*, and *ybtS* mutants were not, and this inhibition was Lcn2 dependent. Therefore, either Gly-Ent or Ybt are sufficient to protect against Lcn2-mediated growth inhibition. However, colonization with the *iroA* mutant induced an increased influx of neutrophils compared to the *entB* mutant and this enhanced neutrophil response to Ent-producing *K. pneumoniae* was Lcn2 dependent. These findings indicate that Lcn2 has both proinflammatory and Fe-sequestering effects along the respiratory mucosa in response to bacterial Ent and may serve as a sensor of microbial Fe metabolism to modulate the host's response appropriately.

## Metal Ion Acquisition As a Determining Factor in the Pathologic Features of Infection

To determine whether *K. pneumoniae* must produce Lcn2-resistant siderophores to cause disease, siderophore production was examined in clinical isolates ($n = 129$) from respiratory, urine, blood, and stool samples through genotyping and liquid chromatography mass spectrometry (Bachman et al. 2011). Three categories of *K. pneumoniae* isolates were identified: Ent(+) (81%), Ent(+) Ybt(+) (17%), and Ent(+) Gly-Ent(+) with or without Ybt (2%). The expression of aerobactin was rare among clinical isolates of *K. pneumoniae*. Ent(+) Ybt(+) strains were significantly overrepresented among respiratory tract isolates ($p = 0.0068$). In *ex vivo* growth assays, Gly-Ent but not Ybt allowed evasion of Lcn2 in human serum, whereas siderophores were dispensable for growth in human urine. In a murine pneumonia model, an Ent(+) strain was an opportunistic pathogen that was completely inhibited by Lcn2 but caused severe, disseminated disease in Lcn2$^{-/-}$ mice. In contrast, an Ent(+) Ybt(+) strain was a frank respiratory pathogen, causing pneumonia despite Lcn2. However, Lcn2 retained partial protection against disseminated disease. Ybt, therefore, is a virulence factor that promotes lower respiratory tract infections through evasion of Lcn2 (Bachman et al. 2011) and leads to worsened survival from pneumonia (Lawlor et al. 2007). In addition to its role in Fe acquisition, Chaturvedi et al. (2012) report that Ybt secreted by uropathogenic *E. coli* facilitates bacterial infection by binding to copper and sequestering Cu(II). The removal of Cu(II) prevents catecholate-mediated reduction to the more toxic form Cu(I), which is able to generate reactive oxygen species and inactivate intracellular iron-sulfur clusters in bacteria.

The siderophores Ent, Gly-Ent, and Ybt are not functionally equivalent and differ in their abilities to promote growth in the upper respiratory tract, lungs, and serum. To understand how Lcn2 exploits functional differences between siderophores, isogenic mutants of an Ent(+) Gly-Ent(+) Ybt(+) *K. pneumoniae* strain were inoculated into Lcn2$^{+/+}$ and Lcn2$^{-/-}$ mice, and the pattern of pneumonia was examined (Bachman et al. 2012). Lcn2 effectively protected against the *iroA ybtS* mutant [Ent(+) Gly-Ent(−) Ybt(−)]. Lcn2$^{+/+}$ mice had small foci of pneumonia, whereas Lcn2$^{-/-}$ mice had many bacteria in the perivascular space. The *entB* mutant [Ent(−) Ybt(+) Gly-Ent(−)] caused moderate bronchopneumonia but did not invade the perivascular space that accumulated transferrin during infection. Accordingly, transferrin or serum blocked Ybt-dependent growth *in vitro*, a result that contrasts with experimental systems using other pathogens and growth conditions (Fetherston et al. 2010). Wild-type *K. pneumoniae* and its *iroA* mutant, which both produce Ent and Ybt, had a mixed phenotype, causing a moderate bronchopneumonia in Lcn2$^{+/+}$ mice and perivascular overgrowth in Lcn2$^{-/-}$ mice. These findings demonstrated that Ent promotes growth around blood vessels that are rich in the Fe-binding protein transferrin, but Ybt does not. Together, transferrin and Lcn2 protect these spaces in the lungs against all types of *K. pneumoniae* tested. Therefore, the way in which iron is acquired can be a determining factor as to where an organism is able to grow and cause disease.

Siderophores are also required for pulmonary infection by *Bordetella pertussis, Burkholderiea cenocepacia, Legionella pneumophila,* and *Yersinia pestis,* and several of these pathogens express multiple siderophores (Brickman et al. 2008; Allard et al. 2009; Fetherston et al. 2010). In the case of *Y. pestis,* which has a complex life cycle with stages of infection involving different tissues, the inability to produce Ybt also affected inflammation in the lungs and, in this instance, shifted an intranasal infection route from a pneumonic to a systemic disease (Fetherston et al. 2010; Lee-Lewis and Anderson 2010). In addition, a *Y. pestis* Ybt mutant was completely avirulent by a subcutaneous route (bubonic plague), although a mutant defective in the Ybt system was fully virulent by an intravenous route (septicemic plague) (Fetherston et al. 2010). This indicates that the Ybt system is not essential for Fe acquisition (or non-iron effects) after *Y. pestis* enters the bloodstream. Ferrous transporters are another example of systems required for Fe acquisition in some host environments but not others. Again, *Y. pestis* provides an example: a *Y. pestis* strain with mutations in two ferrous transporters experienced a significant loss of virulence in a bubonic plague model but was fully virulent in a pneumonic plague model (Fetherston et al. 2012). The same pattern holds true for a strain with mutations in the two known Mn transporters, thus demonstrating that Mn transport mechanisms affect virulence in some host environments but not others (Fetherston et al. 2012). Again, these studies illustrate that the way in which essential metals are obtained can be a determining factor in the tissue tropism for infecting agents.

A recent study also demonstrated the importance of evasion of the Fe-dependent inhibitory effects of Lcn2 in the outcome of bacterial competition and in determining the composition of the microflora (Deriu et al. 2013). The non-pathogenic "probiotic" bacterium *E. coli* strain Nissle, which is equipped with multiple redundant Fe uptake systems, outcompetes *Salmonella* Typhimurium in a mouse model of acute colitis and chronic persistent infection. The success of *E. coli* strain Nissle is dependent on its ability to acquire iron in the gut, since mutants deficient in Fe uptake colonize the intestine but no longer reduce *S.* Typhimurium colonization. *S.* Typhimurium, however, is able to overcome the inhibitory effect of *E. coli* strain Nissle in Lcn2$^{-/-}$ mice. Deriu et al. (2013) concluded that Fe availability impacts *S.* Typhimurium growth and that in this example the beneficial action of probiotic bacteria is mediated by a reduction in intestinal colonization by pathogens like *S.* Typhimurium through competition for this limiting nutrient. Since many Ent-expressing members of the Enterobacteriaceae family normally reside in the gut lumen, a further implication is that inflammation increases the relative role of Lcn2 in modulating the flora in this environment. Interestingly, Nissle resembles uropathogenic *E. coli* strains. Genomic and metabolomic studies suggest that this subset of *E. coli* is generally more fit to colonize the Fe-limited environment of the bladder because of the expression and activity of additional siderophore systems (Henderson et al. 2009).

## Detrimental Effects of Metals on Microbial Interactions

Despite the requirement for metals for normal microbial and host physiology, they may be extremely toxic when present in excessive amounts or under certain environmental conditions. It appears that some organisms may take advantage of this situation and use the toxicity of certain metals for their own competitive success. For example, hydrogen peroxide is produced by *S. pneumoniae* as a byproduct of the activity of pyruvate oxidase (SpxB) under conditions of aerobic growth. Coculture with *S. pneumoniae* leads to a rapid decrease in viable counts of other bacterial species (Pericone et al. 2003). The addition of purified catalase or use of an *spxB* mutant prevents killing of other common inhabitants of the upper respiratory tract (including *H. influenzae, Moraxella catarrhalis*, and *Neisseria meningitidis*) in coculture experiments, suggesting that hydrogen peroxide may be responsible for this bactericidal activity. Production of hydrogen peroxide by *S. pneumoniae* has also been shown to have cytotoxic effects on human epithelial cells in culture and host tissue in animal models of pneumococcal disease. These antimicrobial and cytotoxic effects are thought to occur mainly through DNA damage from hydroxyl radicals (OH$^{\bullet}$) produced via the Fenton reaction: $H_2O_2 + Fe^{2+} \rightarrow Fe^{3+} + OH^{\bullet} + OH^-$. Accordingly, the amount of ferrous iron ($Fe^{2+}$) available to associate with DNA is believed to be a rate-limiting factor in Fenton-reaction killing. At millimolar concentrations of hydrogen peroxide generated by the pneumococcus, killing is thought to involve inactivation of housekeeping enzymes, perhaps through oxidation of active site thiols. The remarkable ability of *S. pneumoniae* to avoid Fenton chemistry and escape lethal damage at the high concentrations of hydrogen peroxide it generates when grown aerobically allows it to outcompete species vying for the same niche (Pericone et al. 2000). There is now clinical and experimental evidence for this effect. As is the case for the pneumococcus, nasal colonization by *S. aureus* is a major predisposing factor for subsequent infection. Recent reports of increased *S. aureus* colonization and disease among children receiving pneumococcal vaccine implicate *S. pneumoniae* as an important competitor for the same niche (Bogaert et al. 2004). Studies in a mouse model showed that expression of catalase by *S. aureus* contributes to the survival of this pathogen in the presence of *S. pneumoniae* during nasal cocolonization (Park et al. 2008). Therefore, iron can mediate interspecies competition by enabling the toxic effects of reactive oxygen molecules produced by one bacterium on its neighbor.

Most antibiotics are derived from the natural products employed by microbes to target other microbes. Although antibiotics act primarily on a number of essential targets of microbial physiology, there is experimental evidence, albeit controversial, that a common effect of antibiotic stress is an increase in levels of reactive oxygen species which triggers damage through the Fenton reaction (Kohanski et al. 2007; Liu and Imlay 2013). There is also a growing appreciation for how microorganisms manipulate the type and amount of potentially toxic metal ions to survive oxidative stress. *E. coli*, for example, can adapt to increased levels of hydrogen peroxide through the exchange of metals (Sobota and Imlay 2011). This mechanism involves Mn import and Fe depletion, converting a key enzyme in the pentose-phosphate pathway from Fenton chemistry susceptible to resistance. However, replacing iron with the wrong metal can also be disastrous. Gallium, a metal structurally similar to iron but unable to perform its redox chemistry, disrupts *P. aeruginosa* Fe metabolism and protects mice from lethal pneumonia (Kaneko et al. 2007). Excess zinc may also be toxic to bacteria. Zinc(II) concentrations are elevated in response to inflammation, and dietary supplementation with zinc has been associated with a decreased incidence of pneumonia in children (Brooks et al. 2005). For the leading bacterial cause of acute respiratory infection, *S. pneumoniae*, Mn(II) is an essential metal, but extracellular Zn(II) inhibits the acquisition of Mn(II) by competing for binding to the solute binding protein PsaA (McDevitt et al. 2011). Although the affinity of PsaA for Zn(II) is far lower, Zn(II)-PsaA is more thermally stable than Mn(II)-PsaA. This suggests that Zn(II) may bind the permease irreversibly inducing Mn(II) starvation. Binding of Zn(II) does not lead to its transport and it does not substitute the organism's requirement for Mn(II). The superoxide dismutase of the pneumococcus contains Mn(II), and the loss of this micronutrient leaves the organism more sensitive to oxidative killing by neutrophils. These observations suggest that host levels of Zn(II) and metal ion competition maybe an important mechanism for innate defense of host mucosal surfaces.

## Conclusion and Future Research Directions

The competition that microbes face for essential metals is severe and multifaceted. Microbes compete among themselves, compete with their hosts, and even exploit host competition factors to inhibit growth of their rivals. Metals themselves compete for binding to microbial proteins and if microbes successfully accumulate substantial metal concentrations, they risk lethal toxicity. Although our understanding of microbial competition for metals is substantial, important questions remain unanswered: What are the pathologic effects of microbial metal theft by pathogens on their hosts? How does competition for metals influence microbiome dynamics and how do metal-based changes in our microbiome affect our health? We have clues to these questions regarding iron, but Mn, Zn, and Cu metabolism appear to be crucial to microbial fitness as well. By unraveling the intricacies of microbial competition for metals, we may discover novel therapeutic approaches to protect us from these microbial pathogens.

# 4

# The Fate of Intracellular Metal Ions in Microbes

Slade A. Loutet, Anson C. K. Chan, Marek J. Kobylarz,
Meghan M. Verstraete, Stephanie Pfaffen, Bin Ye,
Angel L. Arrieta, and Michael E. P. Murphy

## Abstract

Metals are essential for all microorganisms as they are required as cofactors of enzymes that mediate metabolic processes that are indispensable for cellular energy production and growth. Some metals, such as zinc, are readily bound and serve as key structural elements of many macromolecules. Thus, to grow, microorganisms have an essential quota for several metals. The catalytic and other chemical properties of metals that microorganisms value create issues for metal management. Due to their high affinity for amino acids and their reactive nature, uptake, intracellular transport, and storage of metals are mediated by tightly regulated proteins. Protein chaperones function to supply some specific metals to sites of utilization and, in some cases, storage. In particular, iron is difficult to acquire and is stored as a mineral in protein nanocages. Other metals, when present in excess, induce the expression of export systems to maintain a defined intracellular concentration of readily exchangeable metal.

## Introduction

Whether a microorganism is a pathogen or a commensal, dependency on metals is universal. Although metals and metalloids dominate the periodic table, the list of essential metals is short and likely varies between species. The mechanisms by which these metals came to have biological relevance were probably influenced by factors such as their chemical properties and bioavailability. The overall availability of each metal has changed over the course of geological history due to the onset of photosynthesis, which switched Earth from an anoxic to an oxic environment (Catling and Claire 2005). As a result, metals, such as iron (Fe), were sequestered and others, such as copper (Cu) and zinc (Zn), were solubilized. Defining the availability of a metal also depends on the subcellular localization within the cell, such as the bacterial periplasm versus cytoplasm, which have differing metal concentrations as well as oxidative versus reductive environments, respectively. As excessive metal concentrations can be highly toxic, tight control is maintained over the intracellular concentration of metals. Due to this supply limit, a given metalloprotein may not be bound to the metal for which it has the highest affinity but rather it must compete for it with all of the other metalloproteins present. This competition adds a layer of complexity that is difficult to monitor using current technologies.

The metabolic pathways requiring metals are diverse, with metals often found as key cofactors in both essential and nonessential processes (Figure 4.1), including the synthesis of biological molecules (amino acids, DNA, RNA, lipids, and carbohydrates) and energy production (tricarboxylic acid [TCA] cycle, electron transport chain, and photosynthesis). Our understanding

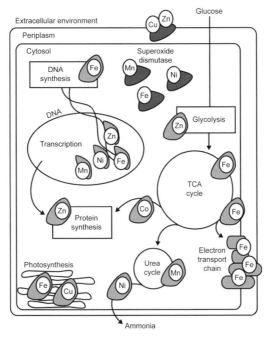

**Figure 4.1**   The major pathways in a bacterial cell that involve one or more metalloproteins (light gray). Examples of the metal ion(s) involved in each pathway are highlighted. Specific examples include ribonucleotide reductase (Fe, DNA synthesis), the Fur-like family (Zn/Ni/Fe/Mn, transcriptional regulation), threonyl-tRNA synthetase (Zn, protein synthesis), class II fructose-bisphosphate aldolase (Zn, glycolysis), aconitase and succinate dehydrogenase (Fe, TCA cycle), arginase (Mn, urea cycle), plastocyanin (Cu, photosynthesis), photosystems (Fe, photosynthesis), and cytochromes and succinate dehydrogenase (Fe, electron transport chain). This partial picture will continue to grow as studies continue to identify metalloproteins or reveal examples of metal promiscuity. In addition, proteins such as superoxide dismutase (dark gray) collectively utilize a variety of metals to perform the same biological function.

of the fate of intracellular metals lies primarily within the detailed but often independent characterization of each protein that comprises the biochemical pathways within the cell.

In this chapter we aim to familiarize the reader with general principles concerning the function of metal ions in bacteria, the movement and storage of metals within bacterial cells, and the strategies of metal detoxification used by bacteria. We note that many gaps exist in the fundamental understanding of these processes in bacteria; in particular, little is known about these processes in relation to infection.

## Forms and Concentration

Metals are trace elements in physiology. The total and readily exchangeable concentrations of specific metals are tightly regulated within the cell but vary greatly from metal to metal. Data on the content of specific metals per cell of many microorganisms are rarely available. The most comprehensive information in the literature is direct measurement of metal content by inductively coupled plasma mass spectrometry (ICP-MS) for *Escherichia coli*, some of which is summarized in Table 4.1. In general, available data stems from organisms that are easy to culture in a laboratory setting. Values obtained from a few species are often generalized without much supporting evidence. Large differences in metal content exist as the ratio of manganese (Mn) to iron can vary by over five orders of magnitude in bacteria (Lisher and Giedroc 2013).

Iron and zinc are the most abundant metals in *E. coli* (Table 4.1). Iron is necessary for almost all forms of life under physiological conditions, it exists primarily in one of two readily interconvertible oxidation states: the reduced $Fe^{2+}$ ferrous form and the oxidized $Fe^{3+}$ ferric form. Bacteria generally require

**Table 4.1** Content in *Escherichia coli* of biological transition metals. Total elemental content reported by Nies (2007) from data by Outten and O'Halloran (2001).

| Element | Ionic form | Content (µM) |
|---|---|---|
| Iron | $Fe^{2+}/Fe^{3+}$ | 180 |
| Zinc | $Zn^{2+}$ | 270 |
| Copper | $Cu^{1+}/Cu^{2+}$ | 18 |
| Nickel | $Ni^{2+}$ | <5 |
| Cobalt | $Co^{2+}$ | <0.5 |
| Manganese | $Mn^{2+}$ | 1.7 |
| Molybdenum | $Mo^{6+}$ | 8 |
| Vanadium | $V^{5+}$ | 77 |
| Tungsten | $W^{6+}$ | no data |

approximately $10^{-7}$ to $10^{-5}$ M iron to achieve optimal growth. The total Fe content of *E. coli* is estimated to be ~200 μM of which 10–30 μM is accessible to a chelator, as determined by electron paramagnetic spectroscopy on whole cells (Yan et al. 2013). Zinc is present in larger quantity than iron (~300 μM) and occurs exclusively as divalent cation $Zn^{2+}$. The free $Zn^{2+}$ concentration, as estimated by Zur and ZntR transcription assays in *E. coli*, is about $10^{-15}$ to $10^{-16}$ M (Outten and O'Halloran 2001); however, the readily exchangeable concentration is much higher (20 pM) and is more relevant to estimating the availability of this metal (Wang et al. 2011a).

Copper is both essential and toxic for many microorganisms. Approximately 20 μM of copper were measured, associated with *E. coli* cells. However, Cu-containing proteins are generally located outside the cytoplasm; thus no cytoplasmic metal is required. Because of the reducing cytoplasmic conditions, $Cu^{1+}$ is likely the dominant oxidation state within the cell. Almost all $Cu^+$ is bound by glutathione and other thiols. In yeast, the free $Cu^+$ in the cytoplasm is virtually nonexistent, and in *E. coli* the concentration is estimated to be $10^{-21}$ M (Changela et al. 2003).

Nickel (Ni), typically used by microbes for anaerobic growth, is found at <5 μM in *E. coli* under aerobic conditions. Total $Ni^{2+}$ in the cell may be increased under anaerobic growth when Ni-containing hydrogenase is expressed. The free concentration is estimated at $10^{-12}$ M based on the affinity of transcriptional regulator NikR in *E. coli* (Chivers and Sauer 2002). As detailed later, Ni- and Cu-trafficking systems have been discovered that explain the low exchangeable concentration of these metals in the cytoplasm.

For other metals, data are limited or nonexistent. For instance, $Co^{2+}$ (total concentration of <0.5 μM in *E. coli*) remains the major free form of cobalt (Co) in microbes, but the cytoplasmic concentration has not yet been studied. Nevertheless, the free Co concentration is likely low due to its toxic competition with other biologically essential metal ions (Okamoto and Eltis 2011). $Mn^{2+}$ (total concentration of ~2 μM in *E. coli*) is imported by microorganisms for use in Mn-specific enzymes, and can also be exchanged with iron in the metal-binding sites of some Fe proteins (Cotruvo and Stubbe 2012). The paucity of data on the overall metal content and speciation within many phyla of microorganisms is remarkable.

## Functions

In biological systems, metals are observed to participate in various types of roles: they can act as signaling molecules, catalysts, or structural elements. Identification of the physiologically and functionally relevant metal in proteins is not straightforward. The favored metal bound to a metalloprotein can, in some cases, be estimated by the observed amino acid ligands and the geometry of the metal site, though mischaracterization can occur due to the promiscuity of metal-binding sites and the similar chemical properties of certain metals. Peptide deformylase is a prime example, emphasizing the need for careful identification of the native metal (Maret 2010). This enzyme was originally purified with bound $Zn^{2+}$ and later extensively characterized with bound $Ni^{2+}$, a form that provided full activity. Subsequent studies, however, demonstrated that $Fe^{2+}$ was bound *in vivo*. Moreover, $Fe^{2+}$-bound peptide deformylase is highly sensitive to inactivation by hydrogen peroxide ($H_2O_2$). During $H_2O_2$ stress, $Mn^{2+}$ import is upregulated and can displace the bound $Fe^{2+}$. $Mn^{2+}$-bound peptide deformylase retains partial activity and is invulnerable to oxidation by $H_2O_2$ (Anjem and Imlay 2012). Species-based metal cofactor specificity has also been observed for proteins such as the superoxide dismutases (SODs), which can collectively utilize manganese, iron, binuclear copper–zinc, or nickel (Banci 2013). In yeast mitochondria, SOD can use either manganese or iron but selectively utilizes manganese, even though Fe concentrations are two orders of magnitude greater (Naranuntarat et al. 2009). Alternatively, isoenzymes utilizing different metals can functionally replace each other in a single organism. For example, NrdAB ribonucleotide reductase is an Fe enzyme essential for *E. coli* aerobic growth, but under periods of Fe restriction, the expression of Mn-dependent NrdEF is induced (Martin and Imlay 2011). Overall, this seemingly conflicting property of metal flexibility and selectivity attests to the finely tuned, but adaptable nature of metal homeostasis within an organism.

As a part of this adaptable nature, metals are involved in signal transduction pathways and are recognized by sensory proteins to maintain metal homeostasis. Changes in metal content can indicate a change in the environment, such as the transition experienced by a pathogen moving from an external environment to inside a host. In addition, host organisms actively sequester metals from bacterial commensals and pathogens alike. Therefore, bacteria must have the ability to sense the abundance of each metal and respond accordingly. Metal homeostasis is controlled by sensory proteins that bind specific metals and regulate uptake, export, or utilization of the metal. A classic example is the Fur-like family of related bacterial regulators—Fur, Zur, Mur, and Nur—which recognize and regulate $Fe^{2+}$, $Zn^{2+}$, $Mn^{2+}$ and $Ni^{2+}$ homeostasis, respectively (Fillat 2014). Metal complexes such as heme can also function as signaling molecules. One example is HrtR from the commensal *Lactococcus lactis*, which is a heme sensor that regulates a heme efflux system (Lechardeur et al. 2012).

In addition to their direct role in regulating metal acquisition, these sensory proteins can also modulate the expression of virulence and survival factors. For example, *Staphylococcus aureus* Fur was discovered to enhance the expression of several immunomodulatory proteins: protein A (SpA), staphylococcal immunoglobulin G-binding protein (Sbi), and extracellular fibrinogen-binding protein (Efb) (Torres et al. 2010).

Deprivation of iron typically elicits a complex response which ultimately results in a metabolic shift to pathways that rely less on iron. In *S. aureus*, this "iron-sparing" response redirects its metabolism from the Fe-requiring tricarboxylic acid (TCA) cycle and respiratory chain to the Fe-independent glycolytic pathway (Friedman et al. 2006). Little is known of the potential metabolic shifts akin to "iron sparing," when bacteria find themselves in environments low in other metals. In some rare cases, select bacteria completely eliminate the need for a particular metal as a metabolic strategy. Notably, *Borrelia burgdorferi*—the only known bacteria that does not directly require iron or produce nucleotides *de novo*—is an obligate intracellular parasite that appears to utilize manganese in key proteins and depends on its (iron-requiring) host for essential nutrients (Posey and Gherardini 2000).

Transition metals (i.e., those elements in the d-block of the periodic table) play essential catalytic roles in microbial metabolic pathways. Of the transition metals, iron is commonly employed because its reduction potential is favorable for biochemical reactions. Iron is typically incorporated into enzymes as free ions, heme, or iron-sulfur (Fe-S) clusters, with the majority of Fe enzymes falling under the oxidoreductase class (Andreini et al. 2008). An essential free Fe-containing enzyme is the NrdAB ribonucleotide reductase, which produces deoxyribonucleotides from ribonucleotides for DNA synthesis and repair (Ando et al. 2011). The TCA cycle enzyme aconitase is a well-known Fe-S cluster enzyme responsible for the isomerization of citrate into isocitrate (Prodromou et al. 1992). Heme iron plays a major role in the electron transport chain as a cofactor in cytochromes, which mediate electron transfer that ultimately leads to the generation of ATP (Kamen and Horio 1970). Enzymes can also require more than one type of iron. For example, succinate dehydrogenase plays a role in both the TCA cycle and the electron transport chain, and contains three Fe-S clusters as well as a heme cofactor (Yankovskaya et al. 2003).

In biological molecules, cobalt is often bound in the center of a cyclic, four pyrrole ring structure (corrin). Derivatization of the corrin ring leads to a family of compounds known as the corrinoids, the most well-known of which is cobalamin (vitamin B12). Methionine synthase utilizes a cobalamin cofactor to transfer a methyl group to homocysteine, thus forming methionine (Drennan et al. 1994). The noncorrin Co enzyme methionine aminopeptidase is also involved in methionine metabolism and catalyzes the removal of the N-terminal methionine from newly synthesized peptides (Ben-Bassat et al. 1987). Methionine aminopeptidase is essential for the maturation, subcellular localization, and degradation of many proteins (Kobayashi and Shimizu 1999), and inactivation of this enzyme has been demonstrated to be lethal in organisms such as *E. coli* (Chang et al. 1989). Despite all of the work that has been done to characterize methionine aminopeptidase as a Co enzyme, some have suggested that iron is the true cofactor inside *E. coli* (Chai et al. 2008).

Zinc is an essential transition metal estimated to be used by 4–10% of proteins encoded by the genome of some organisms (Andreini et al. 2011). In fact, it is the second most abundant metal in characterized enzymes, behind magnesium and slightly ahead of iron (Andreini et al. 2008). The majority of prokaryotic Zn proteins are enzymatic in nature, although the Zn cofactor can participate as either a structural or catalytic component. In addition to acting as a catalytic Lewis acid, zinc is distinct from other common transition metals in that it lacks redox reactivity and is thus an excellent metal for stabilizing negative charges. Not surprisingly, examples of Zn proteins are found in all six major classes of enzymes, with the largest proportion being hydrolases such as alkaline phosphatase and thermolysin.

Nickel is an essential metal in some prokaryotes. For the gastric pathogen *Helicobacter pylori*, two Ni-containing enzymes contribute to its pathogenicity (Eaton et al. 1991; Olson and Maier 2002). Nickel-iron hydrogenase allows for the use of molecular $H_2$ as a substrate for respiration. Urease is an essential factor in stomach colonization; it neutralizes stomach acid through the production of ammonia.

No bacterial Cu-dependent proteins have been observed to be localized to the cytoplasm (Rensing and McDevitt 2013). Thus far, only ten types of Cu enzymes have been identified in prokaryotes, with cytochrome *c* oxidase present in most organisms. In *E. coli*, the major periplasmic Cu protein is CueO, a multicopper oxidase that is part of a Cu-resistance mechanism (Roberts et al. 2002). In cyanobacteria, copper is shuttled into the thylakoid, a specialized compartment with Cu-requiring photosynthetic and respiratory electron transport proteins (Tottey et al. 2005). All other characterized Cu proteins are localized either to the periplasm or to the cytoplasmic membrane with the active, Cu-binding site facing away from the cytoplasm.

In cases where the metal is structural, the selected metals tend to be redox inert and can act to neutralize repulsive negative charges. The most common metal in this capacity is $Mg^{2+}$, which plays a major role in stabilizing the structures of DNA and RNA backbone phosphate groups (Sreedhara and Cowan 2002) and assists in orienting the phosphate groups in nucleoside triphosphate (e.g., ATP, GTP, CTP, TTP) bound to enzymes (Cowan 2002). $Ca^{2+}$ is another common structural metal, but it is primarily exploited by extracellular proteins, polysaccharides, and other cell wall components (Norris et al. 1991). A well-known structural feature containing a transition metal is the Zn finger motif, which mediates DNA- and RNA-binding as well as protein–protein interactions (Krishna et al. 2003). Zinc can also play a structural role in certain Fur proteins, such as those from *E. coli* and *H. pylori*, where it binds to a second, nonregulatory site (Jacquamet et al. 1998; Vitale et al. 2009).

Although the molecular details of metal uptake and efflux are relatively well studied and the list of characterized metal-binding proteins continues to grow, the distribution of such metals within a cell remains largely uncharacterized. Only recently have we begun to characterize the metalloproteome on a global scale with sufficiently high enough resolution to determine such detailed metal distribution information within a subcellular context. A recent study on the pathogen *Bacillus anthracis* revealed that cytoplasmic iron was primarily found in only four major pools: the electron transfer protein ferredoxin, the miniferritin Dps2, two co-eluted SODs (SodA1 and SodA2), and a single unidentifiable pool of metalloprotein(s) (Tu et al. 2012). Interestingly, manganese consisted of a single major pool, which was identified to be SodA1 as well. Through further investigation, Tu et al. revealed that SodA1 consists of a mixed population primarily bound to manganese *in vivo*, with the remaining population bound to iron. In contrast, SodA2 is exclusively bound to iron.

A key question facing metalloprotein research is the relative role of metals between commensal and pathogenic bacteria. Pathogens have been observed to carry a larger genetic toolbox of metal acquisition proteins and metalloenzymes required for pathogenicity and antibiotic resistance. For example, genes encoding receptors for the siderophores yersiniabactin (Ybt) and aerobactin are more common in extraintestinal pathogenic *E. coli* than in commensal strains (Lee et al. 2010). *S. aureus* produces two distinct SODs as compared to the less virulent coagulase-negative *Staphylococcus* spp., which generally have one (Valderas et al. 2002). In addition, many pathogenic Gram-positive bacteria possess FosB, a divalent metal-dependent thiol-S-transferase implicated in fosfomycin resistance (Roberts et al. 2013). The difference between a commensal and a related pathogen, however, may be at the level of expression control rather than gene content, as known genomic pathogenicity islands were identified in nearly 50% of randomly surveyed commensal fecal *E. coli* strains (Li et al. 2010a). A given organism may act as a commensal or a pathogen, depending on signals from its environment. Serotyping and genotyping studies have shown, in the same individual, that both asymptomatic intestinal *E. coli* and uropathogenic *E. coli* are clonally related (Grüneberg 1969; Yamamoto et al. 1997). Further confounding these issues are opportunistic pathogens, which take advantage of negative perturbations to the host defense systems.

Taken together, whether or not pathogens and commensals have different metal requirements remains an open question. They may have the same general metal requirements, since many of the roles played by metals discussed here are conserved among commensals and pathogens. They might also be distinguished by the possession and regulation of metal uptake and detoxification systems. Current techniques do not allow for detailed analyses of metal-requiring processes on a global and dynamic scale. Advances in high-resolution metallomics techniques, such as those discussed by Maret et al. (this volume), hold promise in providing great insight into metal functions and fluxes within a bacterium, and how these change under different environmental conditions. New data will also inform us on intra- and interspecies differences in metal usage. These data have the potential to lead novel tools for infection control, bioremediation, or bioengineering based on bacterial metal-dependent processes.

## Metallochaperones

Metallochaperones are a class of metalloproteins that bind metal ions and move them between uptake pathways, functional sites, storage systems, or detoxification pathways (Figure 4.2). They insert metal ions into other proteins via specific protein–protein interactions. Free metal ions must be quickly bound by the cognate metallochaperones to both facilitate transfer to the correct location and protect the cell from toxicity associated with free intracellular metal ions. The activity of metallochaperone proteins can be divided into three stages: (a) selective binding of the cognate metal ion, (b) identification of and interaction with the desired target metalloprotein, and (c) transfer of the metal ion to the target metalloproteins (Rosenzweig 2002).

In general, metal ions are bound to metallochaperones at exposed sites to facilitate protein-to-protein metal ion exchange. An example is the periplasmic protein CusF: a $Cu^{1+}$ and $Ag^{1+}$ chaperone for the CusCBA metal detoxification system (Mealman et al. 2012). CusF adopts a β-barrel fold and binds either $Cu^{1+}$ or $Ag^{1+}$ ions at a site at one end of the barrel (Xue et al. 2008). For a given metal, chaperones with different protein folds and binding pockets may exist. For example, Cu chaperones use at least four different protein folds and binding pockets (Robinson and Winge 2010). Purified metallochaperones are often poorly selective for binding of the correct metal ion *in vitro*. $Ni^{2+}$ binding by UreE, the metallochaperone for urease assembly, can be outcompeted by $Cu^{2+}$ and $Zn^{2+}$ *in vitro* (Brayman and Hausinger 1996). In a bacterial cell, a number of factors likely contribute to the correct metal selection by metallochaperones (Tottey et al. 2005; Maret 2010). Bacteria maintain a limited metal pool through restriction of the readily exchangeable metal concentration by expressing storage systems and selective metal import and export systems. Compartmentalization within the bacterial cell can co-localize proteins in the presence of certain metals. Some metalloproteins undergo allosteric changes upon binding of only the correct metal ion. Finally, bacteria can alter their metabolism to exploit the most plentiful metals.

Once a metallochaperone has acquired its cognate metal ion, it must identify and interact with the correct target protein. These protein–protein interactions are driven by the factors that influence all protein–protein interactions, such as electrostatic or hydrophobic interactions between exposed surfaces (Reichmann et al. 2007). For metallochaperone–target protein interactions, other common features include a requirement for the correct metal ion and structural similarity between the metallochaperone and the target. The specificity of protein–protein interactions likely contributes to the target metalloproteins binding the correct metal despite energetic constraints. Finally, the metallochaperone must deliver its metal ion to the target protein. Metal transfer often involves ligand exchange reactions, where both proteins use the same ligands to coordinate the metal ion and, in a stepwise fashion, transfer the metal from the metallochaperone to the target. In some systems, such as the transfer

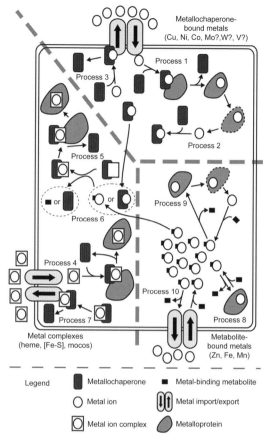

**Figure 4.2**   Metallochaperones are part of a complex set of metal pools that exist to minimize the concentration of free metal ions. The metalloprotein symbol represents proteins with a metal ion as a cofactor, with metal serving a structural role, or with metal being stored. Degraded metalloproteins are represented with dashed outlines. Most, but not all, of the processes illustrated have been experimentally demonstrated. For some metals (top), metallochaperones act to transport metal ions from import systems to target metalloproteins (Process 1). They can also recover metal ions after metalloprotein degradation (Process 2) and transport excess metal ions to export systems (Process 3). Metallochaperones perform similar functions for metal complexes (left). These complexes can be directly imported (Process 4) or they can be synthesized *de novo* (Process 5) with metals obtained from a metallochaperone protein pool or a metabolite-bound pool (Process 6). Metal complexes can also be exported from the cell (Process 7). Some metals (bottom right) are proposed to be bound by small metabolites to buffer the bacterium from free metal ions. The metal-bound metabolites are thought to be in equilibrium with some metal-bound proteins (Process 8). Metal bound to metabolites may bind tightly to metalloproteins and be released only upon protein degradation (Process 9). Theoretically, these metabolites would interact with import and export systems (Process 10). For illustrative purposes these interactions are all being shown as occurring within the bacterial cytoplasm; however, many of these processes also occur in the bacterial cell envelope.

of Ni$^{2+}$ from UreE to the urease enzyme complex (Farrugia et al. 2013), transfer of the metal ion to the target metalloprotein requires the assistance of accessory proteins. Accessory proteins can act as scaffolds to enhance protein–protein interactions; they can provide energy or other enzymatic functions. In the case of the urease complex (Farrugia et al. 2013), UreD acts as a scaffold between the UreABC enzyme and other proteins required for maturation of the enzyme. Ni$^{2+}$ insertion into the urease complex requires GTP hydrolysis, a function provided by UreG. A third accessory protein, UreF, is suggested to enhance the interaction between the GTPase activity of UreG and Ni$^{2+}$ insertion by UreE.

In cells, metal ions can also be found bound to nonprotein cofactors, such as iron bound to protoporphyrin IV (heme) or molybdenum (Mo) bound by a family of related cofactors (known as the Mocos). Metallochaperones exist for these types of complexes: CcmE is a periplasmic heme-binding protein that delivers heme to cytochrome *c* (Schulz et al. 1998), whereas specific chaperones deliver each of the Mocos to their appropriate targets (Neumann and Leimkühler 2011). Another well-known example of a nonprotein cofactor is the widely used Fe-S clusters (Johnson et al. 2005a). In bacteria, at least three different Fe-S biosynthetic clusters exist, with the IscU system being the most well characterized (Vickery and Cupp-Vickery 2007). Although precise mechanistic details are still being characterized, IscU is responsible for building the Fe-S cluster, which is then transferred to an acceptor protein, such as ferredoxin or aconitase, with the assistance of two accessory proteins (HscA and HscB) (Vickery and Cupp-Vickery 2007).

The state of knowledge with regards to metallochaperones for the metals varies. Numerous Cu and Ni chaperones have been described in the literature. Given the prevalence of Fe- and Zn-containing proteins, relatively little is known about metallochaperones for these elements. As proposed elsewhere (see Cavet et al., this volume), due to the large number of zinc, mononuclear iron, and Mn-containing proteins, we speculate that small molecule ligands (e.g., histidine and glutathione) rather than proteins might be used as chaperones for these elements. We believe that other metals used by bacteria in a smaller number of metalloproteins, including cobalt, vanadium, and tungsten, also likely use protein chaperones; however, little data concerning chaperones for these elements are available.

New avenues of metallochaperone research are likely to open up as emerging evidence from metalloproteome studies indicates that a wider variety of metals are incorporated into metalloproteins than previously thought. Metallochaperone research has mainly been confined to a subset of bacteria, particularly those causing disease. Environmental bacteria living in diverse ecosystems likely utilize additional sources of metals and contain novel metallochaperones. Finally, the proposed use of small molecule ligands as chaperones for zinc, manganese, and iron inside the bacterial cell awaits further study.

*S. A. Loutet et al.*

## Detoxification and Cytoplasmic Metal Export

Metals often get into microbial cells via influx pumps for essential elements and must be selectively handled by membrane transport mechanisms, as many are harmful to bacteria. Metals demonstrate toxicity due to their chemical affinity for thiol groups, which can alter enzyme specificity and disrupt cellular functions. Still, some metals (e.g., iron, cobalt, copper, and zinc) are essential micronutrients but can also be toxic at high levels (Bruins et al. 2000). The challenge for the bacterial cell is to maintain a level of homeostasis between metal uptake for nutrition and membrane transport out to avoid toxicity. Microorganisms have adapted by developing a variety of resistance mechanisms, including energy-dependent efflux, enzymatic transformations, sequestration by metal-binding proteins and siderophores, and precipitation of metal sulfides (Figure 4.3). These metabolic responses differ for each metal.

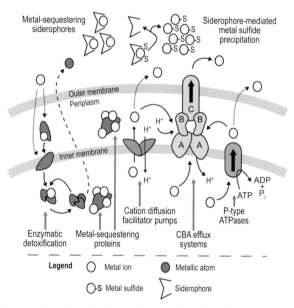

**Figure 4.3**   Examples of mechanisms of metal detoxification and resistance. Enzymatic detoxification (mercury reductase, green) alters a metal to a less toxic form. Mercury reduced to $Hg^0$ is volatile and diffuses out of the cell (dashed line). Periplasmic (SilE, blue) and cytoplasmic proteins (metallothionein, blue) mediate resistance by binding excess intracellular metals. Cation diffusion facilitator family pumps (CzcD, pink), CBA efflux transport systems (CzcCBA, yellow), and P-type ATPases (CadA, orange) are all energy-dependent efflux systems. Siderophores (e.g., pyoverdine) bind metals to lower the extracellular free metal ion concentration and can also participate in metal sulfide precipitation (e.g., pyridine-2,6-bis[thiocarboxylic acid]). For illustrative purposes a Gram-negative bacteria with an outer membrane is depicted: dotted lines illustrate the extracytoplasmic movement of metal ions in Gram-positive bacteria or movement of metal ions through the Gram-negative outer membrane that are poorly understood.

The most frequent, widespread mechanism of metal resistance is energy-dependent efflux, generally without coincident covalent or redox chemistry. Efflux systems fall into a small number of families (Nies 2003; Silver and Phung 2005). These include P-type ATPases, which are single polypeptide determinants with an intermediate phosphorylated by ATP; cation diffusion facilitator pumps that are made up by a single polypeptide chemiosmotic pump; and export systems driven by resistance-nodulation-cell division (RND), which are comprised of three proteins: (a) an inner membrane RND protein, supported by (b) a membrane fusion protein (MFP) that provides a connection through the periplasmic space to (c) a protein belonging to the family of outer membrane factors (OMFs). These three proteins form a complex that can efflux its respective substrate from the cytoplasm, cytoplasmic membrane, or periplasm across the outer membrane to outside the cell. To differentiate this type of efflux mechanism from ATP-driven ABC transporters, the RND-driven export system is also referred to as a CBA efflux system.

Cadmium resistance, for example, is found widely in environmental and clinical isolates for which three types of cadmium efflux mechanisms have been discovered. The CzcD single membrane polypeptide chemiosmotic pump confers resistance by pumping out metal ions directly from the cytoplasm (Anton et al. 1999). The *czc* resistance determinant also encodes a CBA efflux system and contains the genes for the OMF CzcC, the MFP CzcB and the CzcA protein of the RND family (Nies et al. 1989). This efflux system may have the ability to pump metal ions out of both the cytoplasm and the periplasm (Nies 2003) as well as to confer some resistance to $Co^{2+}$ and $Zn^{2+}$ (Nies et al. 1989). CadA, a large single polypeptide P-type ATPase, can also contribute to $Cd^{2+}$ resistance (Nucifora et al. 1989).

P-type ATPases and other transporters for metal efflux have also been found to be involved in extracytoplasmic protein metalation (Arguello et al. 2013). In *Rhodobacter capsulatus* the metalation of the periplasmic protein, $cbb_3$ cytochrome *c* oxidase ($cbb_3$-COX), requires transport of $Cu^+$ through a major facilitator superfamily transporter protein (Ekici et al. 2012). Gonzalez-Guerrero et al. (2010) described two nonredundant $Cu^+$-ATPases, CopA1 and CopA2, in *Pseudomonas aeruginosa*. CopA1 represents a classical $Cu^+$-ATPase for $Cu^+$ efflux, whereas CopA2 has comparably slower transport kinetics and higher affinity for $Cu^+$. Deletion of *copA2* results in a mutant with decreased cytochrome *c* oxidase activity, thus suggesting that the properties of CopA2 are suitable for participation in the assembly of cuproproteins like *ccb3*-COX.

Another metal resistance mechanism that has evolved for bacteria is the enzymatic detoxification of a metal to a less toxic form. Mercury resistance, encoded by the *mer* operon, is a broadly occurring toxic metal resistance system found in Gram-positive and Gram-negative bacteria from environmental, clinical, and industrial samples (Mathema et al. 2011). Bacteria have cleverly developed a way to bind extracellular $Hg^{2+}$ and transport it into the cytoplasm using a series of cysteines on different proteins, termed a thiol "bucket brigade," to active sites on mercuric reductase, while ensuring that no toxic mercury is free within the cell to cause damage (Silver and Phung 2005). In Gram-negative bacteria, there is no outer membrane protein known to be involved in the $Hg^{2+}$ transport system. Instead, a periplasmic MerP protein is thought to relay $Hg^{2+}$ to the inner membrane protein MerT. Once $Hg^{2+}$ is at the inner surface of the cytoplasmic membrane, it is likely transferred to mercuric reductase (MerA) by cysteine-pair to cysteine-pair exchange. Thereafter, $Hg^{2+}$ is reduced to elemental mercury (Furukawa and Tonomura 1972; Schiering et al. 1991), which is volatile and able to diffuse out of the cell (Schelert et al. 2004).

Intracellular sequestration of toxic cations by metal-binding proteins serves as another method of metal resistance. $Cd^{2+}$ and $Zn^{2+}$ are commonly sequestered by cysteine-rich proteins, such as metallothionein (Shi et al. 1992). These small polythiol metal cation-binding proteins function to lower free metal ion concentrations within the cytoplasm and afford a level of resistance. Another example of binding by sequestration is the Sil $Ag^+$ resistance system in which resistance is partly facilitated by a small periplasmic metal-binding protein, SilE (Gupta et al. 1999).

Metal resistance is also mediated through the secretion of siderophores, which are low molecular weight molecules primarily produced for ferric iron acquisition. Siderophores can serve as multifunctional metabolites that are able to bind other metals outside of the cell and protect against metal toxicity. An example of this environmental conditioning is the production of pyridine-2,6-bis(thiocarboxylic acid) (PDTC) siderophore by *Pseudomonas stutzeri* (Zawadzka et al. 2007). This siderophore can form poorly soluble complexes with $Hg^{2+}$, $Cd^{2+}$, $Pb^{2+}$, and $As^{3+}$ and hydrolyze them to form insoluble metal sulfides. Precipitation of metals as metal sulfides using siderophores acts as an environmental detoxification mechanism by restricting the bioavailability of extracellular metals. Conversely, PDTC can also facilitate Zn utilization, as well as Fe uptake, in *Pseudomonas putida* (Leach et al. 2007). Another example of siderophores mediating bacterial tolerance to metals is the production of pyoverdine and pyochelin by *P. aeruginosa* (Braud et al. 2010). Despite their preference for iron, these siderophores are able to bind $Al^{3+}$, $Co^{2+}$, $Cu^{2+}$, $Ni^{2+}$, $Pb^{2+}$, and $Zn^{2+}$ in the extracellular milieu, leading to increased *P. aeruginosa* resistance and decreased intracellular metal accumulation. Uropathogenic *E. coli* (UPEC) uses Ybt to chelate host $Cu^{2+}$ and prevent its reduction to the more bactericidal form, $Cu^{1+}$, thus increasing the Cu resistance of UPEC (Chaturvedi et al. 2012). Importantly, the $Cu^{2+}$-Ybt complex was identified in samples from human patients with active urinary tract infections with UPEC. Though siderophores mediate metal detoxification outside of the cell, they are an intracellular crafted mechanism of resistance. The diversity seen in siderophore chemical composition, the upregulation of siderophore production in response to metals other than iron, the ability of siderophores to bind iron and other metals tightly, the fact that some bacteria make multiple siderophores, and the observation during infections that siderophores play roles in metal binding and detoxification all support the idea that siderophores have evolved to perform multiple physiological functions with regards to homeostasis of iron and other metals (Schalk et al. 2011).

Metal detoxification is a rapidly advancing field of research. *Campylobacter jejuni* has recently been shown to possess a membrane permease for the removal of roxarsone and nitarsone (organic arsenic molecules added to chicken and poultry feed to reduce bacterial infections and increase weight gain) from the cytoplasm (Shen et al. 2014). The permease was specific to these organic arsenic forms and played no role in arsenite or arsenate resistance. *Mycobacterium tuberculosis* produces an extracytoplasmic multicopper oxidase that participates in Cu resistance (Rowland and Niederweis 2013). Bacteria can also precipitate metals as inorganic sulfides, such as nickel sulfide and cobalt pentlandite ($Co_9S_8$) (Sitte et al. 2012). Many more detoxification strategies are being characterized as they are becoming more ubiquitous among bacterial populations in polluted environments and clinical isolates, where metal resistance systems are commonly co-selected for with antibiotic resistance genes due to genetic co-resistance and physiological cross-resistance mechanisms (Baker-Austin et al. 2006). There is growing concern that metal contamination is indirectly selecting for antibiotic resistance, and studies have shown that metal-contaminated environments contain an overabundance of antibiotic resistance genes (Knapp et al. 2011).

## Storage

Iron in excess of that which is needed for cellular homeostasis is toxic and potentially lethal to the cell. Therefore, most organisms, including bacteria, have evolved a strategy that involves the use of proteins of the ferritin superfamily to protect cells from the harmful effects of excess iron (Andrews 2010). Ferritins are the major proteins that bind and store nonheme iron inside cells. The typical ferritin consists of 24 subunits, forming a hollow sphere that takes up soluble ferrous iron and oxidizes it at di-iron ferroxidase centers for storage as a ferric mineral within the central cavity. Mammalian ferritins are composed of two different subunits: the H-chain subunit contains the catalytic ferroxidase center, and the L-chain subunit contains mineral nucleation sites. In bacteria, two ferritin subtypes are found: the heme-containing bacterioferritin (BFR) and the bacterial ferritin. Both types are homopolymers in which the monomer contains the ferroxidase site and the mineral nucleation sites. Both BFR and bacterial ferritin play a role in Fe storage but may also have more specialized functions in Fe detoxification, depending on the organism (Le Brun et al. 2010). Although both could theoretically hold up to 4500 Fe atoms (Crichton and Declercq 2010), when isolated from non-overexpressing sources, BFR holds between 800 and 1600 Fe atoms whereas bacterial ferritin typically stores between 600 and 2300 Fe atoms (Lewin et al. 2005).

Outside the catalytic residues of the ferroxidase site, only a few residues are conserved between ferritin subfamilies (Andrews 2010), and amino acid sequence identities can be as low as 15%. Overall structure, however, is conserved among ferritins and BFR (Crichton and Declercq 2010). The ferroxidase center is located in the center of the monomer, a four helix bundle with a short fifth helix at the C-terminus, and consists of two Fe-binding sites: site A and site B. However, the ferroxidase centers of BFR and bacterial ferritins are distinct in their Fe-coordinating ligand arrangement. In bacterial ferritin, a third Fe-binding site, site C, is located near the ferroxidase center. In the *E. coli* ferritin A, this site is not essential for rapid Fe oxidation but has an effect on the Fe mineralization and Fe movement into the protein cavity (Bou-Abdallah et al. 2014). Residues coordinating to site C are highly conserved in bacterial ferritins, indicating the functional importance of this site (Le Brun et al. 2010).

Although ferritin is the most studied and best understood metal storage protein, little is known about how iron enters and exits ferritin. Iron entry and exit in ferritin is suggested to be through their threefold channels (Treffry et al. 1993). However, ferritins also have B-channels, which are located between two subunit dimers (Carrondo 2003). The roles of the channels in ferritin are not yet clear. Furthermore, the heme groups in BFR do not play a role in the $Fe^{2+}$ uptake but may play an important role in Fe release (Yasmin et al. 2011).

A third Fe storage protein found in bacteria is the Dps (DNA-binding protein from starved cells) ferritin. Dps ferritin forms a 12mer and can store up to 500 Fe atoms (Crichton and Declercq 2010). However, the function of Dps ferritin lies more in protecting DNA against oxidative and mechanical stress as well as enzymatic degradation (Zeth 2012).

Other known metal storage proteins found in bacteria have a much lower storage capacity. For example, MoSto from *Azotobacter vinelandii* is a hexameric Mo storage protein that is functionally related to nitrogen fixation by supplying nitrogenase with molybdenum. It can store more than 100 Mo atoms per hexamer as a polyoxomolybdate cluster in an interior cavity (Kowalewski et al. 2012). Another example is *E. coli* SlyD, which can bind two to seven Ni ions in its unstructured C-terminal region. This protein is proposed to act as a reservoir for nickel, but also contributes to the insertion of nickel into the hydrogenase precursor protein by transferring Ni atoms to the auxiliary protein HypB and modulating its activities (Kaluarachchi et al. 2011).

Ferritin is the most studied and best understood metal storage protein and the only known storage protein with a high capacity of several hundred to thousands of metal ions. MoSto is the only other example that we have come across of a mass storage protein similar to ferritin. In contrast, other known storage proteins can bind few metal ions, and storage by these proteins is considered to be a secondary function.

## Concluding Remarks

Although much progress has been made on the fate of intracellular metal ions in bacteria, many key questions are still outstanding. We know that metal ions play diverse functional and structural roles in bacterial cells but that they can be toxic at high concentrations. Bacteria have evolved machinery to (a) take up metal ions, (b) transport and deliver metal ions to the appropriate locations in cells, and (c) sequester, store, and, if necessary, expel metal ions to maintain an appropriate concentration of metal ions. Of the transition metals, iron, copper, nickel, zinc, manganese, molybdenum, cobalt, vanadium, and tungsten have been shown to be used by bacteria. Bacteria are also exposed to and can detoxify many other toxic transition metals, such as chromium, cadmium, or mercury. This function makes bacteria potential agents for bioremediation.

Despite our advanced knowledge about many metalloproteins, we have yet to identify the complete metalloproteome, even in well-studied bacteria. New technologies should help to identify new metalloproteins and give us a greater sense of the metalloproteome of a given organism or a meta-metalloproteome from a complex, multispecies sample. A well-curated, online resource catalogue of known and predicted metalloproteins would be a welcome resource to metallo-microbiologists. One such platform was the Metalloprotein Database and Browser (Castagnetto et al. 2002), which provided a database of metal-binding sites from protein structures deposited in the Protein Data Bank; however, it is no longer available online. Other sites are available that provide some useful information. METAL-MACiE[1] provides detailed information on the roles played by metals in catalytic mechanisms of approximately 200 metalloenzymes (Andreini et al. 2009). BRENDA[2] provides data on enzyme metal-binding properties curated from publications (Schomburg et al. 2013). We envision a database that provides users lists of experimentally validated and predicted metalloproteins for a given organism of interest. Such a database is essential for the full development of metalloproteomics.

Current data are limited by the bacterial organisms that are commonly studied. We do not know the common trends (if any) in the use, storage, or detoxification of metals that differentiate pathogenic bacteria, human commensal bacteria, or environmental bacteria. As more environmental organisms are described, particularly those living in environments that are contaminated with metals, we will surely identify novel detoxification strategies, but it also seems possible that we will find bacteria using other transition metals functionally. More must also be done to assess the epidemiological risks of environmental metal pollution and how it functions in the maintenance and proliferation of antibiotic resistance.

---

[1] http://www.ebi.ac.uk/thornton-srv/databases/Metal_MACiE/home.html

[2] http://www.brenda-enzymes.org

Finally, much work needs to be done to understand the concentrations and distributions of metals in the cell. ICP-MS has been used successfully in a number of organisms to establish total cellular content of metals (see Maret et al., this volume). As a next step, the distribution of the metals in different pools needs to be determined more accurately. How much of this metal is in readily exchangeable pools? How much is sequestered in storage systems, such as iron in ferritin or molybdenum in MoSto? How do these concentrations vary over time, stage of growth, and in the presence or absence of various nutrient sources? Are there differences between bacteria growing in suspension versus in a biofilm or in the presence or absence of other species of bacteria? In a biofilm, are particular metals sequestered in different regions of the biofilm? For metals with multiple uptake pathways in a given organism, do all uptake pathways feed into all metal pools, or do linkages exist between uptake pathways and cellular pools? The answers to these and similar questions are fundamental to our understanding of the use of metal ions by bacteria in the diverse ecosystems in which they live.

## Acknowledgments

Our work is supported by operating grants from the Natural Sciences and Engineering Research Council of Canada (NSERC) and the Canadian Institutes of Health Research. S.A.L. holds an NSERC postdoctoral fellowship. M.M.V. holds an NSERC Canadian Graduate Scholarship.

# 5

# Common Mechanisms of Bacterial Metal Homeostasis

James A. Imlay

## Abstract

Transition metals are required for the function of nearly half the enzymatic machinery of organisms. This is particularly challenging for bacteria, which move through environments in which metal levels can vary by orders of magnitude. Exacerbating the situation is the fact that metals easily compete for enzyme-binding sites, with inappropriate metallation typically inhibiting enzyme function. Thus microbes work hard to acquire, balance, and sort their metal pools. This chapter surveys the common tactics by which bacteria control intracellular iron (Fe), manganese (Mn), copper (Cu), and zinc (Zn). The focus is on *Escherichia coli*, for which enough information is available to attempt an integrated view. High-affinity import systems are regulated at the level of transcription by specific metal-sensing transcription factors; posttranslational controls have not yet been identified. If these importers are insufficient, then metal-sparing strategies are engaged for iron and zinc, the two metals that are needed to activate essential enzymes. At the other extreme, metal overload can result in chemical injuries (Fe, Zn, Cu) and the mismetallation of noncognate enzymes (Fe, Zn, Mn). Export systems are induced to avoid these outcomes. Underlying the entire situation is the question of whether metals are sorted among enzymes by thermodynamic affinities or whether chaperone systems override binding strengths. At present the author infers that Cu movement may sometimes be chaperone driven, but that the other metals reversibly sample protein binding sites and populate them according to the relative binding strengths of proteins and competing metabolite ligands. This conclusion emphasizes that metal pool sizes must be controlled and balanced.

## Introduction

A microbe can thrive in natural habitats only if it can correctly activate its numerous metalloenzymes. This process is difficult if metals are either under- or oversupplied by the environment. A variety of studies have indicated that mammalian hosts manipulate local metal availability to suppress the growth of invading microbes. Yet long ago bacteria evolved strategies to adapt to fluctuations in metal availability. This review explores how metal deficiency or excess can interfere with enzyme activities, as well as the adaptive measures that bacteria adopt to cope with such stresses. These issues lay the groundwork for considering how this ploy by the host may or may not succeed in blocking microbial growth.

## The Root of the Problem

The challenges of metal homeostasis derive from the fact that contemporary life occurs under conditions that are strikingly different from those of the primordial world in which cellular biochemistry evolved (Anbar 2008; Dupont et al. 2010). That world was anoxic. Iron in its ferrous form was readily available, and its facility at both redox and surface chemistry triggered its recruitment into numerous enzymes. The biochemical capabilities that it provided became the foundations upon which metabolic pathways evolved. Those enzymes and pathways persist today.

Conversely, the anoxic world was one in which reduced sulfur species were stable and abundant. Consequently, soft metals—notably copper—were trapped in insoluble sulfide minerals. Early life forms apparently did not use this metal at all. About 2.8 Gya the newly evolved photosystem II began to generate molecular oxygen. Initially, oxygen was scavenged by reduced $Fe^{2+}$ and sulfur species; it did not begin to accumulate until these were titrated from the seas, a billion years later. By then iron had become much more sparingly available and, conversely, copper was released as a soluble bioavailable species.

Contemporary organisms have thus inherited a requirement for iron that is not easy to satisfy. They feature a relative handful of Cu enzymes, which have apparently all arisen since the great oxygenation event (Ridge et al. 2008). Zinc utilization has also grown (Dupont et al. 2006). The expansion of Zn enzymes was once thought to have arisen from its scarcity in primordial sulfidic environments, but a recent analysis suggests that zinc might always have been bioavailable (Robbins et al. 2013). Indeed, unlike copper, zinc is widely used by, and is probably essential for, current-day anaerobes.

In contemporary environments, metal availability is inconsistent, particularly for organisms that transit between anoxic habitats, which retain the metal content of the ancient world, and oxic ones. It is thus perhaps fortuitous that studies of metal homeostasis began in *E. coli*, a facultative organism that makes its way in both worlds and which therefore must employ multiple strategies to satisfy its metal requirements.

## The General Case

This review will focus on metal usage by *E. coli*. Emphasis will be on the acquisition and control of iron, manganese, copper, and zinc. Subsequent sections outline the ways in which these metals are employed, their routes of import, the hazards of overload, how regulatory proteins track their pool sizes, and the efflux and chaperone systems that cope with excess. Details vary among microbes; however, they follow a general pattern that can be laid out without getting lost in the details. A general discussion highlights the common challenges that organisms face in ensuring proper metallation of client proteins.

The fundamental problem is that although protein surfaces easily discriminate among organic substrates, they have trouble with metals. The divalent transition metals lack shape, have a common charge, and overlap considerably in the coordination geometries that they will tolerate. Nevertheless, they are rarely interchangeable in the enzymes that rely upon them—an indication that actionable differences exist. In redox enzymes these differences arise from the distinct reduction potentials of iron, manganese, and copper. In nonredox proteins the metals exhibit biases in their coordination geometries. Further, softer metals exhibit generally stronger ligand binding than do harder metals, in accordance with the Irving-Williams series: ligand affinities, $Mn(II) < Fe(II) < Co(II) < Ni(II) < Cu(II) > Zn(II)$ (Irving and Williams 1948). Such differences cause variations in catalytic efficiencies when the metals are loaded into enzymes, and they provide the means by which importers, sensors, exporters, and enzymes can (imperfectly) discriminate among them.

## How Does a Cell Provide the Correct Metal to a Divalent Metal-Binding Protein?

This is perhaps the most fundamental problem in metals biology. In principle, two solutions exist. The first is that the protein has a strong kinetic or thermodynamic bias toward the correct metal. The second is that selection occurs at the level of a chaperone, which then guides the metal into a client protein. Both solutions occur.

Cytoplasmic chaperone systems have been verified for copper and nickel (Leitch et al. 2009; Farrugia et al. 2013) but not for the more widely used metals: iron, manganese, and zinc. Might their chaperone systems simply not have been discovered? Perhaps, but this is dubious. A protein-based chaperone typically requires a domain in the recipient protein to serve as its landing site (Schmidt et al. 2000; Padilla-Benavides et al. 2013). These have not been noticed in Fe-, Mn-, and Zn-using proteins, and in any case it would have been evolutionarily cumbersome for such domains to have arisen across a broad expanse of proteins that draw upon a common metal. (In a typical organism, only a few enzymes use copper and nickel, whereas scores may require iron, zinc, and manganese.) Further, the heterologous expression of Fe, Zn, or Mn enzymes from distant organisms is usually successful, which indicates that metal delivery persists. One would have expected that drift in protein–protein recognition would have degraded chaperone-based metal delivery to heterologous proteins. In contrast, heterologous expression of Ni or Cu enzymes is problematic (Natvig et al. 1987).

If chaperones are not involved in delivering zinc or iron to their cognate proteins, then one infers that Zn enzymes tend to acquire zinc in preference to iron, and that Fe enzymes do the opposite, because these are the thermodynamically preferred outcomes in a given cell. At first this seems surprising, given that zinc tends to outbind iron in most proteins.

An example may help. ZntR is a transcription factor that responds to Zn overload. Its $K_D$ for zinc in water is approximately $10^{-15}$ M (Outten and O'Halloran 2001; Ma et al. 2011). It can quickly be deduced that Zn loading occurs by ligand exchange with other solutes, as opposed to the binding of zinc that is water coordinated (i.e., $Zn[H_2O]_n$), and this recognition is critical for thinking about how metals sample binding sites. The maximum second-order rate constant for a reaction in water is $\sim 10^9$ M$^{-1}$ s$^{-1}$; this rate constant means that every encounter between two reactants (say, zinc and a binding site) is productive (the zinc binds). If zinc were exclusively present at $10^{-15}$ M $Zn(H_2O)_n$, then the binding rate would be the product of the rate constant and the concentration: $10^{-6}$ s$^{-1}$. The halftime for binding would be, at best, one week. The amount of aqueous zinc is inadequate to metallate this protein in a workable time frame.

The resolution is that zinc and presumably all metals move inside cells as exchangeable complexes with metabolites and with the surfaces of biomolecules. Thus the amount of zinc that is accessible to ZntR inside an overloaded *E. coli* cell is far higher than $10^{-15}$ M and may approach the total Zn concentration ($10^{-4}$ to $10^{-3}$ M) (Outten and O'Halloran 2001). One might imagine complexes of zinc with glutathione or histidine that, for example, deposit the metal through ligand exchange reactions in the ZntR binding site.

Accordingly, the common statement that "there is no free zinc" (or copper or other metals) inside a cell should be understood as meaning that there is no fully hydrated metal. There are, however, substantial pools of metals that have not been stably incorporated into proteins, which are loosely bound by metabolites. The term "free metal" should really refer to this pool of unincorporated metal, although in frequent usage it has sometimes been confused with fully hydrated metal, which is vanishingly scarce and functionally irrelevant.

However, the metal dissociation constants of proteins, which by convention are measured against water, retain their utility. If ZntR is half-loaded with zinc, then the concentration of aqueous zinc is $10^{-15}$ M but the concentration of a Zn-loaded metabolite might be $10^{-6}$ M. If exchange reactions are quick, then loading times will be short enough such that ZntR can quickly sense a rise in the intracellular Zn pool. Returning to the problem of the thermodynamic distribution of metals, a Zn-dependent protein with a greater affinity for zinc than that of ZntR (say, $K_D$ of $10^{-17}$ M) would, in principle, be saturated with zinc at levels lower than those that occupy ZntR. In this way, ZntR would not trigger the synthesis of Zn efflux systems unless Zn-requiring proteins are already activated.

Iron binds more poorly to proteins than does zinc, but it also binds more poorly to the cellular metabolites. Imagine an Fe-dependent protein with $K_D$ values of $10^{-15}$ M for zinc and $10^{-8}$ M for iron, and a Zn-dependent protein with $K_D$ values of $10^{-18}$ M for zinc and $10^{-7}$ M for iron. The intracellular concentrations of aqueous iron and zinc might be $10^{-6}$ M and $10^{-15}$ M, respectively (matching the $K_D$ values of the metal regulatory proteins, ZntR and Fur; see below). If exchange reactions established thermodynamic equilibrium, the Fe-requiring protein would ultimately be 99% Fe bound and the Zn-requiring protein would be 99% Zn bound, even though both proteins inherently bind zinc better than iron. The metal occupancy would be determined by the balance between the relative availabilities and binding constants of the metals for a given protein.

This analysis depends on the notion that thermodynamic equilibrium is achieved. For this to occur, binding *in vivo* must be quick, and it must be reversible. Can spontaneous metal release into water be sufficiently fast to meet the second criterion, or must something pry out the metal? Consider the first case. For metal release by ZntR to water, $K_D = k_{off}/k_{on} = 10^{-15}$ M. Since $k_{on}$ cannot exceed $10^9$ M$^{-1}$ s$^{-1}$, then $k_{off}$ cannot exceed $10^{-6}$ s$^{-1}$. Again, this implies that spontaneous dissociation into water occurs with a halftime of one week— far too slow for the ZntR regulatory protein to succeed as a dynamic sensor of metal availability. We infer that for this protein to operate as a Zn sensor, the bound zinc must be transferred directly by ligand exchange to other metabolites. That is, metabolites grab zinc and pull it from the protein. A correct formulation of Zn binding by ZntR must be:

$$apo\text{-}ZntR + Zn(L_n) \rightarrow ZntR{:}Zn + nL, \qquad (5.1)$$

where L represents unknown nonaqueous ligands with substantial metal affinity.

This analysis indicates several things. First, for proper metallation, the pools of metals in the cell must be calibrated relative to one another so that each metal competes favorably for cognate proteins but unfavorably for noncognate proteins. It must be the goal of regulatory proteins to set the pools in this way. Second, cellular metabolites must be available to coordinate metals and facilitate both metal binding to and dissociation from proteins. Third, the absolute concentrations of the metal pools inside cells must be high enough so that metalloprotein loading occurs in seconds, not hours.

In most cases we do not yet know the correct values for the intracellular metal levels and for the binding constants of metalloproteins. Presumably, they are indicated by the affinities of the regulatory proteins that tip the cell behavior toward further import or efflux. It is notable that the metal-binding sites of metalloregulators have evolved steric constraints which strongly favor cognate metals. CueR binds copper with high avidity; it does not bind zinc as well (Changela et al. 2003). These preferences are primarily dictated by the geometries of the coordinating residues, and sometimes they are enhanced by allosteric effects which can be imparted by the cognate metals but not by mismatched metals (for an excellent review, see Ma et al. 2009). However, metalloenzymes have less flexibility to evolve these discriminatory features: their structures are constrained by the exigencies of substrate binding and catalysis. Hence, mismetallation is more likely.

Finally, it is important to note that a subset of metalloproteins almost certainly does not achieve binding equilibrium. Superoxide dismutases and proteins with structural Zn atoms, for example, bury their bound metals within the protein so that they are inaccessible to chelators. *In vitro* these metals are released only if the protein is partially denatured. It is unclear whether discrimination against noncognate metals occurs at the level of the association rate or whether noncognate metals fail to trigger protein folding and thus are vulnerable to extraction.

**Iron**

*Chemical Properties and Enzymatic Roles*

Local ligands can tune the electron affinity of iron to a range of physiological potentials, making it a fitting partner in redox reactions. Iron also exhibits little activation energy when it switches between four-, five-, or six-coordinate geometries, a property which, together with its excellence as a Lewis acid, enables it to serve as a surface catalyst. In the most studied bacterium, *E. coli*, iron is by far the most-used transition metal. It serves in the form of heme as a conduit for electrons in cytochrome oxidases, succinate dehydrogenase, sulfite and nitrite reductases, and catalase. Iron-sulfur clusters in [4Fe-4S], [3Fe-4S], and [2Fe-2S] forms are redox-active cofactors in respiratory dehydrogenases (e.g., NADH dehydrogenase I), radical-generating enzymes (pyruvate:formate lyase-activating enzyme), and oxidant-sensing proteins (Fnr). Iron-sulfur clusters can also perform nonredox surface chemistry, binding and activating substrates for dehydration (aconitase); they also can apparently provide protein structure to many enzymes that operate upon nucleic acids (endonuclease III). Finally, lone Fe atoms provide redox-active mononuclear (superoxide dismutase) and binuclear (ribonucleotide reductase) centers, and in their ferrous form they provide substrate binding or activation sites in a wide variety of nonredox enzymes (erythrose-4-phosphate 3-epimerase).

These enzymes are found throughout metabolism: in energy production, amino acid and cofactor biosynthesis, nitrogen and sulfur assimilation, and DNA metabolism. Most bacteria cannot grow when they cannot acquire adequate iron.

*Avoiding Iron Deficiency*

It is an obvious problem that iron is hard to find in contemporary habitats. When iron is abundant, it is typically imported through ferrous Fe importers, such as Feo (Cartron et al. 2006) (Figure 5.1). When iron is scarce several ad hoc solutions come into play. In *E. coli* these tactics are initiated by the deactivation of Fur, an Fe-dependent transcription factor that in its Fe-activated form represses Fe-starvation responses (Hantke 2001). Fur binds a single ferrous Fe atom in a regulatory site with moderate affinity ($K_D = 1$ $\mu$M; Mills and Marletta 2005; Ma et al. 2012), plus a Zn atom in a structural site with high affinity. A dimer of Fe-bound Fur [(Fur:Zn,Fe)$_2$] binds DNA binds DNA and occludes the RNA polymerase binding site of genes that are useful when iron is scarce, thus shutting them off. Fur:Fe displaces protein H-NS from upstream of the gene, encoding ferritin. Since H-NS would otherwise block *ftn* transcription,

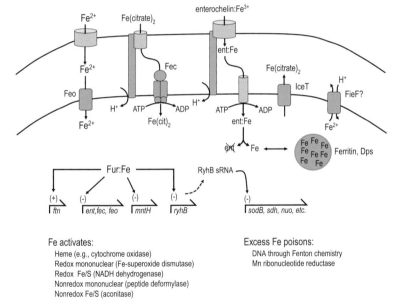

**Figure 5.1** Iron homeostatic mechanisms in *E. coli* K12. Ferrous iron is imported through Feo, citrate-chelated iron through Fec, and siderophore-bound iron through the enterochelin system. The latter two systems depend on TonB to power entry through outer-membrane receptors. Siderophores are then hydrolyzed to release the iron. *E. coli* also expresses receptors (not shown) for siderophores excreted by other organisms. (Additional iron importers, including ones for heme, are found in pathogenic *E. coli* strains.) When iron is sufficient, moderate excess is stored in ferritin, bacterioferritin, or (during oxidative stress) Dps. Two iron export systems, IceT and FieF, have been proposed. Fur is the iron-activated repressor that controls expression of Fe importers, ferritin, the Mn importer MntH, and the sRNA RyhB. During Fe limitation, Mn may substitute for iron in mononuclear enzymes, and RyhB blocks the synthesis of expendable Fe proteins.

Fur:Fe has the effect of positively inducing it (Nandal et al. 2010). Thus, during periods of Fe repletion, the cell stores excess iron, to be drawn upon when Fe levels subsequently decline.

When intracellular iron becomes scarce, Fur is demetallated and thereby deactivated, allowing the engagement of adaptive responses. These responses include the induction of a variety of Fe import systems. Most famously, bacteria excrete siderophores (i.e., small molecules that solubilize ferric iron and deliver it to cells). The binding affinity of siderophores for Fe(III) is so great that after the import of the siderophore-iron chelate, the release of the ferric iron is an energetic problem. Release by ligand exchange to a moderate-affinity metabolite is energetically challenging, even if the latter is abundant. Release to a higher-affinity metabolite, such as citrate, would simply defer the problem. The native siderophore in *E. coli* lab strains is degraded by esterases (Brickman and McIntosh 1992). Lower-affinity siderophores apparently release the iron after its reduction by low-potential electron donors, a strategy that succeeds because the affinity of siderophores for ferrous iron is substantially lower than for the ferric form (Miethke et al. 2011; Wang et al. 2011b).

Pathogenic *E. coli* strains can also acquire their iron from heme, an important Fe source in their host environment (Torres and Payne 1997; Hagan and Mobley 2009). Lab strains, which were isolated from intestinal flora, cannot do this. Variation among the suite of Fe importers is commonly observed in otherwise similar bacteria, as lateral gene transfer is a device that suits bacteria to distinct habitats.

When siderophores are inadequate at acquiring sufficient iron, the cell adjusts further. *E. coli* does so in two ways. The derepression of the RyhB sRNA enables it to block the translation of messages that encode Fe enzymes that are abundant but conditionally dispensable (Masse et al. 2005). Repression of NADH dehydrogenase I, for example, spares the cell all the Fe atoms that would otherwise go into its nine iron-sulfur clusters, while NADH dehydrogenase II (an Fe-free enzyme) carries out the job of NADH reoxidation. The cell loses the proton motive force that NdhI contributes, but essential Fe enzymes (such as the cluster enzymes involved in isoprenoid synthesis; Loiseau et al. 2007) can still be activated. Similarly, succinate dehydrogenase (ten Fe atoms) is not made, prohibiting growth on TCA-cycle substrates like acetate, but growth on fermentable carbon sources remains possible. It is striking that glycolysis, the sole high-titer pathway that is not dispensable under any reasonable condition, contains no metal-dependent proteins.

Interestingly, some other bacteria prioritize the use of limited iron using control systems that are analogous, but not homologous, to RyhB. In *Corynebacteria*, for example, the protein RipA plays the role of RyhB sRNA: RipA is a repressor of Fe proteins and is itself repressed by DtxR when iron is sufficient (Wennerhold et al. 2005). This example underscores the general observation that metal control strategies are broadly distributed even though the specific mechanisms that execute those strategies may vary.

In *E. coli* the other key adjustment to Fe restriction is a shift toward the use of manganese rather than iron in key metalloproteins. MntH, the sole Mn importer, is repressed by Fur:Fe; when iron becomes scarce, the induction of MntH brings manganese into the cell (Kehres et al. 2002a). Manganese probably populates the nonredox mononuclear enzymes that would otherwise rely upon iron. These enzymes require a metal to neutralize the charge of an oxyanionic reaction intermediate, and manganese can do so almost as well as iron (Sobota and Imlay 2011; Anjem and Imlay 2012). Manganese cannot directly substitute for iron in the redox enzymes superoxide dismutase and ribonucleotide reductase, because the polypeptides of those Fe enzymes are configured to poise iron, not manganese, at the proper reduction potential for catalysis. Instead the cell synthesizes Mn-activatible isozymes: the Mn-specific superoxide dismutase and ribonucleotide reductase. Their structural genes (*sodB* and *nrdEF*) are repressed by Fur:Fe and thus are induced only when iron is scarce (Compan and Touati 1993; Martin and Imlay 2011).

One other adjustment to Fe depletion may also exist. *E. coli* contains two aconitases, each of which uses [4Fe-4S] clusters to catalyze their dehydration/rehydration reactions. Strikingly, and unlike clusters in other proteins, the cluster of aconitase B exists in equilibrium with the cellular pool of iron: when iron pools drop, the equilibrium shifts away from cluster stability, apoprotein accumulates and enzyme activity declines (Varghese et al. 2003). Activity does not fall to zero, but citrate levels automatically rise to a higher steady-state to push through the remaining enzyme. Some of the accumulated citrate is excreted. It seems plausible (though not proven) that the excreted citrate traps any available extracellular iron, thereby serving as a short-term emergency siderophore that reenters through the ferric citrate import system (Pressler et al. 1988). The connection between aconitase stability and Fe metabolism has also been seen in other organisms. In *Bacillus*, *Mycobacterium tuberculosis*, and mammals, apo-aconitase similarly accumulates upon Fe limitation and serves as an RNA-binding protein (Banerjee et al. 2007; Volz 2008; Pechter et al. 2013). The cleft vacated by the erstwhile [4Fe-4S] cluster binds conserved elements in mRNAs, stabilizing messages that encode Fe-import proteins and destabilizing those of Fe-storage proteins. There has been some hint that apo-aconitase might do the same in *E. coli* (Tang and Guest 1999).

Some lactic acid bacteria, which typically inhabit Fe-poor environments, have made the fateful commitment to eschew iron dependence (Archibald 1983; Posey and Gherardini 2000). They lack Fe-S and heme proteins, and thus they also lack the respiratory chain and TCA cycle that depend upon them. This compromise permits an independence from iron at the expense of less-efficient energy production. Interestingly, these bacteria commonly contain millimolar levels of manganese, suggesting that their mononuclear enzymes are likely populated by manganese in place of iron. These organisms employ Mn-dependent ribonucleotide reductase and superoxide dismutase. In essence, the Fe-deficiency adaptations that *E. coli* makes are only conditionally constitutive in these other bacteria. As a final twist, these bacteria often employ pyruvate oxidases that release copious hydrogen peroxide into their environment (Pericone et al. 2000). Peroxide is a poison for the Fe enzymes of their competitors (Jang and Imlay 2007; Anjem and Imlay 2012), thereby providing an advantage for the lactic acid bacteria.

The take-home message is this: the central metabolic and biosynthetic pathways that are shared by all organisms evolved in an Fe-laden environment; contemporary organisms have thus inherited a dependence on a metal that is not reliably present. This situation has forced the evolution of ad hoc mechanisms for adaptation to Fe limitation. *E. coli*, an organism that routinely transits from an Fe-rich (anoxic) environment to a frequently Fe-poor oxic one, manifests these.

## Control of Iron Levels: Other Aspects

It is striking that manganese can bind in the regulatory metal-binding site of Fur (Mills and Marletta 2005; Ma et al. 2012). Fur:Mn can repress several members of the Fur regulon, although apparently not all of them. For example, Fur represses synthesis of the MntH Mn importer when either manganese or iron is abundant inside the cell (Kehres et al. 2002a; Ikeda et al. 2005). However, the mangano-superoxide dismutase is only repressed when iron is abundant; when iron is scarce (so that FeSOD cannot be activated) but manganese is abundant, MnSOD synthesis is robust (Pugh et al. 1984). These outcomes make physiological sense, but the physical mechanics of the protein that enable this selective effect are unknown.

IscR is an *E. coli* regulatory protein that controls the synthesis of the Fe-S cluster assembly machinery. It has a cluster binding site, and when [2Fe-2S] is loaded there, IscR substantially represses expression of the Isc assembly system (Schwartz et al. 2001). When cluster demand outstrips assembly, IscR shifts to its apoprotein form, enabling full synthesis of the Isc proteins. Interestingly, apo-IscR additionally acts as a positive transcription factor that induces expression of a secondary cluster assembly machine encoded by the *suf* operon (Yeo et al. 2006). The regulatory pattern makes sense, in that the Suf machinery requires iron levels that are lower than what is needed by the Isc machinery (Outten et al. 2004). The reason that Suf is less fastidious is not known.

Recent studies have revealed that IscR also controls genes that have no obvious association with cluster assembly. These include NrdEF, a Mn-dependent ribonucleotide reductase (Cotruvo and Stubbe 2011; Martin and Imlay 2011). One possibility is that because IscR senses formation of a metal cluster, which can be built with iron but not manganese, it is a more precise sensor of Fe levels than is Fur, which responds to either iron or manganese. It remains to be seen whether this notion is correct.

Fur is widely distributed, but it is not the universal sensor of iron. For example, the Gram-positive bacterium *Bradyrhizobium japonicum* employs the heme-sensing protein Irr as its primary transcriptional activator of Fe-import proteins. When adequate heme accumulates, Irr binds the heme and is converted it to a form that is rapidly degraded by cell proteases, thereby shutting down the synthesis of import systems (Yang et al. 2006). In an apparent analogy to IscR, this system results in specificity for iron. Interestingly, manganese has a secondary controlling effect: when Mn levels are high, manganese binds to Irr and stabilizes it (Puri et al. 2010). The effect is to maintain an Fe:Mn balance inside the cell. The consequence of an imbalance has not been determined.

*Avoiding Too Much Intracellular Iron*

Too much iron is not a good thing. As will be demonstrated, excessive intracellular amounts of most metals are problematic because the excess metal outcompetes other metals for their appropriate binding sites. Iron does this in the limited case of Mn-specific redox enzymes (Whittaker 2003; Martin and Imlay 2011). However, the most recognized effect of excess iron is to drive the formation of hydroxyl radicals through the Fenton reaction:

$$Fe^{2+} + H_2O_2 \rightarrow [FeO^{2+}] \rightarrow Fe^{3+} + HO \cdot \qquad (5.2)$$

Hydroxyl radicals react at nearly diffusion-limited rates with most biomolecules. The most consequential target is DNA (Imlay and Linn 1988). Since hydrogen peroxide is an unavoidable product of flavoenzyme autoxidation in oxic habitats (Imlay 2013), aerobic microbes are at pains to limit hydroxyl-radical formation by controlling the amounts of both reactants: loose ferrous Fe and $H_2O_2$. Deletions of *fur* that derepress Fe-importer synthesis in Fe-rich habitats lead to high rates of DNA damage (Touati et al. 1995). These can be suppressed by the engineered synthesis of ferritins, which lower the amount of free iron.

A complication to oxidative stress is that $H_2O_2$ and superoxide both leach iron from dehydratase Fe-S clusters and mononuclear enzymes, increasing the pool of loose iron (Liochev and Fridovich 1994; Keyer et al. 1995; Anjem and Imlay 2012). Further, they knock iron free from Fur, with the potential effect of inducing Fe importers at the very time when more iron is a bad idea (Varghese et al. 2007). Cells respond in two ways. First, the OxyR transcription factor senses excess $H_2O_2$ and induces higher rates of Fur synthesis, partially compensating for its lower metal occupancy (Zheng et al. 1999). Second, OxyR induces the expression of Dps (Altuvia et al. 1994), a ferritin-like protein that sequesters iron (Ilari et al. 2002). The effect is to down the level of free iron. Mutants that lack *dps* suffer overwhelming damage during periods of $H_2O_2$ exposure (Park et al. 2005).

It is interesting to note that when Fe-starved strains were abruptly supplemented with iron, the intracellular Fe levels rose only modestly: from ~ 20 μM unincorporated iron to ~ 70 μM (Keyer and Imlay, unpublished data). Since the period of Fe starvation strongly induced import systems, what kept Fe levels from sky-rocketing? One possibility is that influx was countervailed by an Fe efflux system. FieF (YiiP) has been proposed to act as a Zn or Fe efflux system (Grass et al. 2005b; Lu et al. 2009). In addition, Frawley et al. (2013) recently reported that MdtD (also known as IceT) acts as an Fe-citrate exporter, although the conditions of its expression are not yet clear. An intriguing alternative is that metal importers may be product inhibited. Control on the level of turnover has not yet been reported for most transition metal importers, but the bacterial MgtE magnesium importer is inhibited when cytoplasmic magnesium binds and induces a conformational shift that closes the pore (Hattori et al. 2009). To date the Zn or Fe efflux pump YiiP provides a rare example of a metal transporter whose turnover is clearly controlled by the allosteric action of its substrate metal (Lu et al. 2009). The fact that we do not know whether metals stimulate or inhibit most transporters comprises an important gap in our understanding of metal homeostatic mechanisms.

## Manganese

### Chemical Properties and Enzymatic Roles

Manganese is a transition element adjacent to iron in the periodic table. Like iron, it tolerates four-, five-, or six-coordinate geometries and can transition between Mn(II) and Mn(III) redox states at physiological potentials. These similar characteristics enable manganese to play many of the same roles as iron and, in fact the metabolism of these metals is intertwined (Figure 5.2).

E. coli expresses only a single Mn importer, MntH, a pump which is powered by the membrane potential (Kehres et al. 2000; Makui et al. 2000). Its close relative, Salmonella typhimurium, has an additional ATP-driven system: SitABC, also known in other bacteria as MntABC (Kehres et al. 2002b). Both the sit and mntH operons are repressed by an Fe-loaded Fur protein, with little expression under routine growth conditions (Kehres et al. 2002a; Ikeda et al. 2005). Indeed, the Mn content of E. coli is very low in nonstressed cells; for example, the Mn-dependent superoxide dismutase (MnSOD) is largely inactive (Anjem et al. 2009). Under these conditions the deletion of mntH does not cause any slowing of growth, even though intracellular Mn concentrations become miniscule. These observations suggest that manganese is specifically imported and employed in circumstances in which iron is unavailable. In fact, the deletion of mntH does block the growth of E. coli during Fe restriction (Grass et al. 2005a).

Regulatory studies revealed that mntH (of both E. coli and Salmonella) is also strongly induced during periods of hydrogen peroxide stress, as its transcription is positively controlled by the $H_2O_2$-sensing OxyR transcription factor (Kehres et al. 2002a). The mntH mutants cannot tolerate extended $H_2O_2$ exposure (Anjem et al. 2009).

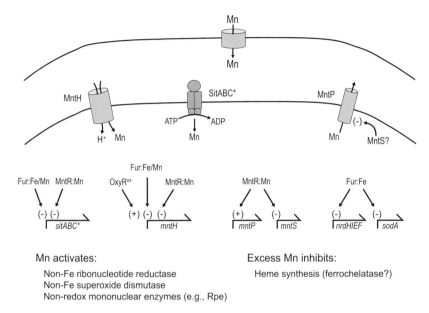

**Figure 5.2**   Manganese homeostatic mechanisms in *E. coli*. Manganese is apparently used only during periods of Fe deficiency or $H_2O_2$ stress. Upon deactivation of the Fur repressor or activation of the OxyR transcription factor, the MntH importer is synthesized and brings Mn into the cytoplasm. SitABC (MntABC) is found in many other bacteria, including the close relative *Salmonella*, but not in *E. coli* (hence the asterisk). Manganese levels are held in check at the transcriptional level by repression of *mntH* by both Mn-charged MntR and Mn-charged Fur. Excess Mn is exported by MntP; when Mn levels fall, MntP synthesis stops, and extant MntP may be inhibited by MntS. Two Mn-specific redox isozymes, Mn superoxide dismutase and Mn ribonucleotide reductase, are induced only during Fe restriction.

Analysis of the enzymes that can use manganese makes sense of these data. *E. coli* contains a number of enzymes in which iron serves as a nonredox co-factor. The cohort of such enzymes has not been adequately identified, because reducing conditions are needed to activate the enzymes with ferrous iron *in vitro*; for this reason some of these enzymes have been mistakenly annotated as using manganese, zinc, or cobalt. These enzymes (e.g., ribulose-phosphate epimerase, peptide deformylase, cytosine deaminase, LpxC) catalyze a variety of reaction types that have in common the formation of an oxyanion intermediate that is stabilized by electrostatic interaction with the divalent ferrous atom (Anjem and Imlay 2012). Lesser activity is exhibited when the enzymes are charged with zinc, which may be reluctant to assume the octahedral geometry of the enzyme:substrate complex, and essentially no activity is provided by magnesium. In contrast, manganese confers turnover numbers that approach those of the Fe-loaded enzymes. Thus the control of MntH synthesis by Fur makes sense if the imported Mn substitutes in these enzymes during Fe scarcity.

This hypothesis is supported by the fact that the structural genes for MnSOD as well as for the Mn-dependent ribonucleotide reductase, NrdEF, are similarly repressed by Fur:Fe (Compan and Touati 1993; Martin and Imlay 2011). These enzymes are induced only when iron is available; that is, when the usual Fe-dependent isozymes (FeSOD and NrdAB) cannot be activated. These are redox enzymes, and direct Mn substitution into the Fe-dependent enzymes cannot work, because the redox potential of manganese in those polypeptide environments is inappropriate for the reaction. Instead, the Mn isozymes are configured to poise manganese at the essential potentials. Thus the overall view is that Mn acquisition is a strategy to maintain the function of mononuclear and binuclear Fe enzymes when iron is unavailable.

The induction of MntH during $H_2O_2$ stress is essential for continued growth; without it, the mononuclear nonredox enzymes are quickly inactivated by the oxidation of the ferrous cofactor by $H_2O_2$ (Sobota and Imlay 2011; Anjem and Imlay 2012). In contrast, manganese does not react easily with $H_2O_2$, and so the Mn-loaded enzymes retain activity when exposed to $H_2O_2$ *in vitro*. It has been inferred that this is the mechanism by which Mn import sustains the activities of these enzymes inside $H_2O_2$-stressed cells. However, direct evidence is lacking, because manganese binds weakly to active sites and dissociates during the process of enzyme recovery from cells. It is notable that lactic acid bacteria, which generate large amounts of $H_2O_2$ via pyruvate oxidase, may be immune to this oxidant because they characteristically maintain millimolar intracellular pools of manganese (Archibald and Fridovich 1981; Daly et al. 2004). It appears that these bacteria have fully committed to the defensive strategy that enteric bacteria resort to only under stressful conditions.

This leads to an obvious question: If iron is often scarce and confers a vulnerability to oxidants, why don't the enterics routinely use manganese? One answer is that Mn-cofactored enzymes are not quite as efficient as Fe-cofactored ones (Anjem and Imlay 2012). Pursuant to the Irving-Williams series, manganese binds ligands more poorly than does iron; thus manganese binds enzymes less efficiently than iron, and in mononuclear enzymes it may also grip the substrate less effectively. A second point is that enteric bacteria would still require iron to populate heme and Fe-S clusters. Manganese cannot substitute. Since enterics must establish intracellular Fe pools in any case, the diversion of some iron to mononuclear enzymes is simple. Finally, enterics are facultative organisms which spend much of their lives in anoxic habitats. Iron tends to be reduced and available in that context. Thus the problems of oxidative stress and Fe scarcity might be relatively rare.

The last point raises the question of whether manganese might be more routinely used by bacteria that dwell in oxic habitats. This is probably the case. *B. japonicum* is an obligate aerobe which, in contrast to *E. coli*, grows very poorly without Mn import; defects arise from the low activities of MnSOD (its sole superoxide dismutase) and its Mn-dependent pyruvate kinase (Hohle and O'Brian 2012). This bacterium has committed to manganese as a cofactor.

Whether the selective pressure for this evolutionary decision arose from the frequency of metal availability or oxidative stress is unclear.

*Avoiding Too Much Manganese*

Returning to *E. coli*, one can ask whether the cell sets upper limits on the amount of manganese that enters the cell. *E. coli*, like many bacteria (Rosch et al. 2009; Sun et al. 2010), has a LysE-family Mn efflux pump (MntP in *E. coli*) that pumps manganese out of the cytoplasm when levels rise too high (Waters et al. 2011). Indeed, *mntP* mutants are poisoned when a surfeit of manganese is provided in growth medium. Specifically, excess manganese poisons heme synthesis, apparently by blocking the insertion of iron into the porphyrin ring (Martin, Waters, and Imlay, unpublished data).

It is typical that bacteria encode both importers and exporters of the same metal. Not surprisingly, the syntheses of both are controlled by the cellular content of the metal. In the case of manganese, this situation is unexpectedly complicated: Mn levels are sensed both by MntR, a Mn-specific member of the DtxR family (Patzer and Hantke 2001; Galsfeld et al. 2003), and by Fur itself, which can form a Fur:Mn complex (Ma et al. 2012). MntR:Mn represses *mntH* and activates *mntP*: when intracellular Mn levels are high, the cell shuts down the synthesis of an importer and activates the synthesis of the exporter. When iron is scarce, repression of *mntH* by MntR:Mn is less effective. Upon MntH induction, the intracellular Mn levels rise quite high: ca. 100 μM, compared to ~ 10 μM under routine conditions (Anjem et al. 2009). Thereafter Fur:Mn complexes form and repress the expression of *mntH* (Kehres et al. 2002a; Ikeda et al. 2005). This system might establish two different Mn set points: a low one when iron is available and a higher one when iron is scarce (or $H_2O_2$ is present). A shift to high manganese in the latter situation makes sense if manganese must occupy mononuclear sites for which it has only moderate affinity. As an added wrinkle, when intracellular Mn levels are low, the synthesis of MntS (a sRNA that encodes a 42-amino-acid protein) is induced (Waters et al. 2011). MntS helps manganese find its way into Mn-using proteins, perhaps by inhibiting the activity of any extant MntP (Martin, Waters, Storz, and Imlay, submitted). When Mn levels rise, MntR:Mn inhibits *mntS* transcription; the effect may be to enable MntP to export the excess.

The ability of Fur to bind manganese in its Fe regulatory site has long been recognized (Ma et al. 2012). Fur:Mn is an effective repressor of many, but perhaps not all, genes in the Fur regulon. When manganese grossly overloads *mntP* mutants, Fur:Mn inhibits the synthesis of Fe importers, and heme synthesis stalls because the Fe levels become too low to sustain it.

In this context we can recognize why manganese is involved in controlling the Fe levels of *B. japonicum*. Irr is an inducer of Fe-import systems, but it is quickly degraded if it complexes with heme, an apparent indicator of Fe sufficiency. Manganese can diminish the affinity of Irr for heme; this has the effect of stimulating greater Fe import if manganese is inside the cell (Puri et al. 2010). Since iron and manganese can problematically compete for some of the same proteins—including ferrochelatase, which synthesizes heme (Martin, Waters, Storz, and Imlay, submitted)—it seems possible that Irr is configured to avoid these conflicts by keeping the two metals in balance with one another. This scenario underscores that the optimal intracellular level of one metal is contingent on the levels of competing metals.

In summary, the regulation of Mn import by Fur, OxyR, and MntR in *E. coli* is configured so that Mn levels rise only when iron is scarce or $H_2O_2$ threatens Fe-cofactored enzymes. The MntP efflux pump serves to remove manganese when its levels rise too high. Both the benefit and threat of intracellular manganese arises from its ability to occupy protein sites that normally acquire iron. In aerobes the evolutionary shift toward the use of manganese may have proceeded further. A key question is whether the Mn-using enzymes in these aerobes have refined their sites so that they are more effective with manganese than with iron.

## Copper

### Chemical Properties and Enzymatic Roles

Copper has an unusual story. Because copper is a soft metal that binds tightly to sulfur ligands, in primordial environments it was trapped in sulfide precipitates (Anbar 2008; Ridge et al. 2008). Its unavailability meant that it was not employed as a cofactor in ancient microorganisms, and in contemporary organisms, it is used as a cofactor only in enzymes that have arisen since the accumulation of molecular oxygen, perhaps 2 Gyr ago.

Further, copper is not used in cytoplasmic enzymes—which, after all, inhabit a cellular compartment that resembles ancient Earth, with high concentrations of sulfur compounds that adhere tightly to cuprous copper. Instead, copper activates a relative handful of periplasmic and membrane enzymes that leverage its redox activity to perform electron-transfer and oxidation reactions. These include monoamine oxidases, superoxide dismutatases, cytochrome oxidases, and plastocyanins (Arguello et al. 2013).

Thus bacteria strive to keep copper out of the cytoplasm and to maintain adequate levels in the periplasm (Figure 5.3). High levels of copper are toxic to bacteria, a trait that has recently been exploited in the manufacture of antimicrobial surfaces, such as hospital doorknobs and catheters. The sensitivity of bacteria to copper depends enormously on whether Cu-binding compounds are present in the environment: while 5 μM copper can poison bacteria in minimal media, 5 mM may be necessary in LB medium (Macomber and Imlay 2009). Presumably the former is a better mimic of natural habitats.

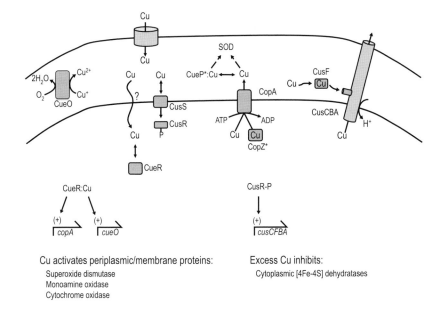

**Figure 5.3**   Copper homeostatic mechanisms in *E. coli*. The few (ca. 5) Cu-dependent enzymes of *E. coli* all receive their copper from the periplasm; there are no cytoplasmic copper enzymes. Copper can slip into the cytoplasm through unknown mechanisms. When it does, the CueR transcription factor detects elevated levels of cytoplasmic Cu and induces the synthesis of the CopA export system and the CueO periplasmic copper(I) oxidase. The latter may diminish Cu influx by eradicating the monocation. Although *E. coli* Cu enzymes apparently acquire Cu passively in the periplasm, excessively high periplasmic copper is sensed by the CusSR two-component system, which triggers synthesis of the Cus exporter. In some bacteria, periplasmic Cu-binding proteins (here, CueP) traffic Cu from the cytoplasmic Cu exporters to periplasmic Cu proteins.

## The Problem with Copper in the Cytoplasm

Toxic doses of copper block particular functions in *E. coli*. Copper exposure impedes the biosynthesis of branched-chain amino acids and the catabolism of TCA-cycle substrates because Cu(I) attacks the solvent-exposed Fe-S clusters of the dehydratases that lie in these pathways (Macomber and Imlay 2009). Copper apparently coordinates the bridging S ligands, thereby displacing iron and ultimately causing full cluster degradation. Workers have also postulated that the redox activity of copper might enable it to participate in Fenton-like reactions that generate toxic hydroxyl radicals, which can damage DNA. This chemistry occurs *in vitro* (Gunther et al. 1995). However, Cu-overloaded *E. coli* did not exhibit higher than normal levels of DNA damage, even when exogenous $H_2O_2$ was supplied (Macomber et al. 2007). The likely explanation

is that cytoplasmic copper predominantly associates with protein and lipid surfaces, away from the DNA, so that its genotoxic effects were small relative to
that of the Fe pool. Copper can also catalyze the oxidation of protein thiols,
although to date this effect has not been demonstrated in live cells.

For most bacteria it is unclear how copper ever enters the cytoplasm. It
seems plausible that Cu(II) might sneak in through metal transporters that
intend to import different divalent metals, and that Cu(I) might ride in through
monovalent (e.g., potassium) systems. In any case, bacteria universally maintain ATP-driven efflux pumps that efflux copper from cytoplasm to periplasm.
These proteins are strongly induced during Cu exposure, and null mutants are
noticeably copper sensitive. Copper toxicity and resistance has been examined in a number of organisms, with *E. coli* and *Enterococcus hirae* among
those which might be regarded as paradigmatic. Synthesis of the *E. coli* exporter, CopA (Rensing et al. 2000), is induced when copper metallates CueR,
a MerR-family transcription factor that in CueR:Cu form activates *copA* transcription directly (Outten et al. 2000). In some organisms (though not *E. coli*),
CopA is apparently fed copper by small cytoplasmic Cu-binding proteins,
which are thus regarded as chaperones (Gonzalez-Guerrero and Arguello
2008). Presumably they sweep copper off the surfaces of the myriad metabolites, proteins, and membranes to which it otherwise sticks. CueR:Cu also
activates expression of *cueO*, a gene that encodes a periplasmic enzyme that
oxidizes Cu(I) to Cu(II) with tetravalent reduction of molecular oxygen to
water (Grass and Rensing 2001; Singh et al. 2004). CueO contributes substantially to Cu resistance. Most workers suspect that Cu(I) penetrates the cytoplasmic membrane more easily than Cu(II) does, so that this action of CueO
lessens Cu influx. Unfortunately, the ability of copper to adhere to cell-surface
molecules is so great that this superficial copper dwarfs cytoplasmic copper,
even in *cueO copA* mutants, thereby precluding accurate measurements of the
levels of cytoplasmic copper.

The measured $K_D$ of CueR for copper is $10^{-21}$ M (Changela et al. 2003).
Its selectivity for Cu(I) arises from linear coordination by cysteine residues,
a geometry that is incompatible with the principle divalent metals. This high
affinity allows CueR to outcompete adventitious Cu ligands. Using the same
argument presented earlier, we can conclude that there is no fully hydrated
Cu in the cell; copper transits from one surface to another through ligand-
exchange processes. Within the cytoplasm the most plausible solubilizers are
thiols (cysteine, glutathione) and amines (histidine, polyamine). Presumably
these or other Cu-binding molecules have enough affinity to extract copper
from CueR, thereby deactivating it, when cytoplasmic Cu levels subside. The
alternatives are that CueR:Cu is deactivated by Cu transfer to an unknown
dedicated protein chaperone, which might in turn transfer it to CopA, or that
CueR is degraded.

*Copper in the Periplasm: Sufficiency and Excess*

*E. coli* and many other bacteria manifest a second pump, CusCFBA, that expels copper from both the cytoplasm and the periplasm into the external environment (Franke et al. 2003). A small Cu-binding protein, CusF, binds excess periplasmic copper and feeds it into the CusCBA transmembrane export complex (Kittleson et al. 2006). Expression of these genes is activated by the two-component CusSR system; the sensor protein is localized in the cytoplasmic membrane and probably directly senses periplasmic Cu levels (Munson et al. 2000). Activation of CusSR requires higher levels of environmental copper than does CueR. Presumably the differences between these two responses provide a window of Cu concentration that enables effective activation of periplasmic enzymes without collateral overloading of the cytoplasm. It is also plausible that high levels of copper directly damage proteins or membranes exposed within the periplasm.

One of the most interesting, unresolved stories involves how copper finds its way to client proteins in the periplasm. Passive metallation is a possibility: superoxide dismutase apoprotein can be activated by simple incubation with copper (Krishnakumar et al. 2004). Indeed, if *Salmonella* is grown with scant copper, superoxide dismutase is synthesized and maintained in an inactive apoprotein form until copper is provided, at which point the enzyme immediately gains activity. It is striking that Cu enzymes, unlike Fe enzymes, are not regulated at the transcriptional level in response to the availability of their cognate metal.

However, in several bacteria it appears that CopA-type cytoplasmic efflux systems and periplasmic chaperones are important for efficient activation of both periplasmic superoxide dismutase and cytochrome *c* oxidase (Swem et al. 2005; Gonzalez-Guerrero et al. 2010; Osman et al. 2013). This implies that copper takes a circuitous route: from the extracellular environment to the periplasm, into the cytoplasm, and then through ATP-driven efflux pumps to periplasmic Cu-binding proteins, which ultimately insert the copper into their client apoproteins. If true, entry of copper into the cytoplasm is requisite for the activation of Cu enzymes. Still, no influx protein has been identified in most of these bacteria. *E. hirae* is an exception (Solioz and Stoyanov 2003).

Why would cells require Cu flow into the cytoplasm to metallate periplasmic proteins? If Cu efflux systems evolved before Cu-requiring proteins—a reasonable idea—then newly evolved periplasmic apoproteins may have found the efflux systems to be the most reliable single source of copper. Periplasmic Cu-binding chaperones may have originally served to sequester copper, after the manner of heavy-metal metallothionines, and subsequently evolved to pluck copper off the export systems and to deposit it onto client proteins. The latter would presumably have acquired chaperone docking sites to make the process maximally efficient.

Copper thus stands alone among metals in several ways that all trace back to the strong affinity with which it binds adventitious ligands. It activates only recently evolved enzymes, which are generally involved in oxygen-dependent processes; it is compartmentalized in the periplasm to avoid reactions between it and exposed Fe-S clusters; and it is trafficked by chaperones to minimize nonproductive associations with biomolecules.

## Zinc

*Chemical Properties and Enzymatic Roles*

The Irving-Williams series indicates that zinc binds ligands with greater avidity than do most transition metals. Zinc is thiophilic, and initial calculations suggested that it was minimally available to the microbes that prevailed in anoxic, sulfur-rich primordial environments (Anbar 2008). A more recent analysis, however, suggests that zinc might not have been so scarce (Robbins et al. 2013). In any case, proteomics analyses indicate that zinc, unlike copper, was employed as an enzyme cofactor in ancient microbes, and it is employed by enzymes in contemporary anaerobes. Its severalfold greater use in eukarya (Dupont et al. 2006) might reflect higher bioavailability in oxic habitats, or it may merely reflect its expansive use in regulatory proteins.

At physiological redox potentials zinc is present exclusively in the divalent Zn(II) state. The most common enzymatic use of zinc is as a Lewis acid that activates water as a nucleophile. In this role, zinc is present in many hydrolases, coordinated in its preferred tetrahedral geometry by three amino acids (e.g., His, Asp, Cys) and a water or hydroxide moiety (Vallee and Falchuk 1993). In some bacterial enzymes (e.g., aspartate transcarbamoylase; Helmstaedt et al. 2001) it plays a structural role. In the latter guise it is bound by four amino acids, often four cysteines, without any open coordination site. Higher organisms exploit zinc in Zn finger structures, wherein the avidity with which it binds $His_2Cys_2$ coordination sites is so great as to organize the protein fold.

Zinc is distinguished from iron, manganese, and copper in that it populates enzymes both in the periplasm and the cytoplasm. One might rationalize the use of zinc in periplasmic proteins by the fact that, like copper, it is a metal that binds proteins tightly. In a compartment in which metals cannot be concentrated, this property might ensure full metallation. In contrast, iron and manganese bind relatively weakly to metal-binding sites, and so their local concentrations must remain high to ensure enzyme activity. Conversely, the thiophilicity of zinc does not match that of Cu(I), and it does not displace iron from Fe-S clusters as readily as does copper (Xu and Imlay 2012). Therefore, substantial levels of zinc can be tolerated in the cytoplasm.

*Ensuring Zinc Sufficiency*

Zinc presumably enters the periplasm by passive movement through porins (Figure 5.4). Based on its binding behavior, one expects the environmental Zn ion to be associated with small organic compounds, and it likely enters biological Zn-binding sites through exchange reactions, without dissociation into a fully hydrated Zn(II) form. Entry into the cytoplasm is catalyzed by both ATP- and pmf-driven Zn importers. These are found throughout the microbial biota, usually with both types present in a single species. *E. coli*, for example, features both the ATP-driven ZnuABC system (Patzer and Hantke 1998) and the proton-driven ZupT importer (Grass et al. 2002). Typically, pmf-driven importers operate at higher turnover number but lower affinity; the converse is true of ATP-driven importers. ZupT is thus likely to be the predominant importer of zinc when zinc is relatively abundant, whereas the ZnuABC system is induced when cytoplasmic Zn levels fall (Wang et al. 2012a).

In *E. coli*, cytoplasmic Zn sufficiency is monitored by Zur, a Fur-family transcription factor with both structural and regulatory Zn-binding sites (Ma et al. 2011). Like other members of this family, the metallated $[\text{Zur:Zn}_2]_2$ form

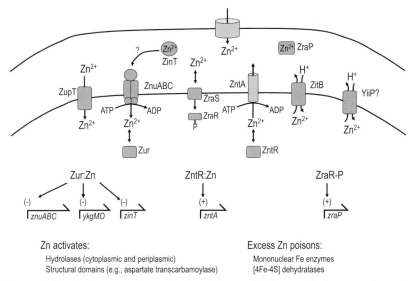

**Figure 5.4**   Zinc homeostatic mechanisms in *E. coli*. Zinc passively enters the periplasm through porins and is pumped into the cytoplasm by ZupT (possibly constitutively) and ZnuABC (during Zn scarcity). Scarcity also triggers the replacement of Zn-binding ribosomal subunits with Zn-independent ones (YkgM and O) as an apparent sparing mechanism. Excess cytoplasmic zinc is sensed by ZntR, which then induces the ZntA exporter to augment the constitutive ZitB exporter. YiiP/FieF may be an additional Zn (or Fe) exporter. Periplasmic zinc proteins apparently bind zinc directly. Excessive amounts of periplasmic zinc are sensed by the ZraSR two-component system, which induces ZraP, a periplasmic protein that may sequester zinc.

acts as a repressor of transcription. It is known to control only three *E. coli* promoters. It represses transcription of the structural genes for the ZnuABC importer, so that this high-affinity, energetically expensive system is induced only when Zn import through ZupT (or other permeases) is inadequate. A *znu* mutant is hypersensitive to Zn deficiency and accumulates less zinc (Patzer and Hantke 1998). This regulatory strategy resembles that for iron.

Zur:Zn also represses YkgM and YkgO (Graham et al. 2009; Hensley et al. 2012). These are Zn-free homologs of Zn-binding ribosomal subunits L31 and L36. During periods of Zn deficiency, the induction of these proteins apparently enables them to supplant the Zn-binding proteins; this action would diminish cellular Zn demand and may actually release "stored" zinc through the degradation of the extant Zn-loaded ribosomal subunits. The sparing effect might be substantial, given the high titer of ribosomal proteins inside the cell. This mechanism of Zn redistribution was first identified in *Bacillus subtilis* and *Streptomyces coelicolor* (Nanamiya et al. 2004; Owen et al. 2007; Shin et al. 2007).

The third Zur:Zn-repressed gene is *zinT*. ZinT is a 25 kDa protein that accumulates in the periplasm and exhibits tight ($K_D \sim 20$ nM) Zn binding (Graham et al. 2009). Its role, however, is unclear. Although researchers have suggested that ZinT might serve as a Zn chaperone, perhaps capturing zinc and delivering it to the Znu importer, *zinT* mutants seem no more sensitive to Zn depletion than do wild-type cells.

These adjustments raise the underlying question: What is the most immediate physiological consequence of Zn deficiency? Whether or not zinc was involved in primordial microbes, in contemporary organisms it is apparently an essential metal. Zinc has been predicted to cofactor ca. 5% of *E. coli* proteins (Andreini et al. 2006b), including essential proteins ranging from RNA polymerase to cell wall amidases. True Zn deprivation is difficult to achieve because the metal taints lab glassware; however, exhaustive efforts by the Poole group have confirmed that Zn deficiency sharply diminishes growth (Graham et al. 2009). Their study did not identify the Zn-dependent enzymes that comprised the growth bottleneck, and it is not clear whether Zn-deficient organisms make metabolic compromises analogous to the RyhB-triggered abandonment of oxidative phosphorylation during Fe deficiency.

*The Hazards of Excessive Zinc*

Zinc has long been recognized as an inhibitor of enzymes *in vitro*. Nanomolar concentrations inhibit a wide variety of enzymes through nonspecific binding to active site His and Cys residues. Perhaps a more avid mechanism of Zn toxicity *in vivo* is through competition with other divalent metals for metal binding sites: on transporters, regulatory proteins, and metal-dependent enzymes. Among transition metals, zinc is particularly problematic because its position on the Irving-Williams series ensures that it binds especially tightly to protein ligands. The prediction then is that excess zinc will disrupt the function of enzymes that work best with other metals.

*E. coli* is strikingly resistant to zinc. This is testimony to the effectiveness of efflux systems, as sensitivity returns when they are deleted (Grass et al. 2001). When sufficient doses of zinc are added to poison *znt* mutants, at least two classes of enzymes are targeted. Zinc destroys the exposed Fe-S clusters of the same dehydratases that copper poisons (Xu and Imlay 2012). Presumably the mechanism is again that the softer metal binds either the coordinating cysteine residues or the bridging inorganic sulfide atoms of the cluster, displacing iron. Zinc is less effective at this effect than is Cu(I), silver, or mercury—again, in accordance with the greater thiophilicity of the latter metals. Manganese, a harder metal, has no effect on these clusters.

Zinc favors tetrahedral coordination environments, and this geometry is achieved by most Fe and Mn mononuclear enzymes. It is common for ferroproteins to acquire zinc during purification; once bound, the zinc does not easily dissociate. Therefore, it is not surprising that high levels of intracellular Zn poisons enzymes that have evolved to use ferrous iron as a cofactor metal. Ribulose-5-phosphate 3-epimerase (Rpe) is an example of such an enzyme (Gu and Imlay 2013). In its catalytic cycle its ferrous atom forms bidentate bonds to its substrate, activating it for reversible deprotonation; the product is then released. During this process the Fe atom shifts from four- to six-coordinate geometry and back. Iron is effective at this chemistry because of its ability to shift its coordination scheme, and manganese can effectively substitute. In contrast, while zinc binds, it furnishes < 5% the activity of iron. The reason is not clear: the role of the metal is to stabilize electrostatically the oxyanionic substrate intermediate, and all divalent metals should be able to do so. One possibility is that iron more easily shifts coordination geometries over the reaction course; another is that iron releases substrate ligands with more alacrity than does a softer metal like zinc. Yet zinc binds far more tightly to the protein: iron dissociates from Rpe with a halftime of a few minutes, while Zn dissociation is negligible in 8 hours. In fact, when *E. coli* is overloaded with zinc, Rpe activity declines, and the recovered enzyme is quantitatively occupied by zinc.

Interestingly, mismetallation of this type is exacerbated by oxidative stress (Gu and Imlay 2013). Both superoxide and hydrogen peroxide can oxidize the ferrous atoms of such enzymes, causing the ferric iron thus formed to dissociate. Remetallation is customarily rapid. However, when such stress is chronic, the repeated dissociation of iron allows zinc many opportunities to compete for the metal-free site, and eventually it wins. Rpe is probably just representative of several mononuclear nonredox enzymes that become mismetallated with zinc during periods of superoxide or peroxide stress. The same effect has been confirmed for 3-deoxy-D-arabinoheptulosonate 7-phosphate synthase, the Fe enzyme that initiates the aromatic biosynthetic pathway. Failure of this enzyme is likely the cause of the collapse of this pathway during oxidative stress (Sobota et al. 2014).

It is intriguing that although zinc binds extremely tightly to these enzymes *in vitro*, zinc is quickly removed from them *in vivo*: when oxidative stress is relieved inside cells, enzymes reacquire iron within 20 min (Gu and Imlay 2013). This observation suggests that something inside the cell helped extract zinc from these sites. Thiol compounds are the most obvious candidates, and indeed, cysteine (but not glutathione) replicated the effect *in vitro*. Cysteine is generally a better metal chelator than is glutathione, because cysteine provides both a thiolate and a nearby primary amine as metal ligands. In glutathione that amine is derivatized; thus glutathione binds metals poorly. The labilization of zinc by cysteine may be a model for how metals are constantly solubilized and guided away from low-affinity sites and toward high-affinity ones *in vivo*. Of course, it is possible that thiolate proteins (i.e., thioredoxins or glutaredoxins) can also serve this purpose. This has not yet been tested.

*Avoiding Zinc Excess*

How does excess zinc enter a cell? The regulation of the *znuABC* genes by Zur offers compelling evidence that the Znu system serves the purpose of Zn transport (Patzer and Hantke 1998). The *znu* genes are not needed under routine growth conditions, indicating that other systems supply adequate zinc. One possibility is that import of zinc and other divalent metals is supported by general divalent importers. Metal importers powered by proton movement, rather than ATP hydrolysis, are generally less particular in their selection of metals, perhaps reflecting the thermodynamic price that must be paid to achieve substrate specificity. ZupT and MntH can each transport a variety of divalent metals, including manganese, cadmium, cobalt, and iron (Grass et al. 2005a; Taudte and Grass 2010). ZupT is generally regarded as a Zn importer: *zupT* overproduction accelerated the import of exogenous zinc, and *zupT* deficiency exacerbated the chelator-sensitivity of *znu* mutants (Grass et al. 2002). The PitA transporter imports divalent cations chelated by phosphate (van Veen et al. 1994); when exogenous Zn levels are high, deletion of *pitA* lessens the intracellular Zn load (Beard et al. 2000). In *Cupriavidus metallidurans*, the expression of both *zupT* and *pitA* was reduced when high levels of zinc were provided (Kirsten et al. 2011). Whether these systems evolved to be broad in their metal selection, or whether their apparent promiscuity is the outcome of extreme experimental conditions, is uncertain.

Nevertheless, it is clear that Zn overimport is a natural phenomenon, as bacteria universally express countermeasures to avoid it. ZntA is a P-type ATPase that exports zinc from cytoplasm to periplasm (Rensing et al. 1997). ZitB, a member of the cation diffusion facilitator family, does the same (Grass et al. 2001). Both are induced when *E. coli* is exposed to high levels of zinc. Careful measurements show that upon abrupt exposure to zinc, ZitB lessens the immediate Zn accumulation, while ZntA has a more pronounced effect at later points in time (Wang et al. 2012a). The implication is that ZitB may comprise a basal export activity, while after-induction ZntA supersedes it.[1]

The induction of *zntA* is stimulated by Zn-bound ZntR (Brocklehurst et al. 1999). The responsiveness to zinc is sharpened by the fact that the Zn-free ZntR is subject to rapid proteolysis (Pruteanu et al. 2007). *In vitro* measurements indicate that the Zn dissociation constant of DNA-bound Zur is $10^{-16}$ M, while that of ZntR is approximately fivefold higher; this suggests that the window between them represents the target Zn activity inside cells (Outten and O'Halloran 2001). Total Zn in *E. coli* is ~ 0.2 mM. One infers that even exchangeable zinc is continuously coordinated by metabolites and the surfaces of biomolecules. As discussed above, aqueous metal provides a standard state for binding-constant measurements but is not regarded as physiologically relevant. By using a modified form of carbonic anhydrase as a Zn sensor, however, the Fierke group determined that the steady-state level of hydrated zinc inside wild-type *E. coli* is actually far higher, about 20 pM (Wang et al. 2012a). Since ZntR is not activated inside these cells—as judged from the fact that *zntA* and other ZntR-controlled genes are not induced—there is an apparent contradiction. One possibility is that the *in vitro* behaviors of either ZntR or the carbonic anhydrase construct did not represent their Zn affinity *in vivo*. Alternatively, Wang et al. considered whether activation might be kinetically determined; that is, that the activity of ZntR may depend on the speed with which it acquires zinc, rather than on its binding equilibrium per se. In principle, rapid activation might require Zn levels far in excess of femtomolar levels. However, they noted that during a post-pulse period of Zn efflux, the ZntR response shut down even while intracellular Zn levels were still in the low nanomolar range, as reported by the carbonic anhydrase construct. Absent additional regulatory wrinkles (or inadequate equilibration by the reporter protein), this result implies that the binding constant of ZntR determined *in vitro* does not apply *in vivo*. This conundrum is currently unresolved, but the work presents a creative experimental design to put questions about Zn homeostasis on a quantitative footing.

Finally, exposure to extracellular zinc activates a pair of two-component systems. First, the ZraS/ZraR system triggers synthesis of a single gene: *ZraP* (Appia-Ayme et al. 2012), which encodes a 15 kD Zn-binding periplasmic protein. Under high Zn conditions, ZraP is reported to bind 70% of the proteome-associated zinc (Sevcenco et al. 2011). Although a chaperone role is possible, the function of ZraP may simply be to sequester or buffer zinc. ZraS differs from ZntR in that ZraS senses periplasmic Zn levels. Sequestration there, of course, could protect both periplasmic and cytoplasmic compartments from overloading. Second, the BaeSR system is also activated by exogenous zinc,

---

[1] Complicating the picture: YiiP (FieF) is another CDF family member. It effluxes either Fe or Zn *in vitro* and is modestly induced by overload of either *in vivo* (Grass et al. 2005b; Lu et al. 2009). Its physiological substrate is uncertain.

and it stimulates the synthesis of proteins that also diminish cytoplasmic Zn levels (Wang and Fierke 2013). Two members of the regulon, MdtABC and MdtD, appear to be pumps, and the most obvious explanation is that they export zinc or zinc complexes. Why the cell would need so many efflux pumps is unclear.

## Summary

Metal metabolism is a major part of cellular biochemistry, and both metal deficits and excesses disrupt physiology. The particular challenge with metals is that they are similar enough that mistakes are made, but different enough that enzyme mismetallation impedes function. This review has attempted to summarize current knowledge of how metals are used, how their intracellular concentrations are controlled, and how cells cope with too much or too little. Perplexing questions remain:

- Are importers controlled at the level of enzyme activity, either by allostery or product inhibition? How about exporters?
- How are metals trafficked through the cell: by ligand exchange with a multitude of metabolites, or with a dedicated few?
- How are metals excised from inappropriate sites? Is the identity of a metal in a protein site determined primarily by binding thermodynamics or kinetics?
- Do optimal metal pool sizes depend on environmental circumstances? If so, how does the cell adjust its homeostatic mechanisms to change the pool size?
- How are metal regulatory proteins configured to resist or cope with metallation by noncognate metals?
- To what extent has evolution adjusted the metals used by particular enzymes to fit the metal availability of the local habitat? What is the nature(s) of these adjustments?

## Acknowledgments

Insightful comments from other participants in the Forum are gratefully acknowledged. Research in the author's lab is supported by GM49640 and GM101012 from the National Institutes of Health.

# 6

# Intervention Strategies for Metal Deficiency and Overload

Fudi Wang and Lihong Zhang

## Abstract

An increasing amount of evidence shows the linkage between metal ion homeostasis and human disease. Deficiency or overload of metal ions play vital roles in many human diseases, including infectious disease. Nutritional supplementation and metal-based drugs have been suggested as potential intervention strategies to develop treatment for various diseases related to metal deficiency and overload. However, there are numerous forms of metal ion supplementation and metal-based drugs with different features. This chapter provides an overview of the recommended dietary allowance, tolerable upper intake levels, and bioavailability of metal elements and offers perspectives on intervention strategies for metal deficiency and overload. Data for analysis were obtained from research articles, reviews, and reports from the World Health Organization; the National Academic Press websites were another principal source of data.

## Introduction

It is well known that some metal ions (iron, zinc, copper, selenium, manganese, molybdenum, nickel, and vanadium) are essential for the proper functioning of living cells. Deficiency of these essential metal ions is often linked with an increased risk for various diseases, including infectious diseases, especially among at-risk populations. Supplementation with metal ions has been shown to prevent, attenuate, and treat a portion of infectious diseases successfully. For example, worldwide, Zn deficiency is responsible for approximately 16% of lower respiratory tract infections, 18% of malaria, and 10% of diarrhoeal disease; Zn supplementation has been recommended by the World Health Organization as the main treatment of choice for diarrhea among children under five years of age (WHO/UNICEF 2004).

Whether essential or not, all metal can be toxic to living cells. Metal overload may cause illness and even death in humans. For example, about 100,000 children born with transfusion-dependent β thalassaemia are currently reliant on regular transfusions, and at least 3,000 die annually in their teens or early twenties from uncontrolled Fe overload (Modell and Darlison 2008). Moreover, Fe overload has been demonstrated to be related to some of the world's most common infections: malaria, HIV-1, and tuberculosis (Sazawal et al. 2006; Boelaert et al. 2007; Prentice et al. 2007; Drakesmith and Prentice 2008). Therefore, it is urgent to consider the most appropriate strategies for prevention and treatment of metal overload.

Government agencies in many countries have been providing nutritional (including essential metal elements) advice to the public for several decades. The aim of this chapter is to give an overview of the recommended dietary allowance (RDA), tolerable upper intake level (UIL), and bioavailability of metal elements and present perspectives on intervention strategies for metal deficiency and overload.

## Recommended Dietary Allowance

RDA is the daily intake level of a nutrient that is considered to be sufficient to meet the requirements of 97% of healthy individuals for sustenance or avoidance of deficiency states. It was developed during World War II by Lydia J. Roberts, Hazel Stiebeling, and Helen S. Mitchell. They surveyed all available data, created a tentative set of allowances for "energy and eight nutrients," and submitted them to experts for review. The final sets of guidelines were accepted in 1941. The committee established by the U.S. National Academy of Sciences to investigate issues of nutrition was renamed the Food and Nutrition Board in 1941. Since then, this board reviews and revises the RDAs every five to ten years.

The reference daily intake or recommended daily intake (RDI) is based on the RDA from 1968. However, in 1994, at the suggestion of the Institute of Medicine (IOM) of the National Academy, RDA became one part of a new broader set of values known as the dietary reference intake (DRI) system (Flo et al. 2004), which consists of the estimated average requirement (Blackwell et al. 2001), RDA, adequate intake (AI), and tolerable UILs. Hence, newer RDAs have since been introduced into the DRI system, though the RDI is still used for nutritional labeling.

### Essential Metal Ions per Individual for
### Populations in Different Countries

The value of RDA for essential metals varies in different countries. For example, the selenium RDA for the Japanese population is much lower than people in other parts of the world. Here we summarize the RDA for people in the United States, Australia/New Zealand combined, China, Japan, and the European Union for iron (Table 6.1), zinc (Table 6.2), copper (Table 6.3), and

**Table 6.1**    Recommended dietary allowances for iron (mg/day) per individual, for populations from different countries: United States, Australia and New Zealand (combined), China, Japan, and the European Union. AI: adequate intake.

| | USA ♂ | USA ♀ | AUS/NZ ♂ | AUS/NZ ♀ | China ♂ | China ♀ | Japan ♂ | Japan ♀ | EU ♂ | EU ♀ |
|---|---|---|---|---|---|---|---|---|---|---|
| 0–6 mon | 0.27 (AI) | | 0.2 (AI) | | 0.3 | | 0.4 | | – | |
| 7–12 mon | 11 | | 11 | | 10 | | 6 | | 6.2 | |
| 1–3 yr | 7 | | 9 | | 12 | | 5.5 | 6 | 3.9 | |
| 4–8 yr | 10 | | 10 | | 12 | | 6.5 | 8.5 | 4.2 | |
| 9–13 yr | 8 | 8 | 8 | 8 | 16 | 18 | 11 | 13 | 9.7 | 21.8 |
| 14–18 yr | 11 | 15 | 11 | 15 | 20 | 25 | 10.5 | 11 | 12.5 | 20.7 |
| 19–30 yr | 8 | 18 | 8 | 18 | 15 | 20 | 7.5 | 10.5 | 9.1 | 19.6 |
| 31–50 yr | 8 | 18 | 8 | 18 | 15 | 20 | 7.5 | 10.5 | 9.1 | 19.6 |
| 50–70 yr | 8 | 8 | 8 | 8 | 15 | 15 | 7.5 | 10.5 | 9.1 | 7.5 |
| > 70 yr | 8 | 8 | 8 | 8 | 15 | 15 | 6.5 | 10.5 | 9.1 | 7.5 |
| Pregnancy: | | | | | | | | | | |
| < 18 yr | 27 | | 27 | | 15 | | 24 | | 30 | |
| 19–30 yr | 27 | | 27 | | 25 | | 24 | | 30 | |
| 31–50 yr | 27 | | 27 | | 35 | | 24 | | 30 | |
| Lactation: | | | | | | | | | | |
| < 18 yr | 10 | | 10 | | 25 | | 13.5 | | 10 | |
| 19–30 yr | 9 | | 9 | | 25 | | 13 | | 10 | |
| 31–50 yr | 9 | | 9 | | 25 | | 13 | | 10 | |

selenium (Table 6.4). These tables provide an overview of the RDA for people in different life stages and gender groups as well as data for pregnant and lactating women.

**Perspectives**

Normal dietary levels of various essential metal ions are required to prevent the occurrence of metal deficiencies. The RDA provides the public nutritional advice. Used properly, it can also inform intervention strategies to address metal deficiency and achieve metal ion sustenance as well as to reduce the risk of some diseases, including infectious diseases.

The important point that we wish to emphasize is that it is necessary for RDA users to have a thorough knowledge of major concepts in the DRI system. For example, estimated average requirements is a concept used to represent the estimated median requirement (half of healthy individuals) and is particularly appropriate for applications related to planning and assessing intakes for groups of persons. RDA is derived from the estimated average requirement

**Table 6.2** Recommended dietary allowances for zinc (mg/day) per individual, for populations from different countries: United States, Australia and New Zealand (combined), China, Japan, and the European Union.

| | USA ♂ | USA ♀ | AUS/NZ ♂ | AUS/NZ ♀ | China ♂ | China ♀ | Japan ♂ | Japan ♀ | EU ♂ | EU ♀ |
|---|---|---|---|---|---|---|---|---|---|---|
| 0–6 mon | 2 (AI) | | 2 (AI) | | 1.5 | | 2 | | – | |
| 7–12 mon | 3 | | 3 | | 8 | | 3 | | 4 | |
| 1–3 yr | 3 | | 3 | | 9 | | 4 | | 4 | |
| 4–8 yr | 5 | | 4 | | 12 | | 5 | | 6 | |
| 9–13 yr | 8 | 8 | 6 | 6 | 18 | 15 | 6 | 7 | 9 | 9 |
| 14–18 yr | 11 | 9 | 13 | 7 | 19 | 15.5 | 8 | 7 | 9 | 7 |
| 19–30 yr | 11 | 8 | 14 | 8 | 15 | 11.5 | 9 | 7 | 9 | 7 |
| 31–50 yr | 11 | 8 | 14 | 8 | 15 | 11.5 | 9 | 7 | 9 | 7 |
| 50–70 yr | 11 | 8 | 14 | 8 | 11.5 | 11.5 | 9 | 7 | 9 | 7 |
| > 70 yr | 11 | 8 | 14 | 8 | 11.5 | 11.5 | 8 | 7 | 9 | 7 |
| Pregnancy: | | | | | | | | | | |
| < 18 yr | | 12 | | 10 | | 11.5 | | 10 | | 7 |
| 19–30 yr | | 11 | | 11 | | 16.5 | | 10 | | 7 |
| 31–50 yr | | 11 | | 11 | | 16.5 | | 10 | | 7 |
| Lactation: | | | | | | | | | | |
| < 18 yr | | 13 | | 11 | | 21.5 | | 10 | | 12 |
| 19–30 yr | | 12 | | 12 | | 21.5 | | 10 | | 12 |
| 31–50 yr | | 12 | | 12 | | 21.5 | | 10 | | 1 |

(EAR) and covers requirements for 97% of the population. UIL is the highest average intake that is likely to pose no risk of adverse health effects to almost all individuals (discussed in detail below), whereas average intake is used when an EAR/RDA cannot be developed; average intake level is based on observed or experimental intakes.

Despite the emphasis on the population basis of the RDA, RDA has often been misused to assess dietary adequacy in individuals. In fact, RDA is a general guide designed to assist the public or nutrition and health professionals in assessing the dietary requirements of individuals. The recommendations are used for healthy people and may not meet the specific nutritional requirements of all individuals.

## Tolerable Upper Intake Levels

Tolerable UILs are defined as the highest level of daily nutrient intake that is likely to pose no risk of adverse health effects to almost all individuals in the general population. As intake increases above the UIL, the risk of adverse

**Table 6.3**   Recommended dietary allowances for copper (mg/day) per individual, for populations from different countries: United States, Australia and New Zealand (combined), China, Japan, and the European Union.

| | USA ♂ | USA ♀ | AUS/NZ ♂ | AUS/NZ ♀ | China ♂ | China ♀ | Japan ♂ | Japan ♀ | EU ♂ | EU ♀ |
|---|---|---|---|---|---|---|---|---|---|---|
| 0–6 mon | 0.2 (AI) | | 0.2 (AI) | | 0.4 | | 0.3 | | – | |
| 7–12 mon | 0.22 | | 0.22 | | 0.6 | | 0.3 | | 0.3 | |
| 1–3 yr | 0.34 | | 0.7 | | 0.8 | | 0.3 | | 0.4 | |
| 4–8 yr | 0.44 | | 1 | | 1 | | 0.4 | | 0.7 | |
| 9–13 yr | 0.7 | 0.7 | 1.3 | 1.1 | 1.8 | 1.8 | 0.7 | 0.7 | 0.8 | 0.8 |
| 14–18 yr | 0.89 | 0.89 | 1.5 | 1.1 | 2 | 2 | 0.9 | 0.7 | 1 | 1 |
| 19–30 yr | 0.9 | 0.9 | 1.7 | 1.2 | 2 | 2 | 0.8 | 0.7 | 1 | 1 |
| 31–50 yr | 0.9 | 0.9 | 1.7 | 1.2 | 2 | 2 | 0.8 | 0.7 | 1 | 1 |
| 50–70 yr | 0.9 | 0.9 | 1.7 | 1.2 | 2 | 2 | 0.8 | 0.7 | 1 | 1 |
| > 70 yr | 0.9 | 0.9 | 1.7 | 1.2 | 2 | 2 | 0.8 | 0.7 | 1 | 1 |
| Pregnancy: | | | | | | | | | | |
| < 18 yr | | 1 | | 1.2 | | 2 | | 0.8 | | 1.1 |
| 19–30 yr | | 1 | | 1.3 | | 2 | | 0.8 | | 1.1 |
| 31–50 yr | | 1 | | 1.3 | | 2 | | 0.8 | | 1.1 |
| Lactation: | | | | | | | | | | |
| < 18 yr | | 1.3 | | 1.4 | | 2 | | 1.3 | | 1.4 |
| 19–30 yr | | 1.3 | | 1.5 | | 2 | | 1.3 | | 1.4 |
| 31–50 yr | | 1.3 | | 1.5 | | 2 | | 1.3 | | 1.4 |

effects (including any significant alteration in the structure or function of the human organism or any impairment of a physiologically important function) increases. Therefore, UIL is used to examine the possibility of excessive intake of nutrients that can be harmful in large amounts. The term "tolerable" indicates a level of intake that can, with high probability, be tolerated biologically by individuals. However, it does not imply acceptability of that level in any other sense, which indicates that upper intake levels do not mean that nutrient intakes greater than the RDA or AI are recommended as being beneficial to an individual.

## Essential Metal Ions per Individual for Populations in Different Countries

The value of the UIL for the essential metal ions varies in different countries. The scientific data used to develop the UIL derive, in fact, from observational and experimental studies of different countries; life stages and gender of the population were also considered to the fullest extent possible. Here we

**Table 6.4** Recommended dietary allowances for selenium (μg/day) per individual, for populations from different countries: United States, Australia and New Zealand (combined), China, Japan, and the European Union.

| | USA ♂ | USA ♀ | AUS/NZ ♂ | AUS/NZ ♀ | China ♂ | China ♀ | Japan ♂ | Japan ♀ | EU ♂ | EU ♀ |
|---|---|---|---|---|---|---|---|---|---|---|
| 0–6 mon | 15 (AI) | | 12 (AI) | | 15 | | 16 | | – | |
| 7–12 mon | 20 | | 15 | | 200 | | 19 | | 8 | |
| 1–3 yr | 20 | | 20 | | 20 | | 9 | 8 | 10 | |
| 4–8 yr | 30 | | 30 | | 25 | | 15 | 15 | 20 | |
| 9–13 yr | 40 | 40 | 50 | 50 | 40 | 40 | 20 | 20 | 35 | 35 |
| 14–18 yr | 55 | 55 | 70 | 60 | 50 | 50 | 30 | 25 | 45 | 45 |
| 19–30 yr | 55 | 55 | 70 | 60 | 50 | 50 | 30 | 25 | 45 | 45 |
| 31–50 yr | 55 | 55 | 70 | 60 | 50 | 50 | 35 | 25 | 45 | 45 |
| 50–70 yr | 55 | 55 | 70 | 60 | 50 | 50 | 30 | 25 | 45 | 45 |
| > 70 yr | 55 | 55 | 70 | 60 | 50 | 50 | 30 | 25 | 45 | 45 |
| **Pregnancy:** | | | | | | | | | | |
| < 18 yr | 60 | | 65 | | 50 | | 29 | | 55 | |
| 19–30 yr | 60 | | 65 | | 50 | | 29 | | 55 | |
| 31–50 yr | 60 | | 65 | | 50 | | 29 | | 55 | |
| **Lactation:** | | | | | | | | | | |
| < 18 yr | 70 | | 75 | | 60 | | 45 | | 70 | |
| 19–30 yr | 70 | | 75 | | 60 | | 45 | | 70 | |
| 31–50 yr | 70 | | 75 | | 60 | | 45 | | 70 | |

summarize the UIL for people in the United States, Australia/New Zealand combined, China, Japan, and the European Union for iron (Table 6.5), zinc (Table 6.6), copper (Table 6.7), and selenium (Table 6.8). These tables provide an overview of the UIL for people in different life stages and gender groups as well as data for pregnant and lactating women.

## Perspectives

The UIL is the highest level of daily consumption that current data have shown to cause no side effects in humans when used indefinitely without medical supervision. It is thus an important part of the intervention strategies for metal overload. Many individuals self-medicate with nutrients for curative or treatment purposes. However, it is impossible to identify a "risk-free" intake level for a nutrient that can be applied with certainty to all members of a population. Despite its inclusion of sensitive individuals (e.g., pregnant and lactating women), the UIL is a general guide for most members of the general population. It should be applied properly, especially for those who live in areas with metal pollution.

**Table 6.5**　Tolerable upper intake levels for iron (mg/day) per individual, for populations from different countries: United States, Australia and New Zealand (combined), China, Japan, and the European Union.

| | USA ♂ | USA ♀ | AUS/NZ ♂ | AUS/NZ ♀ | China ♂ | China ♀ | Japan ♂ | Japan ♀ | EU ♂ | EU ♀ |
|---|---|---|---|---|---|---|---|---|---|---|
| 0–6 mon | 40 | | 20 | | 10 | | – | | – | |
| 7–12 mon | 40 | | 20 | | 30 | | – | | – | |
| 1–3 yr | 40 | | 20 | | 30 | | 25 | – | – | |
| 4–8 yr | 40 | | 40 | | 30 | | 30 | 8.5 | – | |
| 9–13 yr | 40 | 40 | 40 | 40 | 50 | 50 | 35 | 35 | – | – |
| 14–18 yr | 45 | 45 | 45 | 45 | 50 | 50 | 50 | 50 | – | – |
| 19–30 yr | 45 | 45 | 45 | 45 | 50 | 50 | 50 | 50 | 50 | 50 |
| 31–50 yr | 45 | 45 | 45 | 45 | 50 | 50 | 55 | 55 | 50 | 50 |
| 50–70 yr | 45 | 45 | 45 | 45 | 50 | 50 | 50 | 50 | 50 | 50 |
| > 70 yr | 45 | 45 | 45 | 45 | 50 | 50 | 45 | 45 | 50 | 7.5 |
| Pregnancy: | | | | | | | | | | |
| < 18 yr | | 45 | | 45 | | 50 | | 50 | | 50 |
| 19–30 yr | | 45 | | 45 | | 50 | | 50 | | 50 |
| 31–50 yr | | 45 | | 45 | | 50 | | 50 | | 50 |
| Lactation: | | | | | | | | | | |
| < 18 yr | | 45 | | 45 | | 50 | | 50 | | 50 |
| 19–30 yr | | 45 | | 45 | | 50 | | 50 | | 50 |
| 31–50 yr | | 45 | | 45 | | 50 | | 50 | | 50 |

Most metals, whether essential or not, can produce adverse health effects if intakes are excessive. Metal ions can be obtained from any combination of food, water, or nonfood sources (e.g., nutrient supplements and pharmacologic agents). Moreover the setting of the UIL is based on nutrients as part of the total diet. Therefore, nutrient supplements, which are usually taken separately from food, require special consideration due to wide-ranging factors surrounding their intake. As a result, nutrient supplements may produce toxic effects. The addition of essential metal ions to a diet—through the ingestion of large amounts of highly fortified food or nonfood sources such as supplements—may pose a risk for adverse health effects.

## Bioavailability

Bioavailability, one of the essential tools in pharmacology and nutritional science, is a subcategory of absorption and is defined as the fraction of an administered dose of unchanged drug that reaches the systemic circulation. In general, it can be described as absolute bioavailability or relative bioavailability.

**Table 6.6** Tolerable upper intake levels for zinc (mg/day) per individual, for populations from different countries: United States, Australia and New Zealand (combined), China, Japan, and the European Union.

| | USA | | AUS/NZ | | China | | Japan | | EU | |
|---|---|---|---|---|---|---|---|---|---|---|
| | ♂ | ♀ | ♂ | ♀ | ♂ | ♀ | ♂ | ♀ | ♂ | ♀ |
| 0–6 mon | 4 | | 4 | | – | | – | | – | |
| 7–12 mon | 5 | | 5 | | 13 | | – | | – | |
| 1–3 yr | 7 | | 7 | | 23 | | – | | 7 | |
| 4–8 yr | 12 | | 12 | | 23 | | – | | 11 | |
| 9–13 yr | 23 | 23 | 25 | 25 | 37 | 34 | – | – | 18 | 18 |
| 14–18 yr | 34 | 34 | 35 | 35 | 42 | 35 | – | – | 22 | 22 |
| 19–30 yr | 40 | 40 | 40 | 40 | 45 | 37 | 30 | 30 | 25 | 25 |
| 31–50 yr | 40 | 40 | 40 | 40 | 45 | 37 | 30 | 30 | 25 | 25 |
| 50–70 yr | 40 | 40 | 40 | 40 | 37 | 37 | 30 | 30 | 25 | 25 |
| > 70 yr | 40 | 40 | 40 | 40 | 37 | 37 | 30 | 30 | 25 | 25 |
| **Pregnancy:** | | | | | | | | | | |
| < 18 yr | 34 | | 35 | | 35 | | 30 | | 25 | |
| 19–30 yr | 40 | | 40 | | 35 | | 30 | | 25 | |
| 31–50 yr | 40 | | 40 | | 35 | | 30 | | 25 | |
| **Lactation:** | | | | | | | | | | |
| < 18 yr | 34 | | 35 | | 35 | | 30 | | 25 | |
| 19–30 yr | 40 | | 40 | | 35 | | 30 | | 25 | |
| 31–50 yr | 40 | | 40 | | 35 | | 30 | | 25 | |

Absolute bioavailability compares the bioavailability of an active drug in systemic circulation following non-intravenous administration (such as oral, rectal, transdermal, subcutaneous, or sublingual administration) with the bioavailability of the same drug following intravenous administration. It is the fraction of the drug absorbed through non-intravenous administration compared with the corresponding intravenous administration of the same drug. Therefore, a drug given by the intravenous route will have an absolute bioavailability of 100%, whereas drugs given by other routes usually have an absolute bioavailability of less than 100%, due to incomplete absorption and first-pass metabolism.

Relative bioavailability measures the bioavailability of one formulation of a certain drug when compared with another formulation of the same drug, usually an established standard, or through administration via a different route. By definition, when the standard consists of intravenously administered drug, this is known as absolute bioavailability.

**Table 6.7** Tolerable upper intake levels for copper (mg/day) per individual, for populations from different countries: United States, Australia and New Zealand (combined), China, Japan, and the European Union.

| | USA ♂ | USA ♀ | AUS/NZ ♂ | AUS/NZ ♀ | China ♂ | China ♀ | Japan ♂ | Japan ♀ | EU ♂ | EU ♀ |
|---|---|---|---|---|---|---|---|---|---|---|
| 0–6 mon | – | | – | | – | | – | | – | |
| 7–12 mon | – | | – | | – | | – | | – | |
| 1–3 yr | 1 | | 1 | | 1.5 | | – | | 1 | |
| 4–8 yr | 3 | | 3 | | 2 | | – | | 2 | |
| 9–13 yr | 5 | 5 | 5 | 5 | 5 | 5 | – | – | 4 | 4 |
| 14–18 yr | 8 | 8 | 8 | 8 | 7 | 7 | – | – | 4 | 4 |
| 19–30 yr | 10 | 10 | 10 | 10 | 8 | 8 | 10 | 10 | 5 | 5 |
| 31–50 yr | 10 | 10 | 10 | 10 | 8 | 8 | 10 | 10 | 5 | 5 |
| 50–70 yr | 10 | 10 | 10 | 10 | 8 | 8 | 10 | 10 | 5 | 5 |
| > 70 yr | 10 | 10 | 10 | 10 | 8 | 8 | 10 | 10 | 5 | 5 |
| Pregnancy: | | | | | | | | | | |
| < 18 yr | | 8 | | 8 | | 8 | | 10 | | 5 |
| 19–30 yr | | 10 | | 10 | | 8 | | 10 | | 5 |
| 31–50 yr | | 10 | | 10 | | 8 | | 10 | | 5 |
| Lactation: | | | | | | | | | | |
| < 18 yr | | 8 | | 8 | | 8 | | 10 | | 5 |
| 19–30 yr | | 10 | | 10 | | 8 | | 10 | | 5 |
| 31–50 yr | | 10 | | 10 | | 8 | | 10 | | 5 |

## Bioavailability of Different Forms of Metal Elements

Supplements of metal elements are available in a wide variety of forms: inorganic salts, organic salts, amino acid chelates, and yeast form. Inorganic salts (such as sulfates and carbonates) and organic salts (such as citrates and gluconates) are the most commonly used forms. In contrast, the amino acid chelates are formed by hydrolysis of protein. The reaction of the resulting amino acids with an inorganic salt supposedly forms a chelate of the metal with the ligands of the amino acids. The resulting yeast is produced by growing yeast in a nutrient medium containing the inorganic salt. In theory, the yeast absorbs the element by forming a natural chelate between the metal ions and the proteins or amino acids of the yeast.

Table 6.9 summarizes the bioavailability of different forms of iron, zinc, copper, selenium, and manganese in the blood and liver from humans and/or rats.

**Table 6.8**  Tolerable upper intake levels for selenium (mg/day) per individual, for populations from different countries: United States, Australia and New Zealand (combined), China, Japan, and the European Union.

| | USA ♂ | USA ♀ | AUS/NZ ♂ | AUS/NZ ♀ | China ♂ | China ♀ | Japan ♂ | Japan ♀ | EU ♂ | EU ♀ |
|---|---|---|---|---|---|---|---|---|---|---|
| 0–6 mon | 45 | | 45 | | 55 | | – | | – | |
| 7–12 mon | 60 | | 60 | | 80 | | – | | – | |
| 1–3 yr | 90 | | 90 | | 120 | | 200 | | 60 | |
| 4–8 yr | 150 | | 150 | | 180 | | 200 | | 90 | |
| 9–13 yr | 280 | 280 | 280 | 280 | 300 | 300 | 300 | 300 | 200 | 200 |
| 14–18 yr | 400 | 400 | 400 | 400 | 360 | 360 | 400 | 350 | 250 | 250 |
| 19–30 yr | 400 | 400 | 400 | 400 | 400 | 400 | 450 | 350 | 300 | 300 |
| 31–50 yr | 400 | 400 | 400 | 400 | 400 | 400 | 450 | 350 | 300 | 300 |
| 50–70 yr | 400 | 400 | 400 | 400 | 400 | 400 | 450 | 350 | 300 | 300 |
| >70 yr | 400 | 400 | 400 | 400 | 400 | 400 | 400 | 350 | 300 | 300 |
| Pregnancy: | | | | | | | | | | |
| <18 yr | | 400 | | 400 | | 400 | | 350 | | 300 |
| 19–30 yr | | 400 | | 400 | | 400 | | 350 | | 300 |
| 31–50 yr | | 400 | | 400 | | 400 | | 350 | | 300 |
| Lactation: | | | | | | | | | | |
| <18 yr | | 400 | | 400 | | 400 | | 350 | | 300 |
| 19–30 yr | | 400 | | 400 | | 400 | | 350 | | 300 |
| 31–50 yr | | 400 | | 400 | | 400 | | 350 | | 300 |

## Perspectives

Treatment of metal deficiency or overload often involves supplementation of missing metal ions or metal ion chelating agents. Bioavailability is one of the key factors in the assessment of supplementation effects. For dietary supplements, the route of administration is nearly always oral. Therefore, bioavailability influences a nutrient's beneficial effects at the physiological level of intake. It may also affect the nature and severity of toxicity due to excessive intake.

Bioavailability varies from individual to individual. There are many factors that influence the utilization of metal elements, including the concentration and chemical form of the metal elements, the nutrition and health of the individual, the gut flora, and excretory losses. Some metals may be less readily absorbed when they are part of a meal than when they are ingested separately. Most importantly, supplemental forms of some metals (e.g., magnesium) may require special consideration due to their higher bioavailability and may therefore present a higher risk of producing adverse effects than equivalent amounts from the natural form found in food.

**Table 6.9**   Relative bioavailability of different forms of common trace metal elements.
Note: for all studies, the inorganic salt is defined as 100% bioavailable.

| Metal Elements | Model | Forms | Relative Bioavailability (%) Blood | Relative Bioavailability (%) Liver |
|---|---|---|---|---|
| Iron | Rat | Inorganic Salt | 100 | 100 |
| | | Chelate | 57 | 72 |
| | | Yeast | 101 | 121 |
| Zinc | Rat | Inorganic Salt | 100 | 100 |
| | | Chelate | 101 | 129 |
| | | Yeast | 172 | 187 |
| | Human | Inorganic Salt | 100 | |
| | | Organic Salt | 111 | |
| | | Yeast | 175 | |
| Copper | Rat | Inorganic Salt | 100 | 100 |
| | | Organic Salt | 93 | 130 |
| | | Yeast | 124 | 195 |
| | Human | Inorganic Salt | 100 | |
| | | Chelate | 101 | |
| | | Yeast | 144 | |
| Selenium | Rat | Inorganic Salt | 100 | 100 |
| | | Chelate | 60 | 146 |
| | | Yeast | 122 | 226 |
| | Human | Inorganic Salt | 100 | |
| | | Chelate | 122 | |
| Manganese | Rat | Inorganic Salt | 100 | 100 |
| | | Chelate | 111 | 142 |
| | | Yeast | 156 | 163 |

## Implications and Future Areas for Attention

Although metal deficiency and overload have gained worldwide attention, finding effective intervention strategies to prevent and treat the matter is still an arduous task for the government, scholars, and general public.

*Advocacy and training strategies are powerful tools to increase public knowledge of metal homeostasis and decrease the morbidity and mortality related to metal deficiency and overload.*

Indeed, many individuals are self-medicating with nutrients for health or treatment purposes. Although government agencies in many countries have been providing nutritional advice (RDI system) to the public for several decades, most people misuse the data on the RDA, UIL, and bioavailability (discussed above), due to lack of a full understanding of the guidelines, or even without any knowledge of the guidelines. This situation makes it urgent for governments and academic institutions to provide related information, including recent developments in nutritional research, through various publicity approaches such as media, websites, and training programs. To this end, in 2013 we organized the first "Westlake Frontiers in Nutrition Research Training Program" in Hangzhou, China. Designed to provide a perennial platform of exchange for Chinese and overseas nutritional professionals, the program was a huge success. It is hoped that it will become an instrumental component to advance the health of all Chinese people.

*Environmental influences on both metal deficiency and overload cannot be ignored.*

Minamata disease, endemic in Japan, is a typical example of metal overload: large-scale food poisoning is caused by methylmercury. In November 2010, 2,271 patients were officially diagnosed as having Minamata disease; estimates, however, place the number of people from affected areas, who exhibit neurologic signs of methylmercury poisoning, in the tens of thousands (Yorifuji et al. 2013). The bioaccumulation and biomagnifications of heavy metals such as mercury, lead, and cadmium pose a serious, continuous risk for human health because they are nondegradable. Therefore, given the fast growth of the economic industry (e.g., the market of fluorescent lamps that use mercury as an essential component), heavy metal exposure is expected to gain a high degree of public attention.

Keshan disease, an endemic heart disease in China, is a typical example of metal deficiency. Extensive cross-sectional epidemiological studies have shown that low Se concentrations in cereal grains and low Se status of local residents are associated with the occurrence of Keshan disease. Several large population-based intervention trials, using oral administration of sodium selenite tablets, have shown significant reduction in the incidence of Keshan disease (Chen 2012). It is thus imperative to identify deficiencies of essential metal elements in different areas, especially mild levels of metal deficiencies, which are more difficult to recognize than severe and moderate deficiencies. Certainly, data from these endemic diseases provide a scientific basis for identifying the minimum requirement, RDA, or UIL for certain metal elements.

*Metal–metal interaction is an important matter of concern.*

The metabolism and transport of metal ions is a complex process that takes place in numerous transporters in mammals. An example of a typical metal ions transporter can be found in the divalent metal ion transporter 1 (DMT1), which transports not only iron but also zinc, copper, manganese, cobalt, nickel, and the toxic metal ions lead and cadmium. Therefore, any strategy designed to address metal deficiency and overload must take DMT1 into account. Excessive intake or deficiency of one metallic element may interfere with absorption, excretion, transport, storage, function, or metabolism of other metals. Recently, Graham et al. (2012) showed that Fe deficiency—the most common metal deficiency affecting nearly 2 billion people worldwide—may be due to underlying zinc and other trace metal deficiencies. Moreover, Fe deficiency has become a risk factor for cadmium toxicity since it causes increases in tissue cadmium levels (Min et al. 2008). Nutrition and health status may vary from individual to individual, and especially between people living in different areas, due to variations in environmental influence. People obtain metal ions from any combination of food (including highly fortified food), water, and nonfood sources (e.g., nutrient supplements and pharmacologic agents). Imbalances among the concentrations of metal elements may pose a risk for adverse health effects in almost every individual. In addition, the bioavailability and effect of fortified foods or supplements may differ from the natural constituents of foods.

*Regulating the endogenous distribution of metal ions is a vital therapeutic strategy for treating diseases with metal homeostasis imbalance.*

It must be kept in mind that some diseases related to metal deficiency or overload are caused by an inappropriate distribution of metal ions in organs or cell compartments. Using Alzheimer disease as an example, an increasing amount of evidence has demonstrated abundant distribution of Zn ions in the plaques of brains of people with the disease; this indicates an overload of Zn ions in the brain. Metal chelator treatment with clioquinol has provided significant evidence of slowing cognitive deterioration (Adlard et al. 2008). Surprisingly, metal chelator treatment increased the brain Zn level (Cherny et al. 2001); in contrast, low dietary zinc caused a significant 25% increase in total plaque volume in Alzheimer mice using stereological measures (Stoltenberg et al. 2007). Further studies demonstrated that clioquinol and PBT are ionophores that promote the transport of zinc, iron, and copper across cell membranes (Adlard et al. 2008). Furthermore, an imbalance between "soluble" and "insoluble" metal ions (such as $Cu^{2+}$) is also a likely cause for diseases with metal homeostasis imbalance (Faller 2012). Therefore, any strategy for treatment of diseases related to metal deficiency and overload should take this into account.

*Further understanding of metal elements and the mechanisms of metal deficiency or overload is of great importance to the development and design of metal-based drugs.*

Knowledge of metal–metal interactions has been used successfully as a treatment strategy. In the case of Cu overload in Wilson disease, treatment with zinc has been demonstrated as very effective in preventing symptoms. Take iron for example: the identification of hepcidin as a key regulator of Fe absorption and Fe distribution in health and disease has greatly advanced our understanding of Fe homeostasis in humans and, in turn, has promoted the development of drugs aimed at decreasing Fe overload. Hepcidin mimetics, minihepcidins, have been shown to be effective in reducing Fe overload (Ramos et al. 2012).

*Natural plant extracts may provide opportunities for a new intervention strategy to address metal deficiency and overload.*

It is generally more difficult to absorb metal ions (e.g., iron) from plant matter than it is from animal sources. Since ancient times, empirical dietary therapies for treating a wide variety of diseases, including Fe-deficiency anemia, emerged in both traditional Chinese medicine and dietary culture. The contradiction between absorption from plant and animal sources indicates a mechanism that requires analysis. It may account for significant sources of dietary metal and play a key role in regulating the metal homeostasis. To pursue this, we recently screened 16 different medicinal plant extracts used to treat anemia-related disorders in traditional Chinese medicine and identified the extract of Caulis Spatholobi (also called Jixueteng, the stem of *Spatholobus suberectus* Dunn) as a novel, potent hepcidin-encoding gene (HAMP) expression inhibitor. This extract could be modified and optimized into a dietary supplement or a therapeutic option for the amelioration of hepcidin-overexpression-related diseases, including Fe-deficiency anemia (Guan et al. 2013). Of further interest, recent studies in our laboratory on the molecular mechanisms of "black foods" (i.e., foods that are black in color) inducing erythropoiesis have shown that the black soybean extract regulates Fe metabolism by inhibiting the expression of hepcidin (Mu et al. 2014). These findings reveal the potency of natural plants in regulating Fe homeostasis and are bound to attract valuable research into natural plants and their regulation of other metal ions in homeostasis, hence, the prevention and treatment for diseases related to metal deficiency and overload.

In conclusion, metal deficiency and overload have become a major problem affecting billions of people worldwide. Whether metal deficiency and overload are seen as the cause or result of infectious, neurodegenerative, or immune system diseases, intervention strategies offer new insights into the prevention and treatment of these diseases.

First column (top to bottom): Jennifer Cavet, Sascha Brunke, Dennis Thiele, Heran Darwin, Robert Perry, Sascha Brunke, Carol Fierke
Second column: Robert Perry, Heran Darwin, Jeffrey Weiser, Michael Murphy, Jennifer Cavet, Jeffrey Weiser, Dennis Thiele
Third column: Carol Fierke, James Imlay, Anthony Schryvers, James Imlay, group discussion, Michael Murphy, Anthony Schryvers

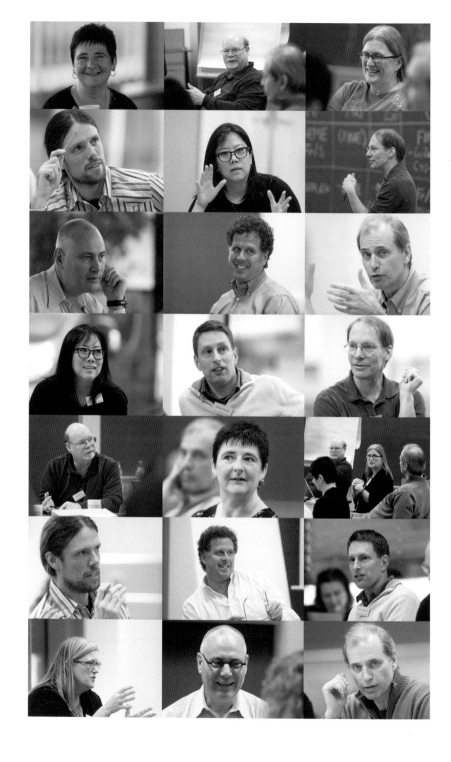

# 7

# Trace Metals in Host–Microbe Interactions

## The Microbe Perspective

Jennifer S. Cavet, Robert D. Perry, Sascha Brunke,
K. Heran Darwin, Carol A. Fierke,
James A. Imlay, Michael E. P. Murphy,
Anthony B. Schryvers, Dennis J. Thiele,
and Jeffrey N. Weiser

### Abstract

Metals play a central role in the outcome of host–pathogen interactions. Microbes must acquire metals for metabolic processes, with nearly a half of all enzymes requiring a metal cofactor for function, yet microbes can be poisoned by metals. The host innate immune defenses are thought to exploit these vulnerabilities to protect against invading pathogens, whereas microbes can respond by employing multiple strategies to maintain their metal homeostasis. An understanding of these microbial strategies combined with knowledge of the diverse metal challenges faced by different microbes in the various host niches could inform the development of much needed new approaches for combating infectious diseases. This chapter summarizes extensive discussions on the interplay of metal ions in host–microbe interactions, from the microbial perspective. The focus is on five key areas, highlighted as requiring a greater understanding: (a) how we define and determine metal availability, (b) the different levels and sources of metals available to microbes in different niches within the host, (c) the effect of the metal status of a pathogen, as derived from its prior environment, on its ability to establish an infection or the severity of disease, (d) the interplay between metals and the microbiota, and (e) how metal restriction and metal oversupply can kill or inhibit the growth of microbes. This chapter provides an overview of current understanding in these areas and raises a number of important open questions in need of future research.

# Introduction

Our discussions addressed the relationship between the metal status of different host niches and the capabilities of different microbes (pathogens and commensals) within these niches to compete for metals and avoid metal poisoning in determining disease outcomes. The best understood microbial systems belong to the bacteria and fungi; hence these organisms formed the basis of the discussions. Four background papers to this Forum informed and contributed greatly to our discussions: Lemire et al. (Chapter 2), Bachmann and Weiser (Chapter 3), Loutet et al. (Chapter 4), and Imlay (Chapter 5).

# Metal Availability

How do we define and determine metal availability in different environments, both within and outside microbial cells? In approaching this question, we focused primarily on intracellular metal availability and how metal-requiring proteins acquire their correct metal cofactors (Figure 7.1).

## Metal Availability outside Microbial Cells

Hosts are suspected of manipulating metal availability in ways that stymie or support the growth of pathogenic and commensal microbes. This concept is difficult to approach and evaluate, because metal availability remains poorly defined and understood. What we consider as bioavailable metal to a pathogen in the host environment may, to some extent, differ depending on the particular pathogen and the array of metal uptake systems and receptors that they possess and express; microbes frequently employ multiple uptake systems, particularly for iron (Fe), to meet their metabolic needs. In addition, the bioavailability of a particular metal within a specific niche is dependent not only on the total metal content, but also on other factors: metal speciation (including oxidation state, mineralization, and the presence of metal-binding ligands), pH, and oxygen levels. The ability of a cell to acquire a given metal may also depend on the concentration of competing metals for expressed transport systems. In terms of trying to address the metal requirements of microbes, there are difficulties in carrying out growth experiments in metal-restricted conditions. The use of chelators to restrict a single metal in microbial growth experiments can be problematic as few chelators are available that are highly specific for a particular metal, and for microbial growth experiments in complex media, alternative practical options are not yet available. A direct assay of the availability of a given metal is not easily accomplished and may be better defined by analyzing the rate at which a given organism is able to accumulate the metal.

Microbial metal-responsive transcription factors act to integrate the expression of cellular metal uptake, export, and sequestration systems with both their

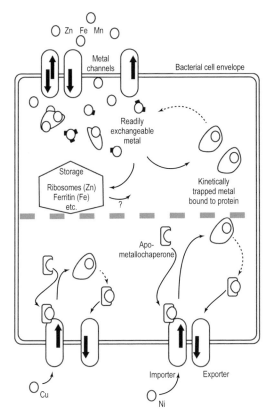

**Figure 7.1** A model for the control of metal availability inside bacteria. Metal channels function to import and export various nutritional metals (circles). These include outer membrane/cell-surface receptors, inner membrane transporters, and transporters that span the entire cell envelope. A readily exchangeable pool of metals (including zinc, iron, and manganese) is thought to exist that is bound to proteins, small metabolites, and membrane surfaces. These metals can be kinetically trapped when bound to some proteins (dashed lines). Metals can also be sequestered for storage (e.g., zinc and iron are stored in ribosomes and ferritin, respectively), which may contribute to the metal buffering capacity of the cell. The metallation status of Zn, Fe, and Mn proteins is thought to be determined by the thermodynamic equilibrium with the readily exchangeable metal pool. For copper and nickel, protein metallochaperones may circumvent thermodynamic competition by delivering cognate metals from importers to their designated proteins (both in the cytoplasm and cell envelope). Excess metal or metal released from protein turnover may also be transported by metallochaperones for efflux.

metabolic needs and environmental metal availability. Metal-sequestering proteins can store metals and allow for their controlled release in cells, whereas transmembrane metal transporters control metal ion uptake into and efflux out of microbial cells. The lack of passive permeation of metal ions across cell membranes means that the active uptake and efflux of metal ions by the transmembrane transporters ultimately determines the intracellular metal levels.

**Metal Availability inside Microbial Cells**

There is still uncertainty as to how proteins acquire the correct metals. Although we currently have tools (e.g., inductively coupled plasma mass spectrometry) that can easily measure the total metal content in microbes (see Matusch et al., this volume), it remains unclear as to what form this metal is in and to what extent it is accessible to metal-requiring proteins. The field has not yet even reached consensus on the speciation of metals in cells and how to define the metal available for binding to high-affinity protein sites in cells.

Another consideration is that metals tend to associate to metal-binding sites of proteins according to the Irving-Williams series. Hence the relative availability of different metals in a cell is likely to determine which metal species associate with a given protein. For example, the concentration and speciation of the Zn and Fe pools within a cell may be controlled to favor Fe binding to an Fe-requiring protein, even though the affinity of the protein for zinc may be higher than that for iron. Alternatively, selection could occur at a kinetic level using a specific metal shuttle (or metallochaperone), thus overcoming thermodynamic constraints. The extent of the involvement of metal shuttles in assisting proteins in acquiring their correct metal cofactors, however, remains a subject of debate.

*What Is the Nature of the Pool of Exchangeable Metal inside Cells?*

In our discussion of the possible nature of the pool of cellular metals available to bind to proteins, it was noted that within cells, metal ions are bound by both high-affinity ligands (such as metalloproteins) and low-affinity ligands (including small molecules and nonspecific binding to macromolecules). However, the field has not yet agreed upon the best way to describe the cellular concentration of metal ions "available" to bind to high-affinity ligands within proteins. Semantically, we dislike the term "free" metal, as it connotes metal bound to nothing but water (fully hydrated metal), which is unlikely to exist within cells. There was, however, general agreement that "available" metals are likely bound to metabolites and adventitious biomolecule surfaces. These metals are likely to be labile: through ligand-exchange reactions, they are accessible to the active metal-binding sites of enzymes. The term "readily exchangeable" metal was put forward as a term to reflect that the ability of metals to populate a binding site is modulated by competing ligands within the cell. Thus, the exchangeable metal pool is buffered by rapid equilibration with other ligands. The extent to which a particular metal is readily exchangeable may differ for different metals. Metals for which we have known metallochaperones (copper [Cu] and nickel [Ni]) should be considered as the least readily exchangeable, whereas manganese (Mn), zinc (Zn), and iron may be considered the most readily exchangeable.

The question then arises: Which molecules are the primary ligands for the pool of exchangeable metal? This is important for modeling metal availability in cells. It is not known if cells modulate the metal-binding capacity of this ligand pool, by increasing or decreasing the concentration of a predominant liganding metabolite, to control the amount or identities of the metals that are available to enzymes. It is likely that the ligands include free amino acids (cysteine, histidine, glutamate) and glutathione; however, they could also include functional groups on the surfaces of membranes, nucleic acids, and proteins. A further consideration is the role and buffering capacity of dedicated metal stores (such as bacterial ferritins) or, for eukaryotic fungal pathogens, vacuoles that have general metal storage capacity or specialized functions (e.g., "zincosomes"; Devirgiliis et al. 2004).

In addition to not knowing the major components of the weak ligand pool in cells, we do not know the size of this weak ligand pool. The kinetics of Zn dissociation from some proteins is faster than would be predicted from simple dissociation rate constants, suggesting that some small molecules facilitate the extraction of metals. It probably follows that these ligands speed the flow of metals between low- and high-affinity binding sites, allowing thermodynamic equilibration to be more rapidly attained. In principle, the size and nature of the weak ligand pool could influence how quickly and specifically various metals populate authentic binding sites in enzymes.

In summary, the nature of the ligands involved in such an important feature of metal homeostasis remains largely unknown. In addition, the importance of this pool of metal ions in allowing pathogens to survive under low metal conditions is still not understood. There are some methods that could be used to evaluate the exchangeable metal pools. Currently, small-molecule fluorescent probes are useful for monitoring calcium and Cu fluxes in cells (Dodani et al. 2011; Davidson and Duchen 2012); a similar approach could potentially be used to monitor other metals in cells, although the probes would need to be in thermodynamic equilibrium (this is often not true for regulators, which may kinetically trap metals). An estimate of the readily exchangeable pool of zinc in *Escherichia coli* has been made by the expression of engineered fluorescent carbonic anhydrase proteins with defined Zn affinity (Wang et al. 2012a). Such an approach might be generalized to other metal pools (e.g., iron and manganese) as well as other microbial species. Protein-based metal sensors are also useful as they can be tagged, but again, their rate of metal exchange must be considered. Another approach would be to use X-ray fluorescence microprobe (XRM) imaging (Fahrni 2007). However, this technique measures only the metal identity and amount; it does not provide information about the metal ligand. For eukaryotic cells, fluorescent ligands and XRM imaging can, however, provide information about the metal compartmentalization in organelles. For a summary of techniques available for the analysis of metals in biological samples, see Matusch et al. (this volume).

*What Are the Native Metals Bound to Enzymes,*
*and How Does One Figure This Out?*

In the published literature, there is substantial uncertainty, and even mis-identification, of the metals that populate specific enzymes. This arises from metal exchange *in vitro*. Mis-identification can lead to a failure to recognize the dependence of certain enzymes and pathways upon the availability of a certain metal. For example, native metal ions may be released from proteins upon cell lysis, followed by binding of an incorrect metal ion. This mechanism is particularly problematic for iron and manganese, which are often replaced by zinc upon cell lysis. Retention of redox sensitive metals, such as ferrous iron, by proteins can frequently be improved by cell lysis under anoxic conditions. Ideally, we would like to identify the metals bound to proteins in live cells. A potential method of doing this would be to use mass spectrometry to identify protein metalloforms *in vivo* (So et al. 2013). However, currently there is a problem of sensitivity: it is not possible to get resolution at the subcellular level, and it is difficult to obtain enough material to measure single metal-protein complexes.

*Do Metalloforms of an Enzyme Differ Depending on Circumstance?*

Some proteins actually have multiple metalloforms *in vivo*. These metalloforms are part of a response to the availability of the metals from a habitat and cellular stores. Less clear is the frequency with which a secondary metalloform actually supplies sufficient enzyme activity *in vivo*. Examples of successful Mn substitution for iron exist (Anjem and Imlay 2012); however, in other cases, full activity is met instead by the expression of a Mn-specific isozyme (Compan and Touati 1993; Cotruvo and Stubbe 2011). Similarly, zinc is capable of replacing nonredox ferrous iron, at least in some cases (and vice versa). For metalloproteins harboring structural metal sites, isozyme substitution can release a metal for general use. An example is Zn release from the substitution of ribosomal proteins (Nanamiya et al. 2004). Many metalloproteins are, however, highly metal specific; the loss of availability of the cognate metal results in loss of activity to the cell. For example, proteins with iron-sulfur (Fe-S) centers and heme are Fe specific, and a lack of iron requires adaption of metabolism. In addition to liberating iron by metal substitution, as described above, microbes may employ an Fe-sparing response that reduces the expression of pathways requiring heme or Fe-S proteins. Example pathways that are repressed are the TCA cycle and sections of the respiratory chain (Masse et al. 2005).

In addition to simply restricting microbial access to essential metals, a hostile host may be able to poison microbes by forcing protein mis-metallation. The microbial metal homeostasis adaptation mechanisms have the potential to mute the possible effect. As such, knowledge of these adaption mechanisms may point to an understanding of how a combination of host metal sequestering and supply systems can be used to control microbes.

*Do Thermodynamics of Binding Sites Control the Metallation Status?*

The metallation status of many Zn and Fe proteins is likely determined by thermodynamic equilibration with the readily exchangeable metal pools in cells. However, the metal status of some proteins likely reflects the kinetic trapping of a metal rather than its thermodynamic equilibration. The trapping of zinc in a Mn periplasmic binding protein provides one example (McDevitt et al. 2011). These differences in the exchange rates of metals may lead to differences in de-metallation behavior. For example, the loss of a metal from a habitat may lead to de-metallation of thermodynamically determined proteins (e.g., some simple Fe and Zn enzymes) by exchange with the cellular ligand pool, but not proteins with a kinetically trapped metal ion (e.g., superoxide dismutase, SOD). This also raises the prospect that the spectrum of under-metallated proteins would differ, depending on whether a protein was de-metallated during metal starvation (SOD would retain its metal) or synthesized during starvation (SOD would not have acquired its metal). It is possible that a variation in Zn affinities of native Zn proteins could constitute a prioritization system under Zn starvation that has been evolutionarily selected. In addition, differences may be seen in the Zn affinities among proteins, if a protein is able to use an alternative metal during Zn deficiency. It is not clear if all proteins are fully metallated under metal-sufficient conditions; the retention of apoenzymes may contribute to the buffering capacity of a cell and may allow the cell to respond to variations in metal content and identity.

*What Is the Involvement of Metal Shuttles (Metal Ligands and Proteins)?*

Protein metallochaperones direct metals to preferred client proteins and circumvent thermodynamic competition. At present, data indicate that nickel and copper are often delivered this way; characterized examples include Cu metallochaperones for Cu, Zn-SOD and caa3-type cytochrome oxidase, and Ni metallochaperones for hydrogenase and urease (Kaluarachchi et al. 2010; Robinson and Winge 2010; Osman et al. 2013). It was noted, though, that *Caenorhabditis elegans* delivers copper to Cu/Zn-SOD without using a metallochaperone (Jensen and Culotta 2005). There are no compelling data to say that iron, zinc, and manganese are handled by metallochaperones, and it appears likely that either there are no protein-based metallochaperones or that redundant systems exist. The role of metallochaperones in protein metallation is an important question, because it may limit the extent to which cellular metal imbalances can lead to protein mis-metallation. Where metal selectivity is dependent on the relative metal concentrations, metal imbalances will lead to mis-metallation. Nickel and copper are delivered to a relative handful of proteins, and so the evolution of a metallochaperone system that includes a receiver domain on client proteins may have been easier. Metallochaperones for iron, zinc, and manganese might also be disfavored if cells have evolved to substitute one metal for another under conditions in which the primary metal is unavailable; a strict metallochaperone system might not allow that latitude.

## Summary

Not all determinants of metal selectivity in cells are yet known. These determinants vary for each metal ion and may change depending on the nutritional environment and pathogen. Currently there are two extreme paradigms for metal selectivity (Figure 7.1). The first stipulates that a metal ion is transported into the cell and immediately transferred to a metallochaperone protein, which delivers the metal to a specific metalloprotein. Most likely, copper and nickel follow this type of pathway in many, but not all, organisms. For metal ions that activate a small number of proteins, these metallochaperone-dependent pathways likely occur. In contrast, other metal ions, such as zinc and iron, do not frequently have identified, dedicated metallochaperone proteins. The metal selectivity in cells for these ions is proposed to depend primarily on the metal affinity of the metalloprotein and the cellular "readily exchangeable" metal concentration, which is determined by both the total metal content and the buffering capacity of the cell. Metal-responsive regulators likely sense this metal pool to modulate the expression of metal homeostatic systems according to cellular needs. These systems control the readily exchangeable metal concentration. In many cases, neither the metal affinity of the proteins nor the readily exchangeable metal concentration in a cell is known, which makes estimation of the native metal ion difficult. Furthermore, the readily exchangeable metal ion concentration in the cell likely varies with metal nutrition and, possibly, cellular metabolites that function as metal buffers. We do not know whether microbes actively manage metal pool speciation to optimize the availability of the appropriate metal for macromolecular incorporation. Under changing metal loads, the metal(s) bound to metalloproteins may also vary. In some cases, the enzymes retain activity with the substituted metal ion, suggesting that this mechanism may potentially be used to address metal scarcity and metal overload. However, the importance of this mechanism during infections is not known and may vary for different microbes.

## Different Levels and Sources of Metals in Different Microbial Niches within the Host

Here we focused on the different potential metal sources available to microbes at distinct locations within the host. At the heart of this discussion was the opinion that the metal sources available to a particular pathogen will vary depending on a variety of factors, including its particular niche within the host, its route of entry, array of metal uptake and storage systems, and strategies for survival within the host.

## Diversity of Ecological Niches for Microbes in the Vertebrate Host

The vertebrate host represents a diverse array of ecological niches for colonizing microbes that vary, for example, in the level of available oxygen, nutrients, metals, metal-binding ligands, and pH. In regard to the availability of metal ions for microbes in these different sites, a primary consideration is the degree to which the availability is due to external sources versus a dependence on host-derived metal ions. For example, microbes that inhabit the gastrointestinal tract may predominantly acquire metal ions provided from the intake of food, whereas microbes that inhabit the skin or upper respiratory tract are primarily dependent on host-derived metal ions. Within the gastrointestinal tract there will also be substantial differences in the nature of the available metal ions in the food, due to the various stages of processing: exposure to acid pH in the stomach, exposure to proteases, and exposure to microbes and microbial products in the lower gut. Metal ions in the form of salts present in food (included as additives) or provided in the form of supplements are modified by the acidic environment of the stomach and influence the subsequent utilization by microbes and uptake by the host.

Although the major differences between environments in different host systems and subdivisions are fairly obvious, the degree to which various "micro-niches" might exist or be created by specific host–pathogen interactions and influence metal availability is less known. Different microbes that can colonize the same region have a different repertoire of metal ion acquisition strategies, and it is not readily apparent whether this is a reflection of inhabiting a distinct niche, accessing different compartments, or a result of microbial interactions. For instance, it is unclear why transferrin receptors are present on *Neisseria meningitidis* and a subset of the "commensal" *Neisseria* species, whereas other *Neisseria* possess a distinct and different repertoire of Fe acquisition strategies (Marri et al. 2010).

## Sources and Forms of Metal Ions in Different Niches

For niches in which the host is the primary source of metal ions, there is a paucity of information regarding the ultimate source or form of available metal ions. For instance, on the mucosal surface of the upper respiratory tract there are no well-described mechanisms for provision of metal ions to the microbes that inhabit that environment. It is generally presumed that glandular cells secrete lactoferrin onto the mucosal surface, but it is normally in the apo form; thus it will not provide a source of iron but will influence the availability and form of any iron that is present. Similarly, the secretion of lipocalin 2 (siderocalin) will capture Fe-siderophore complexes on the mucosal surface but may not represent provision of metal ions to that environment. The secretions from glandular cells contain mucins, which are rich in cysteines, and other constituents that would be capable of complexing metal ions; however, the metal ion content of the secretions has not yet been determined.

The presence of surface receptors on microbes for Fe-containing host proteins or protein complexes and the dependence of some microbial species on these receptors for survival in the host suggest that either these host proteins (transferrin, hemoglobin, hemoglobin-haptoglobin, heme-hemopexin, ferritin) are somehow transported to the mucosal surface, or that the microbes which possess these receptors are capable of accessing or residing in the submucosal space to access these Fe sources. Episodic bleeding or damage and replacement of mucosal epithelial cells are possible sources for these proteins, but whether this would maintain an adequate supply of metal ions is unclear. The recent observation that *Helicobacter pylori* modulates the activity of stomach epithelial cells to bring Fe-loaded transferrin from the submucosal surface to the epithelial surface (Tan et al. 2011) is a demonstration of how microbes could play an active role in accessing host-derived metal ions and influence the form of available metal. Clearly this is an area that requires further investigation, to determine the degree to which this type of phenomenon may impact on the availability and the form of metal ions in various niches in the host.

In the gastrointestinal tract, the form and availability of metal ions will depend substantially on dietary intake (see Ackland et al., this volume). For instance, diets rich in meat will provide a ready source of heme iron that would be a preferred source of iron for both microbes and the host alike. However, the composition of the diet can also reduce the availability of metal ions by altering the form; for example, phytates in grain-rich diets are known to inhibit the uptake of Zn ions (Lim et al. 2013). The form and availability of metal ions can be further modulated through the interplay between microbes and their host. For example, the release of the enterobactin class of siderophores by microbes to complex available ferric iron derived from the lumen of the gastrointestinal tract can be countered by the secretion of host lipocalin 2 (Flo et al. 2004).

**The Intracellular Environment**

The intracellular environment of host cells has a different spectrum of metal sources for pathogens to acquire (Figure 7.2). Furthermore, metal levels will vary between the host cell cytoplasm and the various intracellular compartments. Metal availability to intracellular microbes will depend on the lifestyle of the pathogen (e.g., extra- or intra-phagosomal) and their various strategies to propagate within the intracellular niches; for example, an ability to manipulate host cell Fe homeostasis to increase Fe availability (Cassat and Skaar 2013). The majority of the host heme and hemoproteins are intracellular. In addition, ferrous iron predominates in the cytoplasm. Still the host cell cytoplasm is

complexes (transferrin, lactoferrin, hemoglobin-haptoglobin, and heme-hemo-pexin) are host specific and have only been found in microbes that inhabit the upper respiratory tract or genitourinary tract. Pathogens which propagate within a specific niche in the host tend to have and use the transport systems that are effective within that niche. *Bordetella* use siderophore and heme uptake systems during different stages of upper respiratory tract infections, and there appears to be sequential expression of these systems based on environmental signals (Brickman and Armstrong 2009). In contrast, a study with *Yersinia enterocolitica*, which monitored transcriptional expression of the yersiniabactin system and a heme transporter, found different levels of expression in different organs (blood, liver, spleen); however, both systems seemed to be responding coordinately in these niches (Jacobi et al. 2001). In *Y. pestis,* yersiniabactin is essential in the initial lymphatic spread and/or growth in the regional lymph node following a flea bite. However, after gaining access to the bloodstream, this siderophore is irrelevant to subsequent Fe acquisition and growth. In pneumonic infections, a yersiniabactin mutant is attenuated but still lethal at higher infectious doses. However, the disease shifts from growth in the lungs and pneumonic disease to a septicemic disease (Fetherston et al. 2010; Lee-Lewis and Anderson 2010). The Yfe/Sit and Feo ferrous transporters are not critical during pneumonic infection but are important during bubonic plague. It is not clear whether two additional *Y. pestis* ferrous Fe transporters play a role in the lungs, or whether ferrous Fe sources are irrelevant in the lungs (Fetherston et al. 2012). *In vitro* studies have not shown a role for bacterial heme transporters for intracellular growth in host cells; instead some bacteria use a combination of siderophore and ferrous Fe uptake systems for intracellular Fe acquisition (Runyen-Janecky et al. 2003; Perry et al. 2007).

In contrast to Fe/heme uptake systems, identified bacterial Zn and Mn transporters show much less diversity. They primarily consist of ABC-type transporters, such as ZnuABC for zinc and SitABCD/YfeABCD for manganese, as well as the NRAMP-family Mn transporter, MntH (Hood and Skaar 2012). A number of studies with different pathogens have shown loss of virulence when the Zn or Mn transporters are disrupted, supporting the notion that the host is also limiting for these metals (Kehl-Fie and Skaar 2010). Mutation of the two known Mn transporters (Yfe and MntH) in *Y. pestis* causes a loss of virulence in the mouse model of bubonic plague but not in the pneumonic plague model (Perry et al. 2012), again suggesting that niches have different metal availabilities. The neutrophil-derived protein calprotectin (as well as other S100 family proteins), which chelates manganese and zinc, is one mechanism for withdrawing these metals from the sites of extracellular infections. It is likely that other Mn- and Zn-sequestering mechanisms also exist. Whereas most metal-chelating compounds may primarily act to sequester metals away from microbes, they also have the potential to serve as a source of metals for microbes capable of accessing the metals from them. As such, they may provide some pathogens a competitive advantage; for example. *S. enterica* serovar Typhimurium is able to utilize calprotectin-bound zinc which enables it to outcompete the gut microbiota to colonize the gut and invade (Liu et al. 2012). As a similar strategy, the pathogenic fungus *Candida albicans* secretes its own "zincophore" protein to bind and obtain zinc from the environment (Citiulo et al. 2012).

The question arises as to whether pathogens differ from commensals in having a greater capacity to compete for metals by possessing a greater array of metal uptake pathways. We concluded that there is no evidence to support this; more detailed studies need to be undertaken, including cataloguing the array of systems used by pathogens and commensals in different niches. However, assigning organisms as commensals or pathogens can also be complex. Importantly, when examining metal uptake systems in microbes, multiorganism systems should be considered, as microbes rarely exist in isolation within the host. Furthermore, the extent to which variations in the total metal content of different organ systems (e.g., between the genitourinary tract, upper respiratory tract, and gastrointestinal tract) is influenced by the composition of the microbial communities at these locations and their array of metal acquisition strategies should also be considered.

**Summary**

Whereas we accept that there are likely differences in the available sources of metals to microbes in different locations of the host, beyond the gut we largely do not know what these are: neither the metal levels nor the variety of metal-binding ligands. Direct measurements of metal availability are challenging due to limits of detection as well as difficulties in sampling the various niches, particularly for studies with humans. The use of model hosts (mammalian as well as others, such as zebrafish and *C. elegans*) offer advantages as they permit controlled studies into the effects of diet and other factors on metal sources. A potential strategy to identify and compare the various metal sources within the different host niches would be to catalog (e.g., using metagenomics) the different metal uptake systems in the microbes that naturally inhabit them, rather than focusing on pathogens that are often only in transit through these environments. Knowledge of the substrates for identified metal uptake systems may yield clues as to what is being accessed. (Meta-)transcriptomic approaches can be used to monitor the temporal (and spatial) expression of metal import and export systems; however, the question arises as to whether their expression is being driven by microbial needs or their exposure to host factors in a particular niche. It would be useful to combine knowledge of expression studies of host metal transporters with those of microbial metal-handling systems, which could also be combined with measurements of total metal levels in tissues (e.g., by laser ablation ICP-MS). It also may be useful to compare germ-free versus nongerm-free animals to gain an idea of the effect of resident microbes on metal availability.

# Effect of the Metal Status of a Pathogen, as Derived from its Prior Environment, on its Ability to Establish an Infection or the Severity of Disease

Does the previous environment of a pathogenic microbe (e.g., is it replete or deplete for certain metals) have an effect on its transmission to a host and disease outcome. In other words, can microbes be primed for entry into a host by their metal status?

## Does Preinfection Metal Exposure Impact on Infectivity and Disease Outcome?

Metal availability, whether it is in the essential or toxic range, has a strong impact on the transcriptome and the metabolism of pathogenic microbes. As microbial pathogens change from one environment to the other during dissemination, metal status is retained, at least in the short term, thereby providing a rheostatic physiological parameter of potential importance in infection. As many virulence factors and large-scale metabolic pathways are either dependent on metals for their catalytic activities and/or are under physiological control of metal-sensing systems, microbial pathogens may exhibit very different phenotypes when confronting the host, depending on previous exposure to different metal concentrations. Furthermore, the impact of this prior metal exposure may vary across the different organ systems that impose different metal stresses. Alternatively, the host's nutritional immune strategies might be, at least initially, circumvented by a sufficiently large pool of metals, or metal detoxification systems, in the microbe. This effect is further aggravated by the presence of metal storage systems, such as bacterial ferritins or fungal vacuoles. After a period of metal surplus, starvation can likely be buffered during the early stages of an infection. This seems especially true for opportunistic commensal and environmental pathogens, as they are naturally exposed to metal species and concentrations that are very different from the host. With a sufficiently large pool of metals, growth may continue for several generations in the absence of external sources due to metal partitioning to daughter cells. These few to tens of divisions may be decisive in establishing an infection, or at least in allowing survival until new sources of metals are accessed. Opportunistic commensals may thus serve as a good, biologically relevant model for studying the effect of preinfection metal levels.

An example of an environmentally derived human pathogen is the fungus *Cryptoccocus neoformans*, which in the environment can exist on the leaves of trees and grasses or in bird guano, with low- or high-metal availability, respectively (Heitman et al. 2011). In the environment, the yeast or spore form is aerosolized and rendered available for entry into the lung, the initial site of infection in humans or other mammals. Successful colonization of the lung allows *C. neoformans* to disseminate to the bloodstream and cross the blood-brain barrier, where it causes lethal meningitis, particularly in immune-compromised individuals, but also in seemingly immunocompetent subjects. Therefore, we need to consider how the ability of organisms (such as *C. neoformans* or other pathogenic microbes) to acquire metals or resist metals, at different locations in its life cycle, impacts on a successful primary infection in the lung or other primary infection site. When *C. neoformans* enters the lung during an infection, it is engulfed by alveolar macrophages, which, among other antimicrobial effectors, use Cu toxicity within the lumen of the phagosome as an antimicrobial weapon (Figure 7.2). For a leaf-derived infecting yeast form, the immediate stress arguably should be higher in this model, where the expectation is that the *C. neoformans* is somewhat Cu deficient and has not primed a Cu defense response, which in this case is strongly mediated by the Cu-inducible, Cu-sequestering metallothionein proteins (Ding et al. 2011, 2013). Successful colonization of the lung allows *C. neoformans* to escape from alveolar macrophage surveillance, disseminate to the circulation, cross the blood-brain barrier, and enter the brain where it causes lethal meningitis. In the central nervous system, *C. neoformans* produces melanin as a virulence factor, using the Cu-dependent enzyme laccase (Salas et al. 1996). This need for copper is further driven by well-characterized Cu-dependent Fe uptake permease-oxidase complexes, which serve as a major source of iron for Fe-S cluster biogenesis or as a direct catalytic cofactor for a variety of enzymes (Kronstad et al. 2013). Consequently, as an environmental opportunistic pathogen, *C. neoformans* finds itself transitioning from a Cu overload environment to an environment where Cu acquisition is essential to thrive, once again inverting the balance between external sources and metabolic need.

The acquisition of zinc by fungal and bacterial pathogens is dictated largely by high-affinity Zn importers at the plasma membrane, the transcription of which is induced under Zn deficiency and dampened by Zn satiety. In addition to the integral membrane Zn importers, starvation for zinc leads to the expression of an auxilliary Zn acquisition system, Pra1, in the fungal gastrointestinal tract commensal and pathogen *C. albicans* (Citiulo et al. 2012). Pra1 protein has roles in both Zn binding and immune modulation via direct interaction with the complement system. As zinc plays a critical role in immune competency, Pra1, which binds multiple Zn atoms, could in addition compromise immune function by sequestering zinc. As Pra1 expression is induced by Zn deficiency, Zn levels encountered by *C. albicans* prior to the transition to the pathogenic phase may therefore play a role in the early stages of systemic infection. Furthermore, as with most pathogenic microbes, when *C. albicans* experiences Fe starvation it undergoes a change in carbon metabolism, away from the heavily Fe-dependent TCA cycle and oxidative phosphorylation. Alternative pathways, such as the glyoxylate cycle in fungi, are likely to be more beneficial for survival to the antimicrobial insults in the glucose-poor environment of the phagosome during infection. In fact, *C. glabrata* depends

on xenosiderophores, produced by other fungi, to survive macrophage engulfment after being grown under conditions of low external iron, but it can become independent of siderophore-mediated Fe uptake in macrophages engineered to mimic human Fe-overload disease due to a dysfunctional Fe exporter
ferroportin (Nevitt and Thiele 2011).

In bacterial pathogens, Fe starvation is known to induce the expression of a
plethora of virulence-associated factors, such as hemolysins in *Staphylococcus
aureus* (Schmitt et al. 2012). The 50% lethal dose ($LD_{50}$) of cells prestarved
for iron is accordingly significantly lower. This poses the question of where
these effects may be seen in natural infections, and how they can be correctly
replicated in the laboratory. The precise nature of the changes likely depends
on the type of transmission and, hence, environments encountered (e.g., directly from host to host, via vectors, or entering the host from the environment
or a commensal stage). In *Y. pestis*, the pathogen is transmitted from the blood
via a flea vector to a new host. Inside the insect gut, blood is digested, with
significant changes in the concentration of available iron likely ensuing (Perry
et al. 1993).

Most infection models are based on preculture conditions in the laboratory,
which do not mimic the natural habitat or source from which the infecting
organisms may derive metals in nature. Thus far, data strongly indicate that in
addition to other factors (e.g., temperature, pH, and carbon sources), the metal
supply of precultured pathogens should be taken into account. This will lead to
infection experiments that better simulate the events in nature. As data or estimates on naturally occurring preinfection metal concentrations are not widely
available, it would be informative to test the effect of biologically relevant
metal concentrations on the outcome of laboratory infection experiments.

For pathogens that spend time in the external environment, mechanisms
must exist to allow metal transport to support basic metabolic needs for survival. This challenge may be compounded by potential requirements for elaborating degradative enzymes to liberate environmental metal sources so that the
metals are available to serve as substrates for cell-surface metal import mechanisms. The absence of these mechanisms, or of metal substrates for import,
demand the elaboration of mechanisms to mobilize metals from intracellular
stores such as bacterial ferritin or, in the case of fungal pathogens, from the lumen of vacuoles for copper, iron, or zinc via dedicated transporters. The latter
could serve as a buffer against vastly changing metal concentration, but data on
the role of these buffers (and their capacity) in infections are for the most part
still lacking. Furthermore, several mechanisms are feasible for the pathogen to
avoid other detrimental effects of differing pre- and peri-infection metal concentrations. With respect to metal toxicity, ligand-inactivated transporters may
help in avoiding metal overload after a switch from relative starvation to metal
surplus. The notion is that metal concentrations in microbial populations are
generally Gaussian-distributed and may allow subpopulations with appropriate
metal homeostasis mechanisms to cope with their previous environment. They

may, therefore, achieve "correct" metal concentrations, which allow them to progress more easily with a productive infection.

To determine the nature and effect of the influence of previous metal exposure on infections, several experimental approaches are likely to be informative. For example, *in vivo* competition experiments with deletion or transposon mutant libraries of pathogens grown under different, defined metal preconditions could help to determine the necessary genetic setup that is pivotal to the outcome of the initial infection. The actual metal status of microbes re-isolated from the host after infection could be investigated; in combination with different preculture metal levels, this would give insight into whether or not high (or low) metal levels in the pathogen are kept within the host, so as to provide a selective advantage for growth and dissemination in the host during infection.

## Summary

The ability to acquire or resist metals in a previous environment likely sets the stage for determining, to a significant extent, the fitness of a microbial pathogen for dissemination to additional tissues for virulence. Consequently, understanding the environments from which microbial pathogens are derived is an underappreciated, yet important area for investigation. Moreover, for microbial pathogens that possess multiple systems for metal acquisition, such as the use of ferrous Fe importers and siderophore-mediated Fe uptake, the selection of which mechanisms are used in specific environments likely provide a mechanism for optimally positioning a pathogen for initiating successful colonization of host tissues. Clearly the metal levels of the infecting pathogen influence the expression of many genes, including known virulence factors. However, in laboratory infection experiments, metal levels are not controlled for normally. They may not be simulative of the environment from which the pathogen normally derives (e.g., gut, skin, vector), or they may have little relevance to the levels encountered by the pathogen prior to the initial host infection event. Biological relevance of these experiments may therefore be limited in this respect. In addition, for different pathogens, the metal concentrations that precede infection, as well as their metal status, constitute an area for further investigation. With this information in hand, one could then consider if changes (within biologically relevant ranges) in specific prior metal exposure levels influence the course and/or outcome of an infection. Would different prior exposure levels alter the ability of pathogens to cope with severe changes in metal levels during the initial stages of infection, such as those occurring during an inflammatory response? Are these changes "predicted" by other external cues before the infection? Does prior metal exposure generally serve as a signal in itself for induction of metal-independent virulence factors?

## The Interplay between Metals and the Microbiota

Here we focused primarily on the influence of the microbiota composition on metal availability in different body environments and vice versa. Related topics were also discussed in other groups, with some degree of overlap (see Rehder et al., Ackland et al., and Maret et al., this volume). The complexity of the different microbial communities that exist at different anatomical sites within the body has been highlighted by The Human Microbiome project, supported by the U.S. National Institutes of Health Common Fund (NIH HMP Working Group 2009).

### Metals and the Microbiota

Evidence that a host's microbiota can contribute to human physiology and immune status has been generated from a range of studies. With regard to metals and the microbiota, future research should be aimed at examining (a) whether the microbiota influences the bioavailability of dietary metals and (b) whether dietary or environmental intake of metals influences the structure and function of the microbiota (see Ackland et al., this volume).

Some early work addressed the influence of the microbiota on tissue Fe distribution using germ-free mice (Donati et al. 1969). Thus, the above questions need to be revisited with state of the art sequencing, which provides rich analysis and definition of complex communities, along with new knowledge about how the microbiota influences development of the immune system (Arrieta and Finlay 2012), and susceptibility to colonization by pathogens (Buffie and Pamer 2013). Initial goals should be to discern correlations between the microbiota content and metal availability in the host and, *more importantly*, to determine the underlying mechanisms and consequences of those correlations. It is vital to get beyond simply counting numbers and extend any findings to uncover mechanisms that relate to the microbiota. This would likely include investigations into the meta-transcriptomics and metabolic output of these complex communities in relation to metal homeostasis.

There are already studies that show specific effects of metals in modulating microbial communities and the role of the host in the competition for these micronutrients. For example, the expression of a high-affinity ABC transporter for Zn uptake by *Campylobacter jejuni* is required for its survival in chicken intestines in the presence of normal microbiota, but not when chickens are reared under germ-free conditions with a more restricted microbiota (Gielda and DiRita 2012). The ability to survive was associated with the presence of numerous Zn-binding proteins in the intestines of conventional chicks, which were absent from limited-microbiota chicks. This study demonstrates that the microbiota in the gastrointestinal tract stimulates a reduction in Zn availability and, as such, restricts the growth of bacteria that lack the ability to compete using high-affinity transporters. In this regard, human polymorphisms in Zip4 affect Zn uptake in the small bowel (Lichten and Cousins 2009), but whether or not this is exacerbated or otherwise influenced by the microbiota is unclear. A comprehensive picture of how host and microbial factors in the gut affect metal dynamics in the host is lacking (NIH HMP Working Group 2009). Given the significance of the upper intestine on metal uptake in the body, research on how the microbiota might contribute to this process should focus on the small bowel inhabitants, without ignoring those of the colon and even feces, where much microbiota work related to pathogenesis of infection has been focused.

The influence of any correlations that are discovered on the susceptibility to, or outcome of, infection should be assessed in human populations and model systems to ensure that both clinical correlations and underlying mechanisms are addressed. The burden of metal deficiencies in particular populations (e.g., Zn deficiencies in Pakistan and elsewhere) is a well-recognized issue (Akhtar 2013; Bhutta et al. 2013), and these populations would serve logically as the basis for human-centered research on any correlations with the microbiota. Laboratory models such as the mouse or zebrafish will ultimately be important for understanding basic mechanisms of how diet and microbiota interact. Veterinary research on growth-promoting use of Zn oxide includes, for example, investigations into its effects on stimulating beneficial microbes within the pig ileum (Vahjen et al. 2011). Whether or not this correlates to changes in susceptibility to infection has yet to be determined, but such research might provide data for hypotheses to test in human populations.

Some skin pathologies arise from metal deficiencies (Ackland and Michalczyk 2006), and Zn replacement in otherwise deficient populations has had rapid therapeutic effect on respiratory symptoms, in addition to diarrheal symptoms (Prasad 2013). Thus, research into relationships between the microbiota and metal homeostasis, and their potential effects on infectious disease, should also consider the skin and respiratory microbiota in addition to gut microbiota. It is likely that metal acquisition and utilization by these communities relies on access to host sources, whereas the microbes in the gut could additionally obtain these micronutrients directly from the diet.

A further consideration is the status of the colonized host surface. Inflammatory states will affect the availability of metals, the influx of host defense factors that are dependent on metals, and the composition of the microbiota and metal utilization by these populations. In general, acquisition of metals has been studied in pathogens, or opportunistic pathogens, which are adept at handling the inflammatory states they encounter in the host during disease. Our understanding of metal dynamics in organisms in a strict commensal relationship with their host, and especially complex communities of commensal organisms, is far less complete. Based on estimates of the size and complexity of the microbiota, this population has the potential to act as a significant reservoir/requirement for total metal species associated with a host.

Microbial systems for sensing and acquiring iron, zinc, and manganese appear to be highly conserved. Transcriptome and integrative metagenome and metabolome studies of the microbiota are therefore likely to be informative about whether a host environment is metal replete or deplete.

## Summary

Metals appear to affect the size and composition of the microbiota. There is a growing appreciation for how alterations in the microbiota affect various infectious and noninfectious disease states. As these studies define specific microbial species and factors that impact disease, it will be important to define the role of metals in influencing these effects of the microbiota.

# How Metal Restriction and Oversupply Can Kill or Inhibit the Growth of Microbes

What are the mechanisms by which exposure of microbes to metal excess or metal deficiency can inhibit microbial growth or cause death? When considering this question, we need to keep in mind that excess of one metal may also induce deficiency of a different metal. Hence the interplay between different metals is important.

## How Do Metals Poison Microbial Cells?

In our discussions of the effects of metal restriction and metal oversupply, we considered the effects on a model organism, *E. coli*, so as to lay out the type of information that allows one to focus on this topic.

### The Effects of Metal Restriction

*E. coli* growth fails upon Fe restriction due to loss of heme and Fe-S cluster synthesis. Manganese is used only as a substitute for iron when the latter is unavailable; thus Mn restriction is consequential only in that circumstance. Zinc is much more broadly used, yet restriction has been difficult to study due to trace Zn contamination of culture systems. Copper activates very few enzymes, and these are useful but dispensable (at least in artificial culture); thus restriction is relatively benign. However, it is possible that in certain environments these enzymes become critical; examples are Cu/Zn-SOD to protect against high extracellular reactive oxygen species (Craig and Slauch 2009). In contrast to *E. coli*, other bacteria may rely more heavily on manganese (e.g., *Bradyrhizobium japonicum*; Hohle and O'Brian 2012) and/or less on iron (e.g., *Borrelia burgdorferi*; Posey and Gherardini 2000). Collectively, the impact of metal restriction likely varies from organism to organism, according to how (or if) the organism uses a particular metal. For an individual organism, this may also depend on its immediate environment.

*How an Overabundance of Intracellular Metals Impedes Cell Growth*

Excess iron leads to Fenton chemistry that generates hydroxyl radicals; its major effect is to accelerate mutagenesis. The level of damage, however, does not rise to the point of growth inhibition, let alone death. In *E. coli*, excess manganese blocks heme synthesis by competitively inhibiting ferrochelatase. Since the requirement for heme arises from its use in cytochrome oxidase, Mn overloading blocks growth under oxic, but not anoxic, conditions. Iron can be outcompeted by excess zinc in Fe-using nonredox enzymes. Copper poisons solvent-exposed Fe-S clusters. Additional mechanisms may also exist but have not been elaborated. The targets in *E. coli* are, however, not universal: lactic acid bacteria, for example, lack both heme and Fe-S clusters and are therefore resistant to manganese and possibly copper. Thus, some metals damage narrow subclasses of enzymes, and organisms which lack these may prove substantially resistant. More research needs to be done to understand the mechanisms of metal intoxication of various pathogens. Although *E. coli* has provided invaluable information, it is not a universal model.

*The Effect of Metal Import and Export Systems*

It is notable that genetic mutations in metal import and export systems are often needed to establish metal restriction and metal overloading. Both metal restriction and overloading are common experiences for many microbes. Many biological habitats are metal limited. Conversely, when a metal-limited bacterium moves from a metal-poor habitat to a metal-rich environment, the cytoplasmic metal levels are likely to overshoot, because the extant import systems are not allosterically controlled. This is quickly corrected by the induced synthesis of export pumps, some of which are encoded by plasmids that enable growth in metal-rich habitats (Gutierrez-Barranquero et al. 2013) simultaneously with the repression of import pumps. Transient overshooting is not a problem for the microbe, since the poisoning mechanisms are readily reversed when metal levels fall. Inhibition of heme synthesis and of Fe enzymes is relieved when manganese and zinc dissociate from the enzymes that they are inhibiting; as Cu levels decline, the damaged Fe-S clusters are repaired. Thus, for overloading to have an important effect on bacterial populations, the metal stress would have to be persistent and of a severity that cannot be corrected by homeostatic responses.

Metal importers with surface-exposed metal-binding ligands may be more vulnerable to metal poisoning than cytoplasmic enzymes. The cytoplasm has an abundance of low molecular weight metabolites, such as cysteine, that continuously facilitate the extraction of incorrect metals from inhibited enzymes. However, such compounds are less likely to be present in the periplasm or the extracellular environment to provide similar protection to extra-cytoplasmic metal-binding sites. Thus, for example, the inhibition of a Mn importer by zinc may not easily be reversed; irreversible inhibition of the *Streptococcus pneumoniae* ABC-type Mn importer by Zn binding has recently been reported (Counago et al. 2013). The impact of fluctuations in the bioavailability of one metal can also depend on a second metal, if both are able to perform equivalent functions. For example, because Mn import can correct for Fe deficiency, the absence of both metals can be synergistic. Conversely, since excess zinc competes for the Fe sites of enzymes, excess zinc can exacerbate Fe deficiency.

*Exposure to Metal Surfaces*

Solid metallic copper, Cu(0), or silver is able to kill many/most microbes rapidly through surface contact. This property has been exploited in the design of antimicrobial surfaces (e.g., door handles, Cu pipes, incubator linings, catheters), which reduce the incidence of nosocomial infection. The effect seems dissimilar to what solubilized copper can achieve, but the underlying molecular mechanism of metallic Cu toxicity is currently unknown.

*Nonnutritional Metals*

Nonnutritional metals have been used to treat microbial infection. In the preantibiotic era, toxic compounds such as mercurials and arsenicals were used to treat infections such as syphilis. More recently, silver has been exploited for its antimicrobial properties, for example, in wound dressings (Mijnendonckx et al. 2013). Gallium has also been explored as an antibacterial agent, with some success demonstrated in treating *Pseudomonas aeruginosa* lung infections (Halwani et al. 2008). Metallotherapeutic agents are now being explored to treat parasitic infections, including using ruthenium, rhodium, and gold derivatives of chloroquine as antimalarials (Navarro and Visbal, this volume). However, the antimicrobial effects of these metals are largely unknown.

**Summary**

Since the effects of metals are directed toward the activities of enzymes, metal availability has the greatest impact on growing organisms that must maintain high metabolic fluxes. Actively growing organisms are more sensitive to iron, which can catalyze Fenton chemistry on hydrogen peroxide, a by-product of metabolism. Static biofilms, for example, are less likely to be affected. It appears that the vulnerability of microbes to both metal limitation and metal toxicity is exploited as part of the host's antimicrobial arsenal. Whereas the effects of metal overloading and underloading are usually bacteriostatic, in a host this might be good enough, since nongrowing organisms can then be cleared by the host's immune defenses. For some metals, such as arsenic, the toxic effects are still unknown, and further research is needed to understand these mechanisms.

Knowledge of how metals kill cells can be used to design more optimal metal-based antimicrobial treatments.

## Acknowledgments

We would like to thank the members of the other discussion groups for their contributions to the discussions and writing of this report.

# Host–Microbe Interactions: The Host Perspective

# 8

# Metal Homeostasis during Development, Maturation, and Aging

## Impact on Infectious Diseases

Inga Wessels

### Abstract

This chapter provides a summary of the functions of essential metallic elements in human metabolism and during infectious diseases as well as their homeostasis during development, maturation, and aging. A list of food sources as well as information on the effects of deficiency and excess is provided for each metallic element. As concentrations of metallic contaminants in the environment rise, brief characterizations of nonessential but biologically relevant metallic environmental contaminants have been added. Cases of under-, mal- and overnutrition are increasing worldwide. In combination with decreased nutritional food values, this creates a growing threat for human health, affecting societal and health systems. Potential ways of approaching this problem are suggested and discussed.

## Introduction

Metals enter the environment through natural and anthropogenic means. Sources include natural weathering of Earth's crust, mining, soil erosion, industrial discharge, urban runoff, sewage effluents, pest or disease control agents applied to plants, air pollution fallout, and others. A number of metals are essential for human health, affecting different aspects of human metabolism (Appendix 8.1): cobalt (Co), copper (Cu), iron (Fe), molybdenum (Mo), manganese (Mn), selenium (Se), and zinc (Zn). Deficiency as well as excessive intake can cause severe side effects throughout life, especially during fetal development (Appendix 8.1). Therefore, metal homeostasis is tightly regulated

*I. Wessels*

in the human body. The essentiality of arsenic (As), chromium (Cr), nickel (Ni), and vanadium (V) for human health has been suggested but remains to be proven. Aluminum (Al), cadmium (Cd), and mercury (Hg) do not show any beneficial effect on human health (Vieira et al. 2011) and are generally considered toxic to humans and animals; the adverse human health effects associated with exposure to these metals, even at low concentrations, are diverse and include, but are not limited to, neurotoxic and carcinogenic actions (Castro-Gonzalez and Mendez-Armenta 2008; Jomova and Valko 2011; Tokar et al. 2011; Appendix 8.1).

A well-balanced diet provides sufficient amounts of each element to meet the recommended dietary allowance (RDA) for a healthy person (Table 8.1). Risk groups including neonates, children, and pregnant women; athletes and the elderly may have different needs, which can be met by changing to a special

**Table 8.1** Recommended dietary allowance (RDA) and adequate intakes (*) for essential metallic elements, adapted from the dietary reference intake (DRI) reports (www.nap.edu). RDA for chromium (**) may need adjustment, as recent literature suggests lower values (Vincent 2010). Sources: Panel on Dietary Antioxidants and Related Compounds et al. (2000); Panel on Micronutrients et al. (2001).

| Element | Age (years) | Fe (mg) | Zn (µg) | S (µg) | Cu (µg) | Mn (mg) | Cr** (µg) |
|---|---|---|---|---|---|---|---|
| Infants | 0–0.5* | 6 | 2 | 15 | 200 | 0.003 | 0.2 |
| | 0.5–1 | 11 | 3 | 20 | 220 | 0.6 | 5.5 |
| Children | 1–3 | 7 | 3 | 20 | 340 | 1.2 | 11 |
| | 4–6 | 10 | 5 | 25 | 440 | 1.5 | 13 |
| | 7–10 | 8 | 7 | 30 | 550 | 1.7 | 15 |
| Male | 11–14 | 11 | 8 | 40 | 700 | 1.9 | 25 |
| | 15–18 | 11 | 11 | 55 | 890 | 2.2 | 35 |
| | 19–24 | 8 | 11 | 70 | 900 | 2.3 | 35 |
| | 25–50 | 8 | 11 | 70 | 900 | 2.3 | 35 |
| | 50+ | 8 | 11 | 55 | 900 | 2.3 | 30 |
| Female | 11–14 | 15 | 8 | 40 | 700 | 1.6 | 21 |
| | 15–18 | 15 | 9 | 55 | 890 | 1.6 | 24 |
| | 19–24 | 15 | 8 | 55 | 900 | 1.8 | 25 |
| | 25–50 | 18 | 8 | 55 | 900 | 1.8 | 25 |
| | 50+ | 10 | 8 | 55 | 900 | 1.8 | 20 |
| Pregnant | | 27 | 12 | 60 | 1000 | 2.0 | 29 |
| Nursing | 14–18 | 10 | 13 | 75 | 1300 | 2.6 | 44 |
| | 19–50 | 9 | 12 | 70 | 1300 | 2.6 | 45 |

diet or through the use of supplements. A well-balanced diet may not always be easily accessible. One reason is an overall lack of food in developing countries. Moreover, the nutritional value of food is generally declining due to extensive processing and considerable use of chemical fertilizers, insecticides, and pesticides. The decreasing quality of our food creates an increased need to inform the general public on how to achieve a healthy diet so as to avoid sickness and disease. In addition to the general public, medical practitioners also need to be aware of metal deficiencies and toxicities so that they are able to understand disease symptoms and identify the appropriate diagnosis and treatment.

To provide accurate information, a detailed understanding of the homeostasis of metals in the human body during development, maturation, and aging is necessary. This chapter summarizes recent literature on metal homeostasis for essential metals as well as those thought to be necessary for human metabolism. A brief overview of nonessential metals that are most harmful to human health is also included.

## Essential Metallic Elements

### Cobalt

Cobalt is a metallic element with limited function in higher eukaryotes. The only known function that it has is as a component of vitamin B12, which is incorporated into three classes of enzymes: isomerases, methyl transferases, and reductive dehalogenases. These enzymes participate in reactions essential to DNA synthesis, fatty acid synthesis, and energy production, among other biological processes (Banerjee and Ragsdale 2003; Appendix 8.1).

Cobalt is accumulated primarily in the liver, kidney, pancreas, and heart, with the relative content in skeleton and skeletal muscle increasing with time after Co administration. In serum, cobalt ($Co^{2+}$) binds to albumin, and the concentration of free, ionized $Co^{2+}$ is estimated at 5–12% of the total Co concentration (Simonsen et al. 2012). Cobalt is acutely toxic in larger doses, and cumulative, long-term exposure (even at a low level) can give rise to adverse health effects related to various organs and tissues (see reviews by Barceloux 1999; Lauwerys and Lison 1994). Recent concern has been raised in terms of possible systemic health effects that result from elevated blood Co concentrations in patients with Co-containing hip implants (Paustenbach et al. 2014). Adverse effects may impact the thyroid gland (inhibition of tyrosine iodinase, goiter, and myxedema), lungs (asthma, hard-metal disease), skin (allergic contact dermatitis), and the immune system (Sauni et al. 2010). Cobalt metal and salts are also genotoxic; this is primarily caused by oxidative DNA damage through reactive oxygen species, perhaps combined with inhibition of DNA repair. Of note, evidence for carcinogenicity of Co metal and Co sulfate is considered sufficient in experimental animals but is not yet considered adequate in humans. Interestingly, some of the toxic effects of cobalt have recently been connected to disturbances of calcium metabolism. More research is needed to increase understanding of the mechanisms that lead to the strong toxicity of cobalt in humans.

## Copper

Copper plays a critical role in human metabolism as a cofactor for several cupric enzymes, including cytochrome *c* oxidase, lysyl oxidase, tyrosinase, Cu/Zn superoxide dismutase (SOD), and ferroxidases (Pena et al. 1999; Prohaska and Gybina 2004; Shim and Harris 2003; Appendix 8.1). Copper is especially important for adequate uptake of iron by the body as well as for a functioning redox system (Cabrera et al. 2008; Appendix 8.1).

Copper is a potentially toxic metal because of its role in the redox cycle and in supporting Fenton chemistry, which leads to the production of free radicals (Halliwell and Gutteridge 1984). Therefore, Cu homeostasis is tightly regulated. After being absorbed in the intestine, copper is exported from enterocytes into the bloodstream (Hamza et al. 2003; Nyasae et al. 2007). Membrane transporters for copper include CTR1, DMT1, and the Cu "pumps" ATP7A and ATP7B. Liver ATP7B is particularly important in helping mammals, such as rats and humans, eliminate excess copper efficiently in bile in a relatively non-reabsorbable form. In plasma, copper is primarily transported by ceruloplasmin and albumin (Cabrera et al. 2008). Defects in ATP7A (Menkes disease) or ATP7B (Wilson disease) cause Cu accumulation in organs (liver) and result in severe embryonic malformation or are lethal to embryos (Kambe et al. 2008).

Dietary Cu deficiency during embryonic development can be teratogenic and embryotoxic. Mouse embryos with swollen hind brains and offspring with severe neurological impairment and organogenesis defects in multiple tissues (severe connective tissue abnormalities, skeletal defects, lung abnormalities, etc.) have been observed in the offspring of Cu-deficient dams (Keen et al. 1998). The extent and timing of Cu deficiency dictate the severity and tissue specificity of the effects on the embryo, fetus, and newborn. Proper transfer of copper from the mother to the developing embryo and neonate is of critical importance, if neurological abnormalities and growth retardation are to be avoided (Kambe et al. 2008).

Aging has not been associated with significant changes in the requirement for copper, suggesting that Cu metabolism is robust throughout life. Even hospitalized elderly have not show an increased demand for copper, in contrast to Zn levels, which drop significantly and need to be corrected (Belbraouet et al. 2007).

Measurement of Cu status in humans is difficult. Moreover, many factors (e.g., zinc, carbohydrates, and vitamin C intake) affect Cu bioavailability, thus making it hard to establish a requirement for copper (Table 8.1).

# Iron

Iron is the most abundant transition metal in the human body: approximately 4–5 g are present in a normal human adult (weight of 70 kg). The importance of well-defined amounts of iron for the survival, growth, replication, and differentiation in humans is well established. Iron is an essential component of proteins involved in oxygen transport (Andrews 1999; Appendix 8.1). A deficiency of iron limits oxygen delivery to cells, resulting in fatigue, poor work performance, and decreased immunity (Panel on Micronutrients et al. 2001). Conversely, excess iron can result in toxicity and even death (Corbett 1995).

There are two forms of dietary iron: heme (Fe bound to heme proteins) and nonheme. Sources of nonheme iron are plant foods, such as lentils and beans (Hurrell 1997). Heme iron can be found in animal foods, such as red meats, fish, and poultry, and is absorbed better than nonheme iron. For humans, heme iron, which is derived from hemoglobin in red blood cells, is of great importance as it delivers oxygen to cells.

Iron is mainly absorbed via a transporter protein: the DMT1, which facilitates uptake of other trace metals, with both positive (Mn, Cu, Co, Zn) and negative (Cd, lead) effects. Within the enterocyte, iron is released via ferroportin into the bloodstream where it is then bound by the transport glycoprotein (or transferrin). Approximately 0.1% of the total body iron circulates in bound form to transferrin. Most absorbed iron is utilized in bone marrow for erythropoiesis. About 10–20% of absorbed iron goes into a storage pool in cells of the mononuclear phagocyte system, particularly fixed macrophages, and is recycled into erythropoiesis. This provides a balance between the storage and use of iron in the body.

Iron absorption is regulated by dietary and storage mechanisms. If stores are full, hepcidin is released from the liver, causing enterocytes to retain absorbed iron. A drop in body iron diminishes hepcidin, resulting in release of absorbed iron into circulation by the intestinal mucosa. Diet composition may also influence Fe absorption. Citrate and ascorbate can form complexes with iron that increase absorption, whereas tannates (tea), calcium, polyphenols, and phytates (legumes, whole grains) can decrease absorption (Panel on Micronutrients 2001; Hunt et al. 1994; Samman et al. 2001). Greater Fe utilization during growth in childhood, elevated Fe loss through minor hemorrhages or menstruation in women, as well as a greater need for iron during pregnancy can increase the efficiency of dietary Fe absorption to 20% (Allen 2002; Cogswell et al. 2003; see also Table 8.1).

Iron deficiency is the most frequent nutritional problem in the world, affecting 24% of the global population: approximately 4–10% in developed countries, rising dramatically to about 40% in developing countries (Baran 2004). Pregnant women, women with heavy menstrual losses, preterm and low birth weight infants, older infants and toddlers, teenage girls, and people with chronic infections, inflammatory, or malignant disorders (e.g., arthritis and cancer) are at greatest risk of developing Fe-deficiency anemia because they have the greatest loss or need for iron (Allen 2002; Cogswell et al. 2003; see also Table 8.1). Signs of Fe-deficiency anemia include fatigue, weakness, decreased work and school performance, slow cognitive and social development during childhood, difficulty maintaining body temperature, and decreased immune function. The latter increases the susceptibility to infections, such as glossitis or an inflamed tongue (Appendix 8.1; Allen 2002; Panel on Micronutrients et al. 2001). Aging has been widely documented to be associated with dyshomeostasis of Fe metabolism and regulation in both rodents and humans. This process adversely affects muscle strength, physical performance, cognition, and longevity. Underlying mechanisms remain to be clarified. Iron-related disorders include Alzheimer disease, Parkinson disease, Friedreich's ataxia, and retinal disease. Despite the prevalence and adverse health effects associated with these disorders, the mechanisms are still not well defined and many questions remain to be answered (reviewed in Xu et al. 2012).

Considerable potential exists for Fe toxicity because very little iron is excreted from the body. Excessive iron can accumulate acutely or chronically in tissues and organs. Acute Fe poisoning is mainly seen in children. Toxicity-producing gastrointestinal symptoms, including vomiting and diarrhea, occur with ingestion of 20 mg of elemental iron per kg of body weight. If ca. 60 mg per kg body weight are ingested, systemic toxicity occurs. Early signs of Fe poisoning (within six hours after ingestion) include vomiting, diarrhea, fever, hyperglycemia, and leukocytosis. Later signs include hypotension, metabolic acidosis, lethargy, seizures, organ damage, and coma (Madiwale and Liebelt 2006).

Hereditary hemochromatosis (HHC), due to mutations in the *HFE* gene, is an example of an autosomal recessive disorder of Fe metabolism. For Caucasian populations in Northern Europe, incidence of HHC is between 1:200 and 1:500. Persons with HHC absorb dietary iron at two to three times the normal rate. Iron deposits in many organs and affects their function, presumably by direct toxic effect. The major affected organs are the liver (cirrhosis), heart (cardiomyopathy), pancreas (diabetes mellitus), skin (pigmentation), joints (polyarthropathy), and gonads (hypogonadotrophic, hypogonadism). However, in the absence of a family history or genetic testing, HHC would not be suspected. Therapeutic phlebotomy to remove excess iron is used as treatment. The most common causes of death in individuals with HHC are hepatocellular carcinoma associated with cirrhosis, hepatic failure, and cardiac failure (Crownover and Covey 2013).

## Manganese

Manganese was first found as a constituent of animal tissues in 1913, although a state of Mn deficiency was not described until 1931. Its oxidation state ranges between $-3$ and $+7$. Over time $Mn^{2+}$ (the only form absorbed by humans) is oxidized to $Mn^{3+}$ (the oxidative state) in plasma. The human body contains approximately 10–20 mg of manganese: 25–40% is present in bone whereas 5–8 mg is turned over on a daily basis. Manganese is essential as a cofactor for the metalloenzymes SOD, xanthine oxidase, arginase, galactosyltransferase, and pyruvate carboxylase (Buchman 2012).

Under normal circumstances, dietary manganese is the main route of exposure for most people; however, water and atmospheric contamination can also be an exposure route (Wood 2009). Homeostasis is achieved by the tightly controlled regulation of Mn absorption in the intestine and the inducible biliary excretion of manganese (Yoon et al. 2011). Dietary manganese is absorbed by a diffusion mechanism as well as a transport mechanism, both of which are rapidly saturable. Approximately 6–16% of dietary manganese is absorbed (Buchman 2012); absorption decreases in the presence of a large calcium load. After absorption into the portal circulation, manganese remains either free or bound, preferably to transferrin, 2-macroglobulin, and albumin. All three are rapidly taken up, primarily by the liver but also by the pancreas and kidney. Metabolically active tissues with high numbers of mitochondria and pigmented structures appear to have the greatest concentrations of manganese. Excretion occurs primarily through the bile and, as such, nearly all manganese is excreted in the feces (Buchman 2012).

Despite its essentiality, excessive Mn levels are toxic to the central nervous system. Manganese has been identified as an occupational health hazard for miners, battery manufacturers, and automotive repair workers. Pathological Mn concentrations lead to a neurological disorder, called manganism, which is characterized by early psychotic symptoms, frequently followed by chronic symptoms similar to Parkinson disease (Sidoryk-Wegrzynowicz et al. 2009).

Manganese is essential for proper fetal development and other important aspects of metabolism (Yoon et al. 2011). The findings of two recent studies (see Wood 2009) indicate that lower maternal blood manganese is associated with fetal intrauterine growth retardation, lower birth weight, and higher neonatal morbidity and mortality. Additional basic studies of maternal and fetal Mn physiology are needed.

In experimental animals, Mn deficiency is associated with impaired growth, skeletal defects, reduced reproductive function, abnormal glucose metabolism, and altered lipid and carbohydrate metabolism, whereas excess manganese can induce adverse neurological, reproductive, and respiratory effects (Wood 2009). In the elderly, it has been reported that Mn deposits in the basal ganglia, especially the globus pallidus, and excessive levels of this metal can induce symptoms similar to Parkinson disease (Sidoryk-Wegrzynowicz et al. 2009). In addition, the progression of cognitive decline among the elderly in this study has been associated with increased levels of copper and manganese (Ghazali et al. 2013).

## Molybdenum

Molybdenum was recognized as essential for human xanthine oxidase activity in 1953 and for sulfite oxidase activity in 1971. The concentration of molybdenum in foods reflects levels in the soil and irrigation water in which they were grown. Rich sources include legumes, grains, and nuts. Lower amounts are found in animals, fruits, and vegetables (Eckhert 2012; Appendix 8.1).

Molybdenum is rapidly absorbed and excreted from the kidney, with retention regulated primarily by urinary excretion. Physiologically relevant oxidation states for molybdenum are between +4 and +6. Molybdenum accumulates as the molybdopterin cofactor in the liver, kidney, adrenal gland, and bone at concentrations that range from 0.1 to 1 mg/g wet weight (Eckhert 2012).

Molybdenum serves an essential role in the nitrogen cycle: it is a cofactor of molybdoenzymes which are involved in nitrogen fixation and nitrate reductase, an enzyme required for the conversion of nitrate to ammonia. Another important Mo function in mammalian systems is the transfer of oxygen to a two-electron substrate using one-electron-transferring compounds, such as flavin adenine dinucleotide. Three mammalian hydroxylases are molybdoenzymes (Mendel and Bittner 2006): mitochondrial sulfite oxidase, xanthine oxidase, and aldehyde oxidase.

Molybdenum toxicity has been induced in rats where it was shown to cause renal insufficiency. In rabbits, it induced weight loss and histopathologic changes in the kidney and liver (Eckhert 2012). In humans, a case of Mo toxicity may have occurred in 1961, causing gout-like symptoms and abnormalities of the gastrointestinal tract, liver, and kidneys (Eckhert 2012).

Genetic and nutritional deficiencies of molybdenum have been reported but are rare. Genetic sulfite oxidase deficiency was described, for example, by Irreverre et al. (1967). It resulted from the inability to form the Mo coenzyme despite the presence of adequate molybdenum. The deficiency caused intellectual disability, seizures, opisthotonus, and lens dislocation (Bayram et al. 2013). Molybdenum deficiency resulting in sulfite toxicity occurred in a patient who was receiving long-term total parenteral nutrition. Symptoms were tachycardia, tachypnea, headache, nausea, vomiting, and coma. Laboratory tests showed high levels of sulfite and xanthine and low levels of sulfate and uric acid in the blood and urine. Administered intravenously, daily doses of 300 µg of ammonium molybdate IV caused dramatic recovery (Eckhert 2012).

## Selenium

Selenium is an essential micronutrient and exists in two forms: inorganic (selenate and selenite) and organic (selenomethionine and selenocysteine). Both have dietary sources. Selenium functions through selenoproteins and plays critical roles in reproduction, thyroid hormone metabolism, DNA synthesis, and protection from oxidative damage and infection (Hill et al. 2012; Sunda

2012; Appendix 8.1). Some tissues (e.g., testis, kidney, and bone marrow) synthesize selenoproteins for export and thus have greater requirements for selenium than other tissues.

Intestinal absorption of selenium is not regulated; in plasma, selenium is mostly bound and transported by Se-binding protein 1. In addition, the Se content of the body is regulated by hepatic production of methylated Se compounds, which are excreted predominantly into the urine (Kobayashi et al. 2002).

Skeletal muscle is the major site of Se storage, accounting for approximately 28–46% of the total Se pool (Sunda 2012). Recent changes in the Se metabolism can be analyzed via blood or urine samples; hair or nails provide good sources for long-term tests. The brain must have a reliable supply of selenium to be viable and exhibits high priority over the body's Se supply and retention under conditions of dietary Se deficiency (Steinbrenner and Sies 2013).

Selenium deficiency produces biochemical changes that might predispose people under additional stresses to develop certain illnesses or heart failure (Kucharzewski et al. 2002; Saliba et al. 2010; Appendix 8.1). It is also associated with male infertility and might play a role in Kashin-Beck disease, a type of osteoarthritis occurring in certain low Se areas of China, Tibet, and Siberia (Sunda 2012). Iodine deficiency may be exacerbated by Se deficiency, potentially increasing the risk of cretinism in infants (Sunda 2012). Risks for Se deficiency include populations living in Se-deficient regions, dialysis patients, and individuals with HIV. In preterm babies, low selenium is associated with an increased risk of complications, such as chronic neonatal lung disease and retinopathy of prematurity (Iranpour et al. 2009). Cancer, cardiovascular diseases, cognitive decline, and thyroid disease have also been connected to a disturbance in Se metabolism.

Serum Se concentrations decline with age. Marginal or deficient Se concentrations might be associated with age-related declines in brain function, possibly due to decreases in selenium's antioxidant activity (Shahar et al. 2010). Selenium status should be controlled regularly and corrected through supplementation.

## Zinc

Zinc is an essential metal involved in numerous aspects of cellular metabolism. Required for the catalytic activity of approximately 300 enzymes, it plays a role in immune function, protein synthesis, wound healing, DNA synthesis, and cell division (Haase et al. 2006; Haase and Rink 2013; Appendix 8.1). Zinc also supports normal growth and development during pregnancy, childhood, and adolescence (Maret and Sandstead 2006) and is required for a proper sense of taste and smell (Prasad 2013; Appendix 8.1).

The human body contains 2–3 g $Zn^{2+}$, concentrated primarily in the liver, kidneys, pancreas, eyes, and bone. Daily, 0.1% of body zinc is exchanged (Maret and Sandstead 2006). Because no major storage organs for zinc exist, a continuous nutritional supply is needed to cover $Zn^{2+}$ requirememts . Following its uptake by the small intestine, the distribution of $Zn^{2+}$ is carried out through plasma, where it is bound by proteins, mostly albumin (Scott and Bradwell 1983). Cellular $Zn^{2+}$ is distributed in the nucleus (30–40%), membrane (10%), and cytoplasm (50%). The latter contains membrane-enclosed structures rich in zinc, so-called zincosomes (Haase and Rink 2013). Remaining cytoplasmic zinc is mostly bound to proteins, especially metallothioneins. Zinc homeostasis in the human body is regulated by 14 Zip (Zrt/Irt-like) proteins, which increase the amount of zinc in the cell cytoplasm, and 10 ZnTs (Zn transporters), which decrease cytoplasmic Zn concentrations. There is considerable cell-specific expression of some of the transporters, which are dynamically regulated in response to Zn status and endocrine and cytokine signaling. Expression of these transporters can also regulate signal transduction via the level of intracellular zinc (Haase and Rink 2009).

Although excessive Zn intake is very rare, recent estimates indicate that Zn deficiency affects over 17% of the world's population (Wessells and Brown 2012). The main cause of Zn deficiency is malnutrition; however, disease and aging may also play a role.

Phytates, which are present in whole grain breads, cereals, legumes, and other foods, bind zinc and inhibit its absorption (Prasad 2012). The predominantly wheat diet in the Middle East contains high quantities of phytate and fiber, which reduce Zn and Fe availability increasing the risk for Zn deficiency (Prasad 2012). Symptoms of Zn deficiency include impaired growth and development, impotence, loss of appetite, diarrhea, hypogonadism in males, eye and skin lesions, weight loss, mental lethargy, dermatitis, delayed wound healing, alopecia (hair loss), various neurological symptoms, and impaired effectiveness of the immune system, leading to a higher susceptibility to infections (Wang and Busbey 2005; Maret and Sandstead 2006; Maret 2012; Appendix 8.1). Zinc deficiency has been associated with birth defects and low birth weight, impaired learning, as well as delayed sexual development. Depending on the extent and timing of the deficiency, embryotoxicity may also occur (Kambe et al. 2008). Supplementation studies show a significant 14% reduction in preterm births in women from low-income settings, but no effect on low birth weight (Mori et al. 2012). *Acrodermatitis enteropathica* (mutation in Zip4) is a rare hereditary autosomal recessive disease of Zn deficiency. It leads to severe immunological consequences, including thymic atrophy, decreased lymphocyte counts and function, and death from infections. Mandatory clinical manifestations are skin changes, chronic diarrhea, and alopecia. Treatment with zinc is necessary to maintain life and reverses the symptoms (Haase and Rink 2009).

A decline of Zn status with age has been established, and a correlation between Zn status and immune function in the elderly seems to exist. The question remains whether Zn deficiency is caused by infections that occur more frequently in elderly people, thus leading to a subsequent loss of zinc, or whether aging poses a risk of becoming Zn deficient, thus leading to immunosenescence and increased susceptibility to infectious diseases. Diseases associated with disturbed Zn homeostasis include diarrhea, common cold, age-related macular degeneration, and Cu deficiency (Wintergerst et al. 2007; Caruso et al. 2007; Chong et al. 2007; Whittaker 1998; Willis et al. 2005).

## Metallic Elements with Suggested Essentiality

### Arsenic

Exposure to the metalloid arsenic occurs daily due to its environmental pervasiveness. Arsenic presents as inorganic arsenate (iAsV), in most cases, or as inorganic arsenite (iAsIII), when anaerobic conditions are present in drinking water. Despite arsenic's reputation as a poison, it actually has fairly low toxicity compared to other metals, although chronic exposure raises concern about its carcinogenicity. In fact, arsenic may even be essential and functional in humans in very small amounts, as it has been shown to be essential in rats and other animals. However, beneficial effects in humans have not yet been defined (Mayer et al. 1993).

At least 90% of ingested iAsV and iAsIII are absorbed from the intestine and excreted primarily in the urine. Arsenic is mainly metabolized in the liver, with inorganic arsenic converted to monomethyl- and dimethylarsenicals by As methyltransferase (Lin et al. 2002). It has been reported that concentrations of iAs peak in the liver and kidney one hour after oral administration of iAsV, with dimethylarsinic acid then becoming the predominant form in the liver four hours after administration (Watanabe and Hirano 2013; Kenyon et al. 2005). Even if arsenic is not actively stored, it accumulates in bone, teeth, skin, hair, nails, and internal organs. On average, there is about 10–20 mg of arsenic in the human body; higher amounts may accumulate when kidney function is decreased. Normally, absorption of arsenic is fairly low ($< 5\%$) as most is eliminated in urine and feces.

Arsenic is considered carcinogenic and has been related to the lung, kidney, bladder, and skin disorders. It is also toxic to developmental and reproductive systems (Chakraborti et al. 2004). Immunotoxic, biochemical, and cellular toxicities cause serious diseases such as hyperkeratosis, blackfoot disease, vascular diseases, and cancers (Sakurai et al. 2004).

In several epidemiologic studies (e.g., Bloom et al. 2010), maternal exposure to high concentrations of inorganic arsenic in naturally contaminated drinking groundwater sources has been associated with an increased risk for the spontaneous loss of pregnancies. Decreased fetal weight and malformation have also been reported. In neonates, As exposure causes encephaly, eye defects, renal agenesis, and gonadal agenesis (Domingo 1994). One study in Japan revealed that arsenic as well as mercury and cadmium accumulate in the human body during aging and may play a role in the aging process (Yasuda et al. 2012). So far, no studies on As deficiency have been reported.

## Chromium

Over fifty years ago chromium was proposed to be an essential element for mammals, with a role in maintaining proper lipid metabolism and regulating blood sugar. Over the next several decades, research recommended Cr nutritional supplements for weight loss and muscle development, without knowledge on mode of action (Anderson 1997; Vincent 2010; Appendix 8.1). A timely review by Hua et al. (2012) addresses some of the recent findings regarding the molecular mechanisms of alleviating insulin resistance by chromium, which sheds light on the potential cellular pathways that are affected.

Chromium occurs in any oxidation state from $-2$ to $+6$. Trivalent chromium ($Cr^{3+}$) is the biologically active form, while hexavalent chromium ($Cr^{6+}$) is potentially toxic to humans and carcinogenic. Absorption of $Cr^{3+}$ from the intestinal tract is low (0.4–2.5%), and the remainder is excreted in the feces (Offenbacher et al. 1986; Eckhert 2012). Absorbed chromium is stored in the liver, spleen, soft tissue, and bone (Lim et al. 1983). Diets high in simple sugar can increase Cr excretion, while vitamin C and niacin can enhance absorption (Kozlovsky et al. 1986; Offenbacher et al. 1986). Stress, infections, exercise, pregnancy, lactation, and aging can increase Cr loss or decrease its absorbtion, and might require supplementation (Davies et al. 1997; Lukaski et al. 1996).

Although rare, Cr deficiency causes glucose-handling disorders with diabetes-like symptoms and abnormalities of the motor and sensory nerves. It is, however, easily corrected through supplementation (Jeejeebhoy et al. 1977; Anderson 1995). However, the required value of Cr supplements for diabetic patients (especially type 2) and to correct blood lipid levels and promote weight loss has not yet been established (Masharani et al. 2012).

Deficiences or overload of chromium, from conception through life, are associated with malfunctions, malformations, acute and chronic diseases, and fetal toxicity (Appendix 8.1); the nature of these depends on onset, duration, and degree of the deficiencies. Pregnant women may be at risk for Cr deficiency, but it should possible to cover the required amount by increasing Cr-rich foods in the diet, since supplements can easily result in high amounts of arsenic, which could negatively affect fetal development (Lindgren et al. 1984; Moukarzel 2009).

## Nickel

The essentiality of nickel in higher organisms is questionable. In order of abundance in Earth's crust, nickel ranks as the 24th element. Thus, humans are constantly exposed to this ubiquitous element, although in varying amounts. Due to its abundance, natural Ni deficiency does not occur (Denkhaus and Salnikow

2002). The blood levels of nickel in nonsmokers range from 0.01–0.26 µg/l (Stojanovic et al. 2004). Nickel intake occurs via inhalation, ingestion, and dermal absorption and is a function of bioavailability. Nickel is excreted equally well via urine and feces. Inhaled nickel is selectively concentrated in the lung, followed by heart, diaphragm, brain, and spinal cord tissues (Tjalve et al. 1984). Exposure to high doses of nickel disturbs established cellular homeostasis via changes of intracellular Ca levels and produces oxidative stress. Nickel allergy, in the form of contact dermatitis, is the most common and well-known reaction. Other known health-related effects include skin allergies, lung fibrosis, variable degrees of kidney and cardiovascular system poisoning, and stimulation of neoplastic transformation. The mechanism of the latter effect is currently unknown and the subject of detailed investigation. Epidemiological studies have clearly implicated Ni compounds as human carcinogens based on a higher incidence of lung and nasal cancer among Ni mining, smelting, and refinery workers (Denkhaus and Salnikow 2002). Nickel exposure can result in significant embryotoxic effects in terms of increased resorption rates, decreased fetal weight, delay in skeletal ossification, and a high incidence of malformations (acephalia, ankylosis of the extremity, club foot, and skeletal anomalies) (Lu et al. 1979; Appendix 8.1).

**Vanadium**

Vanadium is a trace element found in living organisms with a potentially essential role. Less than 5% of ingested vanadium is absorbed. Vanadium is rapidly cleared from plasma, accumulates in kidney, liver, testes, bone, and spleen and is able to cross the placenta. Vanadium is excreted primarily through the kidney, with a small amount through bile. Tissues with the highest concentrations include lung, teeth, thyroid, and bone (Eckhert 2012).

Vanadium is a cofactor for several enzymes including haloperoxidases and nitrogenases. In oxidation state 5 it is an analog of phosphorus, and thus an inhibitor against phosphorylases such as the ATPase, protein tyrosine phosphatases, and ribonucleases. Vanadium demonstrates promising antidiabetic properties and thus has been applied as a potential therapeutic (Eckhert 2012).

No human cases of V deficiency have been reported. Vanadium deficiency in goats increased rates of abortion, convulsions, bone malformations, and early death. However, high concentrations are toxic (Nechay et al. 1986). Vanadium is a reproductive toxin that affects males more than females. The International Agency for Research on Cancer lists vanadium as a possible carcinogen based on inhalation studies of V pentoxide in animals.

Vanadate treatment resulted in micrognathia, supernumerary ribs, and alterations in sternebral ossification. Whereas embryolethality was not observed at any dosage level (Carlton et al. 1982), vanadyl sulfate pentahydrate caused maternal toxicity, embryofetotoxicity, and teratogenicity (cleft palate, micrognathia) at all dose levels tested (Paternain et al. 1990; Appendix 8.1).

## Metallic Elements and Infectious Diseases

For any one or more of the trace metals discussed here, dyshomeostasis has long been associated with susceptibility and progression of inflammatory diseases (Suttle and Jones 1989; Katona and Katona-Apte 2008). Incidence of certain inflammatory diseases has been mapped to areas deficient in selenium and zinc (Di Bella et al. 2010). However, descriptions of the underlying mechanisms as well as the mode of action of supplementation strategies are just beginning to emerge.

Trace elements are structural parts and cofactors of a variety of enzymes. Lack of the metal causes alterations or loss of function as a general consequence. Proteins affected can either belong to the host, with a majority being related to immune functions (see Weiss, this volume) or to the pathogen, which is mostly responsible for their proliferation or virulence (Bachmann and Weiser, this volume; Sterritt and Lester 1980; Thurman et al. 1989; Prado et al. 2012; Haase 2013). The later finding suggests that a benefit for the host can be gained from the deficiency; this might be true for an acute translocation of trace metals away from the microbes (Bachmann and Weiser, this volume). However, prolonged deficiency has major, negative consequences for the host, especially for its immune system as described above (see also Weiss, this volume).

Another general symptom of deficiencies in cobalt, copper, molybdenum, iron, selenium, zinc, and vanadium is an increase in reactive oxygen production, due to the fact that the majority of enzymes involved in redox metabolism are metal dependent. Increased levels of reactive oxygen species can induce rapid mutation in RNA viruses, often resulting in a more virulent form. Recent published examples for Se deficiency-related viral mutation are coxsackievirus B3, influenza virus, and poliomyelitis virus (see Harthill 2011). Selenium supplementation decreased the mutation rate and improved the host response, including viral clearance. This is in concordance with the observation that $H_2N_2$, $H_3N_2$, $H_5N_1$, and SARS originated from regions in China where selenium is low. Experiments in mice confirm those observations: Se-deficient mice had higher rates of mutation to more virulent $H_3N_2$ forms than mice with balanced serum selenium. As an underlying mechanism, elevated reactive oxygen levels could be defined. Also, incidences of HIV and Ebola are high in Se-deprived regions in Sub-Saharan Africa (Di Bella et al. 2010; Harthill 2011).

For HIV, deeper insights into the incidents and severity of the disease independent of Se and Zn homeostasis have recently been established. Results of several studies showed that decreased serum selenium as well as serum zinc caused higher incidents, more severe progression, higher bacterial loads, increased susceptibility to secondary infections (such as hepatitis C), mycobacterial infections, and other especially opportunistic infections as well as higher mortality. Benefits from supplementing HIV patients with selenium or zinc are a decreased viral load, less hospitalization, and milder disease progression

(Baum et al. 2010; Harthill 2011). Because of its strong impact on immune functioning, zinc has been linked to all kinds of infectious diseases (for details, see Haase 2013). Zinc supplementation has been repeatedly shown to be beneficial in preventing diarrhea and decreases the incidents of infections in the neonates. Benefits derive from zinc's role in intestinal fluid transport, mucosal integrity, immunity, and the redox metabolism (Berni et al. 2011). Positive effects have been observed for treatment of pneumonia and other lower respiratory infections, malaria, the common cold, leprosies, tuberculosis, leishmaniasis, and sepsis, especially in risk groups such as infants, children, and the elderly. However, results from studies vary considerably and should thus be explored further in more detail (Fischer and Black 2004; Zeng and Zhang 2011; Basnet et al. 2014; Mocchegiani et al. 2013). An interesting example for the interplay of trace elements during inflammation is that zinc can starve pneumonia by blocking the bacterial Mn uptake. Unique mechanisms have been proposed for the positive role of vanadium in preventing inflammatory diseases: supplementation of mice with vanadium prior to LPS injection leads to upregulation of IL-1 antagonist, damping of brain-based proinflammatory cytokine upregulation, and blunting of central communication. Values for human use remains, however, to be established (Johnson et al. 2005b).

Although trace elements are toxic for humans if overdosed, the literature on the beneficial effects of trace metal supplements goes back ages. Ointments containing trace metals (e.g., zinc) have long been used to treat and prevent skin infections; however, benefits from oral supplementation are more recent. Effects are partly due to the support of the immune system but include direct consequences to the microorganism as well. Cobalt is mostly applied to keep surfaces sterile (e.g., in hospitals) due to its high toxicity for microbes. It is also used as an adjuvant for various infectious disease medications. One famous example is the Co chelate complex CTC-96, used to treat herpes, adenovirus, cytomegalovirus, Epstein–Barr virus, and varicella zoster virus (Schwartz et al. 2001b). The potential importance of cobalt for the host defense has been suggested, but remains to be explored in more detail.

The general antimicrobial properties of copper have been described in literature; over 300 publications were already available in 1973. More recent research has focused on defining more than thirty types of Cu-containing proteins across the animal kingdom. Similar to cobalt, most of our current knowledge stems from experiments that analyze the effect of surfaces containing high amounts of copper rather than a function within the host. A few of the recent studies have suggested an association of changes in Cu homeostasis with *Escherichia coli*, methicillin-resistant *Staphylococcus aureus*, *Clostridium difficile*, influenza, adenovirus, and fungi (Prado et al. 2012).

As indicated earlier, not all trace elements have positive effects on the host defense against pathogens. One study in Bangladesh revealed that high intake of arsenic during pregnancy (ingested, e.g., through contaminated drinking water) increases the risk for infections of the lower respiratory tract and the number of deaths in mothers and their infants. It has been suggested that arsenic causes immune suppression and becomes apparent through suppressed antibody formation, T cell proliferation, decreased size of the thymus, impaired macrophage activity, and elevated production of reactive oxygen species (Rahman et al. 2011). Iron overload has negative effects on the immune system as well and can result in increased susceptibility to infectious diseases.

## Nonessential Metallic Pollutants

To summarize metal homeostasis throughout life, let us review some important facts on the impact of nonessential metals on human health.

Mercury is one of the most toxic metals in the environment. It is released through activities in the agriculture industry (fungicides, seed preservatives), by pharmaceuticals, as pulp and paper preservatives, catalysts in organic syntheses, in thermometers and batteries, in amalgams (dental fillings), and in chlorine and caustic soda production (Zhang and Wong 2007). Exposure to high levels of metallic, inorganic, or organic mercury can permanently damage the brain, kidneys, and the developing fetus (Chang et al. 1980; Lindgren et al. 1984; Holt and Webb 1986; Appendix 8.1). The toxicity of mercury depends on its chemical form: ionic < metallic < organic (Clarkson and Magos 2006).

Cadmium is naturally present in the environment: in air, soils, sediments, and even in unpolluted seawater. It is emitted into the air by mines, metal smelters, and industries that use Cd compounds to produce alloys, batteries, pigments, and plastics, although many countries have stringent controls on such emissions. Tobacco smoke is one of the largest single sources of Cd exposure in humans. Absorption of cadmium in the lungs through smoking is much greater than in the gastrointestinal tract, where people are exposed to cadmium through the consumption of plant- and animal-based foods. Seafood, such as mollusks and crustaceans, can also be a source of cadmium (Castro-Gonzalez and Mendez-Armenta 2008). Cadmium accumulates in the human body and can negatively affect the liver, kidney, lung, bones, placenta, brain, and central nervous system (Castro-Gonzalez and Mendez-Armenta 2008). Other damage that has been observed includes reproductive and developmentally toxic, hepatic, hematological and immunological effects; intrauterine growth retardation; and fetal death (Ahokas et al. 1980; Daston 1982; Holt and Webb 1986; Apostoli and Catalani 2011; Appendix 8.1). Interestingly, adverse effects are produced despite limited embryonic and fetal accumulation of the metal (Domingo 1994).

Oral aluminum is ingested through food and drinking water as well as therapeutic preparations administered in large quantities, such as phosphate binders, antacids, and buffered aspirins (Cannata and Domingo 1989). Although the gastrointestinal tract normally represents a barrier to Al absorption, this barrier can be breached under some circumstances. Moreover, it has been demonstrated that concurrent ingestion of Al compounds and some organic dietary constituents (e.g., citric, lactic, and ascorbic acids) causes significant increase in the gastrointestinal absorption of aluminum (Domingo et al. 1991). Aluminum accumulation in the body manifests in impaired neurological development, Alzheimer disease, metabolic bone disease, dyslipidemia (abnormal blood lipids), and even genotoxic activity (Krewski et al. 2007; Hernandez-Sanchez et al. 2013). Of special concern is the intake of large amounts of aluminum by pregnant women. During pregnancy, "dyspepsia" (condition of disturbed ingestion) is a common complaint, and Al-containing antacids are widely used to relieve dyspeptic symptoms. Aluminum can act as a powerful neurological toxicant, provoking embryonic and fetal toxic effects in animals and humans after gestational exposure. Despite this knowledge, over-the-counter patient information leaflets for European antacids vary substantially in terms of warnings that Al toxicity will increase health risk (Reinke et al. 2003). Further studies are needed to clarify the link between Al exposure and disease in humans. Moreover, harmful and toxic doses need to be clearly defined for the public (Krewski et al. 2007).

## Conclusion

The incidence of malnutrition in the world is alarming, as is the increasing problem of obesity. Furthermore, the incidence of deficiency in essential nutrients is on the rise. The World Food Programme estimates that poor nutrition is responsible for 3.1 million child deaths annually (or 45% of all child deaths).[1] The rate of maternal morbidity due to obesity has also increased.

People of all ages are at risk for deficiencies in essential nutrients, even though the metabolism of adults is often tolerant enough to cope with transient dietary deficiencies. The primary groups at risk are pregnant women, fetuses, and the increasing elderly population. Often neglected are people exposed to high psychological and physical stress, including athletes and those who work in leadership positions. (Those groups of people may, however, be generally more health conscious and thus aware of additional dietary needs.)

Balanced nutrition early in life is vitally important; undernutrition during pregnancy and the first two years of life is a major determinant of (a) stunted development and subsequent obesity and (b) incidence of infectious diseases, with possible long-term damage and manifestation of noncommunicable diseases in adulthood (Black et al. 2013). Disturbed metal balances in the elderly result from lifelong exposure to toxic metals as well as years of wear and tear on their metabolism, including enzyme and organ systems. In addition, dyshomeostasis in trace metals, especially deficiencies, strongly impacts immune function throughout life, causing increased susceptibility and more severe

---

[1] http://www.wfp.org/hunger/stats

progression of all kinds of infectious diseases. Nutritional interference should be approached in different ways, depending on the age group. As described, problems in metal homeostasis in the elderly do not always stem from deficiencies or excess, but rather from a disturbance in an enzymatic process. It is thus imperative to identify the reason for the disturbance rather than simply to prescribe supplements. Supplementation in pregnant women should be carefully monitored. Often, changes in the diet are much more efficient than chemical supplementation, as overexposure to supplemental nutrients can be detrimental for the developing embryo.

Recommended dietary allowances are well defined for age groups, yet how can people meet RDAs and live a healthy life? One option is to increase labeling on food and beverages, so as to indicate not only caloric and fat values but also the amounts of (trace) elements. Initial steps to provide more complete nutritional labeling have been taken, but public awareness and education is needed.

The data provided in this review are only a summary of the mass volume of information that has been generated over the last decade. Detailed reviews on the homeostasis for each element, including involved transporters and binding proteins, are available. How can this information be brought to the public? One approach is to integrate nutrition into school curricula, starting at the kindergarten and primary school levels. Such educational approaches have begun in various areas, offering children and their parents the opportunity to prepare meals together. As an example, a detailed action plan for the United States was generated by the White House Task Force on Childhood Obesity[2] and for Germany by the German Obesity Foundation (Müller et al. 2007). Initiatives such as Let's Move! are great examples of an approach that can be taken to raise a healthy generation of children (for study results, see Pirzadeh et al. 2014). Doctors and antenatal exercise groups are also well positioned to provide information to the public. Here, there is often, however, a tendency to prescribe medications, which may not always be the best solution, when alternatives (e.g., a particular diet or a visit to a dietitian) might serve a patient better.

Essential metals are generally regarded as "safe," in particular if taken up via food, which is the best source of necessary elements. However, there is always a risk of overdosage, although overdosage due to high food consumption has barely been described in the literature. In contrast, highly concentrated supplements have the potential to induce allergic or toxic reactions, and studies are lacking on the effects of supplement combinations. Taking several supplements at the same time may neutralize their impact (and have no benefit) or produce negative, synergistic side effects.

In general, there is much confusion as to what constitutes good nutrition—a situation often exacerbated (rather than remedied) by "health websites" and media reports. In addition to creating headlines, the latest "fad diet" often contradicts basic nutritional knowledge that has been trusted for decades, creating

---

[2] www.letsmove.gov

widespread alarm and instant dietary changes. Many such reports are biased and overgeneralized, marked by failure to evaluate fully the current literature in trusted journal publications. Thus the public is left misinformed and potentially ready to make poor dietary decisions. Yet how can people decide which information is accurate?

The pharmaceutical industry has the ability to influence the generation and updating of RDA values. Often, discrepancies exist between values given by the World Health Organization, the U.S. Food and Drug Association, and on product labels. For example, the recommended dose for chromium in healthy individuals (during pregnancy and while nursing) is high, even though research suggests that lower values are sufficient. Several years ago a conjecture was voiced, and taken up by the media, that chromium could mitigate diabetes and aid weight loss. As a result of the subsequent hype and claims for better health, the market for Cr supplements boomed, even though the claim was not substantiated. Obviously it is not in the economic interest of the pharmacological industry to rectify such ill claims.

One approach to help people eat a more balanced diet is to improve the quality of food. This requires reducing the amounts of chemical fertilizers, insecticides, pesticides, etc., as well as improving food processing methods to retain natural nutrients. In addition, people's eating habits need to be scrutinized. In many societies, there is a tendency to eat prepackaged, ready-made meals that are easily and quickly prepared. Such food, however, has typically much less nutritional value. People need to be aware of the negative health impacts that could result from consuming high amounts of processed fast food and be encouraged, instead, to consume fresh food.

Governmental involvement at all levels would be beneficial. To make fresh food more attractive to the consumer, local producers may need support to lower prices for fresh products. Schools, universities, and businesses should also be encouraged to offer more healthy food options.

The available research information is broad. However, studies have concentrated primarily on a single element; interactions between metals, their competition for transporters, and binding proteins have, for the most part, been neglected. Future research must focus on this to elucidate interactions and symbiotic effects.

Overall, societies are becoming increasingly aware of the increase in malnutrition and have begun to search for solutions. Unfortunately, these solutions have centered on prescriptions and supplements. New strategies need to be developed that are more natural and preventive. Up-to-date research should be used to inform and update nutritional recommendations. Medical professionals should be encouraged to update their knowledge regularly and to pass this on to their patients. Different media venues should be used to educate and inform people of all ages. All efforts should be geared toward expanding our understanding on disease and disease prevention, for this is always better, and usually cheaper, than treatment and medication.

**Appendix 8.1** Functions, food sources, and symptoms of deficiency or overload for biologically relevant essential and nonessential metallic elements. GI: gastrointestinal; SOD: superoxide dismutase; TPN: total parental nutrition. Adapted from Dietary Supplemental Fact sheets (http://ods.od.nih.gov/factsheets/list-all/) and Ross (2012).

| | Functions | Food Source | Deficiency | Overload |
|---|---|---|---|---|
| As | No proven physiological function in humans. Known to be essential in rats and other animals | Rice, flour, spinach, grape juice, (saltwater) fish and seafood, grains, drinking water, fertilizers | In animal models, no deficiency reported for humans: myocardial damage, reduced growth, impaired fertility, increased perinatal mortality | Encephalopathy, GI symptoms, skin pigmentation, dermatitis, peripheral vascular diseases, neuropathy, genotoxicity, cancer, anemia, hepatotoxicity |
| Co | Component of vitamin B12, thus involved in DNA synthesis, fatty acid synthesis, and energy production | Depends on content in soil and air, drinking water | Neurological disorders due to vitamin B12 malfunction | Nausea, vomiting, lung diseases, heart diseases, neurological problems, thyroid disorders |
| Cr | $Cr^{6+}$ (industrial pollution): toxic, teratogen, carcinogen $Cr^{3+}$ (food): suggested but unproven: regulating blood glucose levels, involved in protein and fat metabolism | Meats, poultry, fish, beer, whole grains, fruits, vegetables, spices, water | Impaired glucose removal, elevated fatty acids, neuropathy, weight loss, glucose intolerance (disappears after Cr treatment) | Chrome ulcer, nasal septum perforation, chronic renal failure, lung cancer |
| Cu | Component of enzymes in Fe metabolism, involved in activity of cytochrome oxidase, tyrosinase, cerulo plasmin, lysine oxidase, ascorbate oxidase, SOD, amine oxidase | Organ meats, legumes, nuts, seafood/shellfish, seeds, wheat bran cereals, whole grain products, cocoa products, cheese | Anemia, retarded growth, osteoporosis, neutropenia, skeletal abnormalities, decreased pigmentation In premature infants: pallor, decreased pigmentation, superficial veins, skin lesions, diarrhea, neuronal abnormalities | GI distress, liver and renal damage, rheumatoid arthritis, gastric ulcers, cancers, epileptic episodes |

| | Functions | Food Source | Deficiency | Overload |
|---|---|---|---|---|
| Fe | Component of hemoglobin and numerous enzymes; prevents microcytic hypochromic anemia | Nonheme Fe: fruit, vegetables (lentils, beans), fortified bread, grain products/cereal; Heme Fe: red meat, fish, poultry | Tiredness, weakness, dizziness; slow social and cognitive development; easy freezing; decreased immune function or increased susceptibility to infection; glossitis; anemia; tinnitus; headache; cardiac pain or failure | Hemochromatosis, migraine headaches, arthritis, high blood pressure, cancer, heart disease, genetic diseases, GI disorders, diarrhea, nausea, vomiting, constipation, diabetes, preeclampsia, organ damage (cirrhosis of the liver) neurodegeneration, lower IQ in children |
| Mn | Bone and amino acid formation; lipid, protein and carbohydrate metabolism; cofactor of metalloenzymes (e.g., SOD) | Nuts, legumes, tea, seeds, whole grains, seaweed, beans, peas, ginger, coffee | Weight loss, transient dermatitis, nausea, vomiting, changes in hair color and growth, delayed blood clotting, low cholesterol; In neonates: disturbed calcification, demineralization (corrected by Mn supplementation) | Insomnia, depression, delusion, anorexia, arthralgia, weakness, neurotoxicity, mental disorders, muscle tremors |
| Mo | Cofactor for enzymes in catabolism of sulfur amino acids, purines, and pyridines; involved in electron transfer via, e.g., flavin adenine dinucleotide | Legumes, grain products, nuts, lentils, beans, organ meats, soybeans, cauliflower | Not observed in humans, due to TPN; rapid heart and respiratory rates, headaches, night blindness, coma due to genetic defects; severe neurological dysfunction characterized by cerebral atrophy, mental retardation, intractable seizures, and dislocation of ocular lenses | Gout-like syndrome (one reported case of acute supplemental Mb toxicity), insomnia, seizures, psychosis, hallucinations, renal insufficiency, weight loss, changes in liver and kidney |
| Ni | No clear biological function in humans; may serve as a cofactor of metalloenzymes | Grains, vegetables, legumes, meat, poultry, nuts, chocolate, drinking water | Not observed in humans; Pigs and rats: delayed sexual maturity, rough coat, liver abnormalities | Irritation of the respiratory tract, nonspecific symptoms, pulmonary and GI toxicity, pneumonitis, edema, cancer |

**Appendix 8.1 (continued)**

| | Functions | Food Source | Deficiency | Overload |
|---|---|---|---|---|
| Se | Reproduction, thyroid gland function, DNA production, protects from damage caused by free radicals and infection, involved in brain functioning | Organ and muscle meats, seafood, whole grains, eggs, poultry (depending on soil Se content) | Osteoarthritis, dwarfing and joint deformation, muscle pain and tenderness, cardiomyopathy dyschromotrichia, macrocytosis, cancer, thyroid disease, heart disease (Keshan disease) infertility in male, arthritis (Kashin-Beck disease) | Loss of hair and nails, skin lesions and polyneuritis, alopecia, nail changes, garlic breath, nausea, diarrhea, skin rashes, irritability, metallic taste in the mouth, discolored teeth, nervous system problems |
| V | No biological function in humans identified; effect on insulin metabolism suggested | Mushrooms, black pepper, shellfish, parsley, dill seed, vegetable oils, fats, olives, seafood, beer wine, grains | Humans: no reported deficiency Goats: abortion, convulsion, bone malformation, early deaths | Abdominal cramps, diarrhea, hemolysis, increased blood pressure, fatigue, cancer $V_2O_5$: conjunctivitis, rhinitis, pulmonary inflammation |
| Zn | Component > 300 enzymes, 2nd messenger, vital for growth/cell division, fertility, functioning of immune system, taste, smell, appetite, skin, hair, nails, vision | Oysters, crab, lobster, liver, poultry, cheese, fortified cereals, whole grains, red meats, legumes, dairy products | Anorexia nervosa, hypogeusia, retarded growth, delayed sexual maturation, impaired wound healing, skin lesions; defects in reproduction, taste, vision and smell; neurosensory, hormonal, immunological disorders; skin problems; mental irritability, emotional disorders and chronic diarrhea; loss of appetite and hair; impotence; hypogonadism in males, eye lesions | Reduced copper status, nausea, vomiting, loss of appetite, abdominal cramps, diarrhea, headaches, altered Fe function, reduced immune function, reduced levels of high-density lipoproteins |

# 9

# Impact of Metals on Immune Response and Tolerance, and Modulation of Metal Metabolism during Infection

Günter Weiss

## Abstract

Several metals play important roles in host cell and microbial metabolism because they form a part of central enzymes that are essential, for example, for DNA synthesis, cellular respiration, and key metabolic pathways. The availability of these metals differentially impact on host antimicrobial immune responses as well as on microbial defenses against them (Botella et al. 2012). Thus, during infection, host cells attempt to gain sufficient access to these metals or to limit the availability of these factors for microbes; this is thought to play a decisive role in the course of infections. Accordingly, subtle changes in the metabolism of these metals and their distribution throughout the body occur: microbes activate different pathways to secure a sufficient supply of these metals needed for their pathogenicity and proliferation as well as to mount effective defenses against the host immune system.

This review focuses on the role of iron in the host–pathogen interplay. A brief discussion is included on the role of zinc, manganese, and copper for host–pathogen interaction, immune function, and their alteration by the inflammatory response.

## Introduction

Metal ions are pivotal in host–pathogen interactions. This is partly because microbes need metals, such as iron (Fe), zinc (Zn), copper (Cu), or manganese (Mn), for important metabolic processes and proliferation and as central components for defenses against host-mediated radical formation. The basis for the essential function of these metals can be traced back to their ability to accept or donate electrons needed during metabolic processes. Metal accumulation can become toxic, however, due to their ability to catalyze the formation of toxic oxygen and nitrogen radicals, which can intoxicate microbes or damage surrounding cells and tissues. Microbes take up transition metals through multiple pathways, and sufficient acquisition of these metals through pathogens is linked to the pathogenicity and proliferation of microbes. In additional, transition metals (specifically iron) play important roles in antimicrobial host responses, not only by synergistic effects toward antimicrobial radical formation but also by directly affecting immune cell proliferation and antimicrobial immune effector pathways. Thus, the host immune system affects the metabolism of these metals and/or their availability for microbes via the action of cytokines, cellular proteins, or hormones—for which the term *nutritional immunity* has been coined—and plays a decisive role in the course of infection.

## Role of Iron for Immune Cell Plasticity

Iron is an essential metal due to its role as a prosthetic group in several essential proteins and enzymes involved in metabolic processes, mitochondrial respiration, and DNA synthesis. Iron catalyzes the formation of hydroxyl radicals, which then modulate the binding affinity of critical transcription factors, such as HIF-1 or NF-kB, thus affecting gene expression during inflammation (Rosen et al. 1995). Therefore, both Fe overload and Fe deficiency exert subtle effects on essential metabolic pathways as well as on the growth, proliferation, and differentiation of cells. Accordingly, the availability of iron affects the proliferation and differentiation of immune cells, which exploit different pathways to acquire this metal.

The close interaction between iron and immunity is underscored by observations that certain immunological proteins do alter cellular Fe metabolism, as described for β2 microglobulin, HFE (which is a nonclassical MHC-I molecule linked to the majority of cases with human hemochromatosis), tumor necrosis factor receptor (TNF-R), and the natural resistance-associated macrophage protein (NRAMP1). Changes in immune function thus affect Fe homeostasis and vice versa (Weiss 2002).

Lymphocytes have evoked different mechanisms to acquire iron, even under conditions when Fe availability is limited. All lymphocytes subsets, which include B and T lymphocytes as well as natural killer (NK) cells, are dependent on transferrin/transferrin receptor (TfR)-mediated Fe uptake; blockade of this pathway leads to diminished proliferation and differentiation of these cells (Seligman et al. 1992). Accordingly, mitogenic stimuli, such as phytohemagglutinin, increase TfR surface expression on B and T cells. However, lymphocyte subsets differ in their dependence on transferrin-mediated Fe uptake. Induction of experimental Fe overload in rats resulted in a shift in the ratio between T helper (CD4+) and T suppressor/cytotoxic T cells (CD8+), with a relative expansion of the latter. Moreover, even the T helper

(Th) subset responds differently to Fe perturbations. Several subsets of CD 4+ T helper cells are well established in humans; these are termed type 1 (Th-1), Th-2, Th-9, Th-17, and Treg. Each subset produces a typical set of cytokines that regulate different immune effector functions, which cross-react with each other and play a decisive role in host responses to infections.

Whereas Th-1 cells are very sensitive to treatment with anti-TfR antibodies, resulting in inhibition of their DNA synthesis, Th-2 cells are resistant to this procedure. This may be because Th-2 clones exhibit larger chelatable Fe storage pools than Th-1 cells. Thus, Th-1-mediated immune effector pathways are much more sensitive to changes in Fe homeostasis *in vivo* (Thorson et al. 1991). The latter can partly be attributed to a direct regulatory effect of iron on the activity of the central regulatory Th-1 cytokine IFN-$\gamma$ (Nairz et al. 2013).

Monocytes and macrophages are the conductors that orchestrate Fe homeostasis in health and disease; they are thus on the interface between Fe homeostasis and immunity. One reason for this is that macrophages are essential for the maintenance of a sufficient supply of iron for erythropoiesis, which is achieved by recycling iron from senescent red blood cells taken up by macrophages via erythrophagocytosis (Weiss and Schett 2013). In addition, macrophages need iron to produce highly toxic hydroxyl radicals by the enzyme phagocyte oxidase as part of their antimicrobial armamentarium (Rosen et al. 1995). At the same time, macrophages are centrally involved in the diversion of Fe traffic under inflammatory conditions that occur during infection or cancer.

## Alterations of Iron Metabolism in Inflammation

Based on the decisive role of iron for both the host immune system and microbes, it has become clear that Fe metabolism is significantly affected during the course of infection. These alterations of Fe traffic are thought to result from a defense strategy of the body to limit the availability of iron for invading pathogens, for which the term *nutritional immunity* has been coined (Nairz et al. 2010; Cassat and Skaar 2013). This alteration in Fe homeostasis is mediated by cytokines and radicals as well as by acute phase proteins, which originate primarily from the liver. Combined, this mediation leads to retention of iron in macrophages and an impaired Fe absorption from the diet (Weiss and Schett 2013).

The contribution of cytokines to systemic Fe regulation was first confirmed through the observation of sustained hypoferremia in mice injected with TNF-$\alpha$ or IL-1. Hypoferremia was paralleled by hyperferritinemia, which was traced back to induction of ferritin transcription by cytokines in cells of the reticuloendothelial system. In addition, the proinflammatory cytokines IL-1 and IL-6 regulate ferritin expression at the translational level. Iron storage in macrophages is further promoted via increased phagocytosis of erythrocytes.

This occurs when erythrocytes are damaged, as a result of exposure to inflammation-driven radical formation, and are phagocytized via C3bi (CD11b/CD18) receptors, which increase in expression following TNF-α treatment. Accordingly, the application of sublethal doses of TNF-α to mice resulted in a shortening of erythrocyte half-life and a faster clearance of these cells from the circulation via erythrophagocytosis (for a review, see Weiss 2002).

The intriguing relationship between immunity and Fe homeostasis took on a new dimension after the acute phase protein hepcidin was identified as the master regulator of Fe homeostasis (Ganz 2009). The observation that hepcidin-deficient mice injected with turpentine did not develop hypoferremia suggested that hepcidin could be involved in Fe disturbances during inflammation or infection. One underlying mechanism is the induction of hepcidin expression by lipopolysaccharides (LPS), IL-1, IL-6, or IL-22 in hepatocytes. Hepcidin acts on Fe homeostasis upon binding to the only known Fe export protein ferroportin, thereby leading to Fe retention in macrophages and impaired Fe absorption from the diet (Ganz 2009). Accordingly, increased circulating hepcidin concentrations in serum result in reduced circulating Fe levels and increased Fe retention in macrophages, a scenario which should limit the access to iron from circulating pathogens (Ganz 2009; Nairz et al. 2010). In addition, mammalian monocytes and macrophages produce small amounts of hepcidin in response to LPS or IL-6. Although the basal expression is relatively low in comparison to the amount of hepcidin produced in the liver, microbial challenges, such as group A *streptococci* and *Pseudomonas aeruginosa*, can induce a 20- to 80-fold increase of hepcidin expression in these cells through a TLR-4-dependent pathway, whereas IL-6-mediated induction of hepcidin is mediated via STAT3 activation (Nairz et al. 2010; Ganz 2009). Interestingly, hepcidin released by macrophages targets ferroportin in an autocrine fashion, thus promoting macrophage or monocyte Fe accumulation during inflammatory processes. This may be a fast-acting defense mechanism of the innate immune system against invading microbes. Hepcidin targets ferroportin exposed on the cell surface, resulting in immediate blockage of Fe release and reducing the availability of this essential microbial nutrient in circulation.

Effects of hepcidin on Fe homeostasis appear, however, to occur rapidly, but only for a limited duration. This has been confirmed by the observation that injection of LPS results in the induction of hepcidin and development of hypoferremia, which lasted for several hours (Kemna et al. 2005). Thereafter, serum Fe concentrations returned to normal or were even higher than at baseline. Thus, to ensure a sustained modulation of Fe homeostasis under inflammatory conditions and during infection, a concerted action of different signals exerted by cytokines, acute phase proteins, and hormones is mandatory. A central regulatory factor that ensures sustained Fe retention in monocytes or macrophages, as well as reduced expression of ferroportin during inflammation, is IFN-γ. The Th-1-derived cytokine IFN-γ induces ferritin transcription but also affects ferritin translation, which is based on activation of iron regulatory protein (IRP)-binding affinity by the cytokine. This is partly due to the stimulation of nitric oxide (NO) formation by IFN-γ, which then activates IRP-1 binding to the ferritin iron-responsive element (IRE). This leads to an inhibition of ferritin translation, whereas effects to IRP-2 activity depend on the type of cell and NO product (Pantopoulos et al. 2012). Moreover, hydrogen peroxide and superoxide anion modulate IRP-1 activity through a rapidly inducible process involving kinase or phosphatase signal transduction pathways; this results in posttranscriptional regulation of IRE-regulated target genes, such as TfR and ferritin (Recalcati et al. 2010; Pantopoulos et al. 2012). IFN-γ treatment of monocytes blocks the uptake of transferrin-bound iron via downregulation of TfR expression. This is most likely due to induction of a proximal inhibitory factor by IFN-γ, which inhibits TfR transcription. However, IFN-γ induces the expression of divalent metal transporter 1 (DMT1) and acts synergistically with LPS and TNF-α in this respect. This stimulates ferrous Fe uptake into these cells and promotes their incorporation into ferritin (Ludwiczek et al. 2003). At the same time, IFN-γ and LPS induce Fe retention in macrophages by downregulating ferroportin transcription, thus blocking Fe release from these cells (Ludwiczek et al. 2003). Hepcidin formation by macrophages or monocytes may be part of a fast-acting innate immune effector arm aimed at preventing Fe export from macrophages, which is relevant under microbial invasion. The outcome is to reduce circulating Fe concentrations and the availability of this nutrient for pathogens. Thereafter, ferroportin transcription is blocked by IFN-γ or LPS, thus ensuring a prolonged blockage of Fe export.

While anti-inflammatory cytokines (such as IL-4, IL-10, or IL-13) do not affect the suppression of ferroportin mRNA expression by IFN-γ or LPS (Ludwiczek et al. 2003), treatment of murine macrophages with IL-4 and/or IL-13, prior to stimulation with IFN-γ, suppresses NO formation and subsequent IRP activation, which concomitantly enhances ferritin translation. This has also been found to be true in human monocytic cells (THP-1), which do not express detectable amounts of inducible nitric oxide synthase (iNOS). Conversely, TfR mRNA levels increase following pretreatment of IFN-γ-stimulated macrophages with the anti-inflammatory cytokines. This may be referred to as IL-4- or IL-13-mediated antagonization of the inhibitory signal induced by IFN-γ, which inhibits TfR expression by an IRP-independent pathway. In addition, IL-10 and IL-6 may affect macrophage Fe acquisition by stimulating the expression of the hemoglobin scavenger receptor CD163, thus promoting the uptake of hemoglobin-haptoglobin complexes into monocytic cells. The important role of Th-2-derived cytokines for the development of hyperferritinemia under chronic inflammatory processes was confirmed by a clinical study in patients with Crohn disease. In a placebo-controlled, double-blinded study, patients who received therapy with human recombinant IL-10 developed a normocytic anemia preceded by a significant increase in serum ferritin levels;

reticulocyte counts were not, however, affected, compared to placebo-treated controls (Weiss and Schett 2013). Both anemia and hyperferritinemia resolved spontaneously within two to four weeks after IL-10 therapy was terminated. Thus, Th-2-derived cytokines may increase Fe uptake via induction of TfR and CD163, but will also promote Fe storage within ferritin through activated macrophages. In addition, IL-10 stimulates HO-1 expression and activity, thus promoting Fe reutilization from phagocytosed erythrocytes, hemoglobin-haptoglobin complexes, and hemopexin-bound heme, respectively (Gozzelino et al. 2012). In addition, the increased expression of ferritin and the subsequent sequestration of iron within this protein contribute to limiting tissue damage during infection by inhibiting the catalytic action of iron. Thus, overexpression of H-chain ferritin (which harbors ferroxidase activity) results in tolerance to infection by limiting inflammation-induced tissue damage, as shown in animal models of malaria (Gozzelino et al. 2012).

In summary, pro- and anti-inflammatory cytokines and, most importantly, acute phase proteins cooperate at multiple steps to increase macrophage Fe accumulation by stimulating various Fe acquisition pathways in these cells. At the same time, cytokines and hepcidin inhibit Fe export from macrophages by downregulating ferroportin expression. This results in Fe retention within cells of the reticuloendothelial system and Fe-restricted erythropoiesis (Table 9.1).

These processes result in the development of hypoferremia, hyperferritinemia, and Fe-restricted anemia, the latter of which has been termed anemia of chronic disease (ACD) or anemia of chronic inflammation (Weiss and Schett 2013). In a clinical setting, ACD occurs frequently in patients suffering from chronic inflammatory disorders (e.g., autoimmune diseases, chronic infections, malignancies). Although the development of anemia is associated with detrimental effects, especially in relation to cardiac function, quality of life, and growth and mental development, the underlying hypoferremia and the diversion of iron from circulation may also exert potentially positive effects, especially when infections underlie chronic immune activation.

## Impact of Iron on Antimicrobial Immune Effector Function

The development of ACD does not only limit the availability of iron for microbes but can strengthen the immune response directed against invading pathogens. Specifically, Fe loading of monocytes or macrophages inhibits IFN-γ-mediated pathways, such as the formation of TNF-α, reduced expression of MHC class II antigens and ICAM-1, decreased formation of neopterin, and impaired tryptophan degradation via IFN-γ-mediated induction of indole-amine-2,3–dioxygenase (for a review, see Nairz et al. 2010). As a result, Fe-loaded macrophages have an impaired potential, *in vitro* and *in vivo*, to kill various bacteria, parasites, fungi (e.g., *Legionella, Listeria, Ehrlichia, Mycobacterium, Salmonella, Leishmania, Plasmodium, Candida, Mucor*), and

**Table 9.1**    Pathways for regulating Fe homeostasis through cytokines, acute phase proteins, and radicals: interleukin (IL), tumor necrosis factor (TNF), interferon (IFN), divalent metal transporter 1 (DMT1), ferroportin (FP1), nitric oxide (NO), and hydrogen peroxide ($H_2O_2$).

| Factors | Mechanisms |
|---|---|
| TNF-α | Induces ferritin transcription, which promotes iron storage within cells of the reticuloendothelial system |
| | Shortage of erythrocyte half-life (TNF-α) and stimulation of erythrophagocytosis |
| | Inhibits hepcidin formation |
| | Blocks iron absorption from the duodenum |
| IL-1 | Stimulates ferritin transcription and translation and promotes macrophage iron retention |
| | Stimulates hepcidin formation |
| IL-6 | Induces ferritin transcription and translation |
| | Stimulates hepcidin formation |
| | Stimulates CD163 and increases the uptake of hemoglobin-haptoglobin complexes by macrophages |
| | Induces heme oxygenase and heme degradation |
| IFN-γ | Stimulates DMT1 synthesis and increases uptake of ferrous iron into monocytes |
| | Downregulates FP-1 expression, which inhibits iron export from macrophages |
| | Downregulates TfR via induction of a proximal inhibitory signal |
| IL-4, IL-10, IL-13 | Increases TfR expression and transferrin-mediated iron uptake into inflammatory macrophages |
| | Stimulates ferritin translation by inactivating IRP and decreasing NO expression |
| | IL-10 stimulates CD163 and increases the uptake of hemoglobin-haptoglobin complexes by macrophages |
| | IL-10 stimulates heme oxygenase expression and heme degradation |
| IL-22 | Stimulates hepcidin expression |
| NO | Stimulates IRP-1 binding affinity, thus blocking ferritin translation and stabilizing TfR mRNA (feedback regulation with iron; NO formation is affected via modulating iNOS expression) |
| | Induces ferroportin expression via Nrf2 activation |
| | Modulates IRP-2 expression and stability |
| Oxygen radicals | $H_2O_2$ when applied extracellularly stimulates IRP-1 activity with blocking of ferritin translation and stabilizing TfR mRNA |
| | Superoxide anion formed intracellularily inhibits IRP binding affinity |
| Hepcidin | Formed upon stimulation of mice with LPS and several proinflammatory cytokines |
| | Blocks iron egress from macrophages |
| | Inhibits duodenal iron absorption |
| | Exerts autocrine regulation of iron export from inflammatory macrophages |

viruses through IFN-γ mediated pathways. This can partly be attributed to the reduced formation of NO in the presence of iron, since NO is an essential effector molecule of macrophages to fight infectious pathogens and tumor cells. Iron blocks the transcription of inducible NO synthase (iNOS or NOSII), the enzyme being responsible for cytokine-inducible high output formation of NO by hepatocytes or macrophages. In addition, by inhibiting the binding affinity of the transcription factors NF-IL6 and the hypoxia inducible factor-1 to the iNOS promoter iron, iron impairs iNOS inducibility by cytokines (Nairz et al. 2010). According to the regulatory feedback loop, NO produced by activated macrophages leads to an inhibition of ferritin translation, thus linking the maintenance of Fe homeostasis to NO formation for host defense. Through its deactivating effect on IFN-γ function, iron also affects the Th-1/Th-2 balance: Th-1 effector functions are weakened while Th-2-mediated cytokine production (e.g., IL-4 activity) is increased, a condition that is rather unfavorable in an infection (Nairz et al. 2010; Mencacci et al. 1997). Iron overload also has negative effects on neutrophil function: in chronic hemodialysis patients, Fe therapy impairs the potential of neutrophils to kill bacteria, thus reducing their capacity to phagocytize foreign particles (Weiss 2002). By modulating cytokine activities, iron triggers macrophage polarization, and opposite M1 and M2 macrophages differ in contrasting metabolic profiles in regard to Fe homeostasis (Recalcati et al. 2010). Moreover, the induction of M2 polarization along with increased expression of HO-1 has been linked to immune tolerance in infections, specifically in malaria (Gozzelino et al. 2012).

Thus, both Fe overload and Fe deficiency have unfavorable immunological effects *in vivo*. Accordingly, mice kept on an Fe-rich diet presented with a reduced production of IFN-γ, compared to mice fed with a normal diet, and animals that received an Fe-deficient diet showed decreased T cell proliferation (Omara and Blakley 1994). Both Fe-overloaded and Fe-deficient mice had an increased mortality when a sublethal dose of LPS was received, compared to animals with a normal Fe status.

In one study, Fe-deficient children had a reduced incidence of infection accompanied by a higher percentage of CD8+ cells producing IL-6, a more pronounced expression of T cell activation markers on lymphocytes, and an increased formation of IFN-γ, as compared to Malawian children with a normal Fe status (Oppenheimer 2001). This coincides with the observation of an adverse outcome in children who received Fe supplementation, mainly as a result of an increased incidence of severe malaria, bacterial infection, or diarrhea (Sazawal et al. 2006; Soofi et al. 2013). In line with this observation, improved outcomes, but no mortality benefit, were observed in children with cerebral malaria who received the Fe chelator desferrioxamine, which corresponded to antimalarial immune responses. In Africa, an endemic form of secondary Fe overload, caused by the consumption of traditional Fe-containing beer and linked to the presence of a mutation in the ferroportin gene (Gordeuk et al. 2003), is associated with an increased incidence of and mortality from tuberculosis. These latter data are in accordance with *in vitro* findings, which find that changes in intramacrophage Fe availability stimulates the proliferation of mycobacteria and weakens the antimycobacterial defense mechanisms of macrophages. Other infections—ranging from bacterial, viral, and fungal diseases to parasitic diseases, where Fe overload is associated with an unfavorable course of the infection and/or an impaired immune response— have been well summarized (Weinberg 1999).

The importance of iron for the antimicrobial immune response pathways is further underscored by the finding that many innate resistance genes of macrophages act by limiting Fe availability for intracellular bacteria. Macrophages exposed to the intracellular bacterium *S. typhimurium* increase the expression of the Fe export protein ferroportin; this stimulates cellular Fe export and limits Fe availability for intramacrophage bacteria, leading to improved control of bacterial proliferation by macrophages. In part, this is because a reduction of cytoplasmic iron increases the activity of immune effector pathways, such as TNF-$\alpha$, IL-6, IL-12, or NO formation (Nairz et al. 2010). Importantly, part of the antimicrobial activities of the Th-1 cytokine IFN-$\gamma$ and iNOS have been linked to their ability to limit Fe availability in bacteria. Briefly, induction of iNOS by macrophages exposed to intracellular bacteria results in an activation of the transcription factor Nrf2; this stimulates ferroportin transcription, induces the export of iron from *Salmonella*-infected macrophages, and stimulates antimicrobial immune effector pathways. Importantly, the impaired control of *Salmonella* infection in iNOS–/– mice can be completely overcome by treatment with the Fe chelator desferrasirox (Nairz et al. 2013). The crucial role of ferroportin-mediated Fe export for host defense against infections with intracellular pathogens is further supported by the observation that overexpression of ferroportin in macrophages can control the infection with a number of intracellular bacteria, such as *Chlamydia* spp., *Legionella*, *Salmonella*, or *Mycobacteria* (Nairz et al. 2010).

Another immune gene that exemplifies the role of iron in infection is the phagolysosomal protein NRAMP1. The expression of Nramp1 is associated with resistance toward infections in intracellular pathogens such as *Leishmania*, *Salmonella*, or *Mycobacteria* spp., and occurs mainly by shuttling divalent metals across the phagolysomal membrane (Forbes and Gros 2001; Blackwell et al. 2001). Investigations of the RAW264.7 macrophage cell line stably transfected with functional or nonfunctional Nramp1 have demonstrated that macrophages expressing functional Nramp1 exhibit significantly lower iron uptake via TfR and increased Fe release mediated through increased ferroportin expression. Accordingly, as a net effect of the altered expression of Fe transporters, the overall cellular Fe content was lower in macrophages bearing functional Nramp1 (Fritsche et al. 2012). This provides further support for the hypothesis that NRAMP1 expression confers resistance toward intracellular pathogens by limiting the availability of iron to the microbes; a contribution to Fe-mediated formation of toxic radicals has also been discussed (Forbes and Gros 2001). In addition, NRAMP1-mediated alterations of Fe homeostasis stimulate antimicrobial immune effector function, as evidenced by increased formation of NO or TNF-α, whereas expression of the anti-inflammatory cytokine IL-10 is significantly reduced (Nairz et al. 2010). Recent evidence suggests that Nramp1 functionality results in increased formation of lipocalin 2 (NGAL, Lcn2) (Fritsche et al. 2012). Lipocalin 2 is a neutrophil and macrophage-derived peptide that captures Fe-laden microbial siderophores, thus interfering with the acquisition of siderophore-bound iron by specific Gram-negative bacteria, such as *Escherichia coli* or *Klebsiella* spp. (Flo et al. 2004). Moreover, Lcn2 delivers siderophore-bound iron to mammalian cells, which are able to import the complex via Lcn2 receptor. Most interestingly, recent data provide evidence for the existence of mammalian siderophores that are captured by Lcn2, indicating that Lcn2 may be involved in transcellular and transmembrane Fe trafficking in mammals (Pantopoulos et al. 2012).

In addition, Lcn2 expression affects neutrophil recruitment to the sites of infection which, depending on the underlying pathogen, exerts contrasting effects on the outcome of the infection (Warszawska et al. 2013). Interestingly, Lcn2 is also secreted during infection with non-siderophore-producing pathogens, such as *Chlamydia* or *Plasmodia*. This limits Fe availability for *Plasmodia* and impairs erythropoiesis, which further inhibits replication of plasmodia. In addition, following the mechanisms described above, Lcn2 stimulates innate immune responses by limiting Fe availability (Zhao et al. 2012). Similarly, lipocalin 2 may confer resistance to infection by *Salmonella* and *Mycobacteria* spp. in patients suffering from hereditary hemochromatosis. As a consequence of reduced hepcidin formation and increased expression of Lcn2 upon infection, macrophages of these patients are Fe deficient, thus constituting a hostile environment for these pathogens (Nairz et al. 2009).

It is important to note that host-mediated alterations of Fe homeostasis (e.g., via the formation of hepcidin) may directly impact the proliferation of microbes. Hepcidin expression has been shown to affect the proliferation of intrahepatic sporozoites negatively, but it may also increase susceptibility to infection with Fe-dependent pathogens such as *Salmonella* (Portugal et al. 2011). It appears that different regulatory mechanisms are initiated, depending on the type of the infectious pathogens. Although hepcidin induction appears to be a very efficient strategy to limit the availability of iron for extracellular bacteria, since it restricts the nutrient iron within the reticuloendothelial system, this strategy may be detrimental to intracellular pathogens. For intracellular pathogens, multiple pathways (e.g., NOS2, ferroportin formation, NRAMP1) lead to mobilization and export of iron out of macrophages, rendering them Fe deficient; this ameliorates the control of infection with intracellular microbes and positively affects innate immune responses.

## Alterations of Copper, Zinc, and Manganese Homeostasis during Infection

Copper homeostasis is closely linked to Fe metabolism, because the ferroxidases hephaestin and ceruloplasmin (which mediate the oxidation of ferrous to ferric iron and its incorporation into transferrin) are Cu-containing enzymes (Pantopoulos et al. 2012). Thus, Cu deficiency leads to Fe overload and subsequent Fe-mediated tissue damage. In addition, copper plays important roles as a prosthetic group for many enzymes, such as cytochromes, proteins involved in oxidative phosphorylation, and Cu or Zn superoxide dismutase (Hood and Skaar 2012).

As with iron, copper is a redox-active metal iron that is able to catalyze the formation of toxic hydroxyl radicals; Cu accumulation is thus associated with increased antimicrobial toxicity, also termed metal poisoning (Samanovic et al. 2012). Evidence suggests that copper kills microbes via mechanisms that are independent from radical formation (e.g., by displacing iron from Fe-S clusters within enzymes); however, further investigation into these functions is needed. Of note, copper and zinc have been shown to accumulate in phagosomes of macrophages infected with *M. tuberculosis* (Wagner et al. 2005). Proinflammatory cytokines, such as IFN-$\gamma$, induce the expression of the Cu permease Ctrl in macrophages, which results in an increased Cu uptake into macrophages as well as translocation of the P-type ATPase ATP7A to phagolysosomes. This mediates Cu influx into these vesicles and subsequent metal poisoning of bacteria (White et al. 2009). Copper deficiency is, therefore, associated with an increased susceptibility to infections.

The transition metal zinc plays a central role in the function of structural proteins and is essential for immune cell proliferation and differentiation (Liu et al. 2012). Cell differentiation is manifested through the association between Zn deficiency and thymic atrophy, impaired B, T, and NK cell responses, as well as reduced formation of proinflammatory cytokines. Zinc, however, can be used as an antimicrobial weapon to intoxicate microbes. Recent evidence suggests that the granulocyte macrophage colony stimulating factor (GM-CSF) induces the sequestration of zinc in macrophages. Specifically, GM-CSF induced the expression of two Zn transport proteins, leading to accumulation of the metal in the Golgi apparatus which triggered the formation of toxic radicals by virtue of NADPH oxidase, thereby exerting antifungal activity against *Histoplasma capsulatum* (Vignesh et al. 2013a).

Of interest, bacteria need zinc for their pathogenicity and as part of their defense against host-mediated oxidative stress. In randomized controlled trials aimed at improving children's health by avoiding negative effects of Fe and Zn deficiency on growth and mental development, daily dietary supplementation of iron and zinc, in the form of micro-powders, resulted in an increased burden of infections (Soofi et al. 2013). Therefore, Zn sequestration during an infection is considered to represent another branch of nutritional immunity. Components of the S100 protein family bind $Zn^{+2}$, $Cu^{+2}$, and $Mn^{+2}$ (see below), which exert antimicrobial activity (Hood and Skaar 2012). Two of these proteins, S100A8 and S100A9, form a heterodimeric complex named calprotectin. Calprotectin is expressed by neutrophils, where it accounts for up to 50% of cytoplasmic proteins. The secretion of calprotectin is performed primarily by apoptotic neutrophils and associated with extracellular traps. Binding and sequestration of zinc and manganese by calprotectin is suggested to exert antimicrobial activity by weakening the antioxidant defense mechanism of microbes, which need these two molecules to activate their radical detoxifying enzymes. In addition, other S100 proteins, such as S100A12 (calcitermin), can also bind transition metals. Found in human airways, S100A12 exerts antimicrobial activity against several bacteria as well as against fungi or nematodes. The expression of S100 proteins can be induced by IL-17 and IL-22, whereas S100 proteins influence immune function by exerting proinflammatory activity and promoting neutrophil chemotaxis (Hood and Skaar 2012). The S100A7 protein (also termed psoriasin) is secreted by keratinocytes where it exerts antimicrobial actions after binding with zinc. It is important to bear in mind, however, that metal depletion strategies of the host affect pathogenic bacteria as well as the commensal or protective flora. Thus, bacteria which have evolved strategies to outcompete these metal restrictions benefit from a developmental advantage and may thus become more pathogenic (Liu et al. 2012).

As briefly mentioned, Zn sequestration is often accompanied by the capture of manganese, which is needed by microbes as part of the antioxidant defense protein Mn or Zn superoxide dismutase and as a catalytic component of several central proteins (where it can also replace the more redox active metal iron). Like iron, both zinc and manganese are transported by NRAMP1, and limitation of Mn availability within the phagolysosome is considered to be an important mechanism by which macrophages confer resistance toward infection with intracellular pathogens. In addition, NRAMP2 (better known as DMT1) transports a myriad of divalent metal ions across membranes in an ATP- and proton-dependent process. DMT1 expression and Fe transport capacity are increased in inflammatory macrophages (Ludwiczek et al. 2003); however, it has not been investigated thus far whether this is also paralleled by increased accumulation of copper, zinc, or manganese in macrophages and whether or not this strengthens antimicrobial activities. The central role of Mn starvation in antimicrobial activity has recently been underpinned by the finding that calprotectin-mediated Mn restriction causes maximum growth inhibition of bacteria (Damo et al. 2013).

## Conclusion

Transition metals play decisive roles in host–pathogen interactions and affect the outcome of infections, due to their essential nature in pathogen proliferation and microbial resistance mechanisms to oxidative stress. In addition, these metals are important for host immune cell proliferation and differentiation, as well as for mounting an effective antimicrobial immune response.

More efforts are needed to understand metal trafficking between the host and microbe. Specifically, we need to disentangle the multiple roles of these transition metals for innate and adaptive antimicrobial immune responses as well as for microbes. Thus far, most studies have concentrated on evaluating the role of a single metal in host–pathogen interactions, yet the metabolisms of different transition metals are interconnected in multiple ways. To gain new insights into the cross-regulatory interactions of infection, and ultimately *in vivo*, the effects of metals like iron, zinc, copper, and manganese need to be evaluated in parallel in host–pathogen interactions. The resulting knowledge will enable novel therapeutic targets for tackling microbes to be identified and provide insight into how modulation of metal metabolism, on either the host or pathogen site, can positively affect the course of infections.

# 10

# Metal-Based Antiparasitic Therapeutics

Maribel Navarro and Gonzalo Visbal

## Abstract

This review discusses the potential of metal-based compounds to act as safe and affordable drugs in the treatment of important tropical parasitic illnesses such as Chagas disease, leishmaniasis, and malaria. Currently, half the world's population is estimated to be at risk of contracting these vector-borne diseases, and almost one million people die annually from these diseases. No effective vaccine exists to treat these infectious diseases and available treatments are far from ideal. Coordination metal complexes offer potential in the development of new antiparasitic drugs. Indeed, coordination compounds in medicine are a growing and exciting research field, having been used successfully in cancer therapy. As an antiparasitic agent, ferroquine has entered phase II clinical trials against malaria and is an excellent example to encourage the development of antiparasitic metal-based drugs. Insights into the mechanism of actions of metal-based antiparasitic drugs are discussed.

## Introduction

Metals have been used for medicinal purposes since prehistoric and ancient times. Many metals fulfil essential roles in the human body, and deficiency of some metals can lead to disease. Moreover, metals such as iron, zinc, copper, manganese, and cobalt are incorporated into proteins or enzymes which facilitate a number of crucial functions in the body.

It is also well known that metals can induce toxicity in humans. Attention to this undesirable effect was brought to light through Paul Ehrlich's seminal work in 1910 on chemotherapy (the use of drugs to injure an invading organism without injury to the host). Ehrlich's formulation of Salvarsan—an arsenic compound—not only provided a successful treatment for syphilis, it marked the entry of metallotherapeutic agents into broad clinical usage.

Based on the advances in coordination chemistry, a variety of metal-containing drugs have since been proposed, and some have progressed to clinical use. Well-known examples are platinum complexes (cisplatin, carboplatin, nedaplatin, and oxaliplatin) used to treat cancer; gold complexes (auranofin, solganol and myocrisin) used as antiarthritic drugs; silver used as an antimicrobial; and antimony (sodium stibogluconate and meglumine antimoniate) used to treat leishmaniasis. Currently, experimental clinical trials are underway to test several metal-based drugs that are based on titanium, ruthenium, iron, or platinum to treat cancer; bis(ethylmaltolato)oxovanadium(IV) as an antidiabetic drug; and ferroquine to treat malaria (Figure 10.1) (Alessio 2011; de Almeida et al. 2013; Farrell 2002; Guo and Sadler 1999; Thompson and Orvig 2003).

There is growing interest in metal-based drugs with potential application in a variety of therapeutic areas. Most efforts have been focused on developing drugs for cancer therapies, due to the success of cisplatin in the treatment of testicular and ovarian cancer. This success has inspired and led researchers to search for new metal-based chemotherapies for other illnesses, such as parasitic diseases. Unfortunately, though, the use of the metal complexes in the treatment of tropical parasitic diseases has not advanced at the same speed as cancer research.

Parasitic diseases constitute a major public health problem, particularly in the poorest areas of the world. Together they affect about one-third of the world's total population, causing more than one million deaths per year. Most of the available treatments are often toxic, not very effective, expensive, and sometimes difficult to administer. To make things worse, strains resistant to drugs currently in use have emerged (Aguiar et al. 2012; Bhargava and Singh

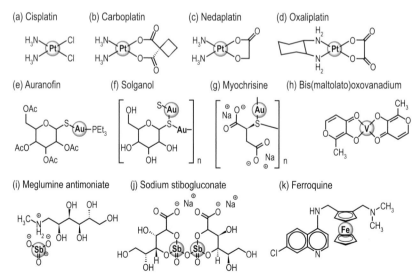

**Figure 10.1** Selected metal-based drugs that are currently used clinically for cancer (a, b, c, d), arthritis (e, f, g), and leishmaniasis (i, j), and in the experimental clinical phase for diabetes (h) and malaria (k).

2012). Thus, there is an urgent need to develop new effective, adequate, affordable, and safe chemotherapies to treat parasitic diseases. Metal-based drugs offer a rich source of effective chemotherapeutic agents against the major protozoan diseases, especially when the drugs are designed to attack specific parasitic targets. Here, we review efforts to discover novel metal-based antiparasitic agents for the treatment of Chagas disease, leishmaniasis, and malaria—important representatives of tropical diseases.

## Metal-Based Therapeutics for Trypanosomatidae

Trypanosomatidae are parasitic protists that cause Chagas disease and various manifestations of leishmaniasis in humans in many tropical and subtropical parts of the world. Even though these infectious diseases constitute a major global health problem, they have been classified as neglected tropical diseases (NTDs), due to the minimal levels of investment, on the part of both public and privates sectors, to develop new drugs for treatment. NTDs are concentrated among the world's poorest populations; worldwide they threaten more than 350 million people, affect up to 20 million, and are responsible for a significant number of deaths annually.

*American trypanosomiasis*, also known as Chagas disease, is endemic throughout Latin America. It is primarily transmitted to humans through the feces of triatomine bugs, also known as "kissing bugs." Occasionally, the responsible parasite, *Trypanosoma cruzi*, is transmitted through contaminated food, blood transfusion, and/or passage from an infected mother to her newborn during pregnancy or at childbirth.

Leishmaniasis is caused by protozoa parasites from over twenty *Leishmania* species and is transmitted to humans through the bite of infected female phlebotomine sandflies. It is currently estimated that 12 million people are infected worldwide.[1] There are three main types of the disease: cutaneous and mucocutaneous leishmaniasis are the most common, and visceral leishmaniasis is fatal if left untreated. An estimated 200,000–400,000 new cases of visceral leishmaniasis occur worldwide each year.

Current treatment for Chagas disease is based on nitroheterocyclic drugs (e.g., nifurtimox and benznidazole), which show significant activity only in the acute phase. The first line of treatment for leishmaniasis relies on pentavalent antimonials: sodium stibogluconate (Pentostam®) and meglumine antimoniate (Glucantime®) are the most representative drugs in use (see Figure 10.1). Although effective, these antimonials can cause severe side effects. When antimonials fail, Amphotericin B, pentamidine, or miltefosine are recommended as a second line of treatment for all three forms of leishmaniasis.

---

[1] http://www.who.int/leishmaniasis/burden/magnitude/burden_magnitude/en/

At present, there is no effective vaccine for either leishmaniasis or trypano-somiasis and, unfortunately, the treatments for trypanosomatid infections are far from ideal. This situation clearly calls for the development of new, effective, and nontoxic antiparasitic drugs. Since most of the drugs currently available for both diseases are characterized by poor efficacy, high toxicity, and increasing resistance, research into metal complexes as potent chemotherapeutic agents against trypanosomiasis and leishmaniasis is, and must remain, a priority.

One promising and attractive approach to the development of metallotherapeutic agents to treat parasitic infection was achieved through the application of metal-drug synergism. This concept consists of designing metal compounds that are based on the coordination of a transition metal into organic compounds with known or potential biologic activity. This modification is important within biological systems, due to the binding capability and reactivity of the transition metals, which are determined by the d-orbitals. These d-orbitals allow the design and preparation of a wide variety of coordination and organometallic compounds with different geometries (coordination spheres), oxidation states (redox potential), and use of diverse kinds of ligands. These geometries lead to metal complexes with enhanced lipophilicity, different kinetic and thermodynamic properties toward biological receptors, and the ability to interact with intracellular biomolecules, etc.

Such combinations can translate into enhanced activity of the parental organic drug. This activity enhancement may be related to the stabilization of the organic drug by coordination to the metal ion, which leads to a longer residence time of the drug in the organism, thus allowing it to reach the biological targets more efficiently. Another important effect of this combination is that it may also result in a decrease in the toxicity of the metal ion, due to complexation with the organic drugs, which makes it less available for undesirable reactions that lead to toxicity. Furthermore, these metallodrugs are capable of affecting multiple parasitic targets simultaneously.

This approach was followed by Sánchez-Delgado and colleagues, and led to the discovery of metal complexes through the coordination of metal-fragment complex to clotrimazole (CTZ) and ketoconazole (KTZ). These ligands, CTZ and KTZ, have been shown to inhibit effectively the growth of the *T. cruzi* parasite. Several metal complexes were achieved using metals such as ruthenium, copper, rhodium, platinum, and gold. All of these metal-CTZs and metal-KTZs were able to inhibit the proliferation of the epimastigotes form of *T. cruzi* considerably better than the CTZ and KTZ ligands. The most active compound of this group of metal-CTZ complexes was $RuCl_2(CTZ)_2$ (Figure 10.2a). This promising metal complex affects the regular function of the sterol biosynthesis when CTZ is liberated and attacks the parasite's DNA through covalent interaction of the Ru motif, thus demonstrating the metal-drug synergistic concept defined above (Sánchez-Delgado and Anzellotti 2004; Navarro et al. 2010; Gambino and Otero 2012).

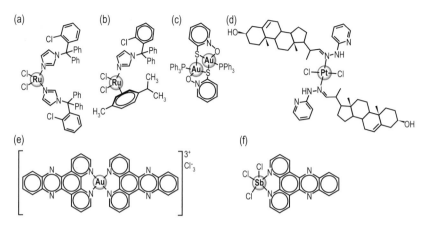

**Figure 10.2** Selected metal-based therapeutic agents for trypanosomiasis (a, b) and leishmaniasis (c, d, e, f).

The Sánchez-Delgado group has continued to use this successful concept and has recently extended it to include the use of ancillary ligands, which provide the leader Ru-CTZ complex with better and desirable physicochemical and biological properties. Accordingly, organometallic Ru-CTZs were developed that displayed high antiparasitic activity *in vitro* against *T. cruzi* epimastigotes and *Leishmania major* promastigotes. Ru[(η⁶-pcymene)Cl₂(CTZ)₂] (Figure 10.2b) was the most promising complex; it increased the activity of CTZ against *L. major* and *T. cruzi*, with no appreciable toxicity to human osteoblasts (Martínez et al. 2012). Similar organometallic compounds have been reported for Ru-KTZ (Iniguez et al. 2013).

Following this approach, the bioactive ligand, 5-nitrofuryl- and 5-nitroacroleine-containing thiosemicarbazones, has been incorporated into Ru, Pt, and Pd complexes, and it was found that Pt(II) and Pd(II) complexes were more active *in vitro* on *T. cruzi* epimastigotes than Nifurtimox and the corresponding free ligand. Another interesting ligand, 2-mercaptopyridine N-oxide (mpo), also coordinated to several metals (e.g., palladium, vanadium, and gold; Figure 10.2c) and showed significantly increased activity compared to mpo sodium salt on epimastigotes of different *T. cruzi* strains. Reported metal-mpo complexes showed a clear correlation between parasite inhibition and NADH fumarate reductase inhibition, thus highlighting this enzyme as the main target of these complexes as well.

Other organometallic compounds of iridium and rhodium with pentamidine (antileishmanial agents) have also been shown to be active against *L. donovani* promastigotes; some were even more active than pentamidine isethionate. A synergistic effect was noted when this complex was administered in combination with pentamidine, amphotericin B, or paromomycin. The Pt(II)-pentamidine complexes appear to be less active than Rh(I) and Ir(I) analogs against amastigotes of *L. donovani*. In addition, nitroimidazole dithiocarba-mates, benznidazole dithiocarbamates, and related ligands coordinated to plati-num, osmium, and rhodium displayed a moderate activity against *L. donovani*.

An interesting approach has been developed using gold(III), palladium (II), and rhenium(V) cyclometallated complexes against *T. cruzi* and three *Leishmania* species: *L. major*, *L. mexicana*, and *L. donovani*. Preliminary data indicate that these metal complexes target parasite cysteine proteases.

Another rational strategy was based on the coordination of sterol hydrazone ligands to platinum (Figure 10.2d). These steroid ligands have been shown to be specific inhibitors of (S)-adenosyl-L-methionine: $\Delta^{24}$-sterol methyl transfer-ase (SMT), an enzyme which catalyzes the incorporation of this alkyl group to produce the main sterol leishmania's parasites (ergosterol and 24-alkylated ste-rol analogs), is necessary for their survival and growth. SMT inhibitors should only affect parasitic cells, without damaging cells from higher eukaryotes, therefore bypassing any undesirable clinical side effect (Visbal et al. 2008).

Other types of metal complexes were developed as antiparasitic agents based on two facts:

1.  The metabolic pathways of kinetoplastid parasites are similar to those present in tumor cells.
2.  Selected antitumor metal-containing complexes, such as cisplatin (functions by binding to DNA and disrupting DNA replication), have been evaluated against *T. rhodiense* and *T. cruzi*.

These results, along with the fact that many antiprotozoal drugs bind to DNA, have led some to propose that, in general, every DNA-interacting compound could be active against parasites (Kinnamon et al. 1979). This motivated us to design DNA metallointercalators that could show activity against some of these pathogenic parasites through their interaction with DNA. This strategy was based on the use of polypyridyl ligands (typically intercalators), such as phen (phenantroline), 1,10-phenantroline-5,6-dione (phendione), dppz (dipyrido[3,2-a:2′,3′-c]phenazine), and dpq (dipyrido[3,2-a:2′,3′-h]quinoxo-line), which were coordinated to copper, silver, gold, palladium, and ruthenium to obtain a series of metal compounds:

- $[Cu(dpq)(NO_3)]NO_3$
- $[Cu(dpq)_2(NO_3)]NO_3$
- $[Cu(dppz)(NO_3)]NO_3$
- $[Cu(dppz)_2(NO_3)]NO_3$
- $[Ag(dpq)_2]NO_3$
- $[Ag(dppz)_2]NO_3$
- $[Cu(dppz)_2]BF_4$
- $[Au(dppz)_2]Cl_3$
- $PdCl_2(Phen)$
- $[Ru(phen)_2phendione](PF_6)_2$.

The biological activity of these metal complexes against *L. (V.) braziliensis and L. (L) mexicana* was evaluated, and all of them showed leishmanicidal activity. This biological activity was higher for the metal-dppz complexes. In addition, the complexes with two coordinated molecules of the planar ligand were more active than those with one. [Cu(dppz)$_2$]BF$_4$, which corresponds to Cu(I) complex, displayed a higher leishmanicidal effect than those observed with Cu(II). In contrast, Ag complexes were less active than complexes of Cu(II), whereas complexes of palladium and ruthenium showed moderate activity. [Au(dppz)$_2$] Cl$_3$ was the most effective complex in the series (Figure 10.2e): its strong *in vitro* activity against *L. (L) mexicana* could be related to its ability to interact with DNA through an intercalative mode. Other DNA metallointercalator (2,2′:6′2″-terpyridine) Pt(II) complexes and analogs have produced remarkable growth inhibition of *L. donovani*. These complexes exploit the intercalative DNA properties of the terpyridine ligand along with the covalent binding ability of the Pt(II) center. Similar complexes using mixed-ligand vanadyl complexes, [V$^{IV}$O(L$_2$-2H)(L$_1$)]—where L$_1$ is a tridentate salycylaldehyde semicarbazone derivative and L$_2$ is dppz as coligand—showed significant activity against *T. cruzi* and were as active as Nifurtimox. A recent report showed [Cu(CH$_3$COO) (dppz)$_2$]CH$_3$COO and [Zn(dppz)$_2$](BF$_4$)$_2$ to have significant activity against a visceratropic *L. infantum* strain and to be more active than the reference drug miltefosine. In addition, their DNA–intercalation interaction correlates with leishmanicidal activity. Trivalent antimony(III) and bismuth(III) complexes with the dppz were synthesized, characterized, and evaluated against the promastigote form of Sb(III)-sensitive and Sb(III)-resistant *L. infantum chagasi* and *L. amazonensis* strains. Both complexes were more effective than dppz alone in inhibiting the growth of *Leishmania* promastigotes. The lack of cross-resistance to the Sb(III)-dppz (Figure 10.2f) complex together with the much lower activity of antimonyl tartrate, SbCl$_3$, and BiCl$_3$ strongly support the model that the metal is not active by itself but rather it improves the activity of dppz through complexation (Benítez et al. 2013; Lizarazo-Jaimes et al. 2012; Madureira et al. 2013; Navarro 2009; Navarro et al. 2007).

Using a different approach, Cu complexes with fluorinated β-diketones were synthesized and tested against promastigotes of *L. amazonensis* and showed inhibition of trypanosomatid-specific trypanothione reductase. It was found that the highly lipophilic and redox activity of these Cu derivatives increased toxicity toward promastigotes (Portas et al. 2012). Copper and zinc with sulfonamides that contain 8-aminoquinoline ligands showed activity against *L. chagasi* and *L. brasilensis* (Everson da Silva et al. 2010).

Interesting results have been reported for Ag nanoparticles (Baiocco et al. 2011) and Au nanoparticles (de Almeida and Carabineiro 2013) in the inhibition of leishmaniasis promastigotes.

In summary, based on the above discussion, it is clear that the presented metal-based drugs are designed to attack important and specific parasitic targets of the *T. cruzi* and *Leishmania*. Due to the well-known complexity of these parasites, these drugs do not have a unique target to attack. Further research and efforts are thus needed to develop a rational design for an affordable and safe drug that will simultaneously attack several specific and/or selective targets in these parasites. Taking into account the metal-drug synergism strategy, metal-based drugs could play an important role in this research and drug design.

## Metal-Based Therapeutics for Malaria

Malaria is a major cause of illness and death in children and adults who live in tropical countries, in particular, Africa. It is one of the world's most ancient diseases and is one of the most devastating parasitic infections known to affect humans. According to the World Health Organization (2013), an estimated 207 million episodes of malaria occurred in 2012 and approximately 627,000 people died. Despite important efforts made in research and the investment in its control, prevention, and treatment, malaria remains a primary cause of mortality and morbidity throughout the Tropics.

Malaria is transmitted to humans through the bite of infected female mosquitoes from more than thirty anopheline species. Five species of parasites of the genus *Plasmodium* are infectious to humans: *P. falciparum, P. vivax, P. ovale, P. malariae*, and *P. knowlesi*. Malaria caused by *P. falciparum* is the most deadly.

The most successful treatment used to be chloroquine (CQ); it was considered the ideal drug, due to its low cost, high efficacy against all species of the *Plasmodium* parasite, and lack of significant side effects. However, CQ-resistant malaria parasites started to emerge in the late 1950s, spreading from Asia to Africa and South America, reducing its efficiency as a first line antimalarial drug and resulting in major setbacks to the effective control of malaria. Fortunately, very effective artemisinin-derivative (dihydroartemisinin, artesunate, and artemethe) drugs replaced chloroquine. However, monotherapy is not recommended for different reasons. Currently, malaria is treated with a combination of two or more drugs that have different modes of action to provide an adequate cure rate and delay development of resistance. Artemisinin-based compounds are combined with drugs including lumefantrine, mefloquine, amodiaquine, piperaquine, and chlorproguanil/dapsone (Sinclair et al. 2009; WHO 2013b). At least three different strategies have been developed to address this public health problem:

1.  The indiscriminate use of insecticides has been discontinued, due to insects' resistance to these chemicals and environmental impact. It should be noted, however, that renewed interest has been shown in the use of indoor residual spraying as a primary vector control intervention to reduce and interrupt transmission in African countries.

2. Vaccination is one of the most effective modes of treatment available, yet despite many efforts, effective vaccines are lacking. At the time of writing this review, encouraging results have been announced for the clinical trial of a new malaria vaccine developed by GlaxoSmithKline, which has shown some effectiveness in children over an 18-month period.

3. The use of chemotherapy, discussed here, focusing on metal-based drugs.

Metal-drug synergism has been exploited to obtain effective antimalarial metal agents. In line with this, chloroquine was modified through the incorporation of a transition metal into the molecular structure. Several metal complexes were synthesized, characterized, and evaluated. The first ones, RhCl(COD)CQ and $[RuCl_2(CQ)]_2$ (Figure 10.3a), demonstrated that coordination to ruthenium is effective in circumventing the resistance of two CQ-resistant strains of *P. falciparum* (FcB1 and FcB2). *In vivo* experiments showed that $[RuCl_2(CQ)]_2$ caused a reduction of the parasitemia by 94% at a concentration equivalent to 1 $ED_{50}$ (50% effective levels) of chloroquine diphosphate. Encouraged by these results, the Sanchez-Delgado group varied the ancillary ligands and overall charge of the complexes, leading to new organometallic Ru-CQ complexes (Figure 10.3b), which showed an enhanced activity against CQ-resistant strains of the parasite.

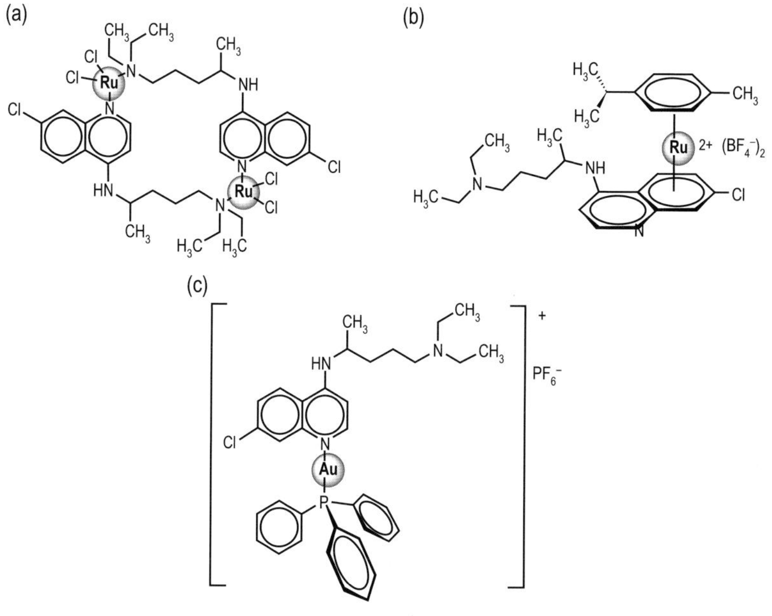

**Figure 10.3** Selected metal-based therapeutic agents for malaria. The main mechanism of the action found for these metal-CQ complexes is the inhibition of the β-hematin formation.

In other efforts to obtain metal complexes of greater efficacy, a Au complex of CQ—[Au(PPh₃)(CQ)]PF₆ (Figure 10.3c)—was synthesized. It caused marked inhibition of the *in vitro* growth of *P. berghei* and was also very effective against two CQ-resistant FcB1 and FcB2 strains of *P. falciparum*, displaying greater activity than the corresponding chloroquine diphosphate.

Motivated by this higher activity, a series of new Au-CQ complexes were developed by coordinating gold to chloroquine with different changes in the structure of the [Au(PPh₃)(CQ)]PF₆ complex. These changes included variations of the phosphine ligand with the purpose of inducing changes in the electronic and steric properties, variations of the counter anion (e.g., nitrate), variations of the Au oxidation state, such as Au(I) and Au(III), or using biologically important ligands such as 1-thio-β-D-glucose-2,3,4,6-tetraacetate. The highest activity in FcB1 and W2 strains was obtained for [Au(PEt₃)(CQ)]PF₆, while Au(III) complexes such as [Au(Cl)₂(CQ)₂]Cl showed excellent activity in strains K1. Chloroquine has been coordinated to other metals such as iridium, platinum, titanium, and copper, which have displayed moderate activities.

To gain insight into the possible mechanism of action of the metal-CQ derivatives, two potential targets of action accepted for the chloroquine have been evaluated: the inhibition of hemozoin (malarial pigment) formation and DNA interaction. Chloroquine is believed to act by concentrating in the parasite digestive vacuole and preventing the crystallization of toxic heme into hemozoin, leading to membrane damage and parasite death. It is uncertain how this drug's mechanism operates, but it is well established that chloroquine forms complexes with hematin in solution and is an inhibitor of β-hematin formation. The main mechanism of the action found for the metal-CQ complexes that were evaluated address the inhibition of β-hematin formation, specifically in interfacing. In terms of Au and Ru concentrations in these drugs, and the likelihood of adverse effects on the patient, Au and Ru complexes have thus far only been tested *in vitro* and *in vivo* in mice. Thus, it is currently not possible to predict the likelihood of adverse effects in humans. More studies are needed before the possible concentration of these potential antimalarial drugs is known.

Using a similar strategy, primaquine, mefloquine, and amodiaquine metal derivatives were prepared and evaluated as antimalarial drugs. These compounds, however, did not show significant reduction in parasitemia.

Another interesting and successful metal-based strategy for malaria treatment involved the introduction of the ferrocenyl moiety into the lateral side chain of chloroquine, known as ferroquine (FQ, SSR97193; see Figure 10.1). FQ is extremely active against both CQ-susceptible and CQ-resistant *P. falciparum*, and is being developed by Sanofi-Aventis; it entered phase II clinical trials in September 2007. In contrast to conventional drugs, FQ is the first organometallic drug: a ferrocenyl group covalently flanked by a 4-aminoquinoline and a basic alkylamine. An extensive investigation was carried out in search of analogs with better activities; indeed a library of ~150 antimalarial complexes has been prepared based on ferrocene-conjugate analogs of known antimalarial drugs, such as artemesinin, atovaquone, mefloquine, and quinine, among others.

Ferroquine was also modified in the secondary and tertiary amines. It was combined with thiosemicarbazones and associated with glutathione reductase inhibitors. Another interesting approach was the study of chloroquine diphosphate associated with ferrocene carboxylic acid via a salt bridge. A ruthenocene analog of FQ was also reported. Mixed CQ and/or FQ metal complexes—[RhCl(COD)L], [Au(L)(C$_6$F$_5$)NO$_3$], and [Au(L)(PPh$_3$)NO$_3$] where L = CQ or FQ—were also synthesized. All of these compounds have shown very promising antimalarial activities, which implies that the presence of the ferrocenyl moiety in these structures causes significant changes that moderate the attack by malaria parasites.

The pharmacokinetic profile of FQ seems to cover (together with appropriate partner) both cure and posttreatment of malaria prophylaxis. The mechanism of action and the induction of resistance to FQ have been studied in detail by Biot and colleagues. Its mechanism of action may be related to a strong inhibition of the hemozoin formation that leads to the accumulation of toxic heme (free or complexed with FQ), and thus to the death of malaria parasite. In addition, possible interactions between the malaria pigment and FQ may destabilize hemozoin, thereby irreversibly damaging the membrane. Evidence was found which shows that FQ accumulates within the digestive vacuole along with sulfur-containing compound(s). As accumulation of sulfur most likely arises from the influx of glutathione and its accumulation, FQ (under the oxidizing conditions of the digestive vacuole) should be capable of undergoing redox reactions, thus causing lipid oxidation. As a consequence, FQ (unlike CQ) might be capable of producing oxidative stress.

Trioxaquines represent a new class of antimalarial agents. These are hybrid molecules that contain two covalently linked pharmacophores: 1,2,4-trioxane, as in artemisinin, and 4-aminoquinoline, as in chloroquine. The first generation of trioxaquines was found to be highly active against CQ-resistant strains of *P. falciparum*. Ferrocene and trioxane derivatives have also been reported, as well as their biological studies which showed that they are active *in vitro* against CQ-resistant *P. falciparum*.

Selected metallodrugs (e.g., cisplatin, auranofin, aurothiomalate, and NAMI-A) have also been evaluated as antimalarial agents. They show different potencies but effectively reduce *P. falciparum* growth *in vitro*, implying high and broad parasite sensitivity to these metals.

Recent reviews have been published on metallopharmaceutics agents developed to fight against malaria parasites (Navarro et al. 2012; Biot et al. 2012; Salas et al. 2013).

Another rational strategy involves the use of Ru-based compounds designed to deliver carbon monoxide and confer robust protection against malaria (Pena et al. 2012). Interestingly, this class of metallodrugs, referred to as

CO-releasing molecules, provide host disease tolerance; that is, they protect the host from developing severe forms of disease without an overt effect on the pathogen itself (Medzhitov et al. 2012).

## Conclusions and Outlook

It is clear that the commercially available drugs for the treatment of leishmaniasis, Chagas disease, and malaria are very limited and far from ideal. There is thus an urgent need to develop new, effective drugs to aid the millions of people suffering from these parasitic diseases, who are waiting for effective, safe, and affordable treatments.

Based on the knowledge that has been gained from analyzing the rationale behind metal-based antiparasitic agents designed to be more active and less toxic than the organic compounds described herein, it is possible to envisage that coordination metal complexes may offer an excellent way to discover and develop new antiparasitic drugs. However, metal-based therapeutics faces two hurdles: not only must they fight against parasitic disease, they must also overcome the prejudice that metals imply toxicity. Metal-based drugs should be treated separately according to their individual biological activity and toxicological properties. This might help attract the attention of pharmaceutical companies and spur more funding for this promising research field.

Undoubtedly, this important area of research needs to be accompanied by firm knowledge and understanding of the biology of these parasites. Fortunately, nowadays, a great number of protein targets have been identified, and novel metal compounds can be designed to attack specific parasitic targets. These advances may have an important impact on the general strategy for the discovery and development of effective metal-based antiparasitic agents with lower toxicity.

The ideal metal-based antiparasitic drug will only be achieved if future work is coordinated. Multidisciplinary groups are needed and should include organic and inorganic synthetic chemists, biologists, pharmacologists, toxicologists, and physicians. Research efforts should be combined and knowledge must be shared. Most importantly, these efforts must be able to rely on financial support from diverse research programs and the pharmaceutical industry.

# 11

# Impact of Lifestyle on Metal Exposure, Homeostasis, and Associated Diseases

George V. Dedoussis

## Abstract

Unhealthy lifestyle factors (e.g., cigarette smoking, excessive alcohol drinking, long working hours, reduced sleep, physical inactivity, obesogenic diets) and psychological stress contribute to cardiovascular disease, cancer, and other causes of mortality in industrialized countries. Many of these factors correlate with alterations in the homeostasis of trace metals, which play an important role in human health and are essential for human antioxidant defense and immune function. Metal levels consumed by humans are influenced by the mineral composition of soil used to grow food as well as weather conditions, the composition of water for irrigation, and agricultural practices (e.g., types and amounts of fertilizers used). In some cases, major sources of trace metals derive from environmental pollution that results from industrial and other anthropogenic activities (e.g., cadmium from agricultural fertilizers). Food processing and packaging also play a role (e.g., aluminum and tin from canned foods). Although some individuals encounter toxic metals mainly in the workplace, for most people primary exposure of toxic and essential metals occurs through diet. The most common foods in our diet that contain metals are fish and seafood (mercury, copper and zinc), vegetables and grains (cadmium, magnesium, and molybdenum), chocolate and coffee (cobalt, copper, and nickel), fruit (lead), nuts (selenium), and mushrooms (vanadium). This chapter discusses the impact that lifestyle has on exposure to metals, homeostasis, and associated diseases.

## Introduction

As of conception and throughout life, humans experience a broad range of physical, chemical, and biological exposures to heavy metals. The health effects of these exposures depend not only on dose but also on how they interact with each other as well as the characteristics of the individual (e.g., age, sex, genotype). Trace metals are ubiquitous environmental pollutants with known toxic properties. Human exposure to these chemicals may occur occupationally, environmentally, or through dietary intake. In the general population, food and water are the most common metal sources, while cigarette smoking is an additional relevant source of exposure to trace metals such as cadmium (Cd) and chromium (Cr). The relationship between chemical elements in rainwater and the frequency of hospitalizations for gastric and duodenal peptic ulcers as well as for chronic myeloid leukemia (CML) was studied on the population of the province of Opole, Poland during the years 2000–2002. A high positive correlation was found between hospitalized cases of gastric peptic ulcers or CML in women exposed to cadmium and lead contained in rainwater (Szygula et al. 2011; Tubek et al. 2011). Gender is a factor that affects the impact of trace metal exposure. For instance, statistically higher amounts of silver (Ag), manganese (Mn), and lead (Pb) have been found in females in some communities. This has been attributed to traditional lifestyles: wearing large amounts of Ag jewelry, cooking with colored Al pots and kitchen utensils glazed with trace metals (Sela et al. 2013). The impact of cooking on trace metal exposure was recently demonstrated through the pan-frying and grilling of fish and shellfish: cooked products had elevated metal concentrations compared to the fresh uncooked specimens (Kalogeropoulos et al. 2012). The cooked marine species studied were shown to be good sources of the essential metals iron (Fe), zinc (Zn), and chromium and also contained low enough levels of the toxic metals cadmium, mercury, and lead so as not to pose a health risk to the consumer.

Fetuses and neonates are especially vulnerable to toxic chemicals because of the immaturity of their detoxification systems. Intake of trace metals per unit of body weight, however, is generally higher in children than in adults (Marti-Cid et al. 2007). A large number of epidemiological studies have associated early exposure to lead, mercury, arsenic (As), and cadmium with infant health effects, including neurological (Wright et al. 2006), developmental (Gundacker et al. 2010), and endocrine disorders (Stasenko et al. 2010). However, micronutrient malnutrition seriously threatens the health and productivity of more than 2 billion people worldwide. Fortification of foods offers one way to address micronutrient deficiencies in a cost-effective manner (Darnton-Hill et al. 2002). In addition, during storage or baking, it does not pose any risk of substantial deteriorative effects on native mineral contents in whole wheat flour—a highly preferred food carrier for the fortification of minerals in the developing world.

Social and environmental epidemiologists underline the synergies between the biochemical environment and the social environment and stress the importance of exploring the role of environmental pollution as a contributing factor in health disparities (O'Neill et al. 2007). The socio-spatial distribution of environmental quality reveals that poor people and deprived communities experience accumulated exposure to multiple, suboptimal environmental conditions (Evans and Kantrowitz 2002): proximity to hazardous waste facilities and busy roads, flood risk, and air quality (Walker and Burningham 2011). For trace metals, negative associations have also been found between socio-economic status and internal concentrations of lead (Elreedy et al. 1999) and cadmium (McKelvey et al. 2007) in adult populations in the United States. The negative relation between socioeconomic status and cadmium or lead (where higher socioeconomic status equals lower exposure) may largely be explained by age, gender, smoking behavior, and the residential area of the adolescent (Morrens et al. 2012).

Hair is considered a suitable biomarker of chronic exposure to many toxic elements (Ag, Al, As, Au, Cd, Cr, Cu, Fe, Hg, Mn, Ni, Pb, Se, Tl, and Zn) and can thus be applied to environmental biomonitoring and forensic medicine (Ochi et al. 2011). This technique was employed in a recent study by Dongarra et al. (2012), conducted in Sicily, and demonstrates how trace mineral levels measured in children's scalp hair varied as a result of environmental contexts. For example, a significant percentage (10–30%) of hair samples taken from one site was found to contain concentrations of aluminum, rubidium, lead, arsenic, and uranium that exceeded the coverage intervals. This is not surprising, since the rocks and therefore soils from this area contain polymetallic sulpho-salt/sulfide mineralizations. Facilitated by the considerable presence of $CO_2$ in solution, the volcano Mount Etna contains concentrations of chromium, antimony, nickel, uranium, and zinc in concentrations that are far higher than those commonly found in Sicilian groundwater (Dongarra et al. 2012).

It is well known that during infection, along with immune system activation, a sequential series of alterations in metabolism occurs, including changes in trace element balance (Corbin et al. 2008). The host's acute response to infection generally includes increased synthesis of metal-binding proteins and a concomitant flux of trace elements between blood and tissues. Necessary for the proper functioning of the immune system, metal ions may have a significant influence on the interaction between bacteria and host. Below I present a short description of the most common trace metals as well as their relation with dietary intake and, when data are available, lifestyle and human activities.

## Arsenic

Human exposure to inorganic arsenic, a known carcinogen, occurs predominately through diet and drinking water. Early in pregnancy, moderate exposure to As-contaminated drinking water has been associated with an increased risk for experiencing nausea, vomiting, and abdominal cramping (Kile et al. 2014). Studies in mice have shown that As exposure during pregnancy reduced the clearance of and exacerbated the inflammatory response to influenza A, and resulted in acute and long-term changes in lung mechanics and airway structure (Ramsey et al. 2013). Long-term exposure to high levels of arsenic is associated with increased risk for cardiovascular disease and mortality, although the risk from long-term exposure to low or moderate As levels (< 100 μg/l in drinking water) is unclear. Dietary exposure to organic forms of arsenic occurs primarily through the ingestion of seafood. Many researchers have reported that urinary dimethylated As levels are increased by seafood intake. In Korea, seaweed is consumed by itself as an ingredient in soup stock and processed foods. Thus, Korean dietary habits may be responsible for the increased urinary dimethylated As levels that have been reported within this population (Lee et al. 2012). Seaweed is also consumed in other Asian countries (e.g., Japan and China). Accordingly, urinary dimethylated As levels may be higher in East Asian countries than in Europe and North America.

## Cadmium

Cadmium, a toxic and carcinogenic heavy metal, is released into the environment as a result of industrial and agricultural activities (Jarup and Akesson 2009). Multiple mechanisms potentially link cadmium with carcinogenesis, including oxidative stress and inflammation (Lag et al. 2010), interference with DNA repair (Asmuss et al. 2000), and alterations of DNA methylation (Takiguchi et al. 2003). Recently it was suggested that HIV-infected patients have higher levels of cadmium in their blood when compared to non-HIV infected individuals, although the cause of this accumulation remains undetermined. Increased levels of cadmium in HIV-infected individuals could contribute to the higher prevalence of chronic diseases among these subjects (Xu et al. 2013). In addition, Cd-induced oxidative stress directly increases the ability of influenza virus to replicate in host cells, thus suggesting that exposure to heavy metals could result in increased severity of virus-induced respiratory diseases (Checconi et al. 2013).

Smoking is a major source for Cd exposure (Bjermo et al. 2013). However, diet can significantly influence Cd uptake. Mollusks, crustaceans, cereals, bread, potatoes, and leafy vegetables have been described as the major dietary Cd sources. Together, vegetables and grains contribute daily, on average, 66% of estimated dietary cadmium. Higher Cd levels have been observed in individuals who consume less discretionary foods (i.e., sweets, bakery products, processed meats, snack foods, etc.) (Bjermo et al. 2013). These individuals may have a healthier lifestyle because of their higher fiber intake, as another observational study (Berglund et al. 1994) demonstrated that high fiber intake inhibited the gastrointestinal absorption of cadmium.

Women are known to be more significantly impacted by Cd exposure than men. Although only approximately 5% of cadmium ingested through food is actually absorbed, Cd absorption is potentiated by low Fe stores. Lower Fe stores of women may, in part, be the reason that women are consistently observed to have higher average urine and blood Cd concentrations (Akesson et al. 2002). Cadmium and Fe homeostasis have been linked by other studies.

For example, plasma ferritin levels were inversely related with cadmium. This is probably due to the up-regulation of transporters caused by low Fe stores influencing Cd absorption (Vahter et al. 2007).

In addition to the gender-specific differential accumulation of cadmium observed by previous studies, Cd levels within the human body are influenced by other biological factors. For example, Cd levels increase with age. This is primarily an effect of the very long half-life at which this element is retained within the human body. A recent study (Ellis et al. 2012) has shown evidence that an NMR-based metabolic profiling strategy in an uncontrolled human population is capable of identifying intermediate biomarkers of response to toxicants at true environmental concentrations. In particular, citrate levels retained a significant correlation to urinary cadmium and smoking status after controlling for age and sex. Oxidative stress (as determined by urinary 8-oxodeoxyguanosine levels) was elevated in individuals with high Cd exposure, thus supporting the hypothesis that trace metal accumulation causes mitochondrial dysfunction.

## Cobalt

Cobalt (Co), an essential element, is a central bonding atom for vitamin B12 (also called cobalamin), which is necessary for the metabolism of folates and fatty acids. The biological functions and activities of cobalt play a role in erythropoiesis, the regulation of various phosphoprotein phosphatases, and as a substitute for zinc in metalloenzymes. Recently, Hoffman et al. (2013) demonstrated that certain Co(II) and Cu(II) metal-based complexes possess antimicrobial action with notable selectivity and marked potency against *Mycobacterium tuberculosis*, including multidrug-resistant strains. These complexes were confirmed to be bacteriocidal and not affected by efflux inhibitors.

In food of animal origin, cobalt is found as cobalamin, whereas in plants it is present in an inorganic form. The gastrointestinal absorption of cobalt in humans is highly variable (18–97%), depending on its chemical form. The highest mean concentrations are found in chocolate (0.139 mg/kg), offal (0.091 mg/kg), and butter (0.046 mg/kg). The mean exposure of a French population to cobalt was estimated at 0.18 μg/kg/day in adults and 0.31 μg/kg/day in children. The main contributor to cobalt intake in adults was coffee (11%). For children, chocolate was the main contributor (12%) (Arnich et al. 2012). While no Co deficiency has been shown in humans, excess Co exposure could be detrimental. In humans, cardiomyopathies were reported in the 1960s in heavy drinkers of beer to which Co had been added as a foam stabilizer. It was calculated that these drinkers had ingested an average of 0.04–0.14 mg Co/kg/ day for several years. However, the risk that has been associated with dietary exposure to cobalt does not seem to constitute a major public health issue with regard to threshold effects.

# Copper

Copper (Cu) is an essential redox active metal that is potentially toxic in excess. Multicellular organisms acquire copper from the diet and must regulate Cu uptake, storage, distribution, and export at both the cellular and organismal levels. Systemic Cu deficiency can be fatal, as seen in Menkes disease patients. Conversely, Cu toxicity occurs in patients with Wilson disease. In addition, Cu dyshomeostasis has been implicated in neurodegenerative disorders such as Alzheimer disease. It has been reported that smoking increases plasma levels of copper and that these levels are positively correlated with Cu/Zn-SOD activity. Both plasma Cu and Cu/Zn-SOD activities have been shown to increase in response to the chronic inflammation of the respiratory tract found in smokers (Northrop-Clewes and Thurnham 2007).

In addition to environmental factors, such as smoking, there are several significant dietary sources of copper. In a recent study, Cu, Mn, Se, and Zn levels were determined in fresh, canned, and frozen fish and shellfish products (Olmedo et al. 2013). The highest concentrations of copper were found in crustacean species (shrimp and prawn), as they have hemocyanin (a Cu-containing protein) which functions as an oxygen transport molecule. Data from the Nutrient Data Laboratory of the U.S. Department of Agriculture indicate that dark chocolate ranges from 1.0 to 1.8 mg Cu/100 g, depending on the content of cocoa solids. Thus 100 g of dark chocolate can provide more than the recommended dietary allowance (RDA) of copper (0.9 mg), and the darkest chocolate can double that amount. Even when diluted with sugar and milk, chocolate can provide an appreciable supplement of copper.

Copper plays an important role in public health. A considerable body of evidence from laboratory-based studies demonstrates that Cu alloys are efficacious against a diverse range of pathogenic microorganisms. Early studies demonstrated a rapid killing of *Escherichia coli* O157, *Listeria monocytogenes*, and methicillin-resistant *Staphylococcus aureus* in the presence of copper (Noyce et al. 2006; Wilks et al. 2006; Warnes et al. 2012). This was followed by observations that both vegetative cells and spores of virulent toxin-producing *Clostridium difficile*, which is responsible for numerous hospital-acquired infections, were destroyed after Cu treatment (Weaver et al. 2008).

It was previously demonstrated that a family of small peptides called trefoil factors (TFFs), implicated in the maintenance of the integrity of gastrointestinal tissue, are able specifically to bind Cu ions at the carboxy-terminus and that Cu binding favors the homodimerization of the peptide, thus enhancing its motogenic activity (Tosco et al. 2010b). The finding that copper can influence expression (Tosco et al. 2010a), biological activity, and structure of TFF1 prompted researchers to use copper to investigate the effect of homodimerization of TFF1 on the interaction between *Helicobacter pylori* and the peptide (Montefusco et al. 2013). Thus, it was demonstrated that the Cu-TFF1 complex promotes *H. pylori* colonization of gastric epithelial cells and a mucus-secreting cell line (Montefusco et al. 2013).

## Iron

The adult human body contains 3–4 g of iron, approximately 70% of which is present in hemoglobin (Hb) in red blood cells and myoglobin in muscle. Iron is instrumental for the transport of oxygen around the body and is an essential component of many enzymes, such as cytochromes, where it plays a role in electron transport, respiration, and hormone synthesis. Iron deficiency affects almost 50% of the population worldwide, making it the most common nutritional deficiency (Zimmermann and Hurrell 2007). Iron-deficiency anemia is the end state of Fe deficiency, and there is a clear gender difference with Fe deficiency being most prevalent among women (Zimmermann and Hurrell 2007). Recently, it was demonstrated that *H. pylori* infection in children influences the serum ferritin and Hb concentrations, markers of early depletion of Fe stores and anemia, respectively (Queiroz et al. 2013). In addition, Fe overload is associated with significant morbidity and mortality. Abnormal accumulation of brain iron has been detected in various neurodegenerative diseases, but the contribution of Fe overload to pathology remains unclear (Rouault 2013).

Good food sources of iron include meat and meat products that contain heme Fe, especially red meat and offal as well as dark poultry meat, oily fish (e.g., tuna and sardines), cereal products (e.g., fortified breakfast cereals), eggs, and dark green vegetables. Since vegetarians do not consume meat, their main sources of iron must come from fortified cereals, soybeans, tofu, lentils, kidney beans, chickpeas, baked beans, and dark green vegetables. Bread, potatoes, and dried fruit are also a useful source of iron. For elderly people, obtaining an adequate supply of iron may be a challenge due to impaired absorption, reduced food intake associated with lower physical activity, and changes in dietary patterns that result in a more limited diet.

In addition to dietary sources impacting Fe stores within humans, other environmental and biological factors affect Fe levels. For example, it is known that serum Fe decreases during active training; this is probably due to the inflammatory response of physical activity (Peeling et al. 2008). Intense physical training can induce a two- to threefold increase in proinflammatory cytokine levels of tumor necrosis factor alpha and interleukin (IL)-1b (Ostrowski et al. 1998) as well as the cytokine IL-6 (Helge et al. 2003). The increase in inflammatory cytokines, especially IL-6, stimulates the synthesis of hepcidin, a key regulator of Fe metabolism (Peeling 2010), thus leading to lower levels of iron and transferrin. In a recent report, Kim et al. (2014) describe the mechanism of Fe homeostasis in response to *Salmonella enterica* var. Typhimurium (*S. typhimurium*) infection, an intramacrophage bacterium. They showed that the estrogen-related receptor $\gamma$ (ERR$\gamma$) modulates the intramacrophage proliferation of *S. typhimurium* by altering host Fe homeostasis, therefore demonstrating an antimicrobial effect of an ERRγ inverse agonist.

## Manganese

Manganese is an essential nutrient involved in the metabolism of amino acids, proteins, and lipids. In excess, however, manganese can be a potent neurotoxicant. Occupational and environmental exposure to airborne manganese has been associated with neurobehavioral deficits in adults and children (Riojas-Rodriguez et al. 2010). Manganese is commonly found in groundwater because of the weathering and leaching of Mn-bearing minerals and rocks into aquifers. Within these waters, Mn concentrations can vary by several orders of magnitude; however, exposure to manganese at levels commonly found in many groundwater sources has been associated with intellectual impairment in children (Bouchard et al. 2011).

Previous studies have reported a relationship between the concentration of manganese in drinking water and the Mn levels present in hair (Bouchard et al. 2007). In addition, it was recently found that the biological samples (scalp hair, blood, and urine) of male HIV-1 patients contained significantly lower concentrations of manganese and chromium compared to control subjects (Afridi et al. 2014). Hence, the lower levels of these trace elements may be predictors for secondary infections in HIV-1 patients. The chemical form of manganese, notably the valence state and solubility, might modify its toxicity (Michalke et al. 2007). Moreover, Mn absorption is decreased in the digestive system with concurrent intake of dietary fiber, oxalic acids, tannins, and phytic acids (Gibson 1994). Gender differences of Mn levels show contradictory results: in Korean populations, men show higher levels compared to women (Lee et al. 2012) whereas in Caucasian populations, women have higher blood Mn levels than men (Clark et al. 2007).

Within a human host, Mn levels are likely to impact microbial growth during infection. It has been shown that manganese is sequestered from sites of infection through the action of a host-derived immune-associated protein known as calprotectin in a murine model of staphylococcal infection (Corbin et al. 2008). The antimicrobial effect of this Mn sequestration is further highlighted by the fact that the staphylococcal Mn acquisition systems MntABC and MntH were required for *S. aureus* survival in mice expressing calprotectin, but were expendable in calprotectin-deficient animals (Kehl-Fie et al. 2013).

## Molybdenum

Molybdenum (Mo) is a trace element and an essential nutrient in the human diet. It is a cofactor for the enzymes xanthine oxidase, sulfite oxidase, and aldehyde oxidase, which are involved in the metabolism of sulfur-containing amino acids, purines, and pyrimidines. A dose-dependent trend between molybdenum and declined sperm concentration and normal morphology has been reported (Meeker et al. 2008). Significant sources of molybdenum (as soluble molybdates) in the human diet are leafy vegetables, legumes, organ meats, grain products, cow's milk, and eggs. The Mo content in food sources varies, depending on the amount that has been taken up from the soil. Before weaning, an infant's primary Mo sources derive from breast milk and infant formula (both cow-milk and soy-based types). In an ongoing study of premature, hospitalized infants, Abramovich et al. (2011) recorded daily intake of formula and breast milk. Based on the intake data and the infants' average weight measured midterm of the hospitalization stay, mean Mo intakes per day and per kilogram bodyweight were calculated. Abramovich et al. (2011) report that the mean Mo content in soy-based and cow-milk formulas intended for the feeding of full-term or premature infants is higher than in human milk. Despite lower bioavailability of molybdenum from formula compared with human milk, the high intake may pose health risks, especially for premature infants due to immaturity of their compensatory mechanisms.

One of the enzymatic functions of bacteria enabled by molybdenum is anaerobic respiration. Anaerobic respiration has been shown to contribute to intestinal disease due to the fact that anaerobically respiring pathogens can outcompete beneficial gut microorganisms when alternative electron acceptors are provided during intestinal inflammation. This process has been disrupted in mutant pathogens with dysfunctional Mo homeostasis (Winter et al. 2013). These findings indicate that dietary molybdenum may play a role in gut disease associated with inflammation-induced dysbiosis.

## Nickel

Exposure to nickel (Ni) increased significantly during the twentieth century because of its common applications (Vahter et al. 2007). Typically, nickel is utilized in metallurgical processes for the production of alloys such as stainless steel (Sharma 2007). The release of nickel into the environment occurs from various sources: metallurgy and refining industries, coal combustion, diesel and fuel oil as well as sewage. Nickel and its compounds are bioaccumulated by the human body through inhalation, ingestion, and dermal absorption. It is considered a carcinogenic agent and is the fourth most frequent contact allergen (Nohynek et al. 2004). Humans are exposed to nickel through food, jewelry, coins, and dental restorations (Vahter et al. 2007). Food which contains considerable amounts of nickel include cacao, dark chocolate, nuts, almonds, soya beans, oatmeal, spinach, tea leaves as well as fresh and dried legumes (Sharma 2007). In addition, Torjussen et al. (2003) report that cigarette smoking is a possible source of Ni exposure and conclude that Ni exposure from smoking is greater than occupational or workplace exposure. Other sources of Ni exposure included photocopiers, PVC and Cu pipes, and amalgam fillings (dental amalgam contains about 50% Hg as well as other toxic metals—Sn, Cu, Ni, and Pd). The literature reports that females more frequently suffer from Ni-induced dermatitis than males (10–20%, 1–5%, respectively) (Picarelli et al. 2011). In a recent study from Poland, Michalak et al. (2012) demonstrated that the type of water-supply system influenced Ni content in hair. The highest content was observed when PVC pipes were present, followed by Cu and finally steel pipes. Gender differences have also been recorded: the hair of females contained statistically higher Ni levels than the hair of males.

One of the most established links between Ni exposure and infection is that of *H. pylori* colonization of the human stomach. The *H. pylori* eradication rate with standard triple therapy is very low. *H. pylori* is known to require the Ni-containing metalloenzymes urease and NiFe-hydrogenase to survive the low pH environment in the stomach. Very recently, the addition of a Ni-free diet to standard triple therapy was shown to significantly increase *H. pylori* eradication rates (Campanale et al. 2014). The reduction of *H. pylori* urease activity due to the Ni-free diet could expose the bacterium to gastric acid and increase the susceptibility of *H. pylori* to amoxicillin treatment.

## Selenium

In terms of its nutritional value and pathophysiological effects, more controversies are associated with selenium (Se) than with any other trace element. The history of its research is a continuous twist between toxicity and essentiality (Stathopoulou et al. 2012). Some studies have suggested a role of selenoproteins in the prevention of chronic degenerative disorders, including Parkinson and Alzheimer diseases, cancer, cardiovascular disease, atherosclerosis, stroke, and infertility. Children with recurrent wheezing were found to have lower hair Se levels than healthy children, thus suggesting a potential link between Se and infection (Razi et al. 2012). In antiretroviral therapy-naive HIV-infected adults, 24-month supplementation with a mixture containing multivitamins and selenium was shown to reduce the risk of immune decline and morbidity significantly (Baum et al. 2013). Concerns, however, have been raised about a possible association between Se supplementation and an increased risk of developing insulin resistance and type 2 diabetes (Sabino et al. 2013).

Dietary Se intake is determined by its content in different foods, the bioavailability of its chemical forms, and the dietary patterns adopted by different populations. The Se content of foods varies according to soil concentration of selenium. Several physicochemical properties of soil (e.g., pH and moisture) can also affect the entrance of selenium into the food chain. Geochemical mapping of selenium has revealed areas that are poor in selenium (e.g., Scandinavia,

New Zealand, certain parts of China) and seleniferous areas (e.g., certain parts of United States, Canada, China and South America). The corresponding dietary intakes vary respectively: from 3 μg/day in Se-poor areas of China to 350 μg/day in Colombia (Rayman 2008). However, the enrichment of soils with Se-containing fertilizers and the use of supplements in animal agriculture have partially overcome low intakes due to Se-poor soils (Combs 2001). Nevertheless, the determination of daily Se intake by food frequency questionnaires is almost impossible because the amount of selenium differs greatly among the same foods, and nutritional tables are unreliable for this trace element. Beef, white bread, pork, chicken, eggs, and fish seem to be the main contributors of selenium in a typical Western diet; Brazil nuts have the highest Se content among all foods (Navarro-Alarcon and Cabrera-Vique 2008). The contribution of fish and shellfish products to the RDA and adequate intakes of copper, manganese, selenium, and zinc range from 2.5% (Mn) to 25.4% (Se) (Olmedo et al. 2013).

## Vanadium

Vanadium (V) is an important trace element responsible for maintaining normal biological systems and body functions in humans. It has been reported that V compounds exhibit an insulin-like function or an antidiabetic effect in rats (Domingo 2002). The best food sources of vanadium are mushrooms, shellfish, black pepper, parsley, dill weed, beer, wine, grain and grain products, and artificially sweetened drinks. Vanadium exists in several forms, including vanadyl sulfate and vanadate. Vanadyl sulfate is most commonly found in nutritional supplements. The average diet provides 6–18 mg per day. Dietary vanadium in excess of 30 mg/kg can alter the amount and diversity of intestinal bacteria in avian broilers, implying that the structure and initial balance in the intestinal microbiota are disrupted (Wang et al. 2012b). These findings could have significant implications to human health because many foodborne infectious diseases originate from the gut microbiota of food animals. If these findings extend to humans, a similar V-induced dysbiosis in the human gut microbiota could lead to intestinal disease. As vanadyl sulfate, vanadium is a trace mineral associated with sugar regulation. It is believed to regulate fasting blood sugar levels and improve receptor sensitivity to insulin (Boden et al. 1996; Schulz et al. 1998). Based on available research, vanadyl sulfate appears to be a useful intervention for type 2 diabetic individuals with insulin resistance.

## Zinc

Zinc is an essential trace element for all organisms, and its content in the human body is 2–3 g. The greatest amount is stored in skeletal muscle and bones:

11% of the total-body zinc is localized in the liver and skin, and only 0.1% is found within the plasma (Tuerk and Fazel 2009). Zinc is present in all food groups, yet the main dietary sources include oysters, red meat, poultry, fish, seafood, legumes, nuts, whole grains, and dairy products. The RDA for zinc is 8 and 11 mg for adult women and men, respectively; however, these values can range from as high as 12–14 mg for women during pregnancy and breast-feeding to as low as 2–9 mg during childhood and adolescence (Trumbo et al. 2001). Zinc homeostasis is regulated via the gastrointestinal tract, including the coordinated functions of many transporters. All Zn transporters have transmembrane domains and are encoded by two gene families: ZnT and Zip (Sandstrom and Cederblad 1980). Zinc homeostasis is impaired in diabetic animals and humans; type 2 diabetes is associated with decreased plasma Zn levels (Jansen et al. 2009). In a European cohort, Marcellini et al. (2006) found that psychological functions were related to Zn deficiency that resulted from a reduced intake and less variety of foods rich in zinc. This phenomenon was more evident in Greece and Poland than in other European countries (Italy and France) (Marcellini et al. 2006). Consistent findings from several Zn supplementation trials in humans and animal models support the idea that zinc offers protection against cellular oxidation and type 2 diabetes (Mariani et al. 2008).

In addition, Zn deficiency may play an important role in susceptibility to infections, since zinc is essential for numerous immune functions (Ibs and Rink 2003). Although nutritional deficiencies are often associated with inadequate food intake and poor dietary quality, many studies have shown that other factors (e.g., intestinal parasites) play an important role as predictors of such deficiencies (Hesham et al. 2004). A consistent change in Zn level in the blood of children infected with *Giardia lamblia* has been noted and eradication of *G. lamblia* led to a significant improvement in the mean serum Zn levels six months after treatment in school children (Quihui et al. 2010). This intestinal parasite causes a generally self-limited clinical illness characterized by diarrhea, abdominal cramps, bloating, weight loss, and malabsorption. However, for reasons that remain obscure, asymptomatic giardiasis with high reinfection rates occurs frequently, especially in developing countries (Cotton et al. 2011).

# 12

# Obesity, Trace Metals, and Infection

Jerome O. Nriagu

## Abstract

Trace metals are required in small quantities for a wide array of metabolic functions in the body. In terms of obesity, they can enhance insulin action through activating insulin receptor sites, serve as cofactors or components for enzyme systems involved in glucose metabolism, increase insulin sensitivity, and act as antioxidants to prevent tissue oxidation. Chronic hyperglycemia causes significant alterations in the status of many trace metals in the body and consequently increases the oxidative stress which can contribute to the pathogenesis of infectious diseases. Whether obese individuals with trace metal deficiency (or toxicity) are at increased risk for infection is a matter of concern in many developing countries, where a growing segment of the population (exposed to traditional health risks) has embraced Western dietary habits. A better understanding of the roles of different trace metals will undoubtedly facilitate the development of new treatment and prevention strategies that can more effectively reduce the silent burden of comorbid obesity and infectious diseases.

## Introduction

This chapter addresses the risk overlap and role of metals at the confluence of First and Third World disease risks. With rapid evolution of the socioeconomic structures and impressive urbanization rates, major chronic degenerative diseases have spread epidemically in many developing countries. We are now witnessing the emergence of a new, highly complex, and challenging pathocenosis in these countries, where comparatively "new" disorders once associated with a "Western" lifestyle (e.g., obesity, diabetes, and immune disorders) coexist rampantly with acute and chronic diseases typical of traditional societies (e.g., malaria, schistosomiasis, viral hepatitis, and other infectious diseases). A matter of critical interest is whether trace metals can play a mediating role when these two nosologic entities are superimposed.

The two strongest selection pressures in human evolution were probably a robust immune response capable of clearing bacterial, viral, and parasitic infection and an ability to store nutrients efficiently to survive times when food sources were scarce (Johnson et al. 2012). These traits have evolved in their relationships over time. Recent studies have shown that the critical proteins necessary for regulating energy metabolism—such as peroxisome proliferator-activated receptors, Toll-like receptors, and fatty acid-binding proteins—also act as links between nutrient metabolism and activation of chronic inflammation in immune cells (Nieman et al. 1999; Keaney et al. 2003; Matsuzawa-Nagata et al. 2008). Expression of these proteins and their metabolism depend on an optimum supply of essential trace elements being available and the absence of large amounts of the toxic metals. Evolutionary selection led to a phenotype characterized by efficient energy storage and the formation of insulin resistance, both of which activate inflammatory cells; this could be considered a protective mechanism that coevolved to repartition energy sources within the body during times of nutritional stress and infection (Johnson et al. 2012; Ruiz-Nunez et al. 2013). The development of insulin resistance could also be considered a survival strategy aimed at reallocating the energy-rich nutrients that result from an activated immune system, limiting the immune response and repairing the inflicted damage, among other things (Ruiz-Nunez et al. 2013). I argue that in ancient times, inflammatory cell activation and insulin resistance were maintained largely by trace metal homeostasis, through regulation by the metabolic cycles of iron and zinc in particular. Modern lifestyles have managed to introduce a number of false inflammatory triggers, characterized by a lack of inflammation-suppressing factors, which have led to an imbalance: energy intake now far exceeds energy output. We have reached a point where a once beneficial adaptive trait has become very detrimental to our health.

The risk factors most commonly proposed for the recent increase in the prevalence of obesity include, but are not limited to, increased availability of energy-dense food items, increased portion sizes (especially in commercially marketed food items), abnormal dietary composition (especially as fast foods), the built environment, and physical inactivity (Poskitt 2014). When an inflammatory disease spreads like an epidemic over a short period of time, it needs to be scrutinized for environmental causes and infectious implications. The changes in environmental exposures and dietary intake from trace metals in Western foods have impacted the obesity epidemic and this deserves some attention. This is especially true considering that systemic low-grade inflammation, altered immune response, and oxidative stress are common features shared by obesity, many infectious diseases, and a dysregulated system of metal homeostasis. What is currently emerging in the scientific literature is that disruption in trace metal homeostasis can impair the immune function of adipose tissue in obesity and, consequently, exacerbate certain infections.

The mediating role of metals in comorbidity of obesity and infectious diseases should not be a matter of "if" but rather a question of "how much."

## Obesity and Infections

Although obesity is a well-documented risk factor for metabolic and cardiovascular problems, its impacts on susceptibility to infectious diseases are just beginning to receive attention (Anaya and Dellinger 2006; Falagas and Kompoti 2006; Smith et al. 2007). Studies in hospital settings report that obese patients are more likely to develop secondary infections and complications such as sepsis, pneumonia, bacteremia, as well as wound and catheter-related infections (Karlsson and Beck 2010). Hospitalized obese patients have been reported to be at increased risk for pulmonary aspiration and community-related respiratory tract infections (Koenig 2001; Jubber 2004). Increased susceptibility to acute respiratory tract infection has been shown to be associated with body mass index (BMI) in overweight children (Jedrychowski et al. 1998). Obese individuals are at increased risk for *Helicobacter pylori* infection (Arslan et al. 2009), and children with increased BMI have been found to be at greater risk of being asymptomatic carriers of *Neisseria meningitidis* (Uberos et al. 2010). Case control studies have shown an increased risk of cellulitis and skin infections in overweight and obese cases (Karppelin et al. 2010; Bjornsdottir et al. 2005). Morbid obesity has been shown to be an independent risk factor for increased severity of infection and death from a recent H1N1 pandemic influenza strain (Morgan et al. 2010). In addition, increased BMI has been associated with greater risk for several other bacterial infections, including periodontal infections, *Staphylococcus aureus* nasal carriage, and gastric infection by *H. pylori* (Herwaldt et al. 2004; Ylostalo et al. 2008). One study found that obesity was significantly associated with herpes simplex virus 1 infection (Karjala et al. 2011). Reported results (Huttunen and Syrjanen 2013) regarding the association between obesity and the risk and outcome of community-acquired infections (e.g., pneumonia, bacteremia, sepsis, and as well as the course of HIV infection) are still equivocal.

Weber et al. (1985) were the first study to describe a relationship between vaccine response and obesity, and they found that higher BMI was the single best predictor of failure to develop detectable antibody to serum-derived hepatitis B vaccine in health-care workers. Further studies have subsequently confirmed the association between obesity and poor antibody response to hepatitis B vaccines (Roome et al. 1993; Wood et al. 1993; Simo-Minana et al. 1996; Young et al. 2001). Other than responses to hepatitis B vaccines, there have been few studies on vaccine efficacy in the obese host. Eliakim et al. (2006) demonstrated that antibody response to standard tetanus immunization was lower in overweight 13-year-olds compared to age-matched controls.

Dinelli and Moraes-Pinto (2008) reported that an obese female remained non-responsive, even following six doses of hepatitis B vaccine. The fact that there has been no published study of BMI in relation to the efficacy of influenza vaccination is a serious oversight. These studies with hepatitis B suggest that vaccine responses in obese individuals may be very different from vaccine responses in lean individuals (Karlsson and Beck 2010). If obese individuals who are immuno compromised do indeed have poor vaccine responsiveness, then they may not be receiving the full benefits of our current immunization protocols.

A number of studies with genetically obese animals consistently find reduced resistance to bacterial and viral infections, consistent with observations in human subjects. These studies often use mouse models lacking leptin (ob/ob), an important adipokine, or the leptin receptor (db/db). Experiments with ob/ob mice have found increased susceptibility to a number of different bacterial infections including *Mycobacterium abscessus*, *Klebsiella pneumoniae*, *Streptococcus pneumoniae*, and *M. tuberculosis* (Wieland et al. 2005; Hsu et al. 2007). Other studies, however, have found no differences in bacterial growth in ob/ob mice challenged with the *K. pneumoniae* and *S. pneumoniae* strains (Mancuso et al. 2002; Wieland et al. 2005; Hsu et al. 2007; Ordway et al. 2008). Experiments with db/db mice have reported increased susceptibility to *S. aureus* and *H. pylori*, and increased susceptibility to *Listeria monocytogenes* has been reported in both ob/ob and db/db mice (Ikejima et al. 2005; Wehrens et al. 2008; Park et al. 2009). Increased susceptibility to viral myocarditis induced by coxsackievirus B468 as well as encephalomyocarditis virus has been reported in studies with ob/ob mice (Kanda 2004). Diet-induced obese animal models have been used to assess the effects of chronic overnutrition, and such studies have yielded confirmatory results. As with the genetically obese model, diet-induced obese mice are more susceptible to bacterial infection, including infection with *Porphyromonas gingivalis* and *S. aureus*-induced sepsis (Amar et al. 2007; Strandberg et al. 2009).

Studies over the past three decades also suggest that some microbes may promote obesity in animals and humans, a phenomenon called "infectobesity" (Dhurander 2011). Germ-free mice are resistant to diet-induced obesity, suggesting that specific microbes may cause adiposities (Backhed et al. 2007; Nathan 2008). Induction of obesity in mice experimentally infected with canine distemper virus was the first report of infectobesity (Lyons et al. 1982; Dhurander 2011). Subsequent studies have shown that several viruses, bacteria, parasites, and scrapie agents can cause obesity in chicken, rodents, and nonhuman primates (Cani et al. 2007). In addition, a number of microbes, including *Chlamydia pneumoniae*, *Selenomonas noxia*, *H. pylori*, and herpes simplex virus 1 or 2, have been associated with human obesity (Dart et al. 2002; Fernandez-Real et al. 2007; Arslan et al. 2009). Adenoviruses are, however, the only human pathogens that are causatively and correlatively linked with animal and human obesity and seem to directly influence the adipose tissue (Hegde and Dhurander 2013).

## Obesity and Trace Metals

Recent studies of early life exposure to environmental chemicals are beginning to provide interesting information on the potentially important role of pre- and perinatal metabolic programming as a risk factor for obesity later in life (Merrill and Birnbaum 2011). A review of metabolic programming and how early life exposure to the "obesogenic" trace metals might be setting the stage for weight gain later in life was recently published by Merrill and Birnbaum (2011). From this review, the two most important obesogenic "metals" that have been identified are organotins and lead. Male mice and male rats exposed to tributyl tin (TBT) during puberty were found to show increased body mass, associated with increased relative fat mass (Makita et al. 2005; Si et al. 2011; Zuo et al. 2011). Two other studies, however, found opposite effects of TBT exposure on the body weights of female rats (Cooke et al. 2004). Cell culture models support a role of developmental exposure to organotins in obesity. TBT also induces adipogenesis in multipotent stem cells of mice and humans, while both TBT and triphenyltin (TPT) induce differentiation of 3T3-L1 adipocytes (Kirchner et al. 2010).

Although some evidence suggests that Pb exposure may also influence the risk of obesity, most of the human data on the association between developmental Pb exposure and obesity is equivocal. Lead levels in the teeth of male and female children in the United States are positively associated with BMI measured at the same time (Kim et al. 1995). A cross-sectional study found no association between blood Pb levels and obesity in 11-year-olds (Merrill and Birnbaum 2011); however, another study of adults showed a marginally significant inverse dose-response relationship between age-adjusted patella Pb levels in adulthood and abdominal obesity (Hu et al. 1998; Park et al. 2006). Results of animal research are consistent with an early-life susceptibility to Pb-associated adiposity and suggests there is a gender effect (Leasure et al. 2008).

While much remains to be learned about early life exposure to obesogenic metals and infectious diseases, numerous studies have reported on the influencing effects of deficiencies in essential trace metals in obese individuals in many parts of the world. A few studies have even suggested that adiposity increases the susceptibility to metal toxicity (Huang et al. 2007; Wildman and Mao 2001; Guerrero-Romero et al. 2006; Komolova et al. 2008). An interesting trend that has been noted is that the rates of obesity are increasing more rapidly in regions of the world where micronutrient deficiencies are more prevalent (Monteiro et al. 2004). This pattern could suggest that (a) the micronutrient deficiencies of individuals in these communities may be contributing to the increase in obesity rates or that (b) the correction of native deficiencies with

Western metal-enriched foods itself is the risk factor for obesity. It is not clear whether such deficiencies in obese individuals are the result of inadequate intake relative to overall body mass and/or are due to alterations in the metabolism and excretion of the trace metals. This question is further complicated by the uncertainty as to how to assess and define the optimal status of trace elements in obese individuals.

Documentation of the influencing factor of Zn status on obesity has come from studies of animal models and human subjects (reviewed by García et al. 2009). A number of epidemiological studies have reported that low Zn intake and low Zn concentrations in blood and other biological fluids are associated with increased prevalence of obesity and diabetes (common comorbid conditions). Obesity has been associated with hypozincemia in Italian (Di Martino et al. 1993), Turkish (Ozata et al. 2002), Thai (Tungtrongchitr et al. 2003), Indian (Singh et al. 1998), and Taiwanese (Chen et al. 1996) adult populations, as well as in Turkish children (Yakinci et al. 1997). A study in Guatemala found that Zn-deficient children were more obese than children with adequate Zn nutrition (Cavan et al. 1993), and a study by Arsenault et al. (2007) reported a higher increase in fat-free mass among a subset of children with mild-to-moderate stunting who received liquid zinc compared to children who were not stunted and who also received zinc.

Zinc is an antioxidant, hence its deficiency has been associated with increased oxidative stress and the inflammatory response in obese individuals (Sprietsma 1999; DiSilvestro 2000; Ozata et al. 2002; Tungtrongchitr et al. 2003; Cunningham-Rundles et al. 2005). Suboptimal Zn intake has been associated with low superoxide dismutase (SOD) activity in overweight and obese individuals (Tungtrongchitr et al. 2003). Another study found that blood concentrations of zinc, SOD, and glutathione peroxidase were significantly lower in obese men compared to a control group (Ozata et al. 2002). The available literature thus implicates Zn deficiency as influencing inflammation. Animal models suggest that Zn deficiency can lead to reduced lean body mass and increased body fat, which may be risk factors for obesity (García et al. 2009). During the initial stage of an infection, levels of zinc (and other essential trace metals) decline rapidly as the metals are redistributed to the point of infection, to boost immunity, and into tissues (especially liver), so as to deny bioavailable trace metals to the infecting pathogens. Furthermore, mobilization of zinc into the cellular compartment may be required to facilitate gene transcription and protein production, including the synthesis of adipocytes (especially leptin and adiponectin), insulin-degrading enzymes, and acute phase proteins (APPs) (Liu et al. 2013). These are also common presentations in obesity.

In obese individuals, Fe deficiency may result from low Fe intake, reduced Fe absorption, and the sequestration of Fe as a result of chronic inflammation (Yanoff et al. 2007; Zimmermann et al. 2008). One of the common pathologic conditions observed in obesity is systemic Fe deficiency and hypoferremia

(Nikonorov et al. 2014). Along with a large number of studies that indicate disturbed Fe homeostasis in obesity, recent data point to a cause–effect relationship between Fe status and obesity-related pathologies (Nead et al. 2004; Pinhas-Hamiel et al. 2003). Although the possibility of obesity-induced Fe-deficient anemia was debated for a long time, this hypothesis has not been confirmed through experimental data (Ausk et al. 2008; Anna et al. 2009). An association between reduced Fe concentrations in human biomarkers and obesity has been reported in a number of epidemiological studies (Seltzer and Mayer 1963; Nead et al. 2004; Chambers et al. 2006; Lecube et al. 2006; Moayeri et al. 2006). An analysis of the NHANES III data showed that children who were overweight or at risk of being overweight were twice as likely to be Fe deficient (Nead et al. 2004); another study of adults found an inverse correlation between serum Fe concentration with BMI, waist circumference, and fat mass in Hispanic women living in the United States (Chambers et al. 2006). A study of obese and nonobese postmenopausal women found significantly higher concentrations of transferrin receptors in serum of the obese women (Lecube et al. 2006). A cross-sectional study of children by Pinhas-Hamiel et al. (2003) found that low Fe concentration in blood and Fe-deficiency anemia were more common in obese children and adolescents than among normal-weight children. Zimmerman et al. (2008) showed that high BMI Z-scores were associated with decreased Fe absorption in women and reported improvement of Fe status in Fe-deficient children following intake of Fe-fortified foods.

The mutual interaction between Fe homeostasis and obesity-related pathogenesis leads to hypoferremia and results in increased adipose tissue Fe content being stored in either adipocytes or adipose tissue macrophages. The inflammation of obesity and obesity-related hepcidin and lipocalin 2 hyperproduction seem to be the most probable cause of obesity-related hypoferremia, since oversecretion of these proteins leads to Fe sequestration in reticuloendothelial system cells (Nikonorov et al. 2014). The latter also leads to increased adipose tissue Fe content, which produces preconditions for adverse effects of local Fe overload. Being a redox-active metal, iron is capable of inducing oxidative stress as well as endoplasmic reticulum stress, inflammation, and adipose tissue endocrine dysfunction. It is presumed to increase the levels of the pro-inflammatory cytokines interleukin 6 (IL-6) and tumor necrosis factor alpha (TNF-$\alpha$), which, in turn, increase the expression of hepcidin (McClung et al. 2009; García et al. 2009). Thus, the disturbance in Fe homeostasis (including both systemic hypoferremia and local adipose tissue Fe overload) and obesity pathogenesis seem to interact mutually in ways that can also influence host–pathogen interactions.

Arsenicism, from intake of inorganic arsenic in water and food, is a major health problem that is found especially in areas with high prevalence rates for infectious diseases and a growing epidemic of obesity (Nriagu et al. 2007). In recent years, increasing epidemiologic evidence from multiple countries supports the role of inorganic arsenic in the development of diabetes (reviewed by Huang et al. 2011; Wang et al. 2014). A recent meta-analysis pooled 17 published articles that reported on 2,243,745 participants and found a 13% increase in risk of type 2 diabetes mellitus for every 100 mg/l increment in concentration of inorganic arsenic in drinking water (Wang et al. 2014). Biologic evidence in support of obesogenicity of arsenic includes the fact that arsenic could affect β cell function and insulin sensitivity through several mechanisms, including oxidative stress, glucose uptake and transport, gluconeogenesis, adipocyte differentiation, and calcium signaling (Tseng 2004; Davey et al. 2007; Diaz-Villasenor et al. 2007; Maull et al. 2012; Douillet et al. 2013). Arsenic can also act as an endocrine disrupter affecting the function of hormone receptors, including glucocorticoid, androgen, estrogen, and thyroid hormone in cell culture and animal models (Bodwell et al. 2006; Davey et al. 2007). In addition, arsenic may also impact diabetes through epigenetic mechanisms, including hyper- and hypomethylation of diabetes-related genes (Smeester et al. 2011; Kuo et al. 2013).

Copper is a pro-oxidant that participates in metal-catalyzed formation of free radicals; together with zinc, copper also acts as a structural and catalytic component of some metalloenzymes (Viktorinova et al. 2009). Copper is necessary for the catalytic activity of Cu/Zn-SOD, which is involved in the protection of cells from superoxide radicals (Viktorinova et al. 2009). Zinc, on the other hand, acts as an antioxidant by protecting the sulfhydryl groups of proteins and enzymes against free radical damage in the body (DiSilvestro 2000). The protective and toxic effects of copper and zinc in the pathogenesis of obesity and diabetic complications have been documented (Walter et al. 1991; Galhardi et al. 2004; Forbes et al. 2008). In particular, the relationships of serum Cu and Zn levels with obesity and diabetes have been extensively studied; results generally show that serum Cu levels are significantly increased (reflecting oxidative status of the adipose) and Zn levels are significantly decreased in obese and diabetic adults (Zargar et al. 1998; Basaki et al. 2012; Ferdousi and Mia 2012; Naka et al. 2013).

Biologically speaking, cadmium and, to a lesser degree, mercury should be of interest in the biology of insulin-secreting β cells, because of their similarity to zinc and the importance of zinc in the physiology of β cells (Afridi et al. 2008; Eddins et al. 2008). Given that zinc is co-secreted with insulin and that β cells have to maintain a high metabolic turnover of zinc, these cells are highly vulnerable to changes in Zn homeostasis (Muayed et al. 2012). Impairment in function of insulin-producing pancreatic β cells has been proposed to be one of the underlying causes of diabetic complication in obesity (Huang and Arvan 1995). The recent study by Muayed et al. (2012) reported that mouse β cells accumulated cadmium in a dose- and time-dependent manner over a prolonged period of time. In this study, Cd uptake led to a functional impairment of β cell function (including inhibition of glucose-stimulated insulin secretion) without inducing general cell toxicity or oxidative stress. The results of such *in vitro* experiments have yet to be validated in human studies.

## Obesity, Trace Metal Homeostasis, and Infection

Modern lifestyles have fundamentally changed the types, amounts, and forms of trace metals to which people are routinely exposed, and the consequences for human health have yet to be fully assessed. A large number of studies suggest that these changes can significantly influence the pathogenesis of obesity and infectious diseases as separate entities (see above). The question as to whether obese individuals with trace metal deficiency or toxicity (growing traits in the developing countries) are at increased risk for infectious diseases has not received much attention. For this review, I have relied on a "weight of evidence" approach to make suggestive inferences.

There are multiple cellular and biochemical pathways in the homeostasis of trace metals which can influence metabolic disorders (including insulin resistance, obesity, and diabetes) and infections. The three potential processes in metal metabolism that can simultaneously influence the pathogenesis of obesity and many infections are:

1.  nutritional trace metal deficiency or excessive exposure to toxic metals, which can compromise immune function;
2.  elevated blood volume as a function of increased adipose tissue mass, which increases the trace metal requirements and can potentially dysregulate the systemic distribution of many metals; and
3.  formation of systemic inflammation and oxidative status common through trace metal homeostasis.

The proposed mechanisms behind obesity and infectious diseases include immune system dysregulation, decreased cell-mediated immune responses, obesity-related comorbidities, respiratory dysfunction, and pharmacological issues (Huttunen and Syrjanen 2013). As to be expected, however, most studies on obesity and susceptibility to infections in humans and animals have focused on the role and functionality of the immune system. The immune system cells and adipocytes show similarities in structure and function, such as the production of various inflammatory mediators (Marti et al. 2001; Huttunen and Syrjanen 2013). Adipose tissue itself has its own immune function and can also interact by secreting adipokines, such as leptin (Nave et al. 2011). In some respect, obesity can be regarded as a violation of the well-balanced system of adipocytes and immune cells, which can lead to a disturbance to the immune surveillance system and dysregulation of the immune response, impairment of chemotaxis, and alteration in macrophage differentiation (Nave et al. 2011; Huttunen and Syrjanen 2013). The homeostatic cycle of many trace metals is closely linked to these processes.

Sepsis, the syndrome of microbial infection complicated by systemic inflammation, provides an exaggerated illustration of the mediating effects of zinc on obesity and infection. An association between obesity and the increased morbidity and mortality from sepsis has been documented in a number of studies (Cheng et al. 2008; Sander et al. 2010), and both conditions share a number of important clinical and pathophysiological features. A characteristic feature of obesity is the induction of a chronic inflammatory state characterized by increased cytokine production by adipocytes or macrophages infiltrating adipose tissue (Oteiza 2012). An exaggerated inflammatory response to microbial infection is a prominent feature of sepsis (Bao et al. 2010b). Adipose tissue secretes proinflammatory adipokines such as interleukin-6, TNF-α, and calcitonin, which are commonly associated with sepsis pathophysiology (Knoell et al. 2009). Adipocytes also express Toll-like receptors, which are responsive to endotoxin; these are also critical factors in sepsis (Andreini et al. 2006a). Another feature of obesity is systemic lipotocixity that results from adiposity, leading to the production of toxic metabolites and overactivation of oxidative pathways (Calvano et al. 2005). Oxidative stress and high lipid concentrations may lead to apoptosis and endothelial dysfunction (Ho et al. 2003; Calvano et al. 2005). Relatedly, Liu et al. (2014) recently made the important observation that Zn deficiency significantly increases mortality in a mouse model of polymicrobial sepsis due to overactivation of the inflammatory response. They showed that during the initial stage of sepsis, Zn deficiency can induce rapid release of cytokines, such as TNFα, IL-1β, and IL-6, which rapidly activate the acute phase response (APR) and lead to the production of APPs. They also report that the upregulation of APR under Zn deficiency was accompanied by enhanced JAK-STAT3 signaling and a corresponding increase in serum amyloid A production. Further, Liu et al. (2014) report that adding zinc to the experimental system reduced the JAK-STAT3 signaling and APR activity, indicating that zinc plays a pivotal role in balancing the host response through the APR and enhanced expression of APPs during the severe infection associated with sepsis.

In recent years, it has become clear that chronic systemic low-grade inflammation, altered immune response, and oxidative stress are the basis for many, if not all, Western diseases centered around the metabolic syndrome (Keaney et al. 2003; Furukawa et al. 2004; Matsuzawa-Nagata et al. 2008; Fernández-Sánchez et al. 2011). These features are also commonly associated with trace metal deficiencies (or toxicity) and infections. The adverse impact of obesity on immunity is particularly striking in tuberculosis, a disease that may have shaped recent human evolution. In premodern times, type 1 diabetes was observed to predispose individuals to tuberculosis (Nathan 2008). It is now becoming clear that obesity-associated prediabetes and type 2 diabetes are risk factors that affect the contagiousness of tuberculosis and prolonged posttreatment of the infection (Alisjahbana et al. 2007; Restrepo 2007; Stevenson et al. 2007). Suppression of the ability to generate interferon (IFN)-α has been implicated in increasing susceptibility (Stalenhoef et al. 2007): IFN-α enhances the antimicrobial capacity of macrophages (Nathan 2008), and deficiencies in its production or signaling underlie most syndromes of susceptibility to myco-bacterial infection (Fortin et al. 2007). In India, the case burden of tuberculosis attributable to obesity and/or diabetes has been estimated to exceed markedly that attributable to infection by HIV (Alisjahbana et al. 2007; Restrepo 2007). Coincidentally, the prevalence of zinc, iron, and other trace metal deficiencies in India is among the highest in the world (see Ackland et al., this volume). Both obesity and deficiencies in trace metals lead to the expression of copious amounts of the inflammatory cytokines seen in tuberculosis patients, and it is most likely that all three conditions share common pathogenic features. The likelihood that the superposition of the growing vulnerabilities of obesity into endemicity of trace metal deficiencies may be involved in the changing pre-sentation of tuberculosis and other infectious diseases in some parts of India cannot be discounted.

A large volume of literature reports that the disruption of the homeosta-sis of redox-active metals (including iron, copper, chromium, cobalt among others) may lead to oxidative stress—a state where increased generation of reactive oxygen species (ROS) overwhelms the body's antioxidant protection and subsequently induces DNA damage, lipid peroxidation, protein modifica-tion, and other effects associated with numerous diseases, including obesity and diabetes and related metabolic syndrome (reviewed by Jomova and Valko 2011). Redox-active metals are quintessentially involved in the formation of superoxide radical, hydroxyl radical (mainly via Fenton and Haber–Weiss reactions), nitric oxide, and other ROS species in biological systems, which can subsequently activate the formation of other organic free radicals. Redox-inactive metals including cadmium, arsenic, lead, and mercury, on the other hand, moderate the biological redox cycles via bonding to sulphydryl groups of proteins and depletion of antioxidant species such as glutathione. An alter-native mechanism leading to the formation of hydrogen peroxide by oxidation of As(III) to As(V) under physiological conditions has been proposed (Mishra and Flora 2008). As a redox-inert metal, zinc occupies a special position among the metals in that it is an essential component of numerous proteins involved in defense against oxidative stress. Under a normal homeostatic mechanism, the metal-induced formation of free radicals is tightly influenced by the action of cellular antioxidants with many low molecular weight antioxidants, such as ascorbic acid (vitamin C), alpha-tocopherol (vitamin E), glutathione, ca-rotenoids, flavonoids, and other antioxidants, being formed which are capable of chelating metal ions, thus reducing their catalytic activity with respect to ROS (Jomova and Valko 2011). The capacity of these metabolites to prevent the harmful effects of hypoxia is limited and can be overwhelmed by habitual intake of energy-dense and antioxidant-poor diet (Ruiz-Nunez et al. 2013).

Some evidence suggests that excessive zinc in energy-dense food causes ex-cessive accumulation of body fat both in rodents and humans, thereby implicat-ing the involvement of zinc in the etiology of obesity (Prentice 1993; Chen et al. 1996; Taneja et al. 1996; 2012). The current understanding of a Zn effect on obesity is that zinc positively modulates secretion of insulin from pancreas and certain adipocites (including leptin, adiponectin) from adipose cells (Song et al. 2009). Zinc deficiency alters Zn transporter expression in adipose tissue (see above) and is associated with reduced serum leptin concentrations in healthy humans and rats (Mantzaros et al. 1998; Baltaci et al. 2005). Obese humans and mice, however, show higher concentrations of circulating leptin hyperleptinemia as well as hyperglycemia and hyperinsulinemia in tandem with lower Zn concentrations (hypozincemia) in blood or adipose tissue, suggesting interesting interrelationships between these factors in obesity (Taneja et al. 2012; Liu et al. 2013). Leptin is essential for normal development of both innate and adaptive immune responses, and the lack of this hormone or its receptor results in severe immune abnormalities and greater susceptibility to viral, bacterial, mycobacterial, and fungal infections (Mancuso 2013). Recent studies show that ob/ob mice exhibit increased pulmonary bacterial burdens and reduced survival following an intratracheal challenge with either *K. pneumoniae* or *S. pneumoniae* (Mancuso et al. 2002; Hsu et al. 2007). The extent to which leptin and other adipokines are involved in mediating the role of zinc and other trace metals in the comorbidity of obesity and infectious diseases is unknown at this time.

## Conclusions

Modern lifestyles have fundamentally changed the types, amounts, and forms of trace metals to which people are routinely exposed, and a growing number of studies suggest that these changes can significantly influence the pathogenesis of obesity and infectious diseases as separate entities. This review uses a weight of evidence approach to suggest that obese individuals with deficiency or toxicity (growing traits in the developing countries) in some trace metals are at increased risk for infectious diseases. Multiple cellular and biochemical pathways are involved in the homeostasis of trace metals, which can influence metabolic disorders (including insulin resistance, obesity, and diabetes) and host–pathogen interactions. Redox-active metals are quintessentially involved in the formation of superoxide radical, hydroxyl radical (mainly via Fenton and Haber–Weiss reactions), nitric oxide, and other ROS species in biological systems, which can subsequently induce DNA damage, lipid peroxidation, protein modification, and other effects associated with numerous diseases, including obesity and diabetes and related metabolic syndrome. The proposed mechanisms linking trace metals to obesity and infection include (a) nutritional trace metal deficiency or excessive exposure to toxic metals, which can compromise immune function; (b) elevated blood volume as a function of increased adipose tissue mass, which increases the trace metal requirements and can potentially dysregulate the systemic availability of many metals to infecting pathogens; and (c) formation of systemic inflammation and oxidative status common through trace metal homeostasis. In truth, our understanding of the trace metal-obesity-infection nexus remains very limited and a fertile area for future research.

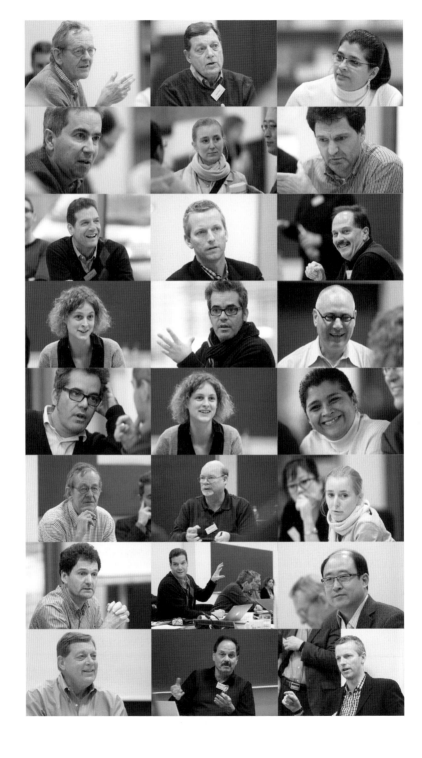

# 13

# Metals in Host– Microbe Interaction

## The Host Perspective

Dieter Rehder, Robert E. Black, Julia Bornhorst,
Rodney R. Dietert, Victor J. DiRita, Maribel Navarro,
Robert D. Perry, Lothar Rink, Eric P. Skaar, Miguel C. P. Soares,
Dennis J. Thiele, Fudi Wang, Günter Weiss, and Inga Wessels

### Abstract

This overview covers the role of the metal ions in infectious diseases, focusing on iron (Fe), copper (Cu), zinc (Zn), and, to a lesser extent, manganese (Mn) and the metalloid selenium (Se). In addition, recommended dietary allowances are addressed, as are metal-based drugs for the treatment of tropical diseases.

The human organism binds essential metals such as iron, manganese, copper, and zinc to specific compounds (including proteins) in order to withhold these metals from invading pathogens ("nutritional immunity"); in this way, metal binding provides resistance to infection. Selenium status can also affect the host–pathogen interaction, but pathogens have mechanisms to counteract this protective potency. As alternative to a withdrawal of metals, microbes can be exposed to particularly high—and thus toxic—levels of metal ions. A secondary protective mechanism stems from the production (by host innate immune cells) of reactive oxygen and nitrogen species; this can also result in host tissue damage. In addition, the gasotransmitters nitric oxide (an oxidant) and carbon monoxide are indirectly involved in side effects (deprotection and protection, respectively, of bound heme) that result from the immune response.

Host-mediated alteration of Fe homeostasis directly impacts on the proliferation of microbes. Depending on the type of pathogen, different regulatory mechanisms can be initiated. Limiting the availability of iron can be an efficient strategy to restrict extracellular bacteria, although such a strategy is detrimental for intracellular pathogens. Iron homeostasis is partly linked to Cu homeostasis. Copper deficiency predisposes mammals to infectious diseases, to some extent as a consequence of a lack of neutrophils induced by inadequate Cu availability or supply. Finally, there is a clear-cut cor-

*D. Rehder et al.*

relation between bacterial infections and Zn removal from serum. More generally, Zn deficiency reduces immune defense against infections, chronic inflammatory disease, and reduced cellular activation, whereas high levels of zinc can hamper effective signal transduction.

Due to the epidemic proportions of tropical diseases (e.g., leishmaniasis, Chagas disease, and malaria) and lack of effective treatment, drugs are being developed that are based on coordination compounds of metals, including copper, iron, ruthenium, and gold. These metals are coordinated to aromatic ligand systems that allow for a stabilization of the drug, during the drug's transport to its target, and eventually intercalation into DNA. For malaria, the increasing resistance of the malaria parasite against the classical drug chloroquine may be overcome by employing ferrocenyl derivatives of chloroquine.

# Introduction

This report focuses on the distribution and function of the essential elements iron, zinc, copper and, to some extent, manganese, and selenium. Molybdenum was excluded because its impact on infectious diseases is hardly known. Also excluded were vanadium, chromium, nickel, and cobalt. Chromium has long been considered to be an indispensable trace metal (Mertz 1993), but from today's point of view, it is unlikely to be essential (Cefalu et al. 2010); there is, however, evidence of its potential to invoke cancer in the +V state, generated from chromate(VI) under physiological conditions (Levina et al. 2009). The essentiality of vanadium has not yet been established. The similarity, however, between vanadate and phosphate strongly suggest a role for vanadate in the regulation of phosphate-metabolizing enzymes, such as phosphatases and kinases (Rehder 2014). An example is the antidiabetic effect of vanadate as a consequence of the inhibition of protein-tyrosine-phosphatase through the coordination of vanadate to the cysteinate in the active site. Cobalt is the central metal in vitamin B12; however, whether external "free" cobalt is a nutritional requirement has yet to be clarified. Finally, nickel does not appear to be directly essential for humans, yet its inalienability for microbes—and thus also for the human microbiome—presupposes an indirect essentiality also for humans. More generally, the consequences of the microbiome for metal availability in the host, and vice versa, remain to be explored.

The essentiality of many transition metals, and of the main group element selenium, presupposes that these elements are available as micronutrients for humans as well as for both symbiotic and pathogenic microbes and parasitic protozoa. In response to an infection, the host can increase the metal concentration up to levels that are toxic for the pathogen or reduce the availability of the essential metal for the invading microbes, using specific metal ion-binding proteins and/ or by withdrawing metal ions from affected cells and tissues. On the other hand, parasitic microorganisms have developed sophisticated mechanisms to cope with metal ion restrictions (Diaz-Ochoda et al. 2014) and overloads.

We begin with an overview of biologically essential elements, in general, and metals/metalloids that are essential for humans and of interest in the host–microbe interaction. We address in some detail the distribution and function of manganese, iron, copper, zinc, and selenium, emphasizing the competition for these elements in the frame of the interaction between the host (the human body) and the invading microbes/parasites. The role of the gasotransmitters carbon monoxide (CO) and nitric oxide (NO) is presented in relation to their interference with bound and free ferrous ions, followed by a brief discussion on dietary allowances for essential metals, as recommended by the World Health Organization (WHO). Finally, we conclude with a discussion of metal-based drugs in the treatment of tropical diseases caused by parasitic protozoa.

## Essential Metals and Metalloids: An Overview

Figure 13.1 shows the periodic table of life elements. To ascertain that neither deficiency nor overload occurs, metal homeostasis must be tightly regulated. Even in the case of intact metal homeostasis, deficiencies are inevitable when a person is subjected to an unbalanced diet. This happens, in particular, in infants, children, pregnant and nursing women, as well as elderly individuals. People who are particularly susceptible to an unbalanced provision (commonly an undersupply) of essential metals and metalloids are those at risk

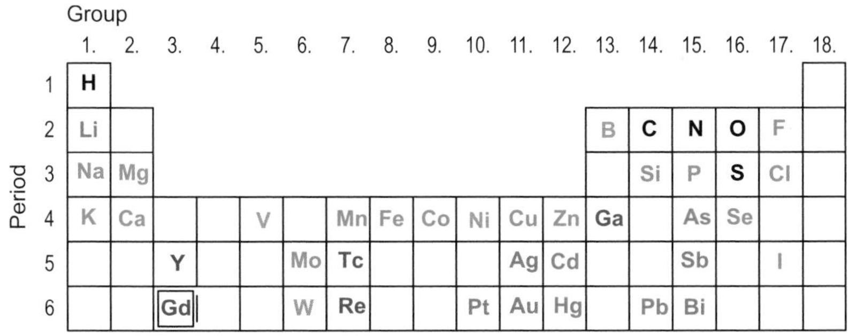

Group

| | 1. | 2. | 3. | 4. | 5. | 6. | 7. | 8. | 9. | 10. | 11. | 12. | 13. | 14. | 15. | 16. | 17. | 18. |
|---|----|----|----|----|----|----|----|----|----|----|----|----|----|----|----|----|----|----|
| 1 | H | | | | | | | | | | | | | | | | | |
| 2 | Li | | | | | | | | | | | | B | C | N | O | F | |
| 3 | Na | Mg | | | | | | | | | | | | Si | P | S | Cl | |
| 4 | K | Ca | | | V | | Mn | Fe | Co | Ni | Cu | Zn | Ga | | As | Se | | |
| 5 | | Y | | | Mo | Tc | | | | | Ag | Cd | | | Sb | | I | |
| 6 | | Gd | | | W | Re | | | | Pt | Au | Hg | | Pb | Bi | | | |

**Figure 13.1** Biologically and medicinally relevant elements. Elements that are demonstrably essential for humans are shown in black (for the buildup of organic compounds) and green. Elements that are essential for only select groups of organisms are noted in gray; toxic metals are listed in red. Metals used in therapy are shown in mauve: Li (bipolar disorder), Ag (wound disinfection), Sb (leishmaniasis, schistosomiasis), Pt (cancer therapy), Au (rheumatoid arthritis), Bi (gastrointestinal disorders). Metals employed in diagnostic techniques (such as positron emission tomography, PET, and magnetic resonance imaging, MRI) are highlighted in blue. Gd is framed, because it is an f-group element. Other metal prescriptions are sporadically used medicinally. For example, lanthanum carbonate is sometimes applied in dialysis to reduce serum phosphate levels (hyperphosphatemia). The essentiality of chromium (e.g., in the form of a hardly defined picolinato-$Cr^{3+}$ complex, the "glucose tolerance factor") has recently been critically scrutinized (Cefalu et al. 2010); Cr has thus not been included.

of undernourishment and/or malnutrition, such as inhabitants of developing countries, people with infections, and, to some extent, vegans.

Recommended dietary allowances (RDAs) for metals, as released and recommended by governmental authorities and the WHO, need to be reviewed and assessed critically in light of the scientific arguments presented in this publication; for detailed discussion of RDAs and relevant tables, see Wang and Zhang (this volume). One problem with RDAs is that speciation (and thus bioavailability) of the respective nutritional element is not considered. Open questions include adverse effects from normal levels of metal supplementation (e.g., iron in relation to copper), in particular with respect to long-term effects, dietary needs, infections, and chronic diseases. Eventually, in setting (upper) limits for the intake of essential metals, differentiation by population should be considered.

Below we provide an overview of the uptake, distribution, and *selected* specific functions of elements essential for humans. Further details on manganese, iron, zinc, and copper, and the metalloid selenium in a broader context are provided by Wessels and Loutet et al. (this volume).

## Magnesium

Magnesium plays a central role in phosphate (and hence energy) metabolism. For example, Mg adenosine triphosphate (ATP)—where $Mg^{2+}$ is coordinated to phosphate, $H_2O/OH^-$, and the carboxylate of Asp or Glu—activates the phosphate-dependent metabolic pathways. Magnesium provides support to endoskeletons, and stabilizes the structure of proteins and polysaccharides.

## Calcium

The majority (about 99%) of calcium is present in bones as hydroxyapatite $Ca_5(PO_4)_3(OH)_{1-x}F_x$ (x ≤ 0.01) and teeth (x ~ 0.1). Calcium also plays a role in muscle contraction/relaxation, blood clotting, enzyme regulation, the gating of $K^+$ channels, stabilization of protein structures, and signal transduction. Extracellular $c(Ca^{2+})$ exceeds intracellular $c(Ca^{2+})$ by a factor of $2.5 \times 10^3$. Three hormones are involved in $Ca^{2+}$ metabolism.

## Manganese

Manganese is associated with the lipid, carbohydrate, and amino acid metabolism. Examples of Mn-dependent enzymes in humans are prolidase, arginase, and mitochondrial superoxide dismutase (SOD). The $Ca^{2+}$-binding protein calprotectin also effectively binds $Mn^{2+}$. $Mn^{2+}$ and $Zn^{2+}$ share some chemical properties; there is, however, no established connection for the competition between these two metal ions.

# Iron

Iron is the most abundant transition metal in the human body. It is critically involved in key physiologic functions, including the transport of gaseous molecules, such as oxygen $O_2$ (hemoglobin), or gasotransmitters, such as NO and CO, electron transport in the mitochodria, and activity of a variety of redox enzymes. Redox enzymes include many that are involved in the formation of free radicals implicated in host defense mechanisms that target pathogens for destruction (e.g., the Fenton reaction). These are commonly based either on heme iron or on iron-sulfur (Fe-S) proteins.

Most iron in the body is recycled; a daily uptake of 1–2 mg suffices for maintenance of Fe homeostasis. A schematic of Fe uptake, distribution, and recycling is illustrated in Figure 13.2. It should be noted that only 20–25% of the bioavailable iron in mammals exists in the form of accessible iron, bound to transferrin, stored inside ferritin, in Fe-S clusters or transiently bound to Fe chaperones and transporters. The remaining 75–80% of bioavailable iron exists inside the protoporphyrine IX ring of heme, the prosthetic group of hemoproteins. Among these, hemoglobin comprises up to 70% of the total pool of heme, thus accounting for the major Fe compartment in mammals. Bioavailable iron can transit from the heme into the labile Fe compartment via a controlled process that relies on heme catabolism by heme oxygenases, as illustrated by the finding that the heme oxygenase-1 isoform, constitutively expressed by hemophagocytic macrophages, is essential to maintain Fe homeostasis (Poss and Tonegawa 1997; Yachie et al. 1999). It becomes apparent therefore that regulation of heme catabolism, allowing for the extraction and recycling of iron into the labile Fe compartment, is essential for the maintenance of Fe homeostasis

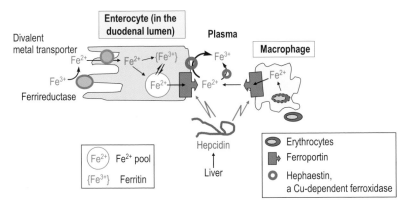

**Figure 13.2**   Uptake of iron and Fe homeostasis. In blood plasma, ferric iron is tightly bound to the transport protein transferrin; ca. 80% of the overall iron is present in the form of heme. The intestinal absorptive cells, termed enterocytes, are located in the duodenal lumen. Hepcidin, a peptide hormone produced in the liver, attains a central role due to its binding to the Fe transporter ferroportin, which *decreases* Fe flow into the plasma by initiating endocytosis and proteolysis of ferroportin.

in mammals (Gozzelino and Soares 2014). Maintenance of Fe homeostasis also relies on the transit of labile iron into the Fe-heme compartment, through de novo heme synthesis, catalyzed by a sequence of eight enzymatic steps completed by the insertion of iron into the proptoporphyrin IX ring, and catalyzed by ferrochelatase. This is essential, for example, for the insertion of Fe-heme into hemoglobin and maintenance of erythropoiesis.

An inadequate supply of iron can lead to anemia and Friedreich ataxia, whereas abundance can result in oxidative stress (due to abnormal Fe deposition) and hemochromatosis.

## Cobalt

Cobalt is the central metal ion ($Co^+$, $Co^{2+}$, $Co^{3+}$) of vitamin B12 and its derivatives. An undersupply of cobalt causes pernicious anemia and results, for example, in damage to nervous tissues. Larger doses of cobalt are acutely toxic. "Free" cobalt, supplied through food, cannot be used in the human physiological system.

## Copper

Copper is present in various redox enzymes, where the metal switches between the oxidation states +I and +II. Copper is also involved in Fe homeostasis (see, e.g., hephaestin in Figure 13.2). Several diseases are connected to Cu imbalance: Wilson disease (Cu overload), Menkes disease (Cu deficiency) and possibly Alzheimer disease (imbalance between "labile" and "tightly bound" Cu). In grazing cattle, molybdate $MoO_4^{2-}$ in soils can immobilize copper and lead to Cu deficiency.

## Zinc

Zinc ($Zn^{2+}$; redox inactive under physiological conditions) is the second most abundant transition metal in the human body and forms the active center of enzymes, including hydrolases, carboanhydrase, and alcohol dehydrogenase. Other Zn-dependent functions are manifest in genetic transcription ("Zn fingers"), in the stabilization of tertiary and quaternary structures of peptides, and in DNA repair proteins. Low molecular mass proteins rich in zinc, the thioneins, store zinc and regulate Zn levels, but can also act as scavengers for toxic $Pb^{2+}$, $Cd^{2+}$ and $Hg^{2+}$ (for an updated view of zinc, see Chasapis et al. 2012).

## Molybdenum

Molybdenum is a constituent of the molybdopterin cofactor in three enzymes in humans: sulfite oxidase (SuOx), xanthine oxidase (XaOx), and DMSO reductase. SuOx is located in the mitochondria, where it catalyzes the oxidation—and thus detoxification—of sulfite (supplied exogenously, or formed in the frame of the metabolism of cysteine and methionine) to sulfate. An inadequate supply of molybdenum causes severe neurological damage in early childhood. XaOx catalyzes the oxidation/dehydrogenation of aldehydes as well as the oxidation of hypoxanthine to xanthine. Dimethyl sulfoxide reductase catalyzes the reduction of dimethyl sulfoxide to dimethylsulfide.

## Selenium

Selenium is an essential micronutrient, present in the body in the form of selenocysteine SeCys and selenomethionine. SeCys serves as a building block in enzymes, such as glutathione peroxidase, and in some molybdopterin cofactors.

## Toxic Elements

The toxicity of cadmium, mercury, and lead results from the ability of these metal ions to form very stable thiocompounds, and thus to denature peptides and proteins through the reaction with cysteine sulfhydryl groups. In addition, Zn metabolism is disturbed when $Zn^{2+}$ is replaced in Zn thioneins. Nickel and aluminum are other possibly nonessential elements that can disrupt metabolic pathways when present in more than trace amounts.

# The Role of Manganese, Iron, Copper, Zinc, and Selenium

## Manganese

*Innate Immunity*

Similar to iron and zinc, mammals bind manganese in an attempt to withhold this transition metal from invading pathogens. The neutrophil-derived protein, calprotectin, chelates both zinc and manganese, removing these metals from sites of infection. Calprotectin is a heterodimer encoded by the genes *S100A8* and *S100A9*, and is one of the most abundant proteins at sites of inflammation. While the relative contribution of Zn and Mn chelation to the inhibition of infections remains to be completely defined, it is clear that Mn chelation by calprotectin is required to inhibit bacterial growth to the greatest extent possible (Corbin et al. 2008) and, as such, to provide resistance to bacterial infections. Moreover, Zn and Mn chelation can inhibit microbial virulence factors that rely on these metals (Liu et al. 2012). The protein S100A12 is also constitutively expressed in neutrophils and has a role in infection and immunity, presumably through Zn binding (Goyette and Geczy 2011). In addition, S100A7 inhibits microbial growth through Zn binding and has an important role in protecting against infections of the skin (Schröder and Harder 2006). Notably, the S100 protein family is comprised of 24 family members, including many metal-binding proteins. This raises the exciting possibility that additional Mn- and Zn-binding components of the innate immune system have yet to be uncovered. In an interesting turn of events, *Neisseria meningitidis*, the causative agent of meningitis, has been reported to produce a protein that binds calprotectin and thus enables the organism to utilize this protein as a nutrient Zn source (Stork et al. 2013). It is likely that bacteria have multiple strategies to circumvent calprotectin-dependent metal binding, but these strategies have yet to be uncovered.

*Transport and Inflammation*

Currently, undefined mammalian compound(s) contribute to Mn chelation. Although some studies have detected manganese bound to transferrin and lactoferrin (Aschner and Gannon 1994), their contribution to withholding manganese from pathogens has not been determined. Mutation of Mn uptake systems in a number of bacterial pathogens results in a loss of virulence in various pathogenesis models (Porcheron et al. 2013). This is further support that chelation of manganese in mammals creates a Mn-deficient environment which pathogens must overcome.

Due to the ubiquitous occurrence of manganese in the diet, daily dietary uptake in industrial countries is higher than the recommended daily requirement. Thus Mn deficiency is extremely rare and has only been shown in experimental models (Roth 2006). Deficiency has been demonstrated in several animal species (e.g., rats, mice, pigs, chicken, and cattle) and can result in several biochemical and structural defects such as poor bone growth, skeletal abnormalities, ataxia, and abnormal glucose tolerance (Santamaria and Sulsky 2010). In human subjects on an experimental low Mn diet, dermatitis, slowed growth of hair and nails, decreased serum cholesterol levels, and decreased levels of clotting proteins have been reported (Finley et al. 2003).

In contrast, toxicity is more common, and chronic manganese overexposure has been shown to correlate with permanently progressing neurodegenerative damage. In a few studies that targeted neuropathological mechanisms, the role of neuroinflammation has been uncovered: Manganese enhances the release of the inflammatory cytokines interleukin-6 (IL-6) and tumor necrosis factor (TNF) from resident macrophages in the brain, i.e., microglial cells which can promote the activation of astrocytes and subsequent release of inflammatory mediators such as prostaglandin E2 and the gasotransmitter NO (Aschner et al. 2009; Filipov and Dodd 2011). In addition, manganese potentiates NO production in cytokine-stimulated astrocytes (Liu et al. 2005).

In biological systems, the most relevant and stable Mn species exist in the form of $Mn^{2+}$ and $Mn^{3+}$. These Mn ions are transported into cells via several mechanisms (e.g., facilitated diffusion and active transport) and transporters for other divalent ions (e.g., $Fe^{2+}$ and $Zn^{2+}$), indicating an interconnection between Mn, Fe, and Zn homeostasis. Manganese is discussed to be transported, among others, via the divalent metal transporter 1 (DMT1), the transferrin receptor (TfR), the divalent metal/bicarbonate ion symporters ZIP8 and ZIP14, various calcium channels, the solute carrier-39 (SLC39) family of Zn transporters, park9/ATP13A2, the Mg transporter hip14, the transient receptor potential melastatin 7 (TRPM7) channels/transporters, homomeric purine receptors (P2X and P2Y), and the citrate transporter (Bowman et al. 2011).

## Iron

*Heme Iron in Host–Microbe Interaction*

There is a key and singular aspect related to Fe metabolism that should be taken into consideration in the context of host–microbe interactions in mammals: the vast majority of bioavailable iron in the affected host is actually contained inside the prosthetic heme groups of hemoproteins. Mechanisms which control host heme synthesis, transport (Yuan et al. 2013), and catabolism (Gozzelino and Soares 2014) should thus play a critical role in the maintenance of host–microbe interactions and in the pathologic outcome of infectious diseases.

Reactive oxygen and nitrogen species produced by host innate immune cells during microbial infections, which confers resistance to infection, can eventually lead to host tissue damage and exacerbate rather than prevent the severity of infectious diseases (Medzhitov et al. 2012). Moreover, inflammatory and immune responses are associated with varying degrees of hemolysis and rhabdomyolysis, and hence with the release of noncovalently bound heme from hemoglobin and myoglobin, generating free heme (Gozzelino et al. 2012). The impact of this event in the deregulation of Fe metabolism during infections should be appreciated, taking into account that the majority of the iron is contained within the heme groups of hemoglobin and myoglobin (Gozzelino and Soares 2014). The redox activity of nonhemoprotein-bound heme, "free heme," is no longer under the control of the amino acids that surround the prosthetic heme groups within the so-called heme pockets of these hemoproteins. Presumably for this reason, free heme is highly pro-oxidant and cytotoxic, exerting proinflammatory effects through the engagement of specific pattern recognition receptors, such as the Toll-like receptor 4 (TLR-4) that is expressed by monocytes/macrophages as well as in endothelial cells (Belcher et al. 2014). Free heme can also exert chemotactic effects via the engagement of G protein-coupled receptors expressed in polymorphonucelar cells. The combination of these effects has a significant and yet unappreciated impact on the outcome of infectious diseases (Gozzelino et al. 2012).

To ensure regulated adaptation of heme transport and catabolism, several stress response systems have evolved to minimize the negative impact caused by the generation of free heme during infection (Gozzelino et al. 2010). These systems are essential to control the proinflammatory, vasoactive and cytotoxicity effects of heme, as well as to sustain systemic Fe homeostasis, avoiding tissue Fe overload, tissue damage, and anemia in the infected host (Soares et al. 2009). The impact of such regulatory pathways has been demonstrated unequivocally for the heme-catabolizing enzyme heme oxygenase-1 (HO-1) in mice, as well as in humans (Yachie et al. 1999), where HO-1 deficiency is associated with impaired Fe recycling, anemia, vascular damage, and depletion of hemophagocytic macrophages (Kovtunovych et al. 2010), presumably driven by heme cytotoxicity (Fortes et al. 2012). Moreover HO-1 deficiency renders infected hosts extremely susceptible to systemic infections, as demonstrated for severe sepsis (Larsen et al. 2012), malaria, and more recently for tuberculosis (Silva-Gomes et al. 2013).

The protective effect afforded by HO-1 expression against systemic infections has been linked to the adaptation of cells to cellular and tissue Fe overload (Gozzelino and Soares 2014). This is demonstrated by the finding that deletion of the ferritin H chain gene, which acts downstream of HO-1 to neutralize the pro-oxidant effect of the iron released from heme catabolism, is strictly required to support the protective effect of HO-1 against systemic infections, as has been demonstrated for malaria.

In the context of systemic infections, the induction of HO-1 expression in the host is essential to provide protection against the cytotoxic effects and presumably the proinflammatory and vasoactive impact of free heme. These salutary effects are essential to reduce tissue damage and hence disease severity, and to support host survival. This host defense strategy, while essential to the survival of an infected host, does not appear to exert a negative impact on the pathogen—a phenomenon referred to as disease tolerance (Gozzelino and Soares 2014).

## Gasotransmitters: The Interaction of Nitric Oxide and Carbon Monoxide with the Heme Group

Gasotransmitters are biologically active molecules produced physiologically by several evolutionary conserved enzymes (Mustafa et al. 2009). These gaseous molecules include nitric oxide, generated by the enzymatic conversion of L-arginine and molecular oxygen to L-citrulline (Figure 13.3a) and catalyzed by different nitric oxide synthases (NOS). Carbon monoxide is generated through the catabolism of heme (Figure 13.3b) and catalyzed by different isoforms of heme oxidases. Hydrogen sulfide ($H_2S$) is produced from cysteine by cystathionine beta-synthase and cystathionine gamma-lyase, but will not be covered in further detail here.

Gasotransmitters share biophysical properties that include lipid solubility, which allows for diffusion across cellular membranes and underlies their intrinsic ability to target, more or less distally, specific intracellular signal transduction pathways without requiring classical cognate ligand/receptor interactions (Mustafa et al. 2009). This occurs, for example, via the physical interaction of gaseous molecules with transition metals (Cooper 1999). This is

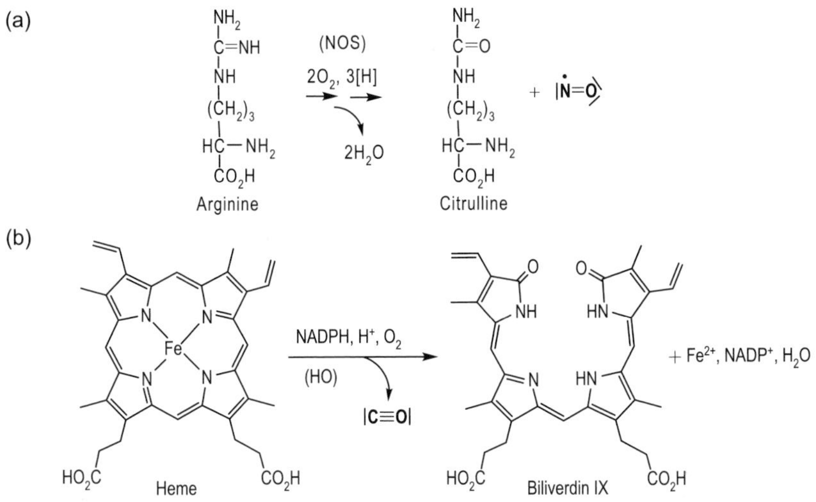

**Figure 13.3** (a) Formation of nitric oxide: NO is catalyzed by nitrogen oxide synthase, NOS, in a two-step process via an [NOH] intermediate. [H] represents reduction equivalents, commonly delivered by nicotine adenine dinucleotide NADPH. (b) Carbon monoxide (CO) forms by oxidative catabolism of free heme, catalyzed by heme oxygenase (HO). A potent inducer for the transcription of the HO-1 gene is nitric oxide.

well illustrated for iron in the context of Fe-S clusters or heme groups within metalloproteins. Briefly, NO or CO binding to $Fe^{2+}$ within Fe-S clusters or in the prosthetic heme groups of metalloproteins can modify the tertiary structure of those proteins and their biological activity, as illustrated, among others, for guanylate cyclase, an enzyme that generates cyclic guanosine monophosphate (cGMP), or for cytochrome-c. Although the signaling pathway for NO includes other well-established mechanisms (e.g., tyrosine nitrosylation), transition metal-mediated signal transduction appears to be a general principle by which gasotransmitters exert their biological effects. While the output of this interaction is specific to each gasotransmitter, this common mechanism illustrates how regulation of the metabolism of transition metals may affect the biologic action of gasotransmitters.

Interaction of gasotransmitters with $Fe^{2+}$ produces additional effects that can be critical for the outcome of infectious diseases. For example, as a pro-oxidant labile-free radical, NO's interaction with $Fe^{2+}$ in the heme group of hemoglobin results not only in tight binding and scavenging of this gasotransmitter, but also promotes the oxidation of hemoglobin (Cooper 1999); this, in turn, can then act in a proinflammatory manner (Silva et al. 2009) to impact the outcome of infectious diseases, as illustrated for sepsis (Larsen et al. 2010; Adamzik et al. 2012). In contrast, the interaction of CO with $Fe^{2+}$ in the heme groups of hemoglobin has the opposite effect: Fe heme oxidation is prevented as is hemoglobin oxidation. Ultimately, this blocks heme release from the globulin chains of hemoglobin (Pamplona et al. 2007; Gozzelino et al. 2010). This latter effect is sufficient in itself to explain the protective effect of this gasotransmitter against the pathological outcome of malaria (Pamplona et al. 2007; Ferreira et al. 2008), the infectious disease triggered by *Plasmodium* infection (Miller et al. 2013). It is likely that in a similar manner to hemoglobin, CO can prevent heme release from other hemoproteins such as myoglobin. Whether this effect of CO also limits the pathologic outcome of other infectious diseases remains to be established, but it is likely to be the case.

*Interplay of Iron Distribution between (Infectious) Microbes and Host Cells*

Infected host cells tend to control the homeostasis of essential metals, either by limiting the availability of metals that are necessary to maintain the physiology and replication of microbes, or by exposing microbes to high (and thus toxic) concentrations of metals directly or indirectly (e.g., by increasing free radical formation). One example is the Fenton reaction: $Fe^{2+} + H_2O_2 \rightarrow Fe^{3+} + OH^- + \cdot OH$. The host immune system affects the availability of essential metal ions for microbes through cytokines (hormonal regulators or signaling molecules). The microbes, in turn, activate pathways to secure a sufficient supply of metal ions.

In the case of Fe homeostasis (cf. discussion in the next section), monocytes and differentiated macrophages (i.e., cells that digest bacteria, dying cells, and senescent erythrocytes) are involved in the regulation of Fe levels and free radical production, including reactive oxygen and nitrogen species. The limitation of the availability of iron for invading pathogens is termed "nutritional immunity." Instantaneous Fe retention by macrophages (and thus restricted availability of plasma iron in the case of an infection) is also induced through binding greater amounts of hepcidin to the ferroportin (Figure 13.2) of macrophages; this switches off the transport protein ferroportin and causes Fe retention in the macrophages and Fe depletion in the (infected) surroundings. In addition, decreased expression of ferroportin, coupled with the inhibition of ferritin (the Fe storage protein) translation, provides a basic means to reduce Fe supply. Inhibition of ferritin translation, in turn, is partly coupled to the stimulation of NO formation. Patients with chronic inflammation, therefore, suffer from Fe deficiency (hypoferremia) and high serum ferritin (hyperferritinemia), and thus develop anemia.

As noted above, bioavailable iron in mammals exists mainly within the hydrophobic methene-bridged tetrapyrrole ring of heme as a prosthetic group in hemoproteins. The most abundant of these are hemoglobin and myoglobin, with another significant pool of ubiquitously expressed hemoproteins formed by cytochromes. Mechanisms controlling host heme metabolism, including heme synthesis, transport (Yuan et al. 2013) and catabolism (Gozzelino and Soares 2014), play a critical role in the maintenance of host–microbe interactions as well as in the pathologic outcome of infectious diseases.

Iron homeostasis is also linked to Cu homeostasis through the Cu-based ferroxidases hephaestin (Figure 13.2) and ceruloplasmin. Thus, Cu deficiency prevents the incorporation of $Fe^{3+}$ into ferritin and provokes an overload of free iron and Fe(hydr)oxide deposits. Comparable to the Fenton reaction (see above), $Cu^+$ can promote the formation of reactive oxygen species (ROS). Cu/Zn superoxide dismutase (SOD) catalyzes the disproportionation (and thus detoxification) of superoxide to peroxide and dioxygen ($2O_2^- + 2H^+ \rightarrow H_2O_2 + O_2$). Thus, Cu deficiency prevents the effective removal of the ROS hyperoxide $O_2^-$. One of the many problems encountered with Zn deficiency points to the same direction. Similar considerations also apply for Mn-dependent SODs.

*Impact on Anti-Immune Effector Functions*

The development of anemia in inflammation and chronic disease not only limits the availability of iron for microbes, it also strengthens the immune response that is directed at invading pathogens. Specifically, Fe loading of monocytes/macrophages inhibits interferon gamma (IFN-γ)-mediated pathways, such as formation of TNF-α, reduced expression of the major histocompatibility complex class II antigens and the intracellular adhesion molecule 1, decreased formation of neopterin, and impaired tryptophan degradation via IFN-γ mediated induction of indole-amine-2,3-dioxygenase (Nairz et al. 2010). As a result, Fe-loaded macrophages have an impaired potential to kill various bacteria, parasites, and fungi (such as *Legionella, Listeria, Ehrlichia, Mycobacteria, Salmonella, Leishmania, Plasmodia, Candida, Mucor*) as well as viruses, *in vitro* and *in vivo* through IFN-γ mediated pathways (see also Cavet et al., this volume). Part of this can be attributed to the reduced formation of NO in the presence of iron, since NO is an essential effector molecule of macrophages to fight infectious pathogens and tumor cells (see above). Iron blocks the transcription of inducible NO synthase (iNOS or NOSII), the enzyme responsible for cytokine-inducible high-output formation of NO by hepatocytes or macrophages. This is attributed to a direct influence of iron on the binding affinities of transcription factors, such as the nuclear factor for the expression of IL-6 or the hypoxia inducible factor-1 (Nairz et al. 2010). According to the regulatory feedback loop, NO produced by activated macrophages activates the iron responsible element (IRE) of the binding function of the iron regulatory protein (IRP-1), leading to inhibition of ferritin translation, and thus linking maintenance of Fe homeostasis to NO formation for host defense. Through its deactivating effect on the IFN-γ function, iron also affects the balance of the thymus helper (Th) cells $T_H1/T_H2$. $T_H1$ effector functions are weakened, whereas $T_H2$-mediated cytokine production, such as the activity of IL-4, is increased, a condition which is rather unfavorable in an infection (Mencacci et al. 1997; Nairz et al. 2010). Iron overload also has negative effects on neutrophil function, as Fe therapy of chronic hemodialysis patients impairs the potential of neutrophils to kill bacteria, thus reducing their capacity to phagocyte foreign particles (Weiss 2002). By modulating cytokine activities, iron also triggers macrophage polarization, and opposing M1 and M2 macrophages differ in contrasting metabolic profiles in regard to Fe homeostasis (Recalcati et al. 2010). Moreover, the induction of M2 polarization along with increased expression of the heme oxygenase HO-1 has been linked to immune tolerance in infections, specifically malaria.

Thus, both Fe overload and Fe deficiency have unfavorable immunological effects *in vivo*. Accordingly, mice kept on an Fe-rich diet exhibited a reduced production of IFN-$\gamma$ as compared to mice fed with a normal diet, whereas animals that received an Fe-deficient diet presented with decreased T cell proliferation (Omara and Blakley 1994). Mortality increased in both Fe-overloaded and Fe-deficient mice when a sublethal dose of lipopolysaccharide (LPS) was received, compared to animals with a normal Fe status.

In one specific study, Fe-deficient children in Malawi featured exhibited a reduced incidence of infection, paralleled by (a) a higher percentage of CD8+ cells[1] which produced IL-6, (b) a more pronounced expression of lymphocytes with T cell activation markers, and (c) an increased formation of IFN-$\gamma$ as compared to children with a normal Fe status (Oppenheimer 2001). This observation coincides with an *adverse* outcome in children receiving Fe supplementation, mainly as a consequence of an increased incidence of severe malaria and bacterial infection (Sazawal et al. 2006), and an *improved* outcome in children with cerebral malaria who received the Fe chelator desferrioxamine, stimulating the antimalarial immune responses. In Africa, an endemic form of secondary Fe overload—traced back to the consumption of traditional Fe-containing beer and linked to a mutation in the ferroportin gene (Gordeuk et al. 2003; Navarro and Visbal, this volume)—is associated with an increased incidence and mortality from tuberculosis. These data are supported by *in vitro* findings which show that changes in intramacrophage Fe availability stimulates the proliferation of mycobacteria and weakens antimycobacterial defense mechanisms of macrophages. Other infections, ranging from bacterial, viral and fungal to parasitic diseases, where Fe overload is associated with an unfavorable course of infection and/or an impaired immune response, have been reviewed (Weinberg 1999).

The importance of iron for antimicrobial immune response pathways is further underscored by the finding that many innate resistance genes of macrophages act by limiting Fe availability for intracellular bacteria. Macrophages exposed to the intracellular bacterium *Salmonella typhimurium* increase expression of ferroportin, which results in a stimulation of cellular Fe export and a limitation of Fe availability for intramacrophage bacteria, and leads to improved control of bacterial proliferation by macrophages. This is partly due to the fact that a reduction of cytoplasmic iron increases the activity of immune

---

[1]  CD8 (CD stands for cluster of differentiation) is a transmembrane glycoprotein; CD8+ is short for cytotoxin T cells with a CD8 surface protein.

effector pathways, such as TNF-α, IL-6, IL-12, or NO formation (Nairz et al. 2010). Importantly, part of the antimicrobial activities of the Th-1 cytokine IFN-γ and iNOS have been linked to their ability to limit Fe availability in bacteria. Briefly, induction of iNOS by macrophages exposed to intracellular bacteria activates the transcription factor Nrf2 (a regulator of the antioxidant defense in macrophages), which stimulates ferroportin transcription, induces the export of iron from *Salmonella*-infected macrophages, and stimulates anti-microbial immune effector pathways. Importantly, the impaired control of *Salmonella* infection in iNOS−/− mice can be completely overcome when mice are treated with the Fe chelator desferrasirox (Nairz et al. 2013). The crucial role of ferroportin-mediated Fe export for host defense against infections with intracellular pathogens is further supported by the observation that overex-pression of ferroportin in macrophages can control the infection by a number of intracellular bacteria, such as *Chlamydia* sp., *Legionella*, *Salmonella*, or *Mycobacteria* (Nairz et al. 2010).

Another immune gene that exemplifies the role of iron for infection is the phagolysosomal protein Nramp1 (natural resistance-associated macro-phage protein 1). Expression of Nramp1 is associated with resistance toward infections by intracellular pathogens such as *Leishmania*, *Salmonella*, or *Mycobacteria* spp. mainly by shuttling divalent metals across the phagolysom-al membrane (Blackwell et al. 2001; Forbes and Gros 2001). Investigations of the RAW264.7 macrophage cell line stably transfected with functional or nonfunctional Nramp1 demonstrated that macrophages which lack functional Nramp1 exhibited a significantly higher Fe uptake via the TfR and, as a conse-quence, an increased Fe release mediated through increased ferroportin expres-sion. Accordingly, as a net effect of the altered expression of Fe transporters, the overall cellular Fe content was lower in macrophages bearing functional Nramp1 (Fritsche et al. 2012). This provides further support to the hypothesis that Nramp1 expression confers resistance toward intracellular pathogens by limiting the availability of iron to the microbes; a contribution to Fe-mediated formation of toxic radicals has also been discussed (Forbes and Gros 2001). In addition, Nramp1-mediated alterations of Fe homeostasis stimulate antimicro-bial immune effector function, as reflected by increased formation of NO or TNF-α, whereas the expression of the anti-inflammatory cytokine IL-10 is sig-nificantly reduced (Nairz et al. 2010). Recent evidence suggests that Nramp1 functionality results in increased formation of lipocalin 2 (also known as sider-ocalin or NGAL) (Fritsche et al. 2012). Lipocalin 2 is a neutrophil (gelatinase-associated) and macrophage-derived peptide which captures Fe-laden micro-bial siderophores, thus interfering with the acquisition of siderophore-bound iron by specific Gram-negative bacteria, such as *Escherichia coli* or *Klebsiella* spp. (Flo et al. 2004). Moreover, lipocalin 2 delivers siderophore-bound iron to mammalian cells that are able to import the complex via a lipocalin 2 receptor. Most interestingly, recent data provide evidence for the existence of mammali-an siderophores (Pantopoulos et al. 2012) that are captured by lipocalin 2, thus

*D. Rehder et al.*

indicating that lipocalin 2 may be involved in transcellular and transmembrane Fe trafficking in mammals.

In addition, lipocalin 2 expression affects neutrophil recruitment to the sites of infection which, depending on the underlying pathogen, exerts contrasting effects on infection outcomes (Warszawska et al. 2013). Interestingly, lipocalin 2 is also secreted during infection with non-siderophore-producing pathogens, such as *Chlamydia* or *Plasmodia*. Concomitantly, lipocalin limits Fe availability for *Plasmodia*, thereby impairing erythropoiesis. Impaired erythropoiesis, in turn, restrains the replication of *Plasmodia*. Thus, through the mechanisms described above, lipocalin 2 stimulates innate immune responses via limitation of Fe availability (Zhao et al. 2012). By a similar mechanism, lipocalin 2 may confer resistance to infection by the intracellular bacterial species *Salmonella* and *Mycobacteria* in patients suffering from hereditary hemochromatosis. As a consequence of reduced hepcidin formation and increased expression of lipocalin 2 upon infection, macrophages of these patients are Fe deficient and are thus a hostile environment for these pathogens (Nairz et al. 2009).

It is important to note that host-mediated alterations of Fe homeostasis (e.g., via the formation of hepcidin) may directly impact the proliferation of microbes. It has been shown that hepcidin expression negatively affects the proliferation of intrahepatic sporozoites, but may also affect the susceptibility to infection with Fe-dependent pathogens, such as *Salmonella* (Portugal et al. 2011). Accordingly, it appears that different regulatory mechanisms are initiated, depending on the type of the infectious pathogens. Hepcidin induction appears to be a very efficient strategy to limit Fe availability in extracellular bacteria, where nutrient iron is restricted within the reticulo-endothelial system. This strategy appears, however, to be detrimental for intracellular pathogens, where multiple pathways lead to the mobilization and export of iron out of macrophages, rendering them Fe deficient—a fact that ameliorates the control of infection with intracellular microbes and also positively affects innate immune responses.

## Copper

Copper is present in a variety of essential redox enzymes such as cytochrome oxidase, Cu/Zn-SOD, and others. Importantly, copper is also a critical cofactor for high-affinity Fe uptake in fungi, Fe efflux from intestinal epithelial cells and macrophages, and Fe loading onto transferrin in mammals (see Figure 13.2 for the interplay of iron and copper).

In mammals, copper is absorbed at the apical surface of the intestinal epithelium primarily by the high-affinity Cu(I) importer Ctr1 in a manner involving cell surface Cu(II) metalloreductase activity. Copper uptake at the apical surface is modulated by Cu-dependent endocytosis of Ctr1, but as high Zn levels can block intestinal Cu absorption, additional Cu transport mechanisms (at the cell surface or at the basolateral membrane) may be involved. Within the cytosol, copper is distributed to enzymes, such as Cu/Zn-SOD, or to the secretory compartment by Cu chaperone proteins CCS (Cu chaperone for SOD) and Atox1 (antioxidant protein 1), respectively. Atox1 transfers copper to the Cu-transporting P-type ATPases, ATP7a, expressed in the intestine, and ATP7b, expressed in the liver and other tissues, for import into the lumen of the trans-Golgi network for loading onto secreted Cu-dependent proteins. Under elevated Cu concentrations, intestinal epithelial ATP7a localizes to the basolateral membrane, where it mobilizes copper into the circulation; consequently, mutations in the *ATP7a* gene cause Menkes disease, an X-linked peripheral Cu deficiency that typically results in death by 2 or 3 years of age. In contrast, mutations in the *ATP7b* gene result in hepatic Cu accumulation: normally, ATP7b excretes biliary Cu, and neuronal dysfunction results from Cu overload.

Copper is clearly required for innate immune cell function in at least two ways. First, copper drives the development of neutrophil myeloid progenitor cells. As the mechanisms for this are as yet unknown, understanding the role of copper in neutrophil development represents a key area for further investigation. As dietary Cu deficiency or cancer chemotherapy lead to neutropenia and predispose mammals to infectious diseases, knowledge in this area is needed to determine dietary or genetic predisposition to infection via inadequate Cu homeostasis or dysfunction of the Cu homeostatic machinery. This is particularly relevant since neutropenia is one of the most sensitive consequences of dietary Cu deficiency. Second, recent accumulating evidence supports a microbiocidal role for copper in the macrophage phagosomal lumen. In response to proinflammatory conditions, expression of both Ctr1 at the plasma membrane and ATP7a (which partially localizes to the phagosomal membrane) is elevated, driving Cu accumulation in the lumen, as ascertained by X-ray fluorescence microscopy studies. RNA iterference-mediated knock down of ATP7a compromises macrophage antibacterial activity, providing strong evidence for the importance of Cu compartmentalization in the phagosome as one of several important host defense mechanisms. Still, the mode by which phagosomal copper is particularly potent in killing microbial pathogens is not well understood. *Mycobacterium tuberculosis* has three independent Cu-resistance pathways that involve the Cu-sensitive operon repressor (CsoR), the mycobacterial Cu transport protein B (MctB), and the regulated-in Cu repressor (RicR) (Shi et al. 2014). Because *M. tuberculosis* is a human-exclusive pathogen, the evolution of this bacterium to possess three Cu-resistance pathways strongly suggests that it encounters toxic levels of Cu in the host and that this may be driving multiple pathways for resistance.

There are varying reports on increased incidence of microbial infection in patients suffering from Menkes disease. However, the precise impact of Cu deficiency on this observation may be obfuscated by the plethora of clinical phenotypes presented in patients that are both a direct or indirect consequence of peripheral Cu deficiency. Future studies will need to elucidate mammalian sources of antimicrobial copper; in particular, ceruloplasmin, an abundant multi-copper oxidase which may play a role in addition to (or perhaps in some instances in place of) ATP7a. Moreover, mice supplemented with copper are better able to control tuberculosis growth (Rowland and Niederweis 2013). In mice, the RicR regulon is required for Cu resistance and virulence (Shi et al. 2014). Copper-resistance mechanisms, via the Cu-specific activation of metallothionein gene transcription, also play a role in *Cryptococcus neoformans* (a fungus) infections (Ding et al. 2013).

## Zinc

*Distribution during Infection*

During bacterial infection zinc rapidly shifts from the serum into the liver (Rink 2011). Zinc uptake and intracellular distribution is mediated by Zn transporters from two families: Zn transporter (ZnT, SLC30A1-10) and Zrt- and Irt-like proteins (ZIP, SLC39A1-14). ZIPs increase cytosolic zinc whereas ZnTs decrease it. Knowledge about the concentration of tissue zinc is incomplete. Serum zinc drops down, since the Zn transporter ZIP14 is upregulated in the liver (Sayadi et al. 2013); this results in tissue Zn accumulation. ZIP14 expression is induced by the proinflammatory cytokines IL-6 and IL-1 (Lichten and Cousins 2009). In other infectious diseases, this shift of zinc has not been directly shown, but since the effect is mediated by cytokines also released during parasitic, viral, and fungal infections, this seems to be a general effect.

On the cellular level, Zn redistribution is more complicated. Some studies have shown that, in macrophages, zinc is accumulated in the cytoplasm, whereas it is depleted in the phagolysosomes. Enrichment of zinc in the phagolysosomes has also been noted. A detailed comparison of the studies revealed that zinc is enriched during bacterial infections but is depleted during infections with protozoa (Haase and Rink 2014). This may imply that the macrophages are able to distinguish between different types of pathogens, and thus choose the appropriate defense mechanism. Since zinc in high concentration is toxic for bacteria (Haase 2013), this would be the obvious approach for this type of infection, whereas Zn deficiency could induce programmed cell death in eukaryotic cells.

*Role in Host Resistance, Susceptibility, and Tolerance*

The essentiality of zinc for the immune system has been known for decades. Zinc deficiency always results in an immune deficiency (Rink 2011). Generally, one has to distinguish between a general effect of zinc on the cell cycle and proliferation, and specific effects toward immune cells. Since the immune system is the organ system with the highest proliferation rate in the human body (e.g., 80 million neutrophils are released from the bone marrow per minute), any micronutrient deficiency with an influence on cell proliferation will reduce the immune response due to leukopenia.

However, several specific effects of zinc on the immune system are known (Rink 2011). The first observation revealed a reduction of the number of T cells due to thymus atrophy. Atrophy of the thymus is induced by a lack in active thymulin, a nonapeptide thymic hormone that is only active in its Zn-bound state (Figure 13.4). Thymulin is involved in T cell differentiation. The influence of Zn deficiency on the B lymphocyte system is less pronounced. There is no effect on mature B cells, whereas the number of B cell precursors is reduced. The number of monocytes/macrophages and dendritic cells is increased during Zn deficiency, since Zn deficiency promotes the differentiation of myeloid cells into monocytes/macrophages as well as dendritic cell maturation. Differentiation of neutrophils, however, is not influenced by Zn deficiency (Haase and Rink 2014).

Furthermore, Zn deficiency results in a proinflammatory phenotype of the immune system, depending on the increased number of macrophages as well as on direct epigenetic effects on proinflammatory cytokine genes (Wessels et al. 2013). Zinc-deficient macrophages produce the proinflammatory cytokines, the interleukins IL-1, IL-6, and TNF-α without a danger signal, normally needed for the induction. At least for IL-1, zinc opens the promoter of the IL-1 gene, leading to an enhanced transcription of the gene (Wessels et al. 2013). Interestingly, the promoter is closed after addition of exogenous zinc, so that the activity of the gene is directly regulated by the cellular Zn concentration.

While the monocytes/macrophages show a chronic inflammatory status due to Zn deficiency, the T helper cell ($T_H1$) system exhibits a reduced capacity, resulting in a decreased production of IL-2 and IFN-γ. These two effects trigger chronic inflammatory diseases and an increased number of infections (Rink

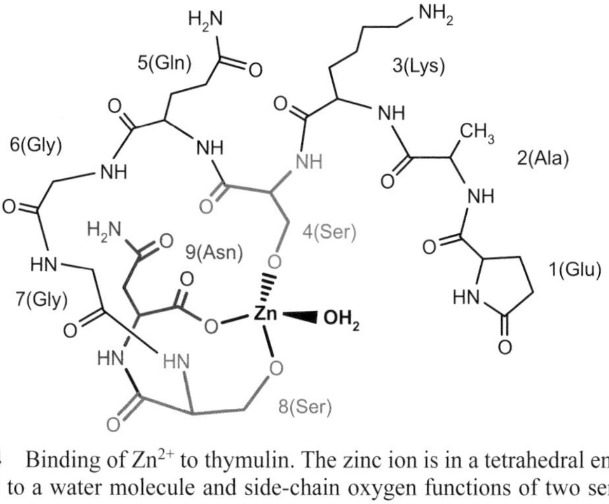

**Figure 13.4**   Binding of $Zn^{2+}$ to thymulin. The zinc ion is in a tetrahedral environment, coordinated to a water molecule and side-chain oxygen functions of two serinates (red and mauve) and one aspartate (blue) of the nonapeptide (after Dardenne and Pleau 1994).

2011). In contrast to the $T_H1$ system, the $T_H2$ system remains almost uninfluenced by Zn deficiency, in regard to cytokine production. However, the signal transduction of IL-4 is diminished in the case of Zn deficiency (Rink 2011; Gruber et al. 2013). Combined, both effects result in $T_H2$ dominance during Zn deficiency. Zinc supplementation restores the $T_H1$ system, inducing a normal production of IL-2 and IFN-γ.

Cellular activation is also influenced by Zn deficiency, since the release of zinc into the cytoplasm is a signal comparable to that otherwise initiated by calcium (Haase and Rink 2009). Zinc signals are generated by TLRs, the T cell receptor, and some cytokine receptors (Haase and Rink 2009, 2014; Rink and Maywald 2014). Therefore, Zn deficiency results in a lack of an appropriate signal of the respective receptor. The function of zinc in the signaling process is not completely understood, but one effect is the inhibition of phosphatases stabilizing the signal induced by kinase activities. Clearly described examples are the mitogen-activated protein kinase phosphatase and PTEN phosphatase and tensin homolog in IL-2 signaling (Haase and Rink 2014). However, signal transducer and activator of transcription STAT-5 phosphorylation in IL-2 signaling is not influenced, showing that zinc has some specificity in its inhibitory capacity. On the other hand, STAT-6 phosphorylation induced by IL-4 is negatively influenced by Zn deficiency, whereas STAT-3 phosphorylation induced by IL-6 is increased (Gruber et al. 2013). A complete picture of the Zn-regulated signaling pathways is still missing, but a summary of the most important pathways is illustrated in Figure 13.5.

Finally, zinc is important for the induction of regulatory T cells (Treg) and for tolerance induction. Zinc stabilizes the Treg-specific transcription factor Foxp3 due to an inhibition of the histondeacetylase sirtuin-1 (Haase and Rink 2014; Rink and Maywald 2014). Normally, sirtuin-1 deacetylates Foxp3 resulting in an ubiquitinylation and degradation of this transcription factor. When sirtuin-1 is inhibited, Foxp3 will not be degraded, eventuating in a regulatory phenotype of the T cells. Therefore, Zn homeostasis is important to maintain the complete capability of the immune system to interact with immune activation or tolerance. Thus, Zn deficiency is not only accompanied by a high frequency of infections, but also by an increase of allergies and autoimmune diseases (Rink 2011).

Excess zinc also exerts negative effects on the immune response, although this is not as stringently defined as Zn deficiency. Whereas slightly increased Zn levels inhibit phosphatases only, unphysiologically high concentrations have been shown to inhibit kinases, thereby interrupting signaling by various receptors. Furthermore, high Zn concentrations decrease the fluidity of membranes and thereby reduce the clustering of receptors normally needed for an effective signal transduction. High Zn concentrations also have negative effects on differentiation and maturation of monocytes/macrophages (Haase and Rink 2009; Rink 2011).

*Therapeutic Effects in Infectious Diseases of Children*

The recognition of the many roles of zinc in human immune and nonimmune defenses against infection, and the increased rates of infectious diseases with severe Zn deficiency syndromes have led to a hypothesis that children with milder degrees of Zn deficiency may be at increased risk of infections. If true, this could result in a large disease burden due to the high prevalence of Zn deficiency and high rates of infectious diseases in low- and middle-income countries. Because of the frequent co-occurrence of Zn deficiency with other nutritional deficiencies, the limitations of determining the Zn status in individuals, and the potential confounding of the relationship with socioeconomic conditions affecting the Zn status and infections, observational studies are not suited to test this hypothesis. Thus, numerous randomized controlled trials, in which the effects of zinc can be segregated, have been conducted. Some of these trials have been focused on the treatment of specific childhood infectious diseases, while others have sought to determine whether daily or weekly Zn supplementation can reduce the incidence of infectious diseases. In all trials where this hypothesis has been assessed, children receiving zinc versus those not receiving zinc is the sole variable between the comparison groups.

Most trials have been done to assess the effect of zinc in treating diarrhea in children. The first definitive trial in India found a 23% (95% Confidence Interval 12–32%) reduction in diarrhea duration (Sazawal et al. 1995). In the nearly two decades since that trial was published, more than a hundred randomized trials of zinc in treatment of diarrhea have been conducted. Overall they confirm that Zn supplementation reduces the diarrhea episode duration by about one quarter (Lamberti et al. 2013). Furthermore, trials done in diarrhea due to specific etiologies have shown a similar effect in childhood illness caused by *Shigella* sp. and *Vibrio cholera*. Clinical trials in health facilities and community-based trials of Zn supplementation for diarrhea treatment have shown that this has some preventive effects also for diarrhea and lower respiratory diseases; the community studies further show a reduction in hospitalizations from diarrhea and pneumonia, and in child mortality (Baqui et al. 2002). These findings resulted in a recommendation, in 2004 from WHO and UNICEF, that zinc (20 mg per day) be used along with fluids to manage all childhood diarrhea. Some, but not all, trials of zinc in the treatment of pneumonia have found benefit, and a recent trial in young infants with probable serious bacterial infection showed a reduction in treatment failure rates with Zn supplementation.

Trials to evaluate the possible preventive effect of daily or weekly Zn supplementation have also been widely done. A recent meta-analysis included 33 comparisons involving almost 17,000 children (Brown et al. 2009). Overall there was a 20% (95% Confidence Interval 10–29%) lower incidence of diarrhea in children who received zinc. A preventive effect of zinc on acute lower respiratory infections has also been demonstrated. Very large randomized controlled trials of Zn supplementation have been carried out in Zanzibar and Nepal (Sazawal et al. 2007; Tielsch et al. 2007). These showed a reduction of 18% (95% Confidence Interval 4–30%) in total mortality in children 12–47 months of age.

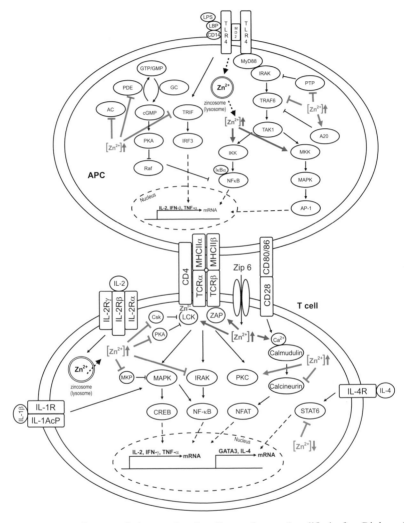

**Figure 13.5** Influence of zinc on the signaling pathways (modified after Rink and Maywald 2014). Top: Zinc interacts with a multitude of signaling pathways in different leukocyte subsets. During the activation of the adaptive immune system, the central interaction (depicted) takes place between antigen-presenting cells (APC) and T cells. Zinc, however, influences the same (as well as some other) pathways in different leukocyte subsets. APCs are activated by pattern recognition receptors, e.g., Toll-like receptors (TLRs). All TLRs, with the exception of TLR-3, generate a Zn signal after stimulation with their specific ligand.

**Figure 13.5 (continued)** For example, the activation of TLR-4 by lipopolysaccharide (LPS) from Gram-negative bacteria is shown to induce a fast Zn release (dotted arrows) from zincosomes. This fast Zn signal (in green) is physiologically required for nuclear factor kappa B (NFκB) activation (solid arrows) as well as for the mitogen-activated protein kinase (MAPK) signaling, both resulting in translocation of the appropriate transcription factors into the nucleus (dashed arrows). However, increasing Zn concentration for a time (e.g., after use of ionophores, highlighted in red) inhibits even TLR-4 signaling (———|). This effect appears to be mediated by direct inhibition of the IL-1 receptor-associated kinase (IRAK), a de-ubiquitination of the tumor necrosis factor receptor-associated factor 6 (TRAF-6) by upregulation of A20, a cyclic nucleotide phosphodiesterase (PDE) inhibition or an inhibition of TIR-domain-containing adapter-inducing interferon-β (TRIF). PDE inhibition results in an increase of cyclic guanosine monophosphate (cGMP). cGMP activates protein kinase A which inhibits RAF directly and NFκB indirectly. Lastly, increased intracellular Zn concentrations persisting for a longer time have the opposite effect due to an inhibition of adenylate cyclase (AC) transcription.

Bottom: On the T cell side, zinc influences the signaling of the T cell receptor (TCR), as well as the signaling pathways of at least IL-1, IL-2, and IL-4. A Zn signal is directly induced by ZIP 6 due to an APC-mediated activation (green) of TCR. This results in augmented ZAP phosphorylation, sustained $Ca^{2+}$ influx, and downstream TCR signaling by binding of the lymphocyte-specific protein tyrosine kinase (LCK). The binding of IL-2 to its receptor (IL-2R) induces a Zn release from zincosomes (dotted arrow). The increased intracellular Zn concentration (red) mediates IRAK inhibition (———|), as described for APCs, and mediates c-Src tyrosine kinase (Csk)/protein kinase A (PKA) inhibition of LCK in TCR signaling. It also induces (solid arrows) a zeta-chain (TCR)-associated protein kinase (ZAP), and protein kinase C (PKC) activity, MAPK signaling, and NF-κB phosphorylation. Lastly, calcineurin (CN) is inhibited by increased intracellular Zn concentrations, avoiding translocation into the nucleus (dashed arrows) of the nuclear factor of activated T cells (NFAT). However, Zn deficiency also influences cytokine signaling in T cells. As an example, phosphorylation of the signal transducer and activator of transcription 6 (STAT6) in IL-4R signaling is decreased during Zn deficiency.Additional abbreviations: IKK, I kappa B kinase; IRF3, interferon regulatory factor 3; MKK, MAPK kinase; PKA, protein kinase A; PTP, protein tyrosine phosphatases; AP-1 activator protein 1; GMP, guanosine monophosphate; GTP, guanosine triphosphate; MKP, MAP-kinase phosphatase; CREB, cyclic adenosine monophosphate response element-binding protein.

*Open Questions*

In this discussion on zinc, ambiguities with respect to Zn homeostasis, the mode of operation of zinc, and Zn supplementation in the case of infectious diseases have been insinuated. To some degree, these open questions also apply to other essential metals. Thus, we briefly summarize core issues that await resolution:

- Is zinc needed for liver metabolism (e.g., in acute phase reaction)?
- Is transient hypozincemia an activation signal for the immune system?
- Does hypozincemia (the withholding of zinc from bacteria) constitute a similar defense mechanism as in iron?
- How does Zn metabolism interact with the metabolisms of iron, copper, and manganese?

- What are the actual molecular targets of zinc within the cell and/or in specific cell types? There are 14 Zn importers (ZIPs, responsible for an *in*crease of cytoplasmatic zinc) and 10 Zn transporters (ZnTs, responsible for a *de*crease of cytoplasmatic zinc); however, their locations (cell type, compartment) are not completely understood yet.
- How are parasites and microbes affected by high or low Zn levels, and what are the mechanisms of the therapeutic effects of zinc?
- How are compartmentalization and speciation of zinc related?
- How do toxic metal ions ($Pb^{2+}$, $Hg^{2+}$, $Cd^{2+}$) "compete" with zinc and interact with Zn-containing enzymes and storage proteins (thioneins)?

## Selenium

*Background*

Selenium is incorporated into a variety of selenoproteins whose functions (e.g., calcium flux, oxidative burst, redox signaling, and effector immune functions) can exert a dramatic impact on inflammation, immunity, and pathogen status (Huang et al. 2012b). Selenium was among the first micronutrients to be characterized in several species for alteration of immune function, including its immunological relationship to other antioxidant-modulating dietary factors (such as vitamin E). In humans, lower Se plasma concentrations have been associated with intensive care unit patients who experience severe infections, increased tissue inflammation, subsequent organ dysfunction, and mortality (Sakr et al. 2007). This general relationship is supported by numerous animal studies, which link Se status to innate immune defenses against pathogens in affected tissues, virulence of certain pathogens, and the risk of immune-mediated organ damage.

*Susceptibility to Viral and Bacterial Infections and to Parasites*

Evidence suggests that Se status and, in particular, Se deficiency can affect the host–pathogen interaction in viral infections. In mouse models, mildly virulent forms of two different viruses, coxsackievirus B3 and influenza, underwent unexpected genetic conversion to highly virulent forms with elevated risk of specific host pathology. The status of the antioxidant selenoenzyme glutathione peroxidase apparently plays a role in this host–pathogen alteration. Examples of similar nutritional–viral pathogenesis interactions appear to occur in humans (Beck et al. 2003).

Evidence suggests that both Se deficiency and supplementation can affect host immunity and resistance to bacterial infections. Selenium deficiency appears to target innate immune cell function, resulting in increased susceptibility to several bacterial diseases. With Se-deficient mice, innate immune-mediated protection was reduced and burdens of *Listeria monocytogenes* were elevated in several tissues over the course of the infection compared with dietary controls (Wang et al. 2009). Selenium supplementation has been reported to protect against chronic bacterial (*E. coli*) prostatitis in a rat model. Alone, selenium reduced bacterial infection and lowered inflammatory cell infiltration of the prostate. In addition, Se supplementation enhanced the effectiveness of antibiotic treatment (Kim et al. 2012).

Selenium also exerts direct effects on bacteria. Organoselenium compounds have been reported to inhibit the formation of biofilms among bacteria such as *Pseudomonas aeruginosa* and *Staphylococcus aureus* (Tran et al. 2009). This has implications for both medical and dental procedures, where Se-based coatings have been applied to polycarbonate medical devices as well as in dental sealants.

Selenium status affects both the host immune response and parasite metabolism. In the nematode infection of *Heligmosomoides bakeri* in mice, adequate Se supplementation affects local tissue $T_H2$ response, resulting in worm expulsion. With Se deficiency, the $T_H2$-driven immune response in tissues is inadequate, glutathione protection is reduced, and the adult worms increase their metabolism, leading to enhanced pathogen success. In this model, dietary restoration of Se levels can rapidly result in an effective host defense and worm expulsion (Smith et al. 2013). Selenium supplementation appears to produce host resistance benefits against trypanosomes. In rats infected with *Trypanosoma bruceri*, dietary Se supplementation beginning two weeks prior to infection resulted in reduced anemia and parasitemias and increased survival intervals (Eze et al. 2013).

Evidence suggests that combined Se and vitamin E deficiency can exert a significant effect on the host immune status and pathogen susceptibility well beyond that of either single deficiency. With *Citrobacter rodentium* infection in mice, double-deficient animals had increased immune cell infiltration of the colon with elevated production of both proinflammatory cytokines and markers of oxidative stress. Bacterial burden was significantly elevated in the double-deficient animals (Smith et al. 2011).

## Recommended Dietary Allowances and Related Intake Levels

The actual guideline for nutritional metal intake for healthy people is the RDA, differentiated according to sex, age, pregnancy, and lactation. Values vary for different countries (United States, China, European Union, Australia). Daily RDAs range between 3–22 mg for Zn, 6–15 mg for Fe, 0.2–1.7 mg for Cu, and 15–200 µg for Se. These guidelines are a source of information for nutritional advice and attempt to reduce the risk of diseases, including infectious diseases related to metal deficiency. For zinc, the missing differentiation in RDAs between the age groups 14–50/70 and >70 years of age comes as a surprise, since the bio-recovery of zinc decreases with age (Chasapis et al. 2012). For iron, the RDA for males appears to be rather high, since just 1–2 mg are excreted daily. Along with RDAs come recommendations which list tolerable upper intake levels (UIL). The UIL defines the highest average daily intake that is likely to pose no risk for adverse health effects, and hence is a tolerable uptake level; however, they are *not* recommended as being *beneficial* to an individual. In particular, the UIL should be considered (and even challenged) in the case of self-medication (e.g., nutritional supplements available in drugstores and supermarkets). Daily UILs range between 10–50 mg for iron, 4–40 mg for zinc, 1–10 mg for copper and 45–450 µg for selenium.

For a detailed overview and corresponding tables of RDAs and UILs in relation to age, sex, and geographical areas, see Wang and Zhang (this volume).

RDAs and UILs do not directly reflect the bioavailability of the metals; that is, to what extent metal ions present in nutrients (and supplements) can actually be disposed of and utilized by an individual. As far as artificial formulations are concerned, absolute and relative bioavailability are distinguished: absolute bioavailability compares bioavailability following nonintravenous versus intravenous application; relative bioavailability compares bioavailability from two differing formulations applied intravenously. Further, bioavailability depends on whether a metal is applied in the form of an inorganic compound, a metal ion coordinated to an organic chelate (e.g., an amino acid), or a conjugate between yeast and an inorganic salt, etc.

In addition, the bioavailability of metals depends on factors associated with characteristics of the respective individual (e.g., age, sex, health, food situation, gut flora). Bioaccumulation and biomagnification of metals can cause nutritional overloads of essential metals/metalloids that are required only in minor amounts, such as copper, molybdenum, and selenium. Furthermore, interaction between different metals can influence their uptake and distribution (e.g., by transporters for divalent metal ions), as discussed above.

## Metal-Based Drugs in the Treatment of Tropical Parasitic Diseases

Metal-based drugs are used therapeutically to treat cancer (cisplatin, carboplatin, and oxaliplatin), arthritis (the gold compounds solganol, myocrisin, and auranofin), and parasitic infections caused by leishmaniasis and schistosomiasis (antimony compounds based an antimonite plus gluconates) (see Navarro and Visbal, this volume). Examples of platinum, gold, and antimony complexes used medicinally are shown in Figure 13.6. In addition, silver and silver compounds are used as disinfectants, and other compounds, such as antidiabetic bis(maltolato) oxidovanadium(IV), have passed phase II clinical tests. Metal-based drugs are otherwise not in common use, and it does not appear that pharmaceutical companies commonly have interest in drugs that contain a metal core.

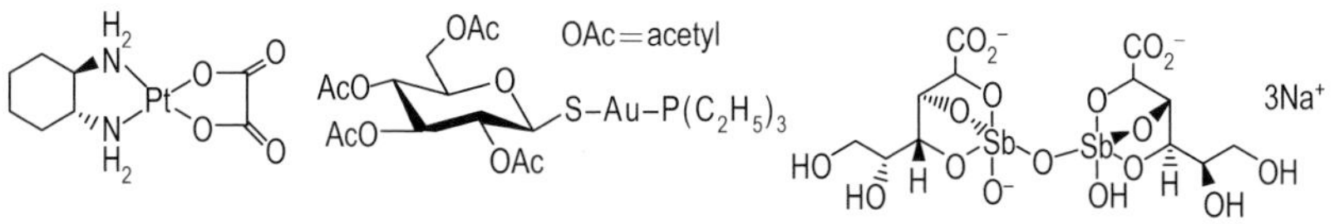

Oxaliplatin                     Auranofin                          Sodium stibogluconate

**Figure 13.6** Examples for coordination compounds of metals that are in medicinal use: oxaliplatin (colorectal cancer), auranofin (rheumatoid arthritis), and sodium stibogluconate (leishmaniasis).

Earlier we addressed the benefits that Se supplementation brings against trypanosomes, organisms which cause sleeping disease and Chagas disease (see also Navarro and Visbal, this volume). Promising *in vivo* and *in vitro* studies have used diverse metal complexes and shown that they are just as effective as antiparasitic drugs in combating leishmaniasis, Chagas disease (*American trypanosomiasis*), amoebiasis, and malaria. These drugs exploit the metal–drug synergism: targeting is more efficient (with respect to the employment of just the organic constituent), and drug stabilization equates to longer residence time. Thus, coordination compounds of ruthenium, copper, rhodium, platinum, and gold (Navarro et al. 2010; Biot et al. 2012), as well as vanadium (an early transition metal; for a review, see Rehder 2012) have successfully been tested for their antimicrobial activity against *Trypanosoma* and *Leishmania* parasites. Examples of efficient ligand systems are hydrazones, semicarbazones, fluorodiketones, sulfonamides, and 8-aminoquinoline. Coordination complexes of copper, silver, ruthenium, and platinum, which contain aromatic or pseudo-aromatic ligands for the potential intercalation in DNA, have shown promising *in vitro* activity against *Trypanosoma cruzi* and *Leishmania major* promastigotes. In many cases, the ligands in this group of complexes derive from ortho-phenanthroline (Figure 13.7), and the action of these complexes suggests a mechanism comparable to that of anticancer drugs.

The increasing resistance of malaria parasites against chloroquine—the classical remedy for malaria infections—has spurred the development of metal (Fe, Au, Ru, and Pt) complexes based on chloroquine and its derivatives. These complexes circumvent resistance against chloroquine by preventing the conversion of hematin to the stable dimer hemozoin:

$$\text{heme} \xrightarrow[\text{Fe}^{2+}]{\text{oxidation}} \text{hematin} \xrightarrow{\text{"dimerization"}} \text{hemozoin} \quad (13.1)$$
$$\text{Fe}^{3+}(\text{OH})\text{–heme}$$

Coupling between two hematins takes place through the formation of coordinative bonds between $Fe^{3+}$ and carboxylate. Hematin, i.e., $Fe^{3+}(OH)$-heme, is generated through the oxidation of heme (containing ferrous iron), which is toxic for the malaria parasite. In addition, ferrocenyl-derivatized amino-chloroquinoline has been shown to function according to a comparable mechanism. For additional details and references, see Navarro and Visbal (this volume)

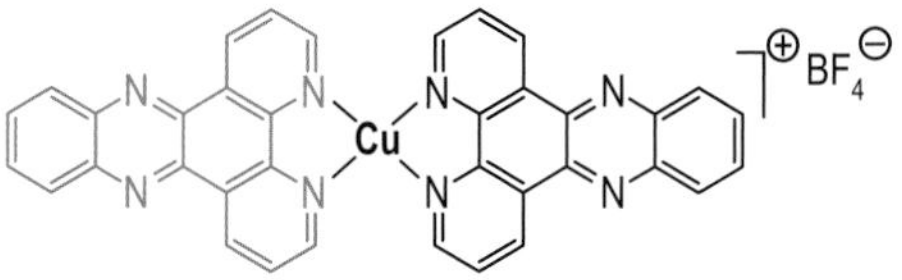

Cu⁺ dipyridophenazine tetrafluoroborate

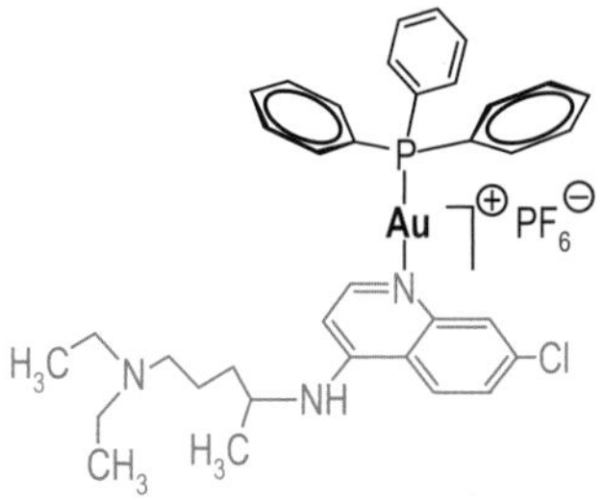

Au⁺ coordinated to (*R, S*)-chloroquine
and triphenylphosphane

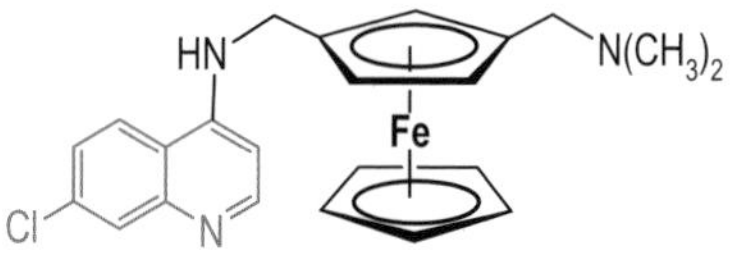

Ferroquine
(Ferrocene is linked to 7-chloroquinoline)

**Figure 13.7**    Three coordination compounds with promising potential in the treatment of tropical diseases: the copper complex with the dipyridophenazin ligand system is active against trypanosomiasis, whereas the gold complex (based on the chloroquine ligand) and ferroquine are active against malaria parasites.

and recent reviews on the development of metallopharmaceuticals to combat malaria (Navarro et al. 2012; Salas et al. 2013).

In conclusion, diverse (transition) metal ions can be used to treat parasitic tropical diseases. The metal commonly functions by stabilizing the active component (the specific ligand in the coordination compound) and by enhancing the drug's activity in the sense that the metal ion improves the drug's lifetime, its target specifity, and the efficacy of binding into the target site. A metal-based drug can also function through the delivery of metal ions to a specific site of action, in particular because the metal switches easily between different oxidation states, such as $Fe^{2+/3+}$ and $Au^{+/3+}$.

# Metals in the Environment as Risk Factors for Infectious Diseases

# 14

# Selenium and Mercury
## Their Interactions and Roles
## in Living Organisms

Tamara García-Barrera

### Abstract

The essential or toxic character of the elements depends not only on their concentration, but also on the chemical form in which they occur. This is the case of arsenobetaine, which has limited biological activity compared to the highly toxic inorganic arsenic. Some elements, however, can counteract the toxic action of others through cooperative, competitive, or availability mechanisms. A good example of this is the protective effect of some chemical forms of selenium (Se) against mercury (Hg) toxicity. The range between deficient and essential dose of selenium is nonetheless narrow, and some chemical forms of selenium are toxic (e.g., selenocystathionine, which is very abundant in *Lecythis minor* and causes hair loss).

Cadmium causes the conversion of xanthine dehydrogenase into xanthine oxidase and abnormalities in urate transporters (hyperuricemia), observed in rats under oxidative stress, but cadmium does not have redox properties. This is because cadmium replaces other metals with redox properties. Another example is that toxicity caused by the presence of arsenic in drinking water in countries like Bangladesh is increased through selenium and zinc (Zn) deficiency detected in the soil.

Clearly, the essentiality or toxic character of trace elements cannot be considered in isolation, since it can be modulated by their interaction with the particular organism (its genome), with other elements, and with biomolecules, and is dependent on dose and chemical form.

## Introduction

Metals play an essential role in the metabolism of living organisms and, in contrast to metabolites, cannot be produced or consumed through biochemical reactions. For this reason, the study of the metabolism of metals lies at an important interface between chemistry and biology. The availability of elements and their specific chemical properties are the promoter forces for the evolution of life on Earth (Thiele and Gitlin 2008). This explains the extremophile organisms and variety of organisms that can live under different geochemical conditions. It is important to consider systems biology in relation to the metabolism of trace metals, in which the metalome is defined as "the distribution of elements, concentration at equilibrium of free metallic ions or free elements in a cellular compartment, cell or organism and refers to the identity and/or quantity of metals/metalloids and their species" (Williams 2001). The systematic study of trace metals requires information about how the organisms detect, incorporate, and use these metals (Thiele and Gitlin 2008). Metallic ions are strongly bound to proteins, which overcomes steric problems, electrostatics repulsions, and other noncovalent interactions that prevent the association with monomeric proteins. The importance of metals in biological systems is revealed by their influence on more than 50% of the proteins as well as by the fact that metalloproteins represent about 30% of the known proteins (Mounicou et al. 2009).

Metalloproteins use the singular properties of metals present in living organisms to develop their function, making life possible. In this sense, the ability of eukaryotic cells to detect and interact with metals is performed through three mechanisms: affinity, allosterism, and accessibility (Waldron and Robinson 2009). Another important factor is the lability of the metal–biomolecule link that promotes the rapid assembly and disassembly of the metal cores as well as rapid association and dissociation of substrates. In this way, metalloproteins consist of kinetically labile and thermodynamically stable units (Lippard and Berg 1994). In addition, the study of complex interactions in cells, where the viscous medium contains high concentrations of other molecules, which stimulate competitive reactions, is mandatory to understand the biological role of metalloproteins in their native environments. Moreover, the regulation of metals in cells differs considerably from that observed *in vitro*, since the metal–biomolecule union is completely modulated by biological molecular filters (Maret 2010). In this way, metallochaperones guide the metals and distribute them among the different enzymes and biomolecules, thus requiring them, at a precise moment, to develop their function and contribute to the metals traffic, homeostasis, signaling, detoxification, and metabolism (O'Halloran and Culotta 2000).

However, elements interact not only with biomolecules but also with other elements or chemical species (García-Barrera et al. 2012). In this sense, some elements or their species can counteract the action of others through cooperative, competitive, or availability mechanisms. A good example of this is the antagonistic effect of selenium on Hg toxicity, first reported in 1967 in an experiment with rats treated with mercury chloride and selenite (Parizek and Ostadalova 1967). Since living organisms are usually exposed to a complex environment in which different elements and their species are present together, these types of interactions complicate even more the panorama of "metallomics." Thus the metabolism of trace elements cannot be considered in isolation.

## The Essentiality of Trace Elements

The classification of essential elements is not absolute because some elements historically considered to be toxic are now classified as essential, such as selenium, chromium (Cocho et al. 1998; Maret and Copsey 2012), or tungsten, which was recently added to the list of metals found in biology (Lippard and Berg 1994). In addition, certain elements have a dual character: they are either essential or toxic depending on their concentration and/or chemical form, which in turn depends on their chemical properties (i.e., selenium or chromium).

The ligands in bioinorganic chemistry are commonly amino acid side chains or constituents of nucleic acids. The coordination depends critically on the three-dimensional folding of proteins and tertiary structures of nucleic acids (Lippard and Berg 1994). Metals, however, can also be bound to prosthetic groups of metalloproteins (i.e., iron-protoporphyrin IX, magnesium-chlorophyll), bleomycin, siderophores, coenzymes (i.e., cobalamin-cobalt), and methylcobalamin. The latter can transfer a $CH_3^-$ ion to Hg, Pb, and Sn salts in aqueous solution, a biomethylation reaction that probably contributes to the toxicity of these elements. Finally, metals can be bound to complex assemblies such as cell membranes, viruses, and intracellular compartments (i.e., ribosome, the mitochondrion and endoplasmatic reticulum) (Lippard and Berg 1994). Another example is the structure defined as "zinc fingers," which is a small protein structural motif characterized by the coordination of one or more Zn ions to stabilize the fold. In this way, some elements (e.g., copper, zinc, cadmium, mercury, and silver) coordinate by proteins through a sulfur atom whereas others (e.g., molybdenum, manganese, iron, cobalt, nickel, copper, and zinc) do so through nitrogen or oxygen atoms. Metabolites of arsenic, selenium, and iodine have a metalloid-carbon covalent bond. Other elements (e.g., aluminum, nickel, and iron) coordinate by small organic ligands. Magnesium, vanadium, iron, cobalt, and nickel coordinate by tetrapyrol ligands; calcium, strontium, barium, lanthanum, and lead form complexes with polysaccharides; and, finally, platinum, ruthenium, chromium, and nickel are coordinated by nucleic acids and their constituents (Schaumlöffel et al. 2005). In selenoproteins (i.e., glutathione peroxidase, selenoprotein P), selenium is strongly bound to the organic moiety since selenocysteine is genetically encoded in these selenoproteins, and thus it is an integral protein constituent.

### Selenium Essentiality and Toxicity

Selenium has antioxidant properties and is used in cancer chemoprevention. It is needed to produce triiodothyronine, which is required for healthy brain and bone development, normal growth, and thermoregulation. At correct levels, selenium has been found to be necessary for proper immune system functioning and has been shown to inhibit the progression of human immunodeficiency virus to acquired inmunodeficiency syndrome (Gergely et al. 2006). Selenium can be incorporated into the diet from several food sources (e.g., yeast, garlic, onions). The daily recommended selenium dose is 21 and 16 μg per day for men and women, respectively (WHO/FAO/IAEA 1996). Due to the narrow range between beneficial and toxic levels of selenium, however, both effects can be elicited. Lower levels can increase the risk of cardiovascular disease and other degenerative diseases, whereas high intake can induce hair loss, nail brittleness and loss, gastrointestinal disturbances, skin rash, garlic breath, fatigue, irritability, and nervous system abnormalities (Gergely et al. 2006). There is, however, some controversy related to the upper limits for Se intake, and while some authors do not report any adverse level for an intake of < 800 μg/day for adults, others report selenosis when Se intakes are ≥850 μg/day (Roman et al. 2014). In this context, the U.S. Environmental Protection Agency has defined an intake limit of 1262 μg/day as the reference at which clinical selenosis appears, whereas the tolerable upper intake level established by the European Community has been set at 300 μg/day (Rayman and British 2004; Roman et al. 2014). For a discussion of the recommended dietary allowance (RDA) and tolerable upper intake levels (UILs) for selenium, as reported by the World Health Organization, see Wang and Zhang (this volume).

It is also well known that inorganic forms of selenium are more acutely toxic than organic forms, such as Se-enriched yeast (Se-yeast), in which selenomethionine (SeMet) is the main species, accounting for 54–74% of total selenium (Rayman and British 2004). The LD50 in rats for Se-yeast has been established by several authors at 37.3 mg/kg, compared with 12.7 mg/kg for sodium selenite, demonstrating that Se-yeast is considerably less acutely toxic than sodium selenite. Histological examination of livers of animals fed Se-yeast revealed up to 50% greater deposition of selenium; however, no corresponding toxicity (e.g., severe hepatotoxicity, cardiotoxicity, splenomegaly) was found in rats fed selenite at levels of 16 μg/day over an eight-week period (Rayman and British 2004). It has been suggested that organic forms of selenium may be more toxic during long-term consumption due to its rapid incorporation into tissue proteins rather than its excretion. In 2002, the EC Scientific Committee on Food expressed concern that organic selenium (e.g., SeMet or Se-yeast) could accumulate in body tissues to toxic levels. However, a large number of studies have shown that Se-yeast can be administered in doses as high as 800 μg per day for lengthy periods without any toxic effects. This lead to the conclusion that there cannot be a continuing rise in tissue selenium and that organic selenium is no more hazardous than supplementation with inorganic selenium. In this way, the conversion of organic Se into $H_2Se$ may be an important regulator of Se bioavailability; this may protect against excessive incorporation of selenium into proteins and prevent toxicity mediated through

**Table 14.1** Lethal doses of the main Se species for $LD_{50}$ mice or rats by intraperitoneal (I), oral (O), or respiratory (R) absorption.

| Compound | Formula | Lethal Dose | Reference |
|---|---|---|---|
| Elemental selenium | Se | 6,700 mg/kg (O) | Cummins and Kimura (1971) |
| Dimethylselenide (–2) | $(CH_3)_2Se$ | 1,600 mg/kg (I) | Al Bayati et al. (1992) |
| Hydrogen selenide (–2) | $H_2Se$ | 0.02 mg/L (R) | Wilber (1980) |
| Trimethylselenonium (–2) | $(CH_3)_3Se^+$ | 49 mg/kg (I) | Wilber (1980) |
| Selenocystine (–1) | $(HO_2CCH(NH_2)CH_2Se)_2$ | 35.8 mg/kg (O) | Sayato et al. (1993) |
| Selenomethionine (–2) | $CH_3Se(CH_2)_2CH(NH_2)CO_2H$ | 4.3 mg/kg (I) 37.3 mg/kg (O, Se-yeast) | Wilber (1980) |
| Selenite (+4) | $SeO_3^{2-}$ | 3.5 mg/kg (I) 12.7 mg/kg (O) | WHO (1987) Vinson and Bose (1987) |
| Selenate (+6) | $SeO_4^{2-}$ | 5.8 mg/kg (I) | WHO (1987) |

reactive oxygen species from excessive intake (Rayman and British 2004). Table 14.1 summarizes the lethal doses of the main Se species for mice or rats by intraperitoneal, oral, or respiratory absorption.

## Mercury Toxicity

Mercury species in the environment are well-established toxicants to human and other organisms. Found in different industrial settings, air, soil, drinking water and food, humans are continuously exposed to Hg species. Divalent inorganic mercury ($Hg^{2+}$) has a high affinity for thiol groups of endogenous proteins and metabolites; thus, it is invariably found in cells, tissues, and biological fluids bound to thiol-containing proteins and metabolites, such as reduced glutathione or cysteine (Andrew et al. 2007). Most likely, $Hg^{2+}$ and $CH_3Hg^+$ bound to cysteine and/or glutathione play important roles in the intracellular transport and disposition of these toxic metal species. Mercury can also produce free radicals that induce protein, lipid, and DNA oxidation (Clarkson 1997). In addition, it is well known that inorganic mercury is linked to some alteration in metabolic pathways, such as energy metabolism, amino acid metabolism, and gut microflora (Wei et al. 2008). Nevertheless, the mechanisms responsible for toxic effects of inorganic mercury in organisms are still not known.

The organic forms of mercury are especially toxic since alkyl mercury is not well metabolized. Due to its high solubility in lipids, organic mercury bioaccumulates and becomes biomagnified through the food chain, thus affecting human health. The World Health Organization sets a maximum tolerable weekly intake of 5 µg/kg of body weight for total mercury, of which no more than 3.3 µg/kg should be present as $MeHg^+$. The guideline level for total mercury in drinking water has been established at 1 µg/l (WHO 1993:51). The European

Commission Regulation 466/2001/EC (amended by Regulation 221/2002/EC) came into effect on April 2002 and sets maximum levels for mercury in bivalve mollusks at 0.5 mg/kg of their wet weight (Moreno et al. 2010).

## Interaction of Mercury and Selenium Species through Biological Mechanisms

### Effects on Toxicity

In general, the simultaneous administration of selenite counteracts the negative impacts of exposure to inorganic mercury, particularly in regard to neurotoxicity, fetotoxicity, and cardiovascular diseases. In humans, a selenite and SeMet-dependent protection against mercury-induced apoptosis and growth inhibition in human cells has been observed. However, other studies reveal that inorganic selenium is ineffective in preventing most of the $MeHg^+$-induced brain biochemical alterations and that alone it is also toxic. The Se:Hg molar ratio is very important since mercury in molar excess over selenium is a stronger inducer of metallothionein levels in some animals (García-Barrera et al. 2012).

As stated previously, selenium can counteract the toxicity of methylmercury, as demonstrated by an *in utero* study of mice exposed to $MeHg^+$ and selenium. The group that was given the lowest amount of selenium and highest dose of $MeHg^+$ was mostly adversely affected in neurobehavioral outcome. In rodents, antioxidant nutrients such as dietary selenium and vitamin E may alter $MeHg^+$ reproductive and developmental toxicity (García-Barrera et al. 2012).

A great number of studies have been carried out related to the protective influence of the selenocompounds against $MeHg^+$ toxicity, especially SeMet. Exposition of $MeHg^+$ in rats resulted in a significant increase in urinary porphyrins and a decrease in motor activity that was counteracted by SeMet (García-Barrera et al. 2012).

### Mechanisms

The following mechanisms have been proposed to explain the interaction between selenium and mercury:

- Selenium provokes the redistribution of mercury to less sensitive organs.
- They compete for the same cleavages.
- Both combine to form Hg-Se complexes.
- Highly toxic Hg species are converted by selenium into less toxic forms.
- Selenium prevents the oxidative stress caused by mercury.

It is believed that a 1:1 Hg-Se compound of low biological availability and activity is formed inside cells, and that cell damage is quite low, even in the presence of very high Hg concentrations, if both elements are present in an equimolecular ratio. This has been stated in studies with marine mammals and humans exposed to high levels of inorganic mercury. In 1978, experiments with marine organisms suggested a direct Hg-Se linkage, and the 1:1 molar ratio of mercury and selenium increment holds true in several species, including humans (García-Barrera et al. 2012). A tissue with a Se:Hg molar ratio higher than 1 is suggested as a threshold for the protective action against Hg toxicity.

The possibility that Hg-Se formation is responsible for the 1:1 molar ratio is supported by experiments which have shown that (a) enzimatically digested liver and plasma fractions with a 1:1 molar ratio release mercury and selenium in insoluble forms and (b) binding to the same plasma protein is preceded with the conversion of selenite to $H_2Se$ in red blood cells (García-Barrera et al. 2012). Selenium can also affect the activities of enzymes cleaving the C-Hg bond in organic mercury compounds. In this way, experiments with rats show an enhancement of PMA (phorbol myristate acetate) cleavage enzymes in liver when sodium selenite is supplemented in drinking water. It has also been observed that $MeHg^+$ exposure exerts an inhibitory effect on paronaxe 1 activity in humans that can be counteracted by selenium. Other hypotheses are that selenium can promote a redistribution of mercury from more sensitive organs (kidney, central nervous system) to less sensitive ones (muscle), that selenium competes for the same receptors, that complexes such as tiemannite or Se-Hg-S are formed, and that $MeHg^+$ conversion into less toxic forms is promoted and oxidative damage prevented. Yang et al. (2002) propose that selenium is involved in the demethylation of $MeHg^+$ in the liver, which results in the formation of inorganic and less toxic Hg compounds (see also García-Barrera et al. 2012).

## Biochemical Interactions

The ability of different Se compounds and selenium incorporated *in vivo* into liver tissue (biological selenium) to form an Hg-Se compound varies and increases in the following order: biological Se < SeMet < selenite. The protective effect of the Se compounds against mercury toxicity might, therefore, follow the same order. Mercury ions can react with thiols (–SH) and selenols (–SeH), which constitute a part of cysteine and selenocysteine. As a consequence, they can be incorporated to proteins, prosthetic groups of enzymes, and peptides. Mercury ions can also react with selenides ($Se^{2-}$) and, with hydrogen selenide, they can form complexes together with glutathione that can be finally bound to selenoprotein P (García-Barrera et al. 2012).

Similar complexes can be formed in other cells with active Se metabolism or during degradation of metal-bonded proteins and metallo(selenoproteins) in lysosomes (biomineralization processes), representing the last step of detoxification. A direct interaction between $MeHg^+$ and the selenol group of glutathione peroxidase has also been reported. However, to explain the reduced activity of the enzyme after $MeHg^+$ exposure, another molecular mechanism has been proposed: cultured cells showed that $MeHg^+$ induced a "Se-deficient-like" condition, which affected the synthesis of glutathione peroxidase thought to be a posttranscriptional effect (García-Barrera et al. 2012).

Mercury vapor shows similar behavior to $MeHg^+$ in relation to its ability to penetrate cell membranes, where it is oxidized in the biological active form ($Hg^{2+}$) by catalase. Such *in situ*-generated ions can react with endogenously generated highly reactive Se metabolites, like $HSe^-$, and consequently a part of the selenium is unavailable for selenoprotein synthesis. Mercury can also provoke the increase of free radicals that induce lipid, protein, and DNA oxidation (García-Barrera et al. 2012).

## Other Interactions

Although the Hg-Se interaction has been widely studied, there are other well-known interactions and other less studied but sufficiently confirmed. One well-studied element is arsenic, which can interact in an antagonistic fashion with zinc and phosphorous and synergistically with cadmium. Likewise, it has been demonstrated in rats that zinc prevents As-induced tissue oxidative stress (Modi et al. 2006), while there is evidence in bacterial systems of arsenic in macromolecules that normally contain phosphorous (Rosen et al. 2011). Otherwise, arsenic and cadmium provoke a more pronounced renal toxicity than exposure to each of the agents alone; they induce lipid peroxidation, expression of glutathione and metallothionein, and redistribution of essential elements.

Zinc, on the other hand, antagonizes testicular damage induced in mice through low doses of mercury (Orisakwe et al. 2001), the teratogenic and embryophatic effects (Gale 1973), and replaces mercury in metallothionein (Day et al. 1984). In rats, zinc also counteracts the hepathotoxicity of cadmium (Rogalska et al. 2011), reduces the Cd-induced metallothionein synthesis (Scheuhammer et al. 1985) and alterations in lipid metabolism (Rogalska et al. 2009), and, in mice, protects against Cd effects on pre-implantation of embryos (Belmonte et al. 1989).

## Analytical Strategies to Study Interactions between Elements

During the last decade, various "-omics" technologies have provided massive information-generating methods to allow comprehensive description of nearly all components within the cell. Genomics has revealed the characteristics of the information contained in the cellular core, which determines cell function and behavior; transcriptomics allows gene expression to be examined; and proteomics analyzes protein synthesis and cell signaling. Nicholson et al. (1999) defined metabonomics as "the quantitative measurement of the dynamic multi-parametric metabolic response of living systems to pathophysiological stimuli or genetic modification." Metabolomics can also be defined as the measurement of all the metabolites in a specified biological sample (Fiehn et al. 2000). Whereas metabonomics provides a means for understanding the variation in low molecular mass metabolites in complex multicellular organisms and their response to change, the "-omics" sciences are concerned with cellular macromolecules. To understand a cell, tissue, or living organism behavior, it is also necessary to consider low molecular mass molecules since they represent the last action mechanism of the organisms. Although metabolomics and metabonomics are the most common strategies for metabolomic analysis, other important approaches (Ogra and Annan 2012) include:

- Metabolite profiling: the identification and quantification of a selected number of pre-defined metabolites, generally related to a specific metabolic pathway.
- Metabolic fingerprinting: high throughput, rapid, global analysis of samples to provide sample classification, usually without quantification and metabolic identification.
- Metabolite target analysis: qualitative and quantitative analysis of one or few metabolites related to a specific metabolic reaction.
- Metabolite footprinting: the study of metabolites in extracellular fluids.
- Metal-metabolomics: the study of metal or metalloid containing metabolites (i.e., selenometabolomics).
- Environmental metabolomics: the comprehensive metabolome analysis of living organisms for the characterization of their interactions with the habitat (see Maret et al., this volume).

As discussed earlier, it is necessary to remember that approximately one-third of all proteins require the presence of metals as cofactors to develop their function (Lobinski et al. 2010). These metals are responsible for catalytic properties or structure of proteins, and their presence in molecules is determined in many cases by the genome (Tainer et al. 1991). Metallomics considers that the identification of a metal cofactor into a protein can greatly assist its functional assignment and help place it in the context of known cellular pathways (González-Fernández et al. 2008). Since chemical species are the specific forms of an element defined to isotopic composition, electronic or oxidation state, and/or complex or molecular structure (Templeton et al. 2000), the defining line between metallomics, metal metabolomics, and chemical speciation is very thin.

In general, genomics can explain "what could happen" in living organisms; transcriptomics can address "what seems to happen"; proteomics looks at "what is provoked so that it does happen"; and metabolomics can explain "what happened in the past and what is happening at the moment." Although metabolomics can be very instrumental in understanding biological systems, other "-omics" are also useful and should be used as well. Under such scenario, metals play essential roles due to their interaction with proteins, metabolites, and other biomolecules (for further discussion, see Maret et al., this volume).

## Acknowledgments

This work was supported by the project CTM2012-38720-C03-01 from the Spanish Ministry of Economy and Competitiveness, and by projects P08-FQM-3554 and P12-FQM-442 from the Regional Ministry of Economy, Innovation, Science and Employment (Andalusian Government, Spain).

# 15

# New Technologies Using Trace Metals of Concern

Jozef M. Pacyna, Kyrre Sundseth, and Elisabeth G. Pacyna

## Abstract

This chapter discusses the occurrence, material flows, technical applications of and pollution by platinum (Pt), palladium (Pd), thallium (Tl), rare earth elements (REEs), gold (Au), silver (Ag), and antimony (Sb), all of which are essential for global economic growth. Modern technology relies on these chemicals for the production of various industrial goods. However, their use releases pollutants into the environment, thus posing a threat to human health.

The impacts of these chemicals on human health are assessed in the context of their linkage to infectious diseases. The consequent environmental damage and political and economic implications of using these chemicals are also discussed.

To reduce environmental emissions and impacts to human health, more efficient cost-effective approaches are needed in mining and production processes. It is suggested that recycling and waste management can be improved significantly in many regions of the world to lessen the environmental impact of using these metals while contributing to a better economic situation. Information on the potential impacts that REEs and technologies using these metals have on infectious diseases is largely missing in the literature. This information gap needs to be closed through forthcoming research.

## Introduction

Waste production, as measured by emission levels of pollutants to the atmosphere, impacts aquatic and terrestrial ecosystems and needs to be minimized, or even avoided, during the production of industrial goods. To this end, new innovative technologies have been designed to address this problem; their implementation, however, is still accompanied by emissions of various pollutants to the environment. This is due primarily to the presence of various chemicals as impurities of raw materials that are used in the production process (i.e., by-product emissions) or to the application of chemicals used to improve the operation of various technologies. Emissions of several trace metals have been well studied over the last three to four decades (e.g., Nriagu and Pacyna 1988; Pacyna and Pacyna 2001; UNEP 2013).

In this chapter, we review information on the application of select trace metals in new technologies to produce industrial goods and the resulting environmental emissions of these metals. High technology and environmental applications of several metals have grown dramatically in diversity and importance over the past four decades. These applications, however, can have an adverse impact on the environment, and consequently on human health.

Our primary focus is to analyze the use and environmental emissions of trace metals with scientifically documented harmful effects on the environment and human health. Wherever heavy metals might affect infectious disease, it is of paramount importance to reduce their release into the environment. Once the most dangerous species, particle sizes, and ways of ingestion are identified, human exposure must be limited. To estimate this exposure and recognize its sources, we provide an overview of overall occurrence, material flows, technical applications of and pollution by platinum, palladium, thallium, rare earth elements, gold, silver, and antimony. Throughout, these metals will be referred to as "metals of concern." Finally, we present an approach that analyzes the costs and benefits of reducing the emissions of these metals to the environment.

## Human Health Impacts

Trace metal toxicology is one of the broadest, rapidly growing fields in toxicology. Metals have served as one of the earliest medicines as well as poisons throughout human history (e.g., Chang 1996). A great number of studies have been conducted to assess the impact of metals in terms of (a) carcinogenesis and genotoxicity, (b) neurotoxicology, (c) renal toxicology, and (d) reproductive and developmental toxicology. In addition, research has been carried out on bioresponses and reactivities to metal toxicity, immunomodulation by metals, and the effects of metals on other organ systems. Over the last two decades, clinical aspects of metal toxicity as well as environmental and human risk assessments have been reported (see, e.g., Chang 1996).

Each metal has a unique mechanism of action with regard to its impact on human health, and these impacts occur primarily on a local scale. We begin, therefore, with a short description of the human health impacts for each metal of concern.

Pure platinum is relatively nontoxic; however, Pt salts give rise to allergic symptoms, including irritation (after short-term exposure) and hypersensitivity of the skin, dermatitis, platinosis, and asthma (a result of long-term exposure). Platinum compounds can also produce toxic effects, including cumulative nephrotoxicity and sometimes neurotoxicity (Van der Voet and de Wolff 1996). Palladium, similar to platinum, is one of 15 metals that can cause allergic contact dermatitis, a form of delayed hypersensitivity reaction of the skin (Kimber and Basketter 1996).

Thallium and its compounds are extremely toxic, and numerous cases of fatal Tl poisoning have been reported (Van der Voet and de Wolff 1996). Large doses of Tl compounds cause acute gastrointestinal symptoms with neurological effects that manifest hours to days after exposure. These symptoms comprise a demyelinating polyneuropathia and may result in mental disturbances (e.g., psychosis, paranoia, and hallucinations). Occasionally, Tl poisoning causes kidney and liver damage. In addition, thallium is a suspected human carcinogen.

Rare earth elements are a set of 17 chemical elements in the periodic table: the 15 lanthanides plus scandium and yttrium. Scandium and yttrium are considered REEs because they tend to occur in the same ore deposits as the lanthanides and exhibit similar chemical properties. Physical growth and development, immune system function, and intelligence can be affected when REEs are present in the environment. Because of this, health response indexes have been devised to measure children's environmental exposure to REEs.

Elemental gold is nontoxic and nonirritating when ingested. Soluble compounds (Au salts) such as Au chloride are, however, toxic to both the liver and kidneys. Common Au cyanide salts (e.g., potassium Au cyanide) are toxic by virtue of both their cyanide and Au content. Rare cases have been reported (Wu et al. 2001) of lethal Au poisoning from potassium Au cyanide. Gold toxicity can be ameliorated through chelation therapy that uses an agent such as dimercaprol. Gold contact allergies affect mostly women. In fact, in 2001, gold was voted the "Allergen of the Year" by the American Contact Dermatitis Society.[1]

Elemental silver is nontoxic to humans; however, its impact on human health is still under debate. Most Ag salts are toxic. In large doses, Ag compounds can be absorbed into the circulatory system, where they become deposited in various body tissues, leading to blue-grayish pigmentation of skin (e.g., Zheng 1996). The eyes can also be affected. Ongoing research is currently searching for information on the toxic effects of nanosilver (e.g., the release of Ag from nanoparticle containing dressing), since nanosilver emissions to the atmosphere have become a new challenge in trace metal studies (Walser et al. 2013).

Antimony and most of its compounds are toxic. The effects of Sb poisoning are similar to arsenic (As) poisoning, although the toxicity of antimony is by far lower than that of arsenic. Fatalities from Sb poisoning are rare, but acute systematic exposure to Sb compounds causes hair and weight loss as well as dry scaly skin. Damage to the heart, liver, and kidneys can occur, and death from myocardial failure may follow. The systemic toxicity of trivalent Sb compounds is significantly less than pentavalent Sb compounds, and this fact is quite important when the use of Sb compounds is considered. A similar toxicity profile is observed for As compounds.

---

[1] http://www.contactderm.org/i4a/pages/index.cfm?pageid=3467 (accessed October 9, 2014)

In Table 17.2, Ackland et al. (this volume) summarize the effects of the above-mentioned trace metals of concern on the immune system and host defenses against infection, as well as their direct antimicrobial properties. However, information on potential impacts of REEs and technologies using these metals on infectious diseases is largely missing from the literature. This gap must be addressed by future research efforts.

## Major Applications

Several industrial sectors use metals of concern throughout production. For many applications, these metals are critical resources that enable modern technologies. As such, ensuring an adequate supply of these metals has become a matter of economics as well as environmental and political concern. Because they are essential for a large and expanding array of high-technology applications, long-term shortage would force significant changes in societal development in various regions of the world.

### Platinum and Platinum Group Metals

Platinum and Pt group metals (PGMs) are critical components for various technologies used in the manufacture of industrial catalysts, automobile catalysts, electronics, glass products, jewelry, dentistry and other applications, including pharmaceutical production. Of the 245 tonnes of platinum sold in 2010, it is estimated that vehicle emission control devices and jewelry accounted for primary usage: 113 tonnes (46%) and 76 tonnes (31%), respectively (Loferski 2011).

Since the early nineteenth century, Pt powder has been used to catalyze the ignition of hydrogen. In automobiles, its use in catalytic converters allows the complete combustion of low concentrations of unburned hydrocarbons from the exhaust into carbon dioxide and water vapor. In the petroleum industry, platinum is used especially in the catalytic reforming of naphthalenes into higher-octane gasoline.

Production of PGMs can be regarded as primary or secondary. Primary production includes mining and smelting processes, whereas secondary production results from the recycling of wastes. Industries which use PGMs have usually developed a closed-loop management of waste with recyclers.

As one of the major users of PGMs, Europe imports its supply in the form of PGM concentrates, refined PGMs, and imported products that contain PGMs (e.g., car catalysts and electronic equipment). PGM flows in Europe have been tracked by Saurat and Bringezu (2008) using substance flow analysis. In 2004, for instance, the EU-25, Norway, and Switzerland imported 113,836 kg of platinum, palladium, and rhodium from South Africa, Russia, Canada, and the United States. Illustrating this flow of PGMs, Figure 15.1 shows the primary uses of these metals, their life cycle, the specific environmental pressures

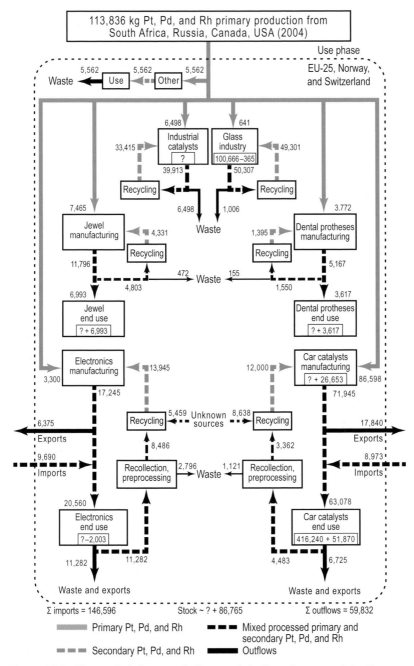

**Figure 15.1**   Flows of platinum, palladium, and rhodium that entered the European Union (EU-25, including Norway and Switzerland) in 2004 are depicted, based on an analysis by Saurat and Bringezu (2008).

created (particularly by secondary production of PGMs), and the recycling rate. This information provides a basis for discussing options to reduce demand for primary PGMs.

Substance flow analysis can also be used to discuss the flow of metals within a given sector. An assessment of Pd, Au, and Ag flows during the preprocessing of waste from electrical and electronic equipment has been prepared by Chancerel et al. (2009). Figure 15.2 shows the flows of these metals during preprocessing of 1 tonne of input in waste electrical and electronic equipment.

**Thallium**

Thallium and its compounds are used mainly in optics, electronics, high-temperature superconductivity, and various medical applications. Because they are harder than other common infrared optics, Tl compounds have been used as infrared optical material. In addition, Tl compounds transmit at significantly longer wavelengths. Thallium is also used to produce high-density glasses.

The electrical conductivity of some Tl compounds changes with exposure to infrared light. As a result, Tl compounds are used to produce photoresistors. They are also used to improve the efficiency of sodium iodine (NaI(Tl)) crystals in scintillation detectors. Finally, one of the most interesting applications of thallium is in the development of high-temperature superconducting materials for applications such as magnetic resonance imaging, storage of magnetic energy, magnetic propulsion, and electric power generation and transmission.

**Rare Earth Elements**

Since 1985, production of REEs has grown rapidly to meet the demand created by new and important applications (see Table 15.1). This sharp increase has been met by China (Figure 15.3), which currently produces over 95% of the world's REE supply, mostly in Inner Mongolia, even though it has only 37% of proven reserves. By 2012, these figures were reported by Bradsher (2010) to have decreased to 90% (production rate) and 23% (proven reserves).

The diverse nuclear, metallurgical, chemical, catalytic, electrical, magnetic, and optical properties of the REEs have led to a variety of applications: from everyday usage (e.g., lighter flints, glass polishing), to high-technology (e.g., phosphorus, lasers, magnets, batteries, magnetic refrigeration) and futuristic applications (high-temperature superconductivity, safe storage and transport of hydrogen for a post-hydrogen economy) (Haxel et al. 2002).

As can be seen from Table 15.1, many applications of REEs are characterized by high specificity. Some of these have led to breakthrough changes in technology. One such example is permanent magnet technology, which uses alloys that contain neodymium, samarium, gadolinium, dysprosium, or praseodymium. In addition, REE magnets have allowed for the miniaturization of numerous electrical and electronic components used in appliances, audio and

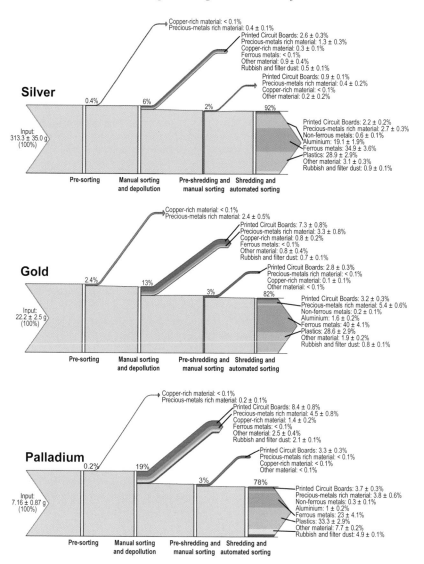

**Figure 15.2**   Flows of silver, gold, and palladium during preprocessing of 1 tonne of input from waste electrical and electronic equipment (from Chancerel et al. 2009; reprinted with permission from John Wiley and Sons).

video equipment, computers, automobiles, communication systems, and military gear (Haxel et al. 2002). REEs are also used in various sustainable energy generation applications (e.g., wind mills, electricity generators), primarily as powerful permanent magnets.

Several REEs are essential in the petroleum industry as fluid cracking catalysts as well as for automotive pollution control as catalytic convertors.

**Table 15.1**  Application of rare earth elements.

| Name | Selected Applications |
|---|---|
| Scandium (Sc) | Al-Sc alloys for aerospace industry components, additive in metal-halide lamps and Hg vapor lamps, radioactive tracing agent in oil refineries, catalyzer in organic chemistry |
| Yttrium (Y) | Yttrium aluminum garnet laser, yttrium vanadate as host for europium in TV red phosphor, $YBa_2Cu_3O_7$ high-temperature superconductors, Yttria-stabilized zirconia, yttrium iron garnet microwave filters, energy-efficient light bulbs, spark plugs, gas mantles, additive to steel, $YAl_3(Ce)$ scintillation detectors |
| Lanthanum (La) | High-refractive index and alkali-resistant glass, flint, LaNi5 hydrogen storage, Ni-metal hybride batteries, camera lenses, fluid catalytic cracking catalyst for oil refineries |
| Cerium (Ce) | Chemical-oxidizing agent, polishing powder, yellow colors in glass and ceramics, catalytic converter for CO oxidation in cars, catalyst for self-cleaning ovens, fluid catalytic cracking catalyst for oil refineries, ferro-cerium flints for lighters |
| Praseodymium (Pr) | High-power magnets, lasers, core material for carbon arc lighting, colorant in glasses and enamels, additive in didymium glass used in welding goggles, ferro-cerium fire-steel (flint) products |
| Neodymium (Nd) | $Nd_2F_{14}B$ magnets, lasers, violet colors in glass and ceramics, didymium glass, ceramic capacitors |
| Promethium (Pm) | Nuclear batteries |
| Samarium (Sm) | $SmCo_5$ and $Sm_2Co_{17}$ magnets, lasers, neutron capture, masers, catalysts, in ceramics and glass |
| Europium (Eu) | Red and blue phosphors, lasers, mercury-vapor lamps, fluorescent lamps, NMR relaxation agent |
| Gadolinium (Gd) | Rare-earth magnets, high-refractive index glass or garnets, lasers, X-ray tubes, computer memories, neutron capture, MRI contrast agent, NMR relaxation agent, magnetostrictive alloys such as Galfenol, steel additive |
| Terbium (Tb) | Dopant materials, green phosphors, lasers, fluorescent lamps, magnetostrictive alloys such as Terfenol-D in naval sonar systems and sensors |
| Dysprosium (Dy) | Rare-earth magnets, lasers, magnetostrictive alloys such as Terfenol-D |
| Holmium (Ho) | Solid-state lasers, wavelength calibration standards for optical spectrophotometers, magnets, colorant in glass |
| Erbium (Er) | Neutron-absorbing control rods in nuclear technology, infrared lasers, vanadium steel, fiber optic technology, photographic filter, medical applications in dermatology and dentistry |
| Thulium (Tm) | Portable X-ray machines, metal-halide lamps, lasers, high-temperature superconductors |
| Ytterbium (Y) | Infrared lasers, chemical reducing agent, decoy flares, stainless steel, stress gauges |
| Lutetium (Lu) | PET scan detectors, high-refractive index glass, lutetium tantalate hosts for phosphors, catalyst in petroleum cracking |

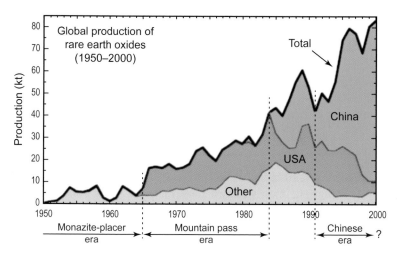

**Figure 15.3**     Global production of rare earth elements (1 kt = 106 kg) from 1950 to 2000 (Haxel et al. 2002).

La-Ni-hydride batteries show greater energy density, better charge-discharge characteristics, and fewer environmental problems in terms of their disposal or recycling.

Another high-technology application of REEs is related to magnetic refrigeration. This type of refrigeration came about after the discovery of the giant magneto-caloric effect in $Gd_5Si_2Ge_2$ by Pecharsky et al. (2003). It is more efficient than conventional gas compression refrigeration and is used in residential, commercial, and automotive air conditioners.

## Gold

According to the Gold Fields Mineral Resources,[2] as of 2012, a total of 174,100 tonnes of gold have been mined throughout human history. Annually (according to 2013 figures), about 2800 tonnes of gold are mined globally for the following primary uses: 50% for jewelry, 40% for coins and ingots, and 10% for industry.

Archaeology has provided evidence of the use of gold in coins in Lydia, Asia Minor as of ca. BC 600.[3] Major industrial applications include the use of gold in toners to shift the color of prints or to increase their stability in photography. In addition, because it reflects electromagnetic radiation (e.g., infrared and visible light as well as radio waves) well, gold is used for the protective coatings on many artificial satellites, in infrared protective faceplates in thermal protection suits and astronaut helmets, as well as in electronic warfare

---

[2]  http://www.gold.org (accessed October 9, 2014)

[3]  http://www.asiaminorcoins.com/gallery/thumbnails.php?album=43 (accessed October 9, 2014)

aircraft. Due to its effectivity in heat shielding, it can be used in automobiles; McLaren Racing Limited, for example, uses a Au foil in the engine compartment of its F1 model. Since it can be manufactured so thin that it appears transparent, gold is also used in the design of some aircraft cockpit windows; passing electricity through it permits de-icing or anti-icing. Finally, gold is used in electronics. Since it is a very effective conductor for electricity, it has been used in the electrical wiring of various high-energy applications.

## Silver

In the Middle Ages, silver and Ag salts were used primarily to produce a strong clear yellow pigment in early stained glass. In the parish church of Le Mesnil-Villeman, Manche, France, evidence of the Ag stain technique is traceable back to 1313 (Marks 1993). Later, silver was used in currency coins, ornaments, and jewelry. More recently, silver has been used in various industrial applications: in electrical contacts and conductors, mirrors, and catalysis of chemical reactions. Some of these electrical and electronic products employ silver because of its superior conductivity (e.g., in cables and wires) and to ensure superior reflectivity of visible light (e.g., mirror production). Silver compounds are used in photographic film as well as in disinfectants, microbiocides, and antibiotics. Control rods of nuclear reactors are routinely made using the $Ag_80In_{15}Cd_5$ alloy; this permits efficient joining of high-absorption cross sections for thermic neutrons (contributions Ag 50 barn, Cd 130 barn, In 10 barn). It also ensures stability during activation, corrosion, and temperature fluctuations: the Ag fraction contributes 50 barn, the Cd fraction 125 barn.

Currently, silver is viewed as one of the "technological nutrients" without which modern society could not function. Therefore, it is of vital importance to quantify cycles of these "nutrients" with indications of their major sources, abundance, and transfer in the environment. A rather large body of information is now available (Rauch and Pacyna 2009), which makes it possible to review Earth's global cycle of silver and seven other chemicals. Figure 15.4 illustrates the flows, stocks, and changes in net stocks of global silver (Rauch and Pacyna 2009).

## Antimony

More than 50% of the world's Sb reserves are located in China. In 2010, about 135,000 tonnes of antimony were produced worldwide, 89% of which derived from China (120,000 tonnes) (Papp et al. 2008).

Major Sb applications include alloys and flame retardants. It is also used as an alloying material for lead and tin, as well as for lead acid batteries: antimony improves charging characteristics and reduces generation of hydrogen. Antimony alloys are also used in the production of bearing metal and solders. Other metallic uses include the production of ammunition, cable covering, and castings.

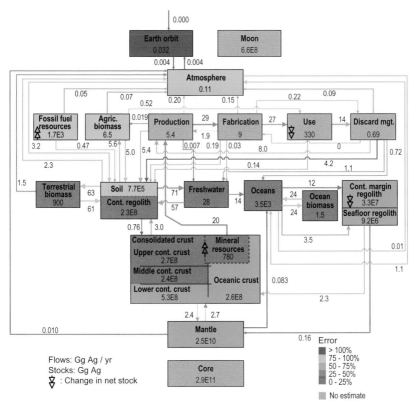

**Figure 15.4** Earth's global cycle of silver (from Rauch and Pacyna 2009, reprinted with permission from John Wiley and Sons).

Trioxide of antimony is used to make flame-proofing compounds and products. These nonmetallic uses include plastic additives in the production of stabilizers, catalysts, ceramics and glass production, and pigment production (Butterman and Carlin, Jr. 2004). Increasingly, antimony is being used in microelectronic applications, where it is being used by the semiconductor industry as a dopant in the production of diodes, infrared detectors, and other devices.

## Environmental Impacts of Production and Application

Ideally, the application of metals of concern in new technologies should improve the efficiency of industrial production without damaging the environment. However, industrial processes (i.e., applications related to both primary and secondary production: mining, smelting, recycling) continue to contaminate the environment with metals and other pollutants (e.g., $CO_2$, sulfur and nitrogen oxides). For example, in 2004, $SO_2$ emissions associated with the production of PGMs used in Europe reached 3% of the total direct $SO_2$ emissions for the EU-15 in 2003. At the same time, reduction of $SO_2$ emissions in Europe resulted in the need to provide sulfur supplementation of soils via fertilizers.

The application of new technologies that utilize metals of concern can, however, benefit the environment by reducing emissions of some contaminants. An obvious example is the reduction of automobile emissions of various gaseous pollutants that was achieved through PGM catalysts, as well as the application of these catalysts in petrochemical industry.

In the following sections, we review information on environmental damage and benefits that have resulted from the application of metals of concern.

## Environmental Damage Caused by the Production

Sources of metals of concern—particularly REEs and PGMs—are placer sand deposits or side elements from ores of other major metals (e.g., zinc, copper, nickel, and lead). Ore mining, refining, and smelting can have serious environmental consequences if not properly managed. Most mining operations occur in underground mines and affect the environment well beyond the immediate area of the extraction site (due, in particular, to sulfur emissions and deposition through acid rain). To reduce aboveground pollution and costs, there is a tendency to sort lumps of ore underground in the mine galleries using automated X-ray analytical techniques. For open pit mines, pollution via dust from carrier ores that are released during digging and milling poses a major concern. Gold, for example, occasionally mined as a trace constituent of arsenopyrit (FeSAs), leads to As exposure, as exemplified around the Kinross Paracatu mine in Brazil.

Two major technological processes are involved in nonferrous metallurgy. The first is the pyrometallurgical process, where roasting is used to split sulfur from the metals in the ores. This high-temperature process is a known source of emissions of various pollutants, including metals of concern to the atmosphere. The second is based on the hydrometallurgical process: ore is dissolved in acid and digested; elements are then differentially precipitated or separated using ion chromatographic techniques, which means that discharges of pollutants to aquatic ecosystems can be expected.

Secondary metal production involves waste recycling that contains various pollutants, including metals of concern. This process usually involves high temperatures, and emissions of contaminants to the atmosphere are very difficult to avoid. Compared to secondary production technologies, primary metal production technologies are much better controlled with respect to the pollutant emissions.

Not all wastes are recycled, however. Significant quantities of metals deposited in wastes can be found in tailing and landfills. This poses a serious problem related to the contamination of terrestrial ecosystems by various contaminants.

Quantification of emissions from metals of concern to the atmosphere, land, and water has been approached only on a limited scale. This information is largely missing from the literature, particularly for emissions on scales larger than local scale (i.e., on national, continental, or global scales). Nriagu and Pacyna (1988) published the first worldwide inventory of antimony, thallium, and 14 other trace elements to air, water, and land. It was estimated that at least one-quarter of all the antimony and thallium produced and used annually at the end of the 1980s ended up as environmental contaminants.

Subsequent to this inventory, the methodology for assessing the charge of metals to the environment, as a result of their production and uses, has improved significantly. Current methodology is based on the application of substance (material) flow analysis and life cycle assessment. Several research groups have been formed to perform analyses. For example, the Stocks and Flows (STAF) Project, from the Center for Industrial Ecology at Yale University, has been involved in evaluating current and historical flows of specific techno-logically important materials, determining available stocks in different types of reservoirs and the flows among the reservoirs, developing scenarios of pos-sible metal use in the future, and assessing metal supply and demand as well as emissions to the atmosphere. Figure 15.5 depicts the flow of metals during these processes and subsequent release to the environment.

Silver was one of the metals analyzed by the STAF program, as shown in Figure 15.4 (Rauch and Pacyna 2009). Earth and its orbital bodies constitute the system boundary, and all flows larger than 1 Mg/yr between reservoirs were explicitly quantified. Mass balance of atmospheric, water, and biomass reservoirs—assuming no net accumulation due to high turnover rates—was ap-plied to estimate flow magnitudes. Estimated uncertainties are absolute errors

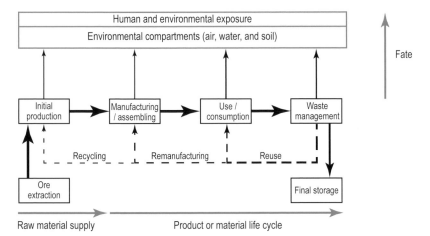

**Figure 15.5** A flow scheme of the releases of pollutants to the environment during various production processes.

calculated by propagation of the estimated or standard errors associated with the source data. The entire exercise provides a diagrammatic representation of Earth's global metal cycles, combining the endogenic reservoirs of the core, mantle, and consolidated crust, the natural exogenic cycles of the pedosphere, hydrosphere, and biosphere, the anthropogenic exogenic reservoirs from production to waste management, and Earth's atmosphere and orbit.

Metals (metal groups) of concern impact the environment in different ways that are related to variations in production/use processes used in various countries. For PGM metals, the total material requirement (TMR), which represents the resource-intensive side of PGM production, is higher for South Africa (over 628,000 tonnes per 1 tonne of extracted PGMs; Saurat and Bringezu 2008) than for Russia. TMR includes wastes from precious metal mining as well as material used to generate the electricity used in mining. Thus, the TMR factor reflects $CO_2$ emissions: the higher the TMR factor, the higher the $CO_2$ emissions. In general, the production of selected metals of concern (e.g., PMGs and gold) requires very high amounts of primary energy, estimated at between 200,000 and 300,000 MJ/kg (UNEP 2013). Thus, large amounts of greenhouse gas emissions can be expected when this primary energy is produced.

A particular hazard related to the production of REEs is mildly radioactive slurry tailings, resulting from the common occurrence of thorium and uranium in the REE ores. However, other resources, such as coal, also contain these radioactive chemicals, resulting in emission of various radioisotopes during the coal combustion for electricity production (needed to produce REEs). In addition, toxic acids are required during the refining process of REEs. Improper handling of these substances may result in significant environmental contamination.

**Negative Implications Related to Usage**

Unfortunately, various applications that use metals of concern negatively impact the environment. As illustrated in Figure 15.5, most of these impacts relate to the disposal of wastes containing these metals. E-wastes (i.e., wastes from electrical and electronic equipment) constitute one important type of waste (e.g., Robinson 2009) and often contain REEs and PMGs compounds, among other trace elements. Concentrations of environmental contaminants found in E-wastes depend on the type of item that is discarded and the point in time when that item was produced. E-waste composition is spatially and temporally heterogeneous. China receives some 70% of all exported E-waste (Liu et al. 2006); significant quantities are also exported to India, Pakistan, Vietnam, the Philippines, Malaysia, Nigeria, and Ghana (Puckett et al. 2005), and possibly to Brazil and Mexico.

Most E-waste currently ends up in landfills (Barba-Gutierrez et al. 2008). From dumpsites where processed or unprocessed E-waste is deposited, E-waste contaminants can enter aquatic systems via leaching. Similarly, following hydrometallurgical processes, disposal of acid into waters or onto soils and the dissolution or settling of airborne pollutants can contaminate aquatic systems.

E-waste contaminants are also dispersed into the air via dust, thus providing a major exposure pathway for humans through ingestion, inhalation, and skin absorption. Atmospheric emissions also occur through metal use in nanotechnology. Good examples are emissions of nanosilver (e.g., Walser et al. 2013) from various applications of nanoparticles in antibacterial materials, antistatic materials, cryogenic superconducting materials and biosensor materials (e.g., Zhang et al. 2006a), and emissions of nanoplatinum and nanopalladium from applications in necessary catalysts for commercially important reactions (e.g., Pauporte et al. 2006).

## Beneficial Implications for the Environment

Major environmental benefits from various applications of metals of concern begin with the employment of high technologies to produce energy and various industrial and agriculture goods. The application of PGMs in catalytic convertors for the automobile industry has reduced emissions of nitrogen oxides ($NO_x$) and NMVOCs (nonmethane volatile organic compounds), although $CO_2$ and $SO_2$ emissions increase slightly during this process due to higher fuel consumption. Still, the use of car catalysts leads to a significant overall reduction of emissions from acidifying and eutrophication agents, whereas the effect on global warming is less relevant (Saurat and Bringezu 2008). The problem, though, shifts from environmental impacts discussed above to impacts that largely affect Earth's surface through the increase in resource extraction and mining wastes. In this context, the overall environmental effect related to the application of PGMs depends on their mode of production. Beneficial effects will be larger if the PGMs are produced from recycling (i.e., through secondary production). However, since recycling rates are still relatively low in many sectors (e.g., electronics, production of catalytic convertors), primary production is needed for the foreseeable future.

PGMs are used as catalyzers not only in the automobile industry but also in other industrial sectors (e.g., in electric power plants, refineries, and the chemical industry) to lower the emissions of NMVOCs and other pollutants. Particularly important is the application of catalyzers in the electricity and heat production sectors, where the application of PGMs to reduce emissions of $NO_x$ is currently regarded as the most modern technology.

Catalytic properties of silver make it ideal to use as a catalyst in oxidation reactions in the chemical industry, where it is used, for example, to produce formaldehyde from methanol. This method of formaldehyde production is regarded as being extremely environmental friendly.

## Political and Economic Implications

The special properties of the metals of concern that we have described explain why these metals are essential for hundreds of applications. Yet despite their necessity, most countries rely on imports to meet their production needs for two reasons: (a) most of the global supply originates from a few exploitable ore deposits and (b) most of the metals are difficult to extract in an economically viable and environmentally sound manner. Due to relatively lower exploitation costs (particularly in terms of labor and regulatory costs) and the transfer of processing technology from Europe and North America to Asia over the last few decades, China has emerged as the major producer of many of these metals (Haxel et al. 2002). This reality (i.e., having a single major provider on a global level) makes geopolitics and trade policies very important factors in the determination of global supply and market price. Additional factors influence market price as well: scarcity, supply-demand balance, stocks and rate of use, market disruptions, market expectations, and the level of speculative versus nonspeculative investments. From 1990–2007, for example, as the observed price of REEs declined, China raised restrictions on exports, which caused prices to increase substantially as of 2007; these restrictions failed in 2012 after threats were made that would have shifted global production (e.g., Haxel et al. 2002; Tse 2011).

Metals of concern are widely used to improve human well-being. Their application is critical in many areas of technology, transport, and defense systems, and, as such, they constitute an important part of the industrial economy. At the same time, the increasing dependency on these metals is a matter of great concern for scientists and policy makers, as future market scarcity becomes likely. New technologies and fast-growing products (e.g., cell phones, computers, electric motors for cars) use many trace metals of concern. The growth of world economies—particularly material-intensive emerging economies and heavily populated developing countries—will drive future demand for these metals. This may lead to a pressure on availability as well as on the value chain of the product, including waste-handling systems. In addition, due to REE use in many defense systems (e.g., some metals are essential for precision-guided missiles, smart bombs, aircrafts, and magnets in defense weapon systems), availability affects national vulnerability.

## Final Comments

Metals of concern are essential for global economic growth. However, many of these metals are difficult to extract in an economically viable and environmentally sound manner. This contradiction needs to be taken into account when the further use of these metals is considered in new modern technologies. In addition, the recycling of waste is a very important issue that must be addressed.

New recycling technologies have been developed that enable better extraction of metals, particularly REEs and PGMs. However, effective recycling has yet to be implemented: in Japan alone, it is estimated that 300,000 tonnes of REEs are currently stored in unused electronics (Tabuchi 2010).

The "true value" of metals, including social and environmental costs and benefits, need to be taken into account when new metals are considered for application. Potential revenues from the entire value chains need to be compared holistically with cost or benefits, assessed according to a life-cycle perspective. To assist analysis, monetary valuation methods need to be employed. Research on mercury provides an example of costs and benefit analysis performance: investment and operational costs to reduce Hg emissions from anthropogenic sources, including the Hg uses, have been compared to damage costs that resulted from Hg pollution of the environment and subsequent human health impacts (Sundseth et al. 2009). It would be worth exploring whether procedures from the Hg costs and benefits analysis could be modified and used to analyze metals of concern.

Future research should find ways to improve the production and use of metals of concern that makes sense, both in economic and environmentally friendly terms. More efficient, cost-effective approaches are needed to mine and produce metals, so that air, water, and soil emissions generated during these processes can be reduced. In addition, energy requirements for primary production constitute a major concern. We need to improve energy efficiency and increase the use of renewable energy sources to reduce environmental impacts related to the use of energy in metal production.

Recycling and waste management can be improved significantly in many regions of the world. This would contribute to a better economy while lowering the environmental impacts of metal's production and use. Recycling rates are increasing but further improvement is needed. System optimization, including a proper product design, offers the ability to do so (e.g., UNEP 2013).

# 16

# The Promise of Nanometals

## Reducing Infection and Increasing Biocompatibility

Mian Wang, Wenwen Liu, and Thomas J. Webster

### Abstract

Conventional metals (e.g., titanium, cobalt-chromium alloys, stainless steel, etc., with micron particulates or micron grain sizes) have a long history of successful use in the body despite the fact that they are non-biodegradable (i.e., they persist in the body for the rest of a patient's lifetime). This could cause a continual inflammatory response and lead to health problems associated with metal compounds or metal ions, especially if such chemistries become separated in particulate form from the bulk metal during use. Recently, research groups have introduced a new classification of metals with nanoscale particulate or grain sizes to decrease traditional metal toxicity, eliminate infection without using antibiotics, reduce inflammation, kill cancer cells, and increase tissue growth. Findings are presented with a mechanistic understanding of how cells recognize and respond favorably to nanomaterials. In contrast to the damage that heavy metals can cause in the body, current innovative approaches use heavy metals formulated at the nanoscale to fight health problems. This chapter summarizes the difficulties associated with the use of metals in the body and discusses how they can potentially be overcome through the use of metallic nanomaterials.

## Toxicity of Metals

Due to their non-biodegradable nature, metal compounds and metal ions have been heavily scrutinized for toxicity in the biomaterial science community. Metals have, however, been widely used successfully for decades in dental, orthopedic, and other medical device applications. In particular, their great strength, ductility, and durability provide excellent properties as bone substitutes. Despite their widespread use in orthopedics, metal ions released from bone biomaterials do possess toxicity and induce some clinical complications.

It is important to keep in mind that all materials are toxic (induce cellular death) at some concentration, and some studies have been completed *in vitro* and *in vivo* to determine metal cytotoxicity (Zhao et al. 2009). There are also clinical reports on the *in vivo* effect of metal ion release (Granchi et al. 2008). Specifically, stainless steel contains more than one kind of metal element which, when considered together, may create even more potential safety problems. Some medical implant alloys may lead to genotoxicity, such as TiAlV and CoCrMo (Gajski et al. 2014). Other studies have also correlated metallic elements with cytotoxicity (e.g., Okazaki and Gotoh 2013). Copper (Cu), zinc (Zn), manganese (Mn), silver (Ag), and aluminum (Al) may all introduce problems as trace elements in the human body. For instance, zinc plays diverse positive roles in biological functions but may adversely influence DNA synthesis, enzyme activity, and hormonal activity (Storrie and Stupp 2005). Most importantly, these metals can lead to significant cytotoxicity when experienced at high doses.

Apart from wear debris generated from surface corrosion and/or mechanical loosening, dissolution of metals after long-term use is another probable cause of metal presence in the body. The prolonged contact of metal alloys with bodily fluids results in gradual corrosion of even the most stable metals. Some implant metallic material components are potentially carcinogenic. The release of soluble metal ions includes aluminum, chromium (Cr), vanadium (V), cobalt (Co), and titanium (Ti) (Daley et al. 2004). Recently, numerous *in vitro* investigations into the impact of metal toxicity toward cells have been established (Daley et al. 2004; Rochford et al. 2012). Among those soluble metals, chromium, cobalt, titanium, chromium, and aluminum have mutagenic actions on tissue-forming cells. However, Cr(VI) and Ni(II) were proved to be carcinogens to humans (Daley et al. 2004). On a genotoxic level, Daley et al. found that metal ions can cause both direct effects, through DNA breakage, and indirect effects, by inhibiting the repair of DNA (Rochford et al. 2012). High concentrations of metals can negatively influence cellular functions and may induce cancer; these concepts are finding increasing agreement (Rochford et al. 2012). As described below, different metal ions have different cytotoxicity mechanisms which must be properly understood in order to develop biometals with decreased toxicity.

**Copper**

Nanoparticles of copper are used in numerous consumer products, from facial sprays to medical devices. Inhaled copper or skin exposure may lead to cytotoxicity. Park et al. (2013) report that copper and its oxides are cytotoxic, possibly even more so when formulated into nanoparticles. Nanoparticles have come under great scrutiny for toxicity concerns since the same volume of nanoparticles of the same chemistry, compared to micron particles, results in increased surface area exposure, which may lead to increased toxicity. Moreover, the nanoparticle size can lead to Cu ion release inside of cells, because they easily cross cell membranes. Karlsson et al. (2008) showed that CuO particles were much more toxic than Cu ions, as CuO particles caused more DNA damage due to oxidative lesions. In neurobiology, copper is the third most abundant transition metal in the human body and brain, with an average neural Cu concentration on the order of 0.1 mM (Gaggelli et al. 2006).

**Zinc**

Zinc is an essential element in the human body and can be used as an anti-bacterial agent. In some research, Zn nanoparticles have been used to modify implants to improve the antibacterial effect (Hu et al. 2012). Zinc, however, is also toxic at high doses in the human body. Zinc inhibits Ca uptake, eventually resulting in reduced total Ca body content in the organism. When Ca reduction is severe enough, an organism will die as a result of hypocalcaemia (Brita et al. 2006). At high concentrations, zinc oxide (ZnO) nanoparticles are toxic to mammalian cells *in vitro* and the human lung *in vivo*; the mechanism of toxicity is poorly understood, and it is not known to what extent sequential nano-bio interfaces play a role (Xia et al. 2008; Palmiter 2004). Both ZnO and zinc are cytotoxic. Some studies have investigated the mechanism of Zn toxicity and proposed that the ZnO particles dissolve to form $Zn^+$. It has also been reported that $Zn^+$ induced a significantly higher rate of cell death than an equivalent amount of zinc in the form of ZnO (Xia et al. 2008; Palmiter 2004). The ZnO dissociation disrupts cellular Zn homeostasis, leading to lysosomal and mitochondria damage and ultimately cell death. Another mechanism of toxicological injury may be through the production of reactive oxygen species (ROS) and oxidative stress (Xia et al. 2008). Dissolution of ZnO raises intracellular $Zn^{2+}$ and is associated with high levels of ROS production (Xia et al. 2008). Palmiter (2004) reports that *in vitro* toxic concentrations of $Zn^{2+}$ typically exceed 10 mg/l. In addition, zinc may inhibit key enzymes in the glycolytic pathway, leading to ATP depletion in cells (Sheline et al. 2000).

**Silver**

Silver is well known for its broad spectrum of antimicrobial activity against Gram-negative and Gram-positive bacteria, fungi, chlamydia, mycoplasma, and certain viruses, especially antibiotic-resistant strains. Many implant surface-modification studies use silver as the antibacterial agent (e.g., Balazs et al. 2004). At suitable doses, it is possible to fabricate coatings with long-term antibacterial characteristics by introducing and controlling Ag release (Zhao et al. 2011). However, silver has a high degree of toxicity. In primary human endometrial epithelial cells, the cytotoxicity of the metal ions is ranked as follows: $Ag^+ > Cu^{2+} > Zn^{2+}$ (Wu et al. 2012). Concentrations of Ag nanoparticles between 5–10 μg/ml induced necrosis or apoptosis of mouse spermatogonial stem cells (Braydich-Stolle et al. 2005). Several studies report different cyto-toxicity concentrations of silver, including 1.6 ppm $Ag^+$ and 36 μmol/l $Ag^+$ for Ag nanoparticles between 5 and 10 μg/ml (Braydich-Stolle et al. 2005; Franck et al. 2004).

## Chromium

Chromium is contained in stainless steel and other orthopedic-related Cr alloys (e.g., CoCrMo). Compared to other metallic implants, it has good properties for corrosion resistance. However, chromium can cause significant cytotoxicity in peripheral blood mononuclear cells, macrophages, osteoblast-like cells, and bone marrow stromal cells. It also can cause an immunogenic effect, which may lead to implant failure (Fleury et al. 2006; Granchi et al. 1998). As such, chromium is not an ideal metal to use in implants, and many industries and researchers are shying away from its use.

## Titanium

Titanium-based dental and orthopedic implants are widely used in clinical settings. It is commonly understood to be a low toxic material due to the oxide that forms on its surface. In fact, there have not been many reports concerning the toxicity of titanium, and most of these studies have focused on Ti alloys (Daley et al. 2004).

## Magnesium

Magnesium is the fourth most abundant mineral found in the human body. It has been intensively investigated for vascular stents and orthopedics, due to its natural ability to biodegrade and because it is a common nutrient for humans. Still, excessive amounts of Mg have been linked to increased risk of cardiovascular disease (Weisinger and Bellorin-Font 1998).

## Use of Metals for Fighting Infection and Inflammation

### Infection

Infection and inflammation are the most common complications caused by implants. They are exacerbated through exposure to heavy metals specifically contained in those implants, the effects of which may persist over the lifetime of the patient, thus, creating a constant potential for infection and inflammation. The presence of an implanted device results in an increased susceptibility to infection for the patient, owing to the creation of an immunologically compromised zone adjacent to the implant. Immune response is influenced by the status of the tissue surrounding the implant, implant design, alignment of implant components, mechanical properties, surface morphology, and wear debris. Bacteria colonization constitutes another cause for concern. Some implant failures are commonly associated with *Staphylococcus aureus* and Gram-negative *S. aureus* (Tillander et al. 2010). Based on clinical statistics, *S. epidermidis*, *S. aureus*, and *Pseudomonas aeruginosa* are common pathogens responsible for medical device infections (Singh et al. 2012). *Escherichia coli*, *Enterococcus faecalis*, and *Enterobacter cloacae* are less frequently encountered (Khosravi et al. 2009). *S. epidermidis* and *S. aureus* (Gram-positive bacteria) as well as *E. coli* and *P. aeruginosa* (Gram-negative bacteria) are the most commonly tested bacteria in medical device antimicrobial research, and recently significant promise has been shown for the use of nanostructured materials to inhibit such bacterial actions (Hetrick and Schoenfisch 2006).

At the cellular level, implant-associated infections result from extensive bacterial adhesion and growth on the implant material surface (Roguska et al. 2012). For a successful implant, tissue integration must occur before bacterial adhesion to the implant materials so that colonization of bacteria at the implant can be prevented. If tissue integration does not occur before bacterial adhesion, the host is unable to protect itself **(Hetrick and Schoenfisch 2006) and** bacterial infection will lead to implant failure quickly after surgery. Peri-implant disease, peri-implant mucositis, and peri-implantitis are complications indicative of implant failure (Bumgardner et al. 2011). Peri-implant infection is a collective term for inflammatory reactions in the soft tissues surrounding implants. Soft tissue surrounding implants will commonly have a reversible inflammatory response, called peri-implant mucositis, whereas soft tissue complications (hyperplastic mucositis, fistulations, and mucosal abscess) seem mainly to have an infectious etiology (Bumgardner et al. 2011).

Loose prosthetic components have been reported to be related to fistulations and hyperplastic mucositis (Sánchez-Gárces and Gay-Escoda 2004). Abscesses can sometimes be seen in relation to food particles trapped in the peri-implantitis, referred to as an inflammatory reaction with a loss of supporting bone surrounding implants **(Norowski and Bumgardner 2009)**. In such cases, adhesive bacteria have the capability to form a biofilm to prevent further desirable tissue formation.

As shown in Figure 16.1, the process of bacterial infection can be separated into three steps (Hetrick and Schoenfisch 2006; Taylor and Webster 2011). The first step is the adsorption of proteins from bodily fluids (such as fibronectin, vitronectin and fibrinogen) onto an implant surface. Depending on the proteins adsorbed, bacteria may subsequently adhere, thus setting up the potential for a device-associated infection. The adhesion of bacteria is generated by the surface adsorption of a bacterial-formed biofilm of macromolecules or organic compounds (Hetrick and Schoenfisch 2006). This second step can be divided into two series based on what happens during and after implant surgery. The primary difference between these two series is whether a special biofilm forms

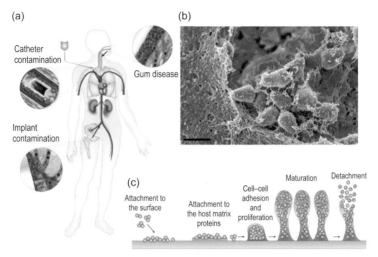

**Figure 16.1** Biofilm pathogenicity in humans is mediated by dissemination and biofilm matrix formation. (a) Possible routes of biofilm dissemination originate from gum disease and catheter or implant contamination. (b) Scanning electron micrographs of biofilm matrix, offering protection of resident bacteria from eradication, imaged from a clinical endotracheal tube identified as *Streptococcus pneumonia*. Scale bar shown is 1 µm. (c) Schematic of biofilm-mediated, device-related infection, starting with bacterial attachment to a device or adsorbed host proteins, leading to biopolymer mediated cell–cell adhesion, maturation, and eventual detachment, which results in the spread of infection. Reprinted from Taylor and Webster (2011) with permission from Dove Medical Press Ltd.

on the implant materials (Taylor and Webster 2011). Padial-Molina et al. (2011) report that implant surface properties (e.g., charge, roughness, morphology, and hydrophobicity) determine the formation of the biofilm, which forms very quickly after implantation. Thereafter, the biofilm affects implant reactions with the host immune system and influences tissue formation and bacterial adhesion. As a result, adhesion of additional bacteria significantly decreases after biofilm formation because the biofilm forms a "capsule" or "microenvironment," which limits interactions with other cells or biological molecules. After the initial attachment of bacteria on the surface of implant materials, bacteria begin to aggregate and accumulate in multiple layers (Vacheethasanee and Marchant 2000). During this process, more protein is secreted by bacteria and absorbed by this biofilm.

As for cellular aggregation and biofilm formation, a microsystem forms on the surface of implant materials, and this can be referred to as the third step (An and Friedman 1998). During biofilm formation, bacteria secrete an exopolysaccharide layer which can prevent microorganism clearance by the immune response. With this protective coating, bacteria in this biofilm have been reported to show a high resistance to antibiotics (Hetrick and Schoenfisch 2006). When a biofilm matures enough, bacteria migrate to the surrounding area or a part of it detaches, moving to the planktonic state within the body fluid to initiate a new cycle of biofilm formation.

Understanding how to minimize infection induced by bacteria has improved over the past decade as a result of improvements in sterilization and surgical equipment cleaning. Although sterilization techniques significantly reduce the chance of infection, new technology is still required to improve medical device bacterial colonization, especially since our standard of care focuses on using pharmaceutical agents, which have quickly led to bacterial mutation and resistance. Passive strategies, including medical device nanostructured surface modification, have significantly reduced the chance of bacterial infection. Another intensely investigated method to improve the antibacterial efficacy of implant materials is to deliver antibiotics underneath the bacteria (i.e., from a surface coating). Common antibiotics that are usually used in this method are vancomycin, tobramycin, cefamandol, cephalothin, carbenicillin, amoxicillin, and gentamicin (Norowski and Bumgardner 2009). The rate and manner in which a drug is released from a coating factor into the effectiveness of the antibiotic; there is concern, however, that such approaches will lead to the development of antibiotic-resistant bacteria. These properties are determined by the matrix into which an antibiotic is loaded or doped (Hetrick and Schoenfisch 2006). Antibiotic release has been widely used in all kinds of coatings. Release strategies from non-biodegradable and biodegradable polymers to carbonated hydroxyapatite are the most representative examples (Price et al. 1996; Stigter et al. 2004). Antibiotics have also been released from porous metals created using anodization, which even without drug release have shown significant abilities to decrease bacteria growth (Figure 16.2).

To date, a common method used to transfer metals into materials to decrease bacterial growth is to coat the metals with polymers. Polymer coatings used for antibiotic delivery include polyurethane and polymethyl methacrylate (Price et al. 1996). Antibiotic release can be prolonged through polyurethane coatings, when an additional thin polymer layer is applied on the top of the antibiotic-loaded polymer (Price et al. 1996). This secondary layer serves as a barrier to drug diffusion, thereby extending the total release duration time. Alternatively, biodegradable coatings can deliver controlled doses of antibiotics. Sustained release is critical for fighting infection due to the persistent nature of bacterial adhesion and functions on medical device surfaces. Similar release profiles have also been obtained from carbonated hydroxyapatite (CHA) coatings. Hydroxyapatite surfaces have strong bonds with bone and have been applied as a promising method for improving long-term implant coatings; when created at the nanoscale, they can decrease bacterial functions. These coatings were premodified via immersion in antibiotic solutions. Although simple, antibiotic-loaded CHA coatings demonstrate very good antibacterial efficacy against *S. aureus*, such bacteria may mutate and form news strains resistant to such antibiotics (Stigter et al. 2004).

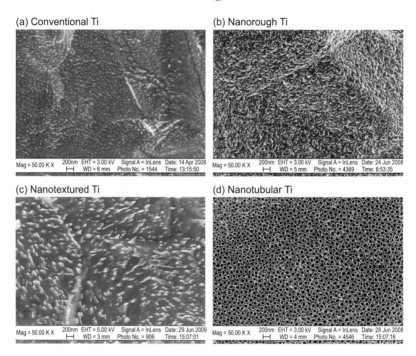

(a) Conventional Ti

(b) Nanorough Ti

(c) Nanotextured Ti

(d) Nanotubular Ti

**Figure 16.2** SEM micrographs of titanium before and after electron beam evaporation and anodization: (a) conventional titanium as purchased from the vendor; (b) nanorough titanium after electron beam evaporation; (c) nanotextured titanium after anodization for 1 min in 0.5% HF at 20 V; (d) nanotubular titanium after anodization for 10 min in 1.5% HF at 20 V. Scale bars = 200 nm. After Puckett et al. (2010), with permission from Elsevier.

For this reason, there is currently much interest in the use of nanostructured surface modification or nanoparticles of metals to fight infection without the use of antibiotics. Specifically, this strategy involves the development of improved antibacterial biomaterials via surface modification, such as changing metallic surface roughness or decorating them with nanomaterials (Roguska et al. 2012; Zhao et al. 2011; Puckett et al. 2010). Altering surface roughness of metallic materials at the nanoscale can significantly increase surface area (and, thus, exposure of the metallic chemistry), leading to changes in net surface energy. This change in hydrophilic properties of the medical device leads to changes in initial protein adsorption and bioactivity, which can influence whether bacteria attach, grow, and form biofilms. For example, for $TiO_2$, it has been reported that novel nanotubes with unique surface energy can be formed on the surface of titanium via an electrochemical reaction (Roguska et al. 2012; Zhao et al. 2011). Apart from surface nanotubes, researchers have also incorporated nanoparticles to decrease bacterial adhesion on implant materials, such as silver, zinc, ZnO, and zirconia ($ZrO_2$) (Huang et al. 2012a; Roguska et al.

2012; Xu et al. 2010; Zhao et al. 2011). These results suggest that nanoparticles known to be antibacterial (such as silver and zinc) combined with common metallic materials can significantly improve the antibacterial performance relative to conventional Ti implant materials. In addition, coating metals with other metals or metal ions is also an effective way to create antibacterial implant materials. As mentioned above, silver and zinc have been reported to act broadly against a wide range of bacteria (Xu et al. 2010; Zhao et al. 2011). The antibacterial properties of silver have been known for centuries as the chemical nature of silver affords antibacterial activity in multiple ways. Biomolecules like proteins and enzymes contain nucleophilic sulfhydryl, hydroxyl, and amine functionalities which can coordinate with Ag cations ($Ag^+$). As a result, $Ag^+$ disrupts the function of bacterial cell membranes and important metabolic proteins or enzymes. This is why silver plays a role in antibacterial adhesion (Zhao et al. 2011). Furthermore, Wang and collaborators have used selenium coatings on numerous materials (including metals) to inhibit biofilm formation on paper towels and polycarbonate medical devices (**Wang et al. 2012c; Wang and Webster 2013**). These studies show that the use of nanoparticle selenium-coated paper towels, polycarbonate, and metallic medical devices creates conditions that do not support the proliferation of bacteria; this increased elimination of bacteria is accomplished without the use of antibiotics, which again could lead to the development of antibiotic-resistant bacteria.

In their attempts to gain a clear understanding of the relationship between the nanostructure of a metal surface and bacterial attachment, Puckett et al. (2010) showed that different roughness values of titanium at the nanoscale can influence bacterial attachment. They investigated the adhesion and growth of *S. aureus*, *S. epidermidis*, and *P. aeruginosa* on conventional titanium, nanorough titanium generated through electron beam evaporation, as well as nanotublar and nanotextured titanium produced by two anodization methods (Figure 16.3). Different nanoscale roughness properties of Ti substrates have already been shown here. Incredibly, without the use of antibiotics, they found that nanorough Ti surfaces were crystalline $TiO_2$ whereas the nanotublar and nanotextured surfaces were amorphous and all decreased bacteria growth. This study provides further knowledge of how to reduce bacteria colonization on metals commonly used in orthopedics through the sole use of nanoscale surface features.

In addition to these efforts concerning modifying the roughness of metals with nanoscale features to decrease bacterial functions, some research has been conducted on the use of metallic nanoparticles to penetrate and then destroy biofilms. Specifically, attention is being focused on superparamagnetic iron oxide nanoparticles (SPION) as a superior nanoparticle chemistry to decrease multiple bacterial infections on demand (and as controlled by an external magnetic source), which is even better than antibiotics or metal salts alone (**Durmus et al. 2013**). This research uses, in a creative manner, a nanoparticle approach: bacterial functions are first stimulated in a biofilm through the

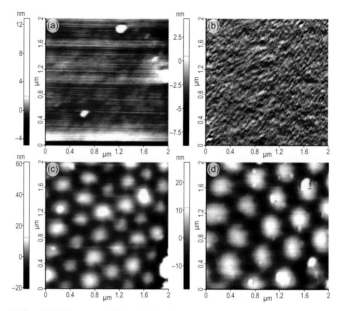

**Figure 16.3**    AFM images of (a) polylactic-co-glycolic acid (PLGA) surfaces created by solution evaporation (nano-smooth), (b–d) PLGA surfaces created using templates of phosphatidylserine nanobeads with a diameter of (b) 23 nm, (c) 300 nm, and (D) 400 nm. After Zhang and Webster (2012a), reprinted with permission.

addition of sugars (such as fructose), which then allows the SPION to enter the biofilm and bacteria to kill them. This research provides breakthrough evidence that SPION may be a promising therapeutic method for on-demand, directed inhibition of bacterial functions.

### Inflammation

In addition to decreasing bacterial functions, metallic nanostructures and nanoparticles have been used to decrease inflammatory responses, which often lead to implant failure. Specifically, after implanted materials react with tissue, the immune response from the body leads to the formation of the complement cascade. The host response ranges from minimal inflammation to chronic inflammation of surrounding tissue to possibly long-term fibrous encapsulation. Several types of immune cells (including leukocytes, neutrophils, macrophages, and other phagocytes) will react to an implant, and this dictates what type of inflammatory reaction results (Rochford et al. 2012). Once a metallic implant comes into contact with a tissue, it can induce monocyte-macrophage activation. When a macrophage attempts to ingest a metallic particle, macrophages will secrete proinflammatory cytokines (such as IL-1β, TNF-α, IL-6, and IL-8), upregulating the transcription factor NFκβ and downstream proinflammatory cytokines (Hallab and Jacobs 2009). Proinflammatory factors, like TNF-α and IL-6 cytokines, are produced by macrophages via the NFκβ pathway. Meanwhile, the proinflammatory cytokine IL-1β has been shown to promote danger signaling in human macrophages (Hallab and Jacobs 2009). Inflammation activation of macrophages to secrete TNF-α, IL-1β, IL-6, and PGE2 stimulate differentiation of pre-osteoclasts into osteoclasts (bone resorbing cells) (Vermes et al. 2001). In this way, osteoclast resorption of bone-surrounding prosthetics may lead to harmful implant loosening; this does not necessarily mean that new bone will form like that which occurs naturally through the stimulation of osteoclast functions (Figure 16.4).

Oftentimes such particles are generated through wear debris from orthopedic implants, but macrophages will also attempt to engulf larger medical device surfaces. The mechanism of implant debris initiating a proinflammatory immune response is still not clear, especially when the role that nanoparticles

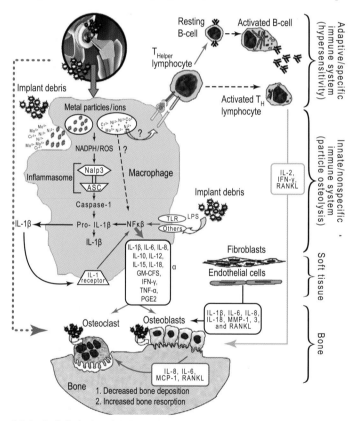

**Figure 16.4** Debris-induced inflammation is primarily mediated by macrophages. Macrophages ingest debris, which results in the release of proinflammatory cytokines that affect local cell types and induce a widening zone of soft tissue damage and inflammation. Reprinted with permission from Hallab and Jacobs (2009).

play in such processes is considered. There is concern that smaller wear debris particles in the nanometer regime will initiate a larger proinflammatory immune response due to a larger surface area to volume ratio; however, some studies have indicated that small enough metallic nanoparticles can even avoid immune system recognition completely.

Apart from the activation of local inflammatory responses, which results in osteoblast deposition, decreasing bone formation, and osteoclast digestion of bone, metallic wear debris has a significant negative influence on mesenchymal stem cell differentiation into functional bone cells (Hallab and Jacobs 2009). Moreover, as the population ages, it can be expected that more patients with osteoporosis will require orthopedic procedures, including arthroplasty. Thus, the toxic consequences of orthopedic wear debris discussed above, in relation to inflammation, need to be closely considered. Adverse outcomes are more likely in osteoporosis patients who require orthopedic procedures (Russell 2013). Thus, some metals and associated wear debris particles will lead to immune reactions or inflammatory reactions that should be considered carefully. In this manner, again, the use of nanometals in orthopedics will result in nanoparticulate wear debris that cannot be recognized by the immune system and may be the future for all metallic-based orthopedic implants.

## Use of Nanometals for Cancer Treatment

It is not possible to discuss the use of metals in orthopedics without mentioning the potential link between metallic wear debris and cancer. Small particles of wear debris (less than 150 nm) can be ingested by cellular endocytosis and pinocytosis processes. Larger particles (more than 150 nm to 10 µm) can be phagocytosed by osteoblasts, fibroblasts, endothelial cells, and, most importantly, macrophages (Hallab and Jacobs 2009). As mentioned, macrophages play an important role in ingesting implant debris and secreting antigens for promoting T cell reactions (Shanbhag et al. 1995; Shanbhag et al. 1998). Once wear debris is ingested by macrophages, a series of biological reactions can occur in the host. Specifically, pathogen antigens are secreted by macrophages and presented to T helper cells. Thereafter, T cells release proinflammatory mediators, which causes wear debris-induced inflammation (Hallab and Jacobs 2009). Finally, this inflammation will lead to implant device loosening.

Most importantly, wear debris and T cell activation can lead to cellular DNA damage (Shanbhag et al. 1998). This has been reported, in animal studies, to lead to a carcinogenic potential of orthopedic implant materials: increases in serum cobalt and chromium concentrations after metallic orthopedic implant insertion have been shown in numerous studies involving rodents, canines, and felines. However, a recent study implies no significant wear debris increases in human leukemia patients after receiving a metallic implant (Hallab and Jacobs 2009). This remains an intensely debated topic, in which numerous researchers believe that metallic implant-induced debris causes bone cancer as a result of DNA damage from reactive oxygen synthesis.

Alternatively, researchers have turned their attention toward nanotechnology to combat cancer. For instance, Zhang and colleagues have investigated various nanopatterned PLGA surfaces with different topographies to explore the ideal material for anticancer implants (Zhang and Webster 2012a, b, 2013). They have found a selective decrease in cancer cell functions pertinent for regenerating healthy bone, lung, and breast tissue in the place of respective resected cancerous tissue, all without the use of chemotherapeutic agents. The mechanism for selectively decreasing such cancer cell functions, while increasing functions of healthy cells, may lie in the fact that nanometer surface features can change selected protein adsorption/bioactivity to inhibit cancer cell functions. Another possible reason is that the stiffer membranes of cancer cells over healthy cells may restrict their attachment on protruding nanorough surfaces (Zhang and Webster 2013) (see again Figure 16.3). This result provides insights into understanding the role of metallic surface nanotopographies in cancer cell interactions. More importantly, it may also lay the groundwork for the next generation of anticancer materials that can selectively decrease cancer cells without the use of chemotherapeutics.

## Conclusions

Metallic prosthetics, particularly corrosion products of metallic implants, do not degrade in the human body and may cause a series of persistent problems over the lifetime of a patient. This chapter addressed numerous problems and diseases associated with the exposure to such metallic materials, such as infection, inflammation, cancer, and toxicity. Although some of these topics are still controversial, it has become clear that nanostructured surface features on metallic implants, as well as metallic nanoparticles themselves, may actually help to decrease infection, inflammation, and cancer. So while some believe that increased surface area to volume ratios can lead to increased metallic nanoparticle toxicity in the body, there may be numerous, yet to be fully explored, options to use metallic nanotechnology in the future to improve the treatment of a wide range of health problems.

---

First column (top to bottom): Leigh Ackland, John Pettifor, Julia Bornhorst, George Dedoussis, Rodney Dietert, Julia Bornhorst, group discussion
Second column: Ellen Silbergeld, Jerome Nriagu, Leigh Ackland, Jozef Pacyna, Jerome Nriagu, Rodney Dietert, Leigh Ackland
Third column: Jozef Pacyna, Rodney Dietert, John Pettifor, Ellen Silbergeld, Julia Bornhorst, George Dedoussis, Jerome Nriagu

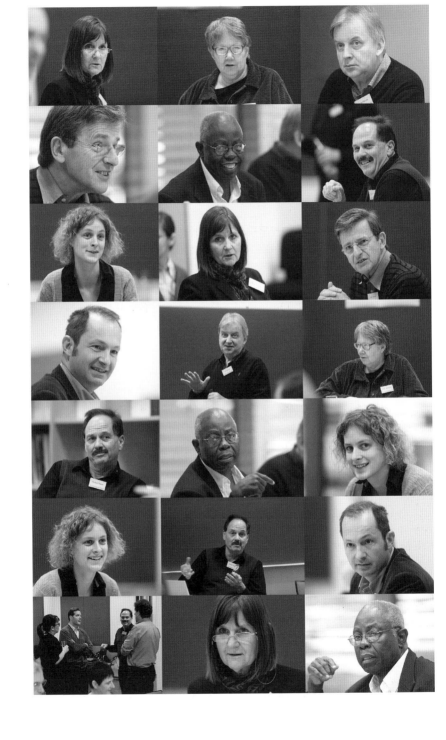

# 17

# Metals in the Environment as Risk Factors for Infectious Diseases

## Gaps and Opportunities

M. Leigh Ackland, Julia Bornhorst,
George V. Dedoussis, Rodney R. Dietert,
Jerome O. Nriagu, Jozef M. Pacyna, and John M. Pettifor

**Abstract**

This chapter aims to provide insights into current knowledge and gaps in our understanding of the influence that trace metals in the environment have on the pathogenesis of infectious diseases. By reducing immune function, trace metal deficiencies may substantially contribute to the global burden of diarrhea, pneumonia, and malaria. Improved methods and biomarkers for assessing the risks of trace metals deficiencies and toxicities are required. Human activities may be contributing to trace metal deficiency in soils and plants, which is a risk factor for infectious diseases in many countries, by exacerbating the preponderance of cereals and cash crops that reduce food diversity and micronutrient intake. Adaptive strategies are needed to reverse these trends. The microbiomes of the body are in the frontline for exposure to metals and crucial in moderating the outcome of host–parasite interactions. Anthropogenic activities have led to increased toxic metal exposure, and effects on human hosts need clarification. Metal toxicities can also impair the immune system and hence increase the susceptibility to infectious pathogens. Climate change affects metal speciation and the build-up of trace elements in the human food chain, with as yet unknown outcomes on infectious disease. Food processing and the use of metallic nanomaterials can alter human exposure to metals in ways that can influence the host–pathogen competition for metals. The effects of metals on human health may also be mediated through modification of the epigenome, conferring drug resistance on pathogenic bacteria and enhancing/reducing human tolerance to infectious parasites. The emerging metals cerium, gadolinium, lanthanum, and yttrium constitute another driver of change in metal exposure and may potentially modulate the immune system with unknown consequences for human health.

## Introduction

Research during the last half century has clearly established that trace metals, whether essential or nonessential, play important roles in a wide variety of processes in living systems and can be a defining factor in the outcome of parasitic infections (Fraga 2005; Winans et al. 2011). From the environmental health perspective, there are currently three anthropogenic drivers of the global biogeochemistry of trace metals that can influence the patterns of infectious diseases by moderating the exposure of human hosts to suboptimal and/ or toxic levels of trace metals:

1. The inadvertent contribution of human activities to the epidemic of trace metal deficiency through modern agricultural practices—a problem that affects over one billion people worldwide and is especially prevalent in developing countries.
2. Worldwide contamination of the environment with toxic but nonessential trace metals through industrial emissions, which have overwhelmed the natural cycles of these elements in many ecosystems.
3. Global change, which tends to increase the bioaccumulation of trace metals in the human food chain.

The first trend is related to the venerated Green Revolution, which promoted selective breeding of high-yielding crops that have low concentrations of zinc and other trace metals (Graham et al. 2012). The unintended consequences of the ongoing changes in trace metal balances in natural ecosystems raise concerns as to whether new efforts in developing countries to increase food production and establish emitting factories will further exacerbate the disparities in the global burden of infectious diseases.

The growing worldwide contamination of the environment with toxic trace metals, such as arsenic, cadmium, lead, mercury, platinum, silver, and thallium, and the bioaccumulation and biomagnifications of these heavy metals up the food chain have been well documented (Nriagu 1984). Since these heavy metals have become so widely dispersed, they have the potential to pose a continuous risk for human and animal health globally over a long time period because they are nondegradable. Increasingly, the riskscape used to evaluate this situation (which includes the coexistence of high levels of toxic metal pollution, the high prevalence of trace metal deficiencies, and the high incidence of infectious diseases) is becoming common in many parts of the world. In addition, the potential for interaction of these risk factors is real, but the consequences for the pathogenesis of infectious diseases have not received much attention.

## Burden of Disease Attributable to Metals and Infections

An assessment of "burden of disease" is widely used in public health to evaluate the aggregate impact that risk factors for a disease have on human health. This is usually considered on a disease-specific basis, such as the contribution of salt to the burden of cardiovascular disease or the contribution of cadmium to end-stage renal disease. By implication, this estimate provides a statement of the expected *reduction* in disease burden that can be predicted by reducing or eliminating exposure to the risk factor (e.g., reducing salt intake). Most diseases have multiple effectors and in the case of infectious diseases, which may be caused by a specific pathogen, involve multiple factors (e.g., prevalence, virulence of the pathogen, transmission, host response) that influence the severity of the disease. Separately, trace metal deficiencies or toxicities and infectious diseases contribute substantially to the global burden of morbidity and mortality. Understanding the role of such factors in disease burden is important to national and international public health investments and programs. Thus, it is important to gain a better understanding of the burden of infectious disease that is attributable to deficiencies in essential metals or excesses of toxic metals; that is, the proportion of the load or burden of infectious diseases that is attributable to metal insufficiency compared to that which is attributable to metal toxicity. A unified global effort to mitigate the high burden of disease attributable to insufficiency and toxicity of trace metals, in relation to infectious diseases, should be considered important for achieving the Millennium Development Goals and should drive future research.

The attributable contributions of metal deficiency or toxicity to the global infectious disease burden have been estimated for only a few metals: zinc, iron, lead, and arsenic. From their dietary trials, Black and colleagues (Caulfield and Black 2004; Black et al. 2008) estimate that Zn deficiency in children less than five years old increases the incidence of diarrheal disease by 1.28 (95% CI 1.10–1.50), pneumonia by 1.52 (95% CI 1.20–1.89), and malaria by 1.56 (95% CI 1.29–1.89). From these relative risks, Zn deficiency was estimated to cause 176,000 diarrhea deaths, 406,000 pneumonia deaths, and 207,000 malaria deaths. The loss of worldwide disability-adjusted life years (DALYs) attributable to Zn deficiency was estimated to be 28 million annually and was ranked fifth among the risk factors for mortality and morbidity. Subsequent analysis by Lim et al. (2012) dramatically revised these estimates downward: in 2010, total mortality due to Zn deficiency was estimated to be 97,330. The revised DALY estimate was 9.14 million; this ranked Zn deficiency 31st among the common risk factors contributing to the global burden of disease (Lim et al.

2012). The variation in estimates, however, underscores the lack of knowledge of the moderating influence of Zn deficiency on infectious diseases.

For 2010/2011, reported annual deaths attributable to Fe deficiency worldwide were estimated to be around 105,000 (Lim et al. 2012; WHO 2013a). Estimated DALYs for this risk range from 46–48 million life years (Lim et al. 2012; WHO 2013a). These estimates were based on Fe-deficiency anemia as the primary outcome measure, with the assumption that common infectious diseases (e.g., hemolytic malaria and parasitic and bacterial infections/infestations such as hookworm, trichuriasis, amoebiasis, and schistosomiasis) contribute to deplete stores of iron and hence result in Fe-deficiency anemia. It must be emphasized that the converse is also true: Fe deficiency is present in these diseases and is thus a risk factor with sequelae that can go well beyond the development of anemia. Because of failure to account for all comorbid effects, most estimates of the contribution of Fe deficiency to disease burden may be grossly incorrect or underreported.

In terms of the contribution of heavy metal toxicities to the global infectious disease burden, in 2010, Pb exposure was estimated to have accounted for 674,000 deaths, and the global DALYs attributable to this risk factor are estimated to be 13.9 million life years (Lim et al. 2012). The most recent assessment by the World Health Organization (WHO) did not rank Pb exposure among the top twenty leading causes of global DALYs (WHO 2013a). The contribution of infections to Pb-induced morbidity on the calculated DALYs is unclear.

A number of studies have estimated the DALYs for As exposure in drinking water in Bangladesh (Lokuge et al. 2004; Ahmed et al. 2005). None, however, has considered arsenic as a risk factor for any of the water-related infectious diseases (e.g., cholera, helminth infections, schistosomiasis, and trachoma) that coexist widely with elevated levels of arsenic in local drinking water. The significance of arsenic on risk for infectious diseases remains, therefore, to be established.

Our ability to assess the metal-attributable fraction of the infectious disease burden is severely limited by lack of information on (a) infectious disease endpoints that can be influenced by metal exposures, (b) distribution of exposure to each metal in the population and the effects of coexposure to more than one metal, and (c) etiological effect sizes for the relationships between metal exposure and disease outcome (WHO 2013a). It is hoped that this chapter will draw attention to the need for epidemiological studies to collect these types of information.

A study has been done on small-scale gold miners in watersheds of the Tapajos in Amazonian Brazil who were coexposed to high incidence of infective mosquito bites and elevated levels of methylated mercury (MeHg) from consumption of contaminated fish (Silva et al. 2004; Silbergeld et al. 2005). Increased risks for malaria (diagnosed by thin smear) were found in miners from downstream settlements exposed to MeHg compared to miners in similar ecosystems that did not use mercury (diamond and emerald miners). High prevalence of endemic malaria exists in many regions of Latin America, Asia, and Africa where intensive artisanal small-scale gold mining is widespread. These settings provide opportunities to conduct epidemiological studies to assess the relationships between metal exposure and malaria.

Animal models of infectious disease have provided insights into the effect of mercury on infectious diseases. Studies have included mercury and malaria in mice (Silbergeld et al. 2005), coxsackievirus B3 (CVB3) and mercury (Nyland et al. 2012), and listeria and both cadmium and lead (Simonet et al. 1984; Kowolenko et al. 1991). These studies have consistently reported that metal preexposures increase the severity of disease in mice. The study of mice infected with CVB3 showed a disturbed Hg balance in the intestine, serum, and brain, as well as infection-induced changes in metallothionein 1 (MT1, a metal-binding/-transporting protein) in the intestine, liver, and brain (e.g., Frisk et al. 2008). This observation was presumed to be a normal response in common infections and the underlying mechanism for the reported findings of Hg changes in blood and tissues. Such results from animal studies (Koller 1975; Beck et al. 1994; Frisk et al. 2007, 2008; Ilbäck et al. 2007) point to serious consequences when infected individuals are concomitantly exposed to potentially toxic metals, such as mercury in their environment.

**Coexposures Involving Metals**

While metals and their impact on risk for infectious disease are often studied on a one metal and one disease basis, humans are more likely to be exposed to mixtures of metals from their diet and environment. The issue becomes more complex in terms of risk assessment since metals may compete for uptake, distribution, and/or use among the host's immune cells and pathogens. As a result, antagonistic or synergistic effects may operate locally or systemically. Table 17.1 illustrates some examples of reported interactions among and between metals and other frequently encountered environmental factors. This list is not intended to be exhaustive. Among the interactions described in Table 17.1, three patterns are apparent:

1. Metals may act synergistically to cause toxic effects on the immune system. In mice, lead and arsenic caused a greater immunotoxic effect when administered together than when singly administered (Bishayi and Sengupta 2006).

2. In many cases, exposure to toxic heavy metals can result in significant local or systemic deficiencies of nutritionally required metals.

3. Nonmetal factors are also important in coexposure. For example, both dietary fat and dietary protein (source and percentage) can modulate risk of metal-induced host toxicity.

**Table 17.1** Select examples of that can affect the host, including immune–microbe interactions.

| Metal | Additional Environmental Risk Factor | Outcome |
|---|---|---|
| Arsenic | Selenium | Selenium protects against some immuno-toxicity (for basal immune profiles) but does not prevent As-mediated oxidative damage |
| Arsenic trioxide | Genistein | Increased oxidative potential |
| Cadmium | Lead | Dose-dependent interactions for oxida-tive-driven neurological outcomes that varies based on developmental window of prenatal coexposures |
| Cadmium | Lead | Antagonism of the metals for suppres-sion of adult hepatic antioxidant enzyme activities |
| Cadmium | Selenium | Selenium alters Cd tissue distribution and protects against Cd-promoted innate im-mune oxidative tissue damage |
| Copper | Zinc | May synergize to inactivate the exposed Fe-S cluster of key bacterial dehydratase enzymes |
| Lead | Maternal diet (protein differences) | Partial immune protection |
| Lead | Arsenic | Increased dose sensitivity of macrophages |
| Lead | High fat diet | Increased blood Pb levels |
| Lead | Iron | Fe deficiency increases Pb absorption |
| Lead | Selenium | In adults, higher Pb levels appear to pre-dispose for Se deficiency |
| Selenium | Vitamin E | Some sparing against oxidative damage |
| Iron | Aluminum | Reduced Fe levels in lymphoid tissues |
| Iron | Gallium | Reduced Fe availability |
| Iron | Cobalt | Reduced Fe availability |
| Iron | Copper | Copper influences Fe recycling in macrophages |
| Manganese | Zinc | Interaction in innate immune, calprotec-tin-mediated host defense |
| Vanadium | Magnesium | Magnesium protects against Vd-associat-ed, oxidative-induced anemia |
| Zinc | Excessive alcohol | Zn deficiency for macrophages |
| Zinc | Lead | Replaces zinc in critical enzymes |
| Zinc | Cadmium | Replaces zinc in critical enzymes |

**Potential for Leveraging Information from Current Population Studies**

Considerably more information is required to establish with certainty the role that heavy metals (deficiencies or excess) play in the pathogenesis, morbidity, and mortality of infectious diseases globally. However, some existing and ongoing studies can be used to obtain data on associations between deficiency of metals and infectious diseases. These include the National Health and Nutrition Examination Survey (NHANES) in the United States, the National Children's Studies (NCS) in many countries and regions, and the EU ZINCAGE study. In a recent cross-sectional study, Xu et al. (2013) used NHANES 2003–2010 to compare exposures to heavy metals (including cadmium, lead, and total mercury) in HIV-infected and non-HIV-infected subjects in the United States. They found that HIV-infected individuals had higher concentrations of all heavy metals than the non-HIV infected group. HIV status was significantly associated with increased blood cadmium ($p = 0.03$) after adjusting for age, sex, race, education, poverty income ratio, and smoking. However, HIV status was not statistically associated with lead or mercury levels after adjusting for the same covariates. Xu et al. concluded that exposure to cadmium was a contributing factor to the higher prevalence of chronic diseases (e.g., cardiovascular diseases) among HIV-infected subjects.

A study based on the Korea National Health and Nutrition Examination Survey (KNHANES) from 2009–2010 explored the additive effects of metals on metabolic syndrome, a constellation of cardiovascular risk factors, including central obesity, hypertension, dyslipidemia, and impaired glucose tolerance (Moon 2013). Although the effect of individual heavy metals (specifically lead, mercury, and cadmium) on metabolic syndrome was weak, the combined heavy metal exposure affected metabolic syndrome more synergistically than individual exposure in the general Korean population. Together, the NHANES and KNHANES studies suggest that metals and infections give rise to similar comorbidities in the form of metabolic syndrome.

Currently, the NCS in the United States is examining the effects of the environment—broadly defined to include factors such as air, water, diet, noise, family dynamics, community and cultural influences—and genetics on the growth, development, and health of children across the United States. The NCS study follows children from before birth until 21 years of age. The goal of the study is to improve the health and well-being of children and to expand understanding of the role that various factors have on health and disease. There should be enough information in the resulting data base to permit the assessment of possible comorbidities attributable to coexposure to trace metals and pathogenic organisms. Another large study that is currently underway is the Japan National Study on Children and the Environment, which has already enrolled over 100,000 infants. It is similar in design to the NCS in terms of methods, data collection, and biosampling in a longitudinal design and can be used similarly to assess comorbidities from metal–pathogen interactions.

## Metal Sufficiency, Deficiency, and Toxicity within the Context of Infections

The lack of clarity in the definitions of deficiency, susceptibility, and toxicity of metals in relation to infectious disease leads to difficulties in determining these parameters. Here we wish to highlight the main issues involved. For further discussion, see Rehder et al. (this volume).

### Conflicts in Principles and Methods Used to Determine Sufficiency and Deficiency of Essential Trace Elements

Different principles and methods have been used by various governmental agencies to establish (a) recommendations designed to protect the public from the toxic effects of trace metals (including essential ones) and (b) advisable safe intakes aimed at protecting the public from the adverse effects of deficiency. This has often resulted in conflicting recommendations. To highlight one example, consider the recommended dietary allowances (RDAs)—established by the U.S. Food and Drug Administration (FDA) and the U.S. National Research Council to ensure adequate nutritional intake of trace metals to maintain normal physiological functions—and the reference dose (RfD) or daily exposure levels—set by the U.S. Environmental Protection Agency to protect the public from trace metal toxicity: Because of uncertainties inherent in toxicity evaluation, RfDs must often include uncertainty factors to provide sufficient margin of safety (especially for vulnerable groups). This, in turn, can bias the RfD estimate toward the low side. For mercury in fish, the current RDA is substantially higher than the RfD; this has led to conflicting fish consumption advisories in the United States and created public confusion. Such conflicts point to the need for new principles and methods in the assessment of risks of essential trace metals: nutritional and toxicological information must be considered in a balanced way (WHO 2002). Such a unified approach should provide a coherent framework for assessing the moderating effects of trace metals on infectious diseases.

### Biomarkers to Establish Links between Metal Exposure and Infectious Disease

Biomarkers, defined as an indicator of some biological state or condition, reflect changes in the organism's metabolism in response to an exposure (or lack thereof). Biomarkers have greatly expanded the scope of epidemiological and toxicological research by providing insights into events that couple exposures and diseases or dysfunctions. In addition, they inform knowledge of events within the organism that connect changes in exposure with changes in health. This approach allows us to test hypotheses as to the processes of pathophysiological response and generates useful information on early signals of adverse effects associated with exposures. Figure 17.1 illustrates the metal pathways that link metal exposure to infectious disease. To the standard model (Silbergeld and Davis 1994), we have added the microbiome at the interface between the external exposure and the internal dose to denote the importance of microbial events in absorption. Each point on the diagram represents a potential biomarker.

The concept of body metal status (i.e., whether the body contains amounts of metals that are sufficient for optimal biological processes) is not well defined, yet it is central to the development of RDAs (Aggett 1991). In assessing metal status, the question of whether subjects are deficient, at risk of being deficient, have adequate body levels, or are experiencing metal toxicity cannot often be answered simply, particularly if the metal (such as zinc) has numerous biological functions. A common host response during acute bacterial, viral, and parasitic infections is an increase in the synthesis of metal-binding proteins in several target organs involved in the infectious process (Beisel 1998; Ilbäck et al. 2004). This may result in significant changes in the dynamics and concentrations of both essential and nonessential trace elements in blood and tissues that are used as biomarkers (Beisel 1998; Ilbäck et al. 2003). A significant amount of work has been done on disease-related redistribution of the essential trace elements following an infection, and a number of proteins that can serve as metal carriers have been identified: Fe-binding ferritin, divalent metal transporter 1 (DMT1), Cu-binding ceruloplasmin, and Zn-binding MT1–MT4 (Beisel 1998; Nordberg and Nordberg 2000; Ilbäck et al. 2004). Since trace elements are required for host defense processes, a flux of trace elements between blood and other tissues, including the tissues that are involved in the disease, is usually orchestrated during active infection (Beisel 1998; Frisk et al. 2007). Although less is known about infection-induced changes in nonessential trace elements, changes have been described that may not be favorable to the host:

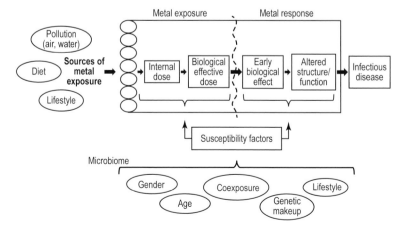

**Figure 17.1** Metal pathways that link metal exposure to infectious disease.

an increased redistribution of cadmium from the liver to the kidneys (Ilbäck et al. 2004), increased Hg concentration in red blood cells (Frisk et al. 2007), or increased loading of arsenic, cadmium, copper, and zinc into the brain (Ilbäck et al. 2007). Biomarkers provide important information about metal status in different tissues and organs with respect to deficiency or toxicity, and they assist in establishing the impact of metal deficiency on infectious disease.

## Global Trends in Trace Metal Deficiency with the Potential to Impact on Infectious Diseases

Trace metal deficiency in soils and plants is a risk factor for infectious diseases in many parts of the world. From 190 major agricultural soils, it is estimated that 49% are deficient in zinc, 31% deficient in boron, 15% deficient in molybdenum, 14% deficient in copper, 10% deficient in manganese, and 3% deficient in iron (Sillanpää 1982; Graham et al. 2012). In general, soils associated with trace metal deficiencies include neutral and calcareous soils, intensively cropped soils, paddy soils and poorly drained soils, sodic and saline soils, peat soils, soils with high available phosphorus and silicon, sandy soils, as well as highly weathered acid and coarse-textured soils; these types of soils are widespread in many parts of the world (Singh 2008; Lyons and Cakmak 2012). Low availability of zinc and other trace metals in such soils is one of the most widely distributed stressors in world agriculture, especially in southeast Asian countries and Australia (Brennan and Bolland 2006; Singh 2008; Lyons and Cakmak 2012). More than 85% of the cereal-growing areas in India are affected by low zinc (Singh 2008). Cereals and wheat grown in such soils are liable to be deficient in zinc and other trace metals, leading to low crop yields and decreased nutritional quality of the food (Bouis 2003; Cakmak et al. 2010).

The preponderance of cereals and cash crops in modern cropping systems and worldwide adoption of high-yielding cultivars have combined to reduce our food diversity and micronutrient intake in ways that can impact the immune system (Govindaraj et al. 2011; Graham et al. 2012). Today, production of various wild, traditional, or ancient food crops, which are genetically very diverse and may be rich in trace elements, has been largely displaced by crops of the modern agricultural system (Welch and Graham 2005; Birner et al. 2007; Graham et al. 2012). The latter has contributed to a decrease in cereal prices and an increase in price for legumes, fruits, vegetables, and animal and fish protein; this has led to the so-called "hidden hunger" or micronutrient deficiency brought about by these less nutritious cereal crops becoming more affordable and available (Cakmak et al. 2010). Among widely cultivated food crops with high-yield capacity, wheat plays a particularly important role in daily energy intake (especially in the developing countries), accounting for about 50% of daily energy intake in many Central Asian and Middle Eastern countries (Lyons and Cakmak 2012). Such high-yield wheat cultivars are poor sources of micronutrients, especially zinc and iron, and are rich in anti-nutritional compounds such as phytic acid and phenolic compounds, which reduce biological availability of zinc and iron in the human digestive tract (Graham et al. 2012). The factors which lead to a reduced availability of trace elements in crops occur in areas of the world with high incidence of infectious diseases.

**Food Systems Approach to a "Greener Revolution"**

Until recently, micronutrient deficiency was primarily viewed as a soil or (to a lesser extent) plant problem. More importantly, though, it needs to be addressed as a human health problem—one that impacts susceptibility to infectious diseases.

The unintended consequences of the Green Revolution, which promoted micronutrient deficiencies in the human population (reviewed by Bouis et al. 2012; Graham et al. 2012), has prompted a growing call for agricultural technologies that can sustainably meet the increasing food demands of the world's expanding population while providing adequate supplies of bioavailable trace elements and micronutrients for public health. Conceptual models have been advanced for such food systems, including a farm-to-fork approach that is focused on cropping systems and their abilities to support balanced human nutrition in sustainable ways (Welch et al. 1997; Lyons and Cakmak 2012). This approach aims to increase diversity (re-diversification) of cropping systems, particularly with respect to indigenous fruits, vegetables, and pulses, and developing trace metal dense cultivars of staple crops. In addition, it advocates finding a more effective means of using the iron and zinc contained in cereal brans (which are often removed during food preparation) and developing appropriate technologies to preserve and store foods (Coombs 2000; Welch and Graham 2012; Thompson and Amoroso 2013). Such new stategies need to address simultaneously the demand of the growing human population for food and a balanced nutrient output, in the context of environmental, economic, and social sustainability. Such a "greener revolution" differs from the traditional concept of agriculture, which measures its success in terms of crop production (bushels per acre yields) or cost in dollars per year; indeed, the new system would expand that view to include measures of impact on human nutrition and health.To provide improved trace element nutrition and potentially lessen the risk for infectious diseases, a greener revolution must include adaptive strategies to reverse micronutrient deficiencies.

**Metal Pathways and Metals in the Microbiome**

"Exposure" to metals occurs outside the organism through, for example, air and water pollution, diet, or lifestyle (cigarette smoking is a major source of exposure to lead and cadmium). The metals in an exposure pathway (Figure 17.1), such as air, water, and food, are then presented to the organism primarily through inhalation, ingestion, or dermal contact. Processes of absorption mediate transfer of metal-containing substances into the internal environments of the organism. As illustrated in Figure 17.1, the microbiome (vertically stacked circles) is situated at portals of entry, such as the gut and skin, at the boundary of the organism.

## The Importance of the Microbiome

The microbiome is a microbial community within a specified niche (e.g., within an organ system or ecologic space) or a community of all microbes, chemicals, and inputs/outputs related to the microbial system. This field of study received a great boost in 2007, when the National Institutes of Health initiated the Human Microbiome Project with the intent of surveying and characterizing the microbes that reside at different body sites (Turnbaugh et al. 2007). The seminal report on microbes from 18 body sites in over 240 healthy volunteers revealed the complex nature of the human microbial inhabitants and the incredible amount of both intra- and interpersonal variation in the communities that inhabit the human body. Nonetheless, how the availability of critical trace elements influences the biotic composition and distribution at each site has yet to receive any attention.

Some microbiomes (e.g., the skin, gastrointestinal tract, and lung) reside at the portals of host exposure to the environment. In the schematic model of biomarkers of exposure and outcomes (Figure 17.1), these microbiomes may represent a front line for exposure to metals, whether via inhalation, ingestion, or dermal route. It is the place where the human host first encounters microbiota and environmental sources of metals. In the following, we introduce a modified exposure–outcome biomarker model to include the microbiome as a significant early stage component affecting host exposure and immune-related host defense. A potentially critical target of heavy metal exposures during development is disruption of complete attainment of the normal adult human microbiome. The processes involved may include interactions that take place in the microbiome (gut but possibly others such as oral and lung), in terms of metabolizing the trace metals as well as removing toxic heavy metals from the organism prior to absorption through the epithelial layer.

*Gut Microbiome*

The gut has the largest microbial community in the human body and contains at least two orders of magnitude more genes than are found in the human genome (Reid 2010). Microorganisms in the human gut microbiome have developed coping strategies to transform a toxic metal into a less harmful form or to bind the metal intra- or extracellularly, so as to prevent harmful interactions within the host cell (Diamond et al. 1998; Monachese et al. 2012).

The gut microbiota can influence two processes pertaining to metals: (a) detoxification in relation to the removal of drugs, mutagens, and other harmful agents from the body, and (b) detoxification to prevent the entry of damaging compounds into the body (Berhane et al. 1994). Detoxification occurs in the human intestinal tract, liver, and kidneys where microbes reduce or moderate the forms and concentrations of toxic metals (Ibrahim et al. 2006). Gut microbiota may also have a major role in binding metals, preventing their entry to the body and thus protecting the host. The extent of detoxification depends on the route of entry, the foodstuff consumed, and the types of host microbiota (Sun et al. 2012). The effects of gut microbiota on the sequestration and detoxification of toxic metals and the extent that these microbes provide protection to the human host remain an area for systematic investigation. One recent study has shown that perturbations in the gut microbiome composition of mice can lead to gut microbiome phenotypes that significantly affect As metabolic reactions, including reduction, methylation, and thiolation (Lu et al. 2013). While some of the observed associations between changes in trace metals, microbiota composition, and disease condition may be no more than epiphenomenal, the critical role of safe and essential levels of trace metals in maintaining a healthy gut ecology must nevertheless be recognized.

An interesting idea of employing certain members of the gut microbiota to reduce metal toxicity in humans was recently proposed (Monachese et al. 2012; Marco and Tachon 2013). Lactobacilli and possibly other bacterial types used in the food industry or as probiotics have the ability to bind and sequester metals and prevent their entry into human organs (Ibrahim et al. 2006). Such "bioremediation" of the human body using microbiota-modifying approaches has several advantages:

- They do not require expensive technology or infrastructure.
- They can be based on locally produced foods, such as yogurt made in the home or community.
- Local acceptance is assured.

This intervention strategy potentially represents an affordable option for billions of people around the world who are being chronically exposed to toxic metals in their environment (Reid 2010). The potential for the human microbiome to be modulated has applications to some clinical conditions, such as ulcerative colitis (Torres et al. 2013), and may be applicable to other diseases including infectious diseases.

*Oral Microbiome*

The human oral cavity is heavily colonized by microorganisms, including viruses, protozoa, fungi, archaea, and bacteria. Unlike the commensal microbiota found at other body sites, which seemingly live in harmony with the host, the normal microbiota of the mouth is responsible for the two most common diseases of humans: dental caries and periodontal diseases (Wade 2013). It has long been recognized that caries is an infectious and transmissible disease that can be moderated by trace metal deficiency or excess in the oral cavity. No specific microorganisms or properties of microorganisms are solely responsible for the initiation and progression of caries. Of the key bacteria in saliva samples, mutans streptococci are probably the most cariogenic microorganisms because of two special features: (a) their high acidogenic and aciduric capacity and (b) their ability to produce extracellular polysaccharides, resulting in the adhesion of dental plaque on tooth surfaces (Larmas 1993). Both processes can be affected by trace metals. Another important group of bacteria is the salivary lactobacilli, which indicate the presence of a caries-type oral environment and are predictors of the progression potential of the lesions (Larmas 1993). Trace metal deficiency and excess have been found to inhibit the growth of these and other plaque species (He et al. 2002). The strongest evidence for stimulatory effects of trace metals on caries prevention comes from the anticalculus and anticaries effects, antibacterial activity, and antiplaque efficacy of many trace metals which have been repeatedly shown in human and animal studies (Lynch 2011). Although a number of human studies have reported significant positive associations between trace metal levels in teeth and saliva and dental caries (Blanusa et al. 1990; Burguera et al. 2002), there are still open questions regarding the mechanisms of pro-caries action and the effects of trace metals on the microorganisms in terms of caries promotion.

Trace metals can influence the differentiation of oral mucosa (Meyer et al. 1981) and the aggregation and adhesion characteristics of dental caries-associated microorganisms (Boosz et al. 1983). The oral microbiome is a unique system for understanding the role of trace metals on its ecology and how the microbiome affects the fate and effects of the metals. There is clearly a need for methodologies that can be used to test the cariogenic properties of the trace metals and how the forms of metals in saliva relate to the diversity and composition of cariogenic bacteria in the oral cavity.

**Influence of Genetic Factors**

Some of the more common polymorphisms (> 5%) involve genes that also play a role in the immune response to infections (e.g., interleukin 6). There are also genes known to regulate toxicokinetics and toxicity of toxic metals, such as arsenic, mercury, and lead. The natural resistance-associated macrophage proteins (Nramp1 and 2) are proton-dependent solute carriers of divalent metals such as $Fe^{2+}$ and $Mn^{2+}$ (Slc11a1 and 2). Their expression in both resting and microbicidal macrophages, which metabolize iron differently, raises questions about the Nramp mechanism of $Me^{2+}$ transport and its impact in distinct phenotypic contexts (Cellier 2012). NRAMP1, vitamin-D receptor, and tumor necrosis factor α (TNF-α) gene polymorphisms have been associated with susceptibility to infectious diseases, but the results have been inconsistent (Merza et al. 2009). In addition to NRAMP, polymorphisms in other metal-related genes have been associated with toxicity effects of metals. For lead, the most significant (and prevalent) gene is that encoding the enzyme δ-aminolevulinic dehydrase (ALAD). The ALAD protein is a significant binding site for lead within the erythrocyte and thus regulates erythrocyte:plasma toxicokinetics for lead. A common polymorphism in the ALAD gene (G177C) can alter plasma Pb concentrations significantly, by 1.66-fold (Montenegro et al. 2006). Another example is the gene that expresses metallothionein. Metallothioneins are a family of intracellular proteins that bind metals and may provide protection against metal toxicity (e.g., zinc, copper, and cadmium). A study in Chinese populations found that a mutation in the gene that encodes MT1A (a Cd-binding form of the protein) was associated with significant increases in blood cadmium and urinary β-2 microglobulin, which is a biomarker of renal toxicity (Lei et al. 2012).

## Gender, Metals, and Infections

Gender (as distinct from genetics) is also associated with essential metal status, toxic metal levels, and infectious disease. In some cases this involves gender-specific differences in diet and behavior. Infectious disease incidence is often male biased. Two main hypotheses have been proposed to explain this observation. The physiological hypothesis emphasizes differences in sex hormones and genetic architecture, whereas the behavioral hypothesis stresses gender-related differences in exposure. The population-level predictions of these hypotheses have yet to be thoroughly tested in humans. After puberty, disease incidence is male biased in cutaneous and visceral leishmaniasis, schistosomiasis, pulmonary tuberculosis, leptospirosis, meningococcal meningitis, and hepatitis A. Severe dengue is female-biased, and no clear pattern is evident for typhoid fever. For most diseases, male bias emerges during infancy, when behavior is unbiased but sex steroid levels transiently rise. Behavioral factors likely modulate male-female differences in some diseases (e.g., the leishmaniases, tuberculosis, leptospirosis, or schistosomiasis) and age classes. The immune system is known to be biased by gender, with genetics, hormonal status, and other factors contributing to male-female differences. As a result there are differences between men and women in terms of infection and severity of many infectious diseases as well as postinfection sequelae (McClelland and Smith 2011).

To date, few studies have examined sex differences in immune response to metals. Silva et al. (2005) report on the effects of prenatal exposures of BALB/c mice to HgCl on the ontogeny of the immune system. Immune function was assessed by collection of cells from lymph nodes, spleens, and thymus from postnatal day 11 through 60 and studied in male and female mice. Organ-specific effects were observed on maturation. At maturity, females and males differed in terms of effects: in females there was an overall decrease in

ConA-stimulated cytokine release from cells *ex vivo*, whereas in males, there was an overall increase in release (both compared to unexposed mice of the same strain and gender). Similar gender-specific effects after *in utero* exposure to HgCl were reported by Pilones et al. (2009).

Growing evidence indicates gender differences in susceptibility to disease infection and in response to metal exposure. However, limited attempts have been made to examine the relationships between these two factors in the pathogenesis of infectious diseases among males versus females. More studies are required to understand the basis of the differences in metal metabolism between males and females.

## Impacts of Metals in the Environment on Infectious Diseases

Mining, smelting, and widespread use of metals to support the expansion of human industrial activities have led to an exponential increase in the amounts of heavy metals that are released into the atmosphere, water, and soil. Anthropogenic inputs have overwhelmed the natural biogeochemical cycles of many elements in many ecosystems (Nriagu 1984). As a consequence, all life forms on Earth are being exposed to a wide range of toxic metals in the environment, which they might not have encountered previously in their evolutionary cycle. As a matter of necessity, many organisms have evolved unique mechanisms which allow them to survive and, in some instances, reduce the toxicity of metals in their environments. The extent to which such coping strategies can be used by pathogens to moderate the influence of new metal compounds on their interactions with human host is a matter that has received little study.

### Sources and Emissions of Toxic Metals

Most of the available information on sources and emissions of toxic metals relates to mercury, lead, cadmium, and arsenic, which are emitted from both anthropogenic and natural sources. For these metals, information is available on geochemical cycling and pathways in the environment as well as on uptake into biota, including the food chain. The most recent and accurate information available is for mercury. The major anthropogenic sources of Hg emissions at present and expected in the future derive from coal combustion, followed by release of mercury as a result of artisanal gold mining and production (Pacyna et al. 2010; UNEP 2013). As much as 2000 metric tons of mercury are emitted annually from anthropogenic sources, and similar amounts are being released from natural sources, including the reemissions of mercury from land and water surfaces (Pacyna et al. 2010). Nonferrous metal smelting and other industrial processes are the main emission sources for the remainder of the abovementioned metals.

An important group of metals in the environmental context consists of other well-known metals, such as vanadium, nickel, copper, zinc, chromium, silver, antimony, gold, thallium, rare earth elements (REEs), and the platinum group of metals (PGMs). Major emission sources, applications, and exposure pathways of all of the abovementioned metals are presented in Appendix 17.1, which also includes information on the possible impact of metals on the immune system as well as their antiviral and antimicrobial properties. As listed in Appendix 17.1, proximate sources of human exposure to toxic metals are not limited to direct consumption of contaminated food but can include inhalation of contaminated air and other specific practices (e.g., tobacco smoking) as a major source of exposure to lead and cadmium. Even though most countries have removed Pb additives from automotive fuels, crude oil still contains substantial amounts of naturally occurring lead. As a result, some unleaded gasoline may contain up to 15 mg/l of this element. It should be noted that emissions of many metals, particularly mercury, occur at local and regional scales, especially in the developing countries with high rates of endemic diseases, such as malaria, leishmaniasis, and dengue.

## Metal Emissions and Lung Infection

Particulate matter exposures are associated with increased risks for human infections, and this association is so rampant that, historically, particle-related disease was frequently, but erroneously, regarded as a variety of infection (e.g., coal workers' pneumoconiosis was previously referred to as "miners' consumption" and "miners' phthisis") (Ghio 2014). Once inhaled, particles are deposited in the nose, pharynx, larynx, trachea, bronchi, and distal lung. It is not by coincidence that the respiratory tract is the system most frequently infected after particulate exposure. Exposures to particles from mining and smelting, fossil fuel combustion, biomass burning, metallurgical works, transportation-related emissions, agricultural work, cigarette smoking, work, environmental tobacco smoke (ETS), wood stoves and gas stoves, as well as ambient air pollution have all been associated with an increased risk for respiratory infections (Ghio 2014). For instance, particulates from cigarette smoking, biomass burning, mining, smelting, and ETS have been linked to an elevated risk for tuberculosis, atypical mycobacterial infections, and meningitis. One possible explanation for particle-related infections is that the surfaces of airborne particulates, especially from anthropogenic sources, are enriched in essential trace elements. Particles deposited in the respiratory tract thus represent a reservoir of essential trace elements which the infective pathogens can exploit to meet their metabolic needs. In addition, particulate surfaces contain nonessential metals (mercury, cadmium, arsenic, beryllium, and manganese) which can increase the risk for infection through moderating the immune response. As an example, elevated levels of serum lead and mercury and low levels of zinc and selenium have been associated with recurrent wheezing in children (Razia et al. 2011). Children with recurrent wheezing are much more susceptible to respiratory tract infections than healthy children, and trace metals could significantly influence the pathogenesis of the recurrent wheezing.

Changes in energy sources (so-called energy mix), manufacturing, and new technologies are changing the physical and chemical characteristics of the aerosols emitted, and hence their effects on human respiratory health (Pacyna and Pacyna 2001). In addition, we are experiencing a geographic shift in terms of where metals are emitted most intensively: from North America and Europe to Asia. These changes have resulted in significant risk overlap in the developing countries and have involved a juxtaposition of metal hazards from modern industries and the so-called traditional hazards typically associated with infectious diseases. Such risk overlap can contribute both directly and indirectly to global health disparities.

## Global Drivers of Change in Metal Exposure

### Climate Change

The twentieth century has witnessed an era of unprecedented, large-scale anthropogenic changes to the natural environment which have influenced the emergence and spread of infectious diseases. Recent studies (Jia et al. 2010; Li et al. 2012; Stern et al. 2012) have shown that climate change is already having a significant impact on many aspects of the transport pathways, speciation, and cycling of trace elements in many ecosystems. How the overwhelming modification of the natural cycles of the trace elements by human activities feeds into this global change/infectious disease link has not received much attention. In this regard, the effects of changes in trace metal levels (to deficiency or subtoxic levels) on the establishment and spread of indirectly transmitted, vector-borne anthroponoses (e.g., malaria, dengue fever, yellow fever) has to be of special interest. We need to understand to what extent the trace metal nutriture in changing ecosystems can influence the vector–pathogen link in the transmission chain. In this sense, it would be good to know how the nonhuman life cycle of the pathogens would respond to changes in trace metal exposures that are driven by climate change.

More generally, climatic change and heavy metal stress can influence various processes in plants, including growth, physiology, biochemistry, and yield, and can hence pose a threat to food security (see review by Rajkumar et al. 2013). Elevated atmospheric $CO_2$ levels have been shown to enhance biomass production and metal accumulation in plants and have been linked to the ability of plants to support greater microbial populations and/or protect the microorganisms against the impacts of heavy metals (Li et al. 2010b; Guo et al. 2011; Kim and Kang 2011). Climatic change can influence metal bioavailability in soils and consequently affect plant growth by moderating the function and structure of plant roots and diversity and activity of rhizosphere microbes (Sardans et al. 2008; Rajkumar et al. 2010). Better understanding of how plant–metal interactions respond to climatic change is essential in developing high-yielding crops that can tolerate multistress conditions without accentuating the toxic metal levels and compromising future food security.

## Food Processing

Another issue that affects human intake of both essential and toxic metals is food processing. Cooking can be a source of exposure to toxic metals (e.g., from the cooking water) as well as a cause of depletion of essential metals from food. Certain ceramic cookware, for example, has been associated with Pb exposure, and some cooking methods may deplete the essential metals in foods (Villalobos et al. 2009). Processing of grains including wheat, rice, and sugar substantially lowers their trace element concentrations. The process of milling rice and wheat removes the bran which contains the major portion of zinc (Borresen and Ryan 2014). Loss of trace elements in refining of wheat to produce white flour results in a 78% loss of zinc, 16% loss in selenium, 86% loss of manganese, and 68% loss of copper; white sugar contains 40 times less zinc than raw sugar, and nearly 6 times less copper (Schroeder 1971). Removal of the essential trace metals during food processing is likely to reduce the immune-boosting capacity of the diet and increase the consumer's susceptibility to infectious diseases.

## Metals in Infant Nutrition

An infant's gut is particularly sensitive to colonization patterns as inherent intestinal defense mechanisms are immature, and immature intestinal epithelial cells are known to have exaggerated inflammatory responses to both commensal and pathogenic bacteria (Mshvildadze and Neu 2010). Since the core microbiota formation is dependent on exposure to the microbes that first colonize the gastrointestinal tract ("founder species"), the establishment of a "healthy" microbiota in the first days of life after birth is expected to be critical for normal development. It is expected that the trace metals status would be one of the important moderating factors that may reduce the normal commensal microbiota colonization and impair beneficial stimulation of gastrointestinal mucosal development as well as innate and adaptive immune responses. During the first one to two years of life, the microbiome of a healthy human infant evolves toward a typical adult microbiota (Palmer et al. 2007; Dave et al. 2012). Infants, in particular neonates, are reported to be at a higher risk from insufficiency of essential metals or from exposure to toxic levels of metals. The role of trace metals on the dysbiosis and metabolic programming during this highly vulnerably period in the development of their gut microbiome should be presumed to be important, but is unknown at this time.

Recent studies have shown that human milk, instead of being sterile, presents a continuous supply of commensal, mutualistic, and/or potentially probiotic bacteria to the gut microbiome of an infant. These bacteria can contribute to the reduction of the incidence and severity of infections and maturation of the immune system in the breastfed infant, among other functions. The introduction of early formula feeding, either exclusively or in combination with continued breast-feeding, reduces or negates the protective benefits of breast-feeding, as is occuring in countries where mixed feeding practices in infants less than six months have become commonplace. The WHO has reported that only one-third of infants worldwide were exclusively breast-fed during the first six months of life in 2009, the majority receiving some other food or fluid in the early months (WHO 2009). In terms of essential metals, levels in infant formulas have been reported to be from 3–100 times higher than the concentrations found in breast milk, depending on the particular metal. For example, three times higher levels of zinc have been found in infant formulas (based on cow milk) than breast milk and 100 times higher levels of manganese in infant formulas (based on soy milk) (Aschner and Aschner 2005). The high concentrations, due to the fortification of formulas with these essential metals, have been justified in the past because of differences in their bioavailability in infant formulas compared to breast milk. However, currently there is less clarity, and the levels of fortification need to be reassessed in light of the low intake of these elements in the breast-fed infant and the possible deleterious consequences of metal overload which could influence host infections (Ljung et al. 2011; Bornhorst et al. 2013) The high intake of zinc with infant formula may account for the difference in the gut microflora of breast- and formula-fed infants, and the differing microbiome phylotypes may account for the increased susceptibility of formula-fed infants to infectious agents.

*Metals in Fast Foods*

The gut microbiota of people in the Western World is significantly different (reduced in diversity) from that of people who live in rural villages in developing countries and are habituated to traditional lifestyles (Bengmark 2013). This difference is usually attributed to the fact that the great majority of ingredients in the industrially produced foods consumed in the West are absorbed in the upper part of the small intestine, and thus of limited benefit to the small intestinal and large bowel microbiotas. Lack of proper nutrition, including safe and essential levels of trace metals for gut microbiota, has been implicated in dysfunction of gut ecology, dysbiosis, chronically elevated inflammation, and the production and leakage of endotoxins through the various tissue barriers and hyperactivation of the immune system (Mshvildadze and Neu 2010; Quigley 2013). In addition, heat- and storage-related treatments can result in the formation of the so-called advanced glycation end products and advanced lipoxidation end products in such foods as dairy products (especially powdered milk, which is frequently used in industrially produced foods), deep-fried foods, grilled meat and poultry, smoked and cured foods, as well as coffee. Consumption of such foods, which are often the main constituents of fast foods, has been linked to inflammation and immune system modulation (Bengmark 2013).

Fast foods have been reported to provide concentrated calories but decreased levels of micronutrients (Bowman and Vinyard 2004; Wimalawansa 2013). Regular consumption of such foods can induce a dysbiosis in the gut bacteria that synthesizes and converts a variety of compounds to impact the physiology, immunity, and presumably the susceptibility or resistance of human individuals to infection. Exposure to elevated levels of nonessential metals and/or suboptimal amounts of essential trace metals due to consumption of fast foods clearly has the potential to impact the gut microbiota and susceptibility to infections in profound ways. Thus more research needs to be focused on this topic.

**Epigenetic Effects of Metals**

Epigenetics is a term that encompasses events in the genome which affect gene expression without direct changes in gene structure, such as deletion or mutation. These events can be heritable. During the early stages of pre- and postimplantation development of the zygote, programmed silencing and/or activation of specific events is key to normal ontogeny (Christensen and Marsit 2011). DNA methylation is the most widely studied epigenetic marker. Epigenetic changes, which may be stable mechanisms or have some plasticity, are likely to emanate from the environment; thus it is important to characterize the role of environmental exposures in epigenetic alterations. Existing evidence that implicates the role of environmental factors on epigenetic changes comes from studies of diseases such as cancer and adverse reproductive/developmental events. A contribution of heavy metal emissions to human health may be mediated though epigenetic effects that affect susceptibility or response to infection. The flexibility of epigenetic responses is a critical mechanism of both innate and adaptive immune responses in which gene expression is rapidly altered to respond to the presence of an antigen or other stressor, as well as accomplishing the achievement of the mature immune response repertoire (Kondilis-Mangum and Wade 2013).

Evidence of the epigenetic effects of metals on infection is illustrated by data which shows that Zn deficiency *in vitro* increases interleukin (IL)-1β and TNF-α mRNA and protein, which is associated with increased accessibilities of IL-1β and TNF-α promoters in Zn-deficient cells (Wessels et al. 2013). The cellular basis of the chromatin-remodeling process induced by Zn deficiency is, however, not clear.

Arsenic is the most frequently studied metal, in terms of its effects on the methyl donor pool, as it is progressively metabolized to a mono- and a dimethyl species (see review by Reichard and Puga 2010). Early life exposure to arsenic has been linked to altered immune function in children in Bangladesh, where children exposed to arsenic via contaminated groundwater have an increased incidence of respiratory infections and reduced thymic function (Winans et al. 2011).

Other metals for which epigenetic effects have been reported include nickel, cadmium, and chromium VI (Salnikow and Zhitkovich 2008; Arita and Costa 2009). Exposure to diesel exhaust particles, often enriched in heavy metals, is associated with an increase in global hypomethylation and hypermethylation of the promoter of several genes, including *IFN-γ* and *FOXP3* (Liu et al. 2008; Brunst et al. 2013). Diesel exhaust particles were shown to induce *COX-2* expression through histone modification of H4 near the *COX-2* gene promoter (Cao et al. 2007). As *IFN-γ* and *FOXP3* are involved in the immune response and *COX-1* is proinflammatory, exposure of bronchial epithelium to metal-containing particulate matter may have an impact on susceptibility to respiratory infection (see above). It is likely that other metals may have significant epigenetic effects.

Available information shows that pathogens and heavy metals can activate or suppress gene expression through epigenetic modifications, and these changes can last throughout life (Ho et al. 2012). The epigenetic targets of some heavy metals are often similar to those of pathogens and include changes in (a) DNA methylation patterns, either at the global or the individual gene level; (b) the histone code, affecting histone methylation, acetylation, ubiquitination, and phophorylation; and (c) miRNA expression (see review by Ho et al. 2012). Whether these epigenetic changes are enhanced or suppressed during coexposure to metals and infective pathogens is unknown at the present time.

## Metalliferous Nanoparticles and Infections

Nanotechnology has been applied in the food sector and is used for various purposes such as food supplements, functional food ingredients, and food packaging (Sonkaria et al. 2012; Chen et al. 2014). Opportunities to exploit and develop nanomaterials have resulted in a large number of patents worldwide. Nanomaterials can be found in the form of uncomplexed metals, inorganic metals, and carbon-based compounds. Inorganic nanoparticles of silver, titanium, aluminium, and zinc oxide are used for numerous applications. Silver nanoparticles, for example, are utilized due to their antimicrobial properties. Silver zeolites are used in beverage containers (EFSA Panel on FEC 2011). However, concerns are rising about the hazardous risks that these may have on human health, especially in terms of long-term effects (Magnuson et al. 2011; Sonkaria et al. 2012). To date, there is little information on the release of metals from nanomaterials, largely due to the fact that there are no requirements for disclosure of nanotechnology use and the failure of agencies to develop rigorous testing rules for specific applications. In Europe, for example, titanium nitride nanoparticles are intended to be used as an additive in polyethylene terephthalate. In 2011 the European Food Safety Authority evaluated the safety of these nanoparticles and concluded that there is no safety concern for the consumer if the nanoparticulate substance used does not exceed 20 mg/kg for a particular application (EFSA Panel on FEC 2012).

In addition to applications in commercial products, nanotherapy aimed at using the chemical and physical characteristics of metallic nanomaterials for the treatment of infectious disease at the molecular level constitutes an active area of research. The small-sized particles are characterized by a high surface area, unique physicochemical properties, and surface charges which enhance their effective antimicrobial action (Weir et al. 2008). Antibacterial nanoparticles consisting of silver, gold, iron, zinc, copper, and titanium or their oxides have been featured in a number of studies and have been found to be effective against *Staphylococcus aureus*, *Escherichia coli*, *Pseudomonas aeruginosa*, and HIV virus (Sundar and Prajapati 2012). The antimicrobial mechanisms of nanomaterials are basically unknown but the commonly proposed pathogenic impacts are said to be dominated by inflammation-driven effects, including photocatalytic production of reactive oxygen species (which damage cellular and viral components), degradation of the bacterial cell wall or membrane, interruption of energy transduction, inhibition of enzyme activity, and DNA synthesis (Weir et al. 2008; Sundar and Prajapati 2012). Metal oxide nanoparticles have been shown to have different inflammatory footprints, implying different hazards in terms of pathology, risks, and risk severity (Chao et al. 2012). The availability of metals in nanoparticles is influenced by the zeta potential, solubility, the immune response associated with inflammation and hypoxic conditions, as well as degradation of macromolecules within inflammatory foci (Nizet and Johnson 2009; Chao et al. 2012). The limited information available suggests that current applications of metal-based nanomaterials can influence susceptibility to infectious diseases, judging by the effects of different metals on infective pathogens. Most of the studies relate to engineered nanomaterials, and there is currently little information on the effect of natural nanomaterials ("colloids") on disease infection.

### Emerging Metals

Emerging metals constitute another driver of change in metal exposure. Among the rare earth metals (Table 17.1), four deserve special attention relative to reported immune and/or microbial effects: cerium, gadolinium, lanthanum, and yttrium. Cerium has been reported to have both immunomodulatory and direct antimicrobial effects. Cerium nitrate has been used as an antibiofilm agent on hospital catheters and shown to significantly reduce biofilm formation by *Candida albicans* (Cobrado et al. 2013). Additionally, cerium helps to restore cell-mediated immunity among immunosuppressed burn patients (Peterson et al. 1985). Gadolinium chloride stimulates the innate immune system and, in particular, modulates macrophage cell population. It appears to signal through

TLR4 and TLR7 receptors on macrophages, increasing the production of several profibrotic or proinflammatory cytokines, chemokines, and growth factors (Wermuth and Jimenez 2012). However, pretreatment of rats with gadolinium chloride prior to bile duct ligation can also reduce Kupffer cell numbers and function in the liver as a means of reducing the risk of septic shock (Jones et al. 2013). Exposure of mice to lanthanum chloride inhibits production of proinflammatory (IL-1 and TNF-α) cytokines (Guo et al. 2011). The metal appears to act by inhibiting activation of NF-kappa B. Yttrium exposure has been reported to elevate humoral immunity while concomitantly producing a deficit of CD8+ T lymphocytes (Zhang et al. 2006b). Both traditional as well as comparatively new groups of metals (e.g., rare earth metals, titanium) contribute to this new category of human exposure. Information on immunomodulation relative to risk of infection by these compounds is becoming available (Appendix 17.1).

**Direct Impacts of the Environment on Host–Parasite Interactions**

From an ecological perspective, the processes by which metals in the environment could possibly impact host–pathogen interactions in a direct manner include (a) the changing pathogenicity of parasites and the emergence and spread of drug resistance and (b) changing of host resistance to the pathogen.

*Metals and Drug Resistance in Bacteria*

Antimicrobial resistant infections are considered the most critical global pathogenic threat to human health, according to recent reports by the WHO and Centers for Disease Control and Prevention. Newly emerging resistant strains are increasingly likely to be multidrug resistant (Jones et al. 2013). For this reason, identification of pressures that contribute to the dissemination of resistance is a high priority in biomedical and basic research.

Metals may be one source of pressure for resistance selection and dissemination. There is evidence for co-packaging of metal- and drug-resistant genes on transmissible genetic elements among bacteria (Baker-Austin et al. 2006). It has been suggested that environmental conditions of increased metal concentrations of both toxic and essential metals could contribute to the emergence and spread of drug resistance within environmental microbial systems (Bednorz et al. 2013). Specific to methicillin-resistant *S. aureus*, Cavaco et al. (2010) reported that cadmium and zinc drive co-selection for methicillin resistance in *S. aureus* through horizontal transfer of plasmids containing both *mec* and *czr* (Cd/Zn-resistance) genes. For this reason, there is increased concern that antimicrobial-resistance genes function as environmental pollutants (Martinez 2009).

*Modification of Host Tolerance*

The human host employs two nonmutually exclusive strategies in response to an infection: the ability to limit parasite burden (resistance) and the ability to limit the harm caused by a given burden of parasites (tolerance). From an ecological perspective, resistance protects the host at the expense of the parasite, whereas tolerance saves the host from harm without having any direct negative effects on the parasite (Ayres and Schneider 2012). This distinction is useful because it recognizes the important fact that hosts can sometimes be quite healthy despite high parasite burdens or, conversely, die with parasite loads that are tolerated by others; in fact, pathogen burden and health are not always well correlated (Schneider and Ayres 2008; Ayres and Schneider 2012; Medzhitov et al. 2012). Although these two components together determine how well a host is protected against the effects of parasitism, studies of human host defense have to date focused primarily on resistance; the possibility of tolerance and its implications have been largely ignored (Miller et al. 2006). The role that trace metal homeostasis might play in human tolerance mechanisms has been completely overlooked.

The mechanisms by which metal homeostasis increases the host's tolerance to invading pathogens have yet to be explored in detail. The following mechanisms may be involved:

- The production of reactive oxygen species and toxic free radicals.
- Inducible mechanisms such as the heme/HO-1 system (deficient for the *Hmox1* gene), which has been shown to provide tolerance for *Plasmodium* and polymicrobial infections (Seixas et al. 2009; Larsen et al. 2010) The expression of the Fe-sequestering protein ferritin H chain in mice and ferritin in humans has also been found to be associated with reduced tissue damage irrespective of pathogen burden (confer tolerance) following infection of mice with *Plasmodium* (Gozzelino et al. 2012).
- Activation of toll-like receptors, which can induce the production of cytoprotective and tissue repair factors to maintain epithelial integrity and homeostasis (Rakoff-Nahoum et al. 2004).
- Dietary imbalance in trace metal intake (Ayres and Schneider 2009).
- Phagocytosis-dependent microbial containment (Deretic and Levine 2009; Rashed 2011; Chifman et al. 2012).

When these and related mechanisms are sufficient to prevent major disruptions in physiological functions of the host after exposure to a parasite, infections remain asymptomatic.

The interaction of immune defense and tolerance mechanisms in protecting the human host against the pathophysiological effects of parasites has not been studied (Medzhitov et al. 2012). What is clear is that morbidity and mortality may result from the failure of tolerance mechanisms, even in the presence of effective resistance. This would normally be indicated by hosts that present different morbidity or mortality profiles at comparative parasitemia. The distinction between failed resistance and failed tolerance is critically important in terms of the choice of therapeutic strategies. When failed tolerance is the underlying factor, boosting immunity and reducing pathogen burden (using drugs) may be ineffective, whereas enhancing tolerance (e.g., with trace metal intervention) may have salutary effects. Drug interventions that target the tolerance pathways may also be more desirable when immune defenses are either inefficient, compromised, or cause excessive immunopathology. Boosting tissue tolerance should be a particularly useful strategy in the case of pandemic diseases that cause morbidity and mortality worldwide, such as malaria, tuberculosis, and HIV—infectious diseases for which pathogen control through vaccination or antimicrobial drugs is currently unattainable (Medzhitov et al. 2012). Trace metal-related intervention holds some promise in this regard.

## New Approaches to Epidemiological Studies

Whole-genome methods have led to the unprecedented discovery of robust associations between genetic markers and susceptibility to disease and have improved the understanding of infectious disease biology by revealing the crucial host–pathogen interaction sites (Khor and Hibberd 2012). Success in mapping the human genome and the realization that genetics can only account for a limited fraction of the etiology of diseases has led to the development of the complementary concept of the "exposome," defined as the measure of all the exposures of an individual during a lifetime and how those exposures relate to health (Buck Louis and Sundaram 2012). Exposomics (the study of the exposome) focuses on simultaneous assessment of exposures that may originate from external and internal sources. External exposures may be from the environment, diet, or behavior, whereas internal environmental exposures stem from bodily functions and processes that govern homeostasis. Assessment of internal exposures focuses on chemicals and biomarkers and relies primarily on high-throughput molecular "omics" technologies: genomics, metabonomics, lipidomics, transcriptomics, and proteomics. Strategies in internal exposure assessment involve the use of (a) biomarkers to determine exposure, effect of exposure, disease progression, and susceptibility factors; (b) technologies that generate large amounts of data; and (c) advanced informatics to find statistical associations between exposures, effect of exposures, and other factors such as genetics with disease (Miller and Jones 2014). External exposures, in contrast, involve measurements related to environmental stressors using common approaches, such as survey instruments, geographic mapping and remote sensing technologies, direct reading instruments, personal exposure sensors, and laboratory-based analysis (Vrijheid et al. 2014). Exposomics thus represents a new and exciting approach to improve, integrate, and consolidate exposure data for use in environment-wide association studies to identify associations between health outcomes and biomarkers of exposures, biomarkers of response, or patterns of disease.

Progress in the study of the nexus of trace metals and infectious diseases will clearly require new research paradigms for transforming how we think about exposures (internal and external), health, and disease; new research design; and new strategies for collecting and interpreting data. Exposome represents a good framework for assessing the effects of coexposure to metals and infective pathogens in that the paradigm is aimed at (a) accurate and reliable measurement of many exposures in the external environment, (b) measuring a wide range of biological responses in the internal environment, and (c) addressing the dynamic and life course nature of the exposure (Miller and Jones 2014). Exposome adopts a holistic approach to understanding the environmental determinants of disease, the mechanism by which these exposures interact with lifestyle behaviors, and delays in the manifestation of effects. Building the exposome for metals and pathologies of infectious diseases will require an integration of approaches, including environmental measurements and validated biomarkers. Below we propose approaches that could be used to address some of the major gaps in our knowledge of how metals impact on infectious disease within the exposome framework. We emphasize that many challenges still remain in developing the exposome concept into a workable approach for epidemiological research (Vrijheid et al. 2014).

## Longitudinal and Cross-Sectional Studies in Areas with Overlapping Risks

Many parts of the world experience coincident exposures to trace metal deficiency/toxicity and endemic communicable diseases. High prevalence rates of As poisoning associated with high levels of arsenic in groundwater have been reported in many areas that have a high incidence of communicable diseases. Similar opportunities exist with respect to mercury (artisanal mining communities), lead (communities around base metal mining and smelting operations), and selenium (communities where soils are highly enriched in this element). The fact that soils with unusual concentrations of toxic metals are depleted in zinc and other microelements could provide an opportunity to explore the combined effects of Zn deficiency and toxic metal exposure on the pathogenesis of infectious diseases. Different types of study design offer the possibility of collecting exposure information from candidate communities:

- A cross-sectional study could be used to collect exposure data from a few people in great detail and determine what additional information is needed to validate hypothesized exposure-biomarker relationships.

- Case control studies could be used to look at exposures that have occurred relatively recently, when no relevant biologic samples may be particularly relevant.
- A cohort study (involving a group with a common set of characteristics over time) could be considered the gold standard in assessing exposure characteristics to ascertain the influence of metals on disease infection.

## Inhalation Exposures to Toxic Metals and Infectious Disease

The lung is a unique microbiome for exposomic study. Real time modeling of exposure to airborne metals from pollutants using technologies that track the absorption and distribution of inhaled metals from airborne particulate matter within the body would give novel insights into how metals interact with the body and its microbiome at different interfaces. Data from such studies would provide information about how potentially toxic metals may influence respiratory and other infectious diseases.

## Biomarkers that Provide Better Representation of Body Metal Status

Many of the body compartments that are sampled to provide estimates of body metal status do not indicate overall body metal status. As discussed earlier, these include, for example, blood, urine, hair, feces, sweat, and saliva. The "blood exposome" and its connection to disease was recently explored using human blood concentrations for 1,561 small molecules and metals along with their sources, evidence of chronic disease risks, and numbers of metabolic pathways (Rappaport et al. 2014). Similar studies could be done with the other biological samples. The resulting data could then be combined and metabolic profiling (metabonomics/metabolomics) used to define an individual's metabolic phenotype, which is influenced by metal exposure, diet, lifestyle, genotype, and disease pathology; this could also reveal intermediate biomarkers for disease risk that reflect adaptive response to exposure. Implementation of such exposomic research will require the development and refinement of analytic methods capable of handling the diverse array of biomakers and also other exposures for which there are no known or measurable biomarkers. Such analytic approaches can lead to a more comprehensive understanding of trace metal status in the context of environmental exposures and how changes in trace metal status relate to human health across the lifespan.

## Use of Stable Isotopes to Study Uptake and
## Distribution of Metals by the Body over Time

In biomedical research, radioactive trace metals are first combined with other elements to form chemical compounds. The labeled compounds are taken internally, either orally or intravenously. Once administered to the patient (or volunteer), the radioactive compounds are localized to specific organs or cellular receptors. This characteristic behavior makes it possible to determine the translocation of a metal to the infected organ(s) as well as to image the extent of a disease process in the body. Since these images are based on cellular function and physiology, rather than on physical changes in the tissue anatomy, they provide important insights on actual metabolic cycle and pharmacokinetics of an element. Radioisotopes can thus be used to assess the effect of disease state on systemic redistribution of a trace metal. A mass balance of the administered radionuclide can be used to estimate the bioavailability and absorption rate across the gastrointestinal tract. Because of concerns for health effects of the radionuclide, dietary exposure studies increasingly rely on stable isotopes of the elements. The diet (or food component) is spiked with a known stable isotope and the changes in the isotope fingerprint are monitored to estimate the excretion and bodily retention rates. This method has been used with success to estimate dietary exposure to zinc, lead, mercury, and other metals with more than one abundant stable isotope.

The identification of peptides that result from posttranslational modifications is important in understanding normal pathways of cellular regulation as well as assessing exposure and identifying damage from a toxic metal. Because of their low abundance in proteomes, effective detection of modified peptides by mass spectrometry typically requires enrichment to eliminate false identifications. Polacco et al. (2011) described a new method of high-resolution mass spectrometry for identifying peptides with Hg-containing adducts based on the influence of mercury's seven stable isotopes on peptide isotope distributions. They showed that the pattern of peak heights in isotope distributions from primary mass spectrometry single scans was able to identify Hg adducts with sensitivity and specificity greater than 90%. Summing peptide isotope distributions across multiple scans improved specificity to 99.4% and sensitivity above 95%, which made it possible to detect unexpected Hg modifications. Polacco et al. (2011) suggest that the method can also be used to detect several less common elements, including the essential element, selenium, as selenocysteine in peptides. This study and others with radioisotopes suggest that the isotopes of metals (radioactive or stable) can be an important tool ("isotopeomics") in exposome research. For a discussion on the applicaton of isotopes for analysis of metal body distribution, see Maret et al. (this volume).

## Conclusions

In this chapter we have tried to provide insights into current knowledge and gaps in understanding of the interplay between trace metals in the environment and disease infection. The contributions of metal deficiencies to the global burden of infectious diseases is substantial for zinc and iron but less defined for other metals. How emerging metals will relate to emerging pathogens, and hence influence the disease burden, is a matter that deserves further research. Despite considerable research that is taking place separately on trace metals and infectious pathogens, little is currently known about the interactions between these two key determinants of health, especially in host microbiomes where direct coexposure occurs. A number of global trends have been identified that have the potential to upset the natural host–pathogen–metal nexus, including climate change, Western-style food processing, increasing reliance on infant formula, consumption of fast foods, and commercialization of products with metalliferous nanomaterials. From an ecological perspective, the two main processes by which the environment can directly impact host–pathogen interactions are (a) the changing pathogenicity of parasites with the emergence and spread of drug resistance and (b) the changing of host resistance to the pathogen. The specific mechanisms involved in each process are essentially unknown. In many parts of the world, the levels of trace metals in soils and local food chain are closely associated with the body burden of the metals and sometimes the health of local communities.

Failure to ascertain the environmental component of disease etiology stems, to a large extent, from limitations in our ability to assess the environmental exposures (which have traditionally been measured using questionnaires and geographical mapping) and tackle multiple exposures. A new exposure paradigm is needed that can integrate many external and internal exposures from different sources over the life course. Exposomics or environment-wide association studies offers one approach that can be used to gain a better handle on the environmental component essential to improving our understanding of the predictors, risk factors, and protective factors in complex interactions between trace metals, the environment, and infective pathogens. An understanding of the effects of such individual (and environmentally determined) exposomes on susceptibility to disease infection would be useful in developing appropriate intervention strategies to reduce burden of infectious diseases in many parts of the world.

## Acknowledgment

We thank Ellen Silbergeld for her input and guidance during the Forum.

**Appendix 17.1** Emission sources, selected applications, exposure pathways, and immune effects of elements. Exposure pathways: A, air (inhalation of contaminated air); F, food (consumption of contaminated food); W, water (drinking of water); T, tobacco (tobacco smoking); M, mouth (hand-to-mouth).

| Element | Major Atmospheric Emission Sources and Select Applications | Exposure Pathways | Effects on Immune System and Host Defenses Against Infection | Direct Antimicrobial Properties |
|---|---|---|---|---|
| Iron (Fe) | *Anthropogenic sources*: production of steel and iron, combustion of fossil fuels, production of cement, waste disposal, use of steel and iron. *Natural sources*: reemission from soil and water surfaces, volcano eruptions | A, F, W | Both Fe deficiency and overload produce significant immune impairment and increased risk for certain categories of infections. Effective Fe homeostasis is critical in both macrophage function and Th balance. Th1 cells are more sensitive to suboptimal iron levels than Th2 cells (see Weiss, this volume) | Tranferrin-based Fe supra-accumulation can starve bacteria and fungi. Fe depletion also inhibits biofilm formation and enhances the activity of certain antibiotics. Fe analogs, such as gallium, also interfere with bacteria enzyme function |
| Aluminum (Al) | *Anthropogenic sources*: Al production, various uses of aluminum, combustion of coal, waste disposal. *Natural sources*: reemission from soil | A, F, W | Al targets primarily macrophages and T cells subchronic overload of AlCl suppresses spleen function Al adjuvants stimulate an inflammatory response which appears to produce adverse outcomes in susceptible individuals (e.g., macrophagic myofasciitis) | Aluminum oxide nanoparticles have demonstrated potential as antibacterial agents |
| Zinc (Zn) | *Sources*: Combustion of fuels, production of cement, non-ferrous and ferrous metals, waste incineration | A, F, W | Absence of Zn severely affects immune response; numerous investigations (e.g., Haase and Rink 2014) indicate not just a single function for zinc but a wide range of different roles | ZnO nano particles have antibiotic activity |
| Copper (Cu) | *Sources*: combustion of fuels, production of nonferrous and ferrous metals, waste incineration | A, F | Apoptotic reduction of CD4+ T cells Immunosuppression Oxidative damage and cellular depletion of lymphoid tissues Enhanced colonization by *Helicobacter pylori* | Cu(II) complexes of bis-thiosemi-carbazones inhibit human *Neisseria gonorrhoeae* |
| Chromium (Cr) | *Sources*: combustion of fuels, production of cement, nonferrous and ferrous metals, waste incineration | A, F, W | Related to oxidative states and redox forms, Cr impairs lung host defenses against bacteria Induces allergic contact dermatitis | α-diimine Cr(III) complexes inhibit both Gram-positive and Gram-negative bacteria |

**Appendix 17.1 (continued)**

| Element | Major Atmospheric Emission Sources and Select Applications | Exposure Pathways | Effects on Immune System and Host Defenses Against Infection | Direct Antimicrobial Properties |
|---|---|---|---|---|
| Manganese (Mn) | *Sources*: combustion of fuels, production of cement, nonferrous and ferrous metals, waste incineration | A, F, W | Mn enhances the release of inflammatory cytokines interleukin-6 and TNF-α from microglial cells that can promote the activation of astrocytes and subsequent release of inflammatory mediators such as prostaglandin E2 and nitric oxide | Insufficient information |
| Mercury (Hg) | *Sources*: fossil fuel combustion, artisanal Au mining and production, production of cement, nonferrous and ferrous metals, chlor-alkali, waste incineration | A, F, W | Immune bias toward Th2 responses<br>Increased risk of viral infection-associated autoimmunity<br>Potential to induce mast cell dysfunction<br>Impairs immune development | Antibacterial properties probably via inhibited respiration |
| Lead (Pb) | *Sources*: combustion of fuels, production of cement, nonferrous and ferrous metals, waste incineration | A, F, W, M, T | Immune bias toward Th2 responses<br>Inflammatory dysfunction<br>Elevated risk of infection-related mortality among patients on maintenance hemodialysis | Antibacterial properties against select Gram-positive and Gram-negative bacteria |
| Cadmium (Cd) | *Sources*: combustion of fuels, production of cement, nonferrous and ferrous metals, waste incineration | A, F, W, T | Prenatal Cd disrupts signaling among thymocytes and reduces T cell numbers later in life<br>Chronic exposure produces inflammatory dysfunction and risk of lung damage<br>Promotes influenza virus proliferation by altering redox state | The composite, CdTe-TiO₂, exhibits antibacterial properties against both Gram-positive and Gram-negative bacteria |
| Arsenic (As) | *Sources*: combustion of fuels, production of cement, nonferrous and ferrous metals, waste incineration | A, F, W | CD4+ T cell-associated immunosuppression combined with elevated risk of innate immune driven-chronic inflammation<br>Compromised airway barrier function and increased risk of respiratory infections | As(III)-containing Schiff bases display antibacterial activity against *Escherichia coli* |

| Element | Major Atmospheric Emission Sources and Select Applications | Exposure Pathways | Effects on Immune System and Host Defenses Against Infection | Direct Antimicrobial Properties |
|---|---|---|---|---|
| Vanadium (V) | *Sources*: combustion of fuels, production of cement and nonferrous metals, waste incineration | A, F, | Disrupted mucosal immunity<br>Reduced thymic dendritic cell function<br>Airway inflammation | V chloroperoxidase inhibits enterococcal biofilm formation. |
| Nickel (Ni) | *Sources*: combustion of fuels, production of cement, nonferrous and ferrous metals, waste incineration | A, F, W | Metal-associated hypersensitivity<br>Potent activator of dendritic cells<br>Signaling via the TLR 4 pathway | Antibacterial properties against select Gram-positive and Gram-negative bacteria |
| Antimony (Sb) | *Sources*: combustion of fuels, production of cement, nonferrous and ferrous metals, waste incineration | A, F | Pentavalent antimony complexes activate macrophages for ROS and NO attack against parasites | Antimony is a preferred agent against leishmaniasis, probably acting in concert with immune effects |
| Selenium (Se) | *Sources*: combustion of fuels, production of cement, nonferrous and ferrous metals, waste incineration | A, F | Deficiency increases risk of certain viral, bacterial, and parasitic infections<br>Increase risk of organ pathology and failure | Organsoselenium inhibits the formation of certain bacterial biofilms |
| Molybdenum (Mo) | *Sources*: combustion of fuels, production of cement, nonferrous and ferrous metals, waste incineration | A, F | Enhanced protection against the nematode parasite *Trichostrongylus colubriformis*<br>Higher levels produce apoptosis and compromise lymphoid tissue architecture | Antibacterial properties against select Gram-positive and Gram-negative bacteria |
| Beryllium (Be) | *Sources*: combustion of fuels, production of cement, nonferrous and ferrous metals, waste incineration | A, F | Induction of airway granulamatous inflammation via innate immune cells, Th1-directed responses, and a dysfunctional dysfunctional CTLA-4 pathway<br>Increase respiratory infections associated with chronic beryllium disease | Insufficient information |
| Gallium (Ga) | *Sources*: Al production, nonferrous metal (mostly Zn) production, combustion of coal | A, F | Gallium arsenide impairs macrophage antigen processing and produces both local inflammation and system immunosuppression<br>Gallium nitrate can restrict the growth of *Mycobacterium tuberculosis* inside macrophages and protect the lung | Gallium interferes with Fe metabolism and has both bacteriostatic and bactericidal properties<br>Gallium nitrate has antibacterial activity against *Rhodococcus equi* |

304

**Appendix 17.1 (continued)**

| Element | Major Atmospheric Emission Sources and Select Applications | Exposure Pathways | Effects on Immune System and Host Defenses Against Infection | Direct Antimicrobial Properties |
|---|---|---|---|---|
| Cobalt (Co) | *Sources*: combustion of fuels, production of cement, nonferrous and ferrous metals, waste incineration | A, F, W | Co-alloy particles can trigger innate immune response via the TLR4 signaling pathway. Potent activator of dendritic cells. Cobalt protoporphyrin reduces the macrophage burden of *Trypanosoma cruzi* during infection | Cobalt Schiff base complexes possess broad-spectrum antibacterial activity. Certain Co(II) complexes have activity against *M. tuberculosis* |
| Tin (Sn) | *Sources*: combustion of fuels, production of cement, nonferrous and ferrous metals, waste incineration, various uses | A, F, W | Organotins (e.g., tributyltin) cause thymic atrophy and apoptosis of immune cells. Suppression of both humoral and cell-mediated immunity result including reduced host defense against bacteria. | $SnO_2$ nanostructures exhibit surfactant-promoted antibacterial activity. $SnO_2$ nanowires inhibit herpes simplex-1 infection. Certain Sn complexes exhibit anti-leishmanial activity |
| Gold (Au) | *Use*: jewelry, photography, electrical appliances, electronics, satellites | A, F | Associated with potential autoimmunity involving mast cell dysfunction. Au salts can be allergic sensitizers | Anti-leishmanial activity of Au nanoparticles. Antibacterial biofilm activity of Au nanocomposites |
| Silver (Ag) | *Use*: color and stained steel, coins, ornaments, jewelry, electrical appliances, catalyzers, cables, wires, mirrors | F | Potential promoter of autoimmunity in susceptible populations. May involve mast cell dysfunction | Antibacterial action against Gram-negative bacteria. Anti-leishmanial activity of Ag nanoparticles. Biofilm inhibition of Ag nanocomposites |
| Boron (B) | *Use*: dopant in semiconductor industry, sodium perborate in bleaching, borax component in fiberglass, in glass and ceramics, reagents in chemical industry | F, W | Benzoxaborole analogs inhibit proinflammatory cytokine responses via inhibition of toll-like receptor signaling | Several B-containing antibacterials inhibit Gram-negative bacteria via inhibition of bacterial leucyl tRNA synthetase |
| Thallium (Tl) | *Use*: optics, electronics, superconductivity, medical applications | F | Insufficient information | Insufficient information |

| Element | Major Atmospheric Emission Sources and Select Applications | Exposure Pathways | Effects on Immune System and Host Defenses Against Infection | Direct Antimicrobial Properties |
|---|---|---|---|---|
| Uranium (U) | *Use:* nuclear reactors, colorant in glass | F, W | Immune bias toward Th2 responses with reduced anti-microbial function of macrophages | |
| Platinum (Pt) | *Use:* catalysts, electronics, glass industry, dentistry, jewelry | A, F | Pt chemotherapeutics enhance dendritic cell activity via a STAT-6 pathway Hypersensitivity reactions are common. | Pd complexes of polyamides containing sulfones have antifungal and antibacterial activity |
| Palladium (Pd) | *Use:* catalysts, electronics, glass industry, dentistry, jewelry | A, F | Reported respiratory and dematological sensitizer Causes occupational asthma Causes some Th-associated cytokine alterations both *in vitro* and *in vivo* | Greater inhibitory activity of Pd nanoparticles against *Staphylococcus aureus* than toward *E. coli* |
| Rhodium (Rh) | *Use:* catalysts, electronics, glass industry, dentistry, jewelry | A, F | Reported to cause allergic contact dermatitis | Rh-metal complexes have reported antitrypanosome activity |
| Scandium (Sc) | *Use:* light Al-Sc alloys for aerospace components, additive in metal-halide lamps and Hg vapor lamps, radioactive tracing agent in oil refineries | F | Insufficient information | A component of laser treatments that has shown antibacterial activity |
| Yttrium (Y) | *Use:* yttrium aluminium garnet laser, yttrium vanadate as host for europium in TV red phosphor, high-temperature superconductors, Y-stabilized zirconia, yttrium iron garnet microwave filters, energy-efficient light bulbs, spark plugs, gas mantles, additive to steel | F | Elevates components of humoral immunity while concomitantly producing a deficit of CD8+ T lymphocytes | Yttrium fluoride nanoparticles inhibit colonization by *E. coli* and *S. aureus* Y(III) complex containing 1,10-phenanthroline as a ligand has shown antibacterial activity |
| Lanthanum (La) | *Use:* high refractive index and alkali-resistant glass, flint, hydrogen storage, battery-electrodes, camera lenses, fluid catalytic cracking catalyst for oil refineries | F | Inhibits innate immune cell production of pro-inflammatory cytokines upon bacterial stimulation | Lanthanum calcium manganate is inhibitory for *Pseudomonas aeruginosa* La nanoparticles may have application as a phosphate starvation strategy against bacteria |

**Appendix 17.1 (continued)**

| Element | Major Atmospheric Emission Sources and Select Applications | Exposure Pathways | Effects on Immune System and Host Defenses Against Infection | Direct Antimicrobial Properties |
|---|---|---|---|---|
| Cerium (Ce) | *Use:* oxidizing agent, polishing powder, yellow colors in glass and ceramics, catalyst, ferro-cerium flints for lighters | F | Cerium oxide nanoparticles accelerate wound healing | Cerium nitrate has been used as an antibiofilm agent on hospital catheters |
| Praseo-dymium (Pr) | *Use:* magnets, lasers, core material for carbon arc lighting, colorant in glasses and enamels, additive in didymium glass, ferro-cerium fire-steel (flint) products. | F | Insufficient information | Insufficient information |
| Neodym-ium (Nd) | *Use:* magnets, lasers, violet colors in glass and ceramics, didymium glass, ceramic capacitors | F | Insufficient information | Incorporated into some antibacterial nanparticles |
| Prome-thium (Pm) | *Use:* nuclear batteries | F | Insufficient information | Insufficient information |
| Samarium (Sm) | *Use:* magnets, lasers, neutron capture, masers | F | 153Sm lexidronam used in stem cell transplantation with no drug-attributed adverse effects | Sm(III) ions enhance the antimicrobial activity of enrofloxacin. |
| Europium (Eu) | *Use:* red and blue phosphors, lasers, mercury-vapor lamps, fluorescent lamps, NMR relaxation agent | F | Insufficient information | Used for imaging of antimicrobials |
| Gado-linium (Gd) | *Use:* magnets, high refractive index glass or garnets, lasers, X-ray tubes, computer memories, neutron capture, MRI contrast agent, NMR relaxation agent, magnetostrictive alloys, steel additive | F | Targets macrophage cell populations possibly with signaling via TLR receptors Specifically depletes Kupffer cells | Insufficient information |

| Element | Major Atmospheric Emission Sources and Select Applications | Exposure Pathways | Effects on Immune System and Host Defenses Against Infection | Direct Antimicrobial Properties |
|---|---|---|---|---|
| Terbium (Tb) | *Use*: green phosphors, lasers, fluorescent lamps, magnetostrictive alloys | F | Insufficient information | Insufficient information |
| Dyspro-sium (Dy) | *Use*: magnets, lasers, magnetostrictive alloys | F | Insufficient information | Dy(III) complex containing 1,10-phenanthroline (phen), $[Dy(phen)_2(OH_2)_3Cl]Cl_2 \cdot H_2O$ has antibacterial activity via bacterial DNA binding |
| Holmium (Ho) | *Use*: lasers, wavelength calibration standards for optical spectrophotometers, magnets | F | Used in lasers for anti-inflammation (e.g., arthritis) treatments | A series of Ho(III) complexes have reported activity against *S. aureus* |
| Erbium (Er) | *Use*: infrared lasers, vanadium steel, fiber-optic technology | F | Associated laser phototherapy appears to promote gingival wound healing | Associated with laser phototherapy against herpes simplex virus infections as well as root canal-associated *Candida albicans* infections |
| Thulium (Tm) | *Use*: portable X-ray machines, metal-halide lamps, lasers | F | Insufficient information | Insufficient information |
| Ytterbium (Yb) | *Use*: infrared lasers, chemical reducing agent, decoy flares, stainless steel, stress gauges | F | Insufficient information | Yb(III) complexes have antibacterial activity via DNA binding |
| Lutetium (Lu) | *Use*: scan detectors, high refractive index glass, lutetium tantalate hosts for phosphors | F | Insufficient information | Lu(III) complexes have reported antibacterial activity |

# Methods and Technologies for Analyzing Trace Metals in Biological Systems

# 18

# Emerging Strategies in Metalloproteomics

Peter-Leon Hagedoorn

## Abstract

The impact of changing metal ion concentrations on infection with a pathogenic microorganism has been established in several cases. To understand the molecular basis of the interplay between metals in the host and the pathogen in infectious diseases, metalloproteomics may prove to be a very powerful approach. Metalloproteomics is the comprehensive analysis of all metal-binding and metal-containing proteins in a biological sample. Strategies in metalloproteomics can be divided into experimental and computer-based approaches.

Samples that have been analyzed using metalloproteomics strategies are cell lysates, subcellular fractions, and recombinantly expressed proteins from structural genomics platforms. Samples can be enriched in metal-binding protein by using immobilized metal ion affinity chromatography (IMAC). Subsequently, metalloproteins have been separated using either 2D electrophoresis or 2D liquid chromatography (LC). Resolved proteins have been further analyzed for metals and protein content. Inductively coupled plasma mass spectrometry (ICP-MS), X-ray absorbance or fluorescence and autoradiography of radioactive metal isotopes have been used to determine the metal content, and different soft ionization mass spectrometry techniques and SDS-PAGE have been used to determine or quantify protein content. Computer-based strategies have been developed to predict metalloproteomes from genomes based on information from literature resources and different genomic and protein structural databases.

Many of the methods presented here are comprehensive in nature. The interplay of computer-based and experimental strategies in metalloproteomics will significantly advance the field in the near future.

## Introduction

The term metallome was originally introduced by the Oxford professor R. J. P. Williams to refer to the free metal ion pool in the cell (Williams 2001). Today, the metallome is defined more broadly (even covering nonmetal elementals) and can be viewed as the comprehensive analysis (structure, function, and interactions) of all metals and metal species in a cell or tissue type (Mounicou et al. 2009). This includes semi-metals (e.g., Se), free metal ions, metal–DNA interactions, and metalloproteins. Metalloproteomics, on the other hand, is the comprehensive analysis of all metal-binding and metal-containing proteins in a biological sample. Thus, it is a subset of the metallome.

Strategies in metalloproteomics can be divided into experimental and computer-based approaches. Experimental approaches usually involve a combination of protein separation and metal analysis techniques (Figure 18.1). Computer-based approaches involve bioinformatics tools to predict, ideally, the whole metalloproteome of an organism or group of organisms based on

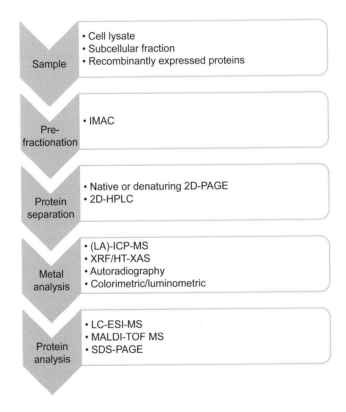

**Figure 18.1** Schematic overview of experimental metalloproteomic strategies. IMAC: immobilized metal ion affinity chromatography; 2D-PAGE: two-dimensional polyacrylamide gel electrophoresis; 2D-HPLC: two-dimensional high performance liquid chromatography; (LA)-ICP-MS: (laser ablation) inductively coupled plasma mass spectrometry; XRF: X-ray fluorescence; HT–XAS: high throughput–X-ray absorbance spectroscopy; LC-ESI-MS: liquid chromatography–electrospray ionization–mass spectrometry; MALDI-TOF MS: matrix assisted laser desorption–time of flight mass spectrometry; SDS-PAGE: sodium dodecyl sulfate–polyacrylamide gel electrophoresis.

genomic information, protein structural information, and biochemical information available in databases.

In this chapter, several experimental and computer-based strategies are presented that have emerged in recent years. In addition, relevant biochemical information is presented that has been obtained using these methods, and specific advantages and disadvantages of the different methods are discussed.

# Experimental Metalloproteomics

## Metal-Binding Protein Fractionation Using Immobilized Metal Ion Affinity Chromatography (IMAC)

IMAC is well known, in the nickel ion bound form, for the isolation of his-tagged proteins. IMAC can be used for other applications as well (Cheung et al. 2012). The method is based on a resin that contains metal ion-chelating groups, such as nitrilotriacetic acid or iminodiacetic acid. Such materials can be charged with different metal ions in a manner that still makes coordination by amino acid residues from metal binding proteins possible. These proteins with high affinity to the chelated metal ions bind and can be eluted using a pH gradient or a competitive ligand, such as EDTA or imidazole. IMAC has been used to enrich metal ion-binding proteins for proteomic investigations. In one instance, Ni-IMAC was used in combination with 2D-PAGE to identify Ni-binding proteins that may be related to metal-specific allergic contact dermatitis (Thierse et al. 2008). Another example is the combination of Ni- and Co-IMAC in combination with mass spectrometry (MS) to identify putative Ni- and Co-binding proteins from *Streptococcus pneumoniae* (Sun et al. 2013).

In a metalloproteomic workflow, IMAC can be used prior to further separation with 2D-PAGE or 2D-LC and subsequent protein identification. The advantage of IMAC is that it is relatively inexpensive and straightforward and can be implemented in high-throughput liquid-handling workflows. Important disadvantages are the occurrence of false positives (e.g., histidine-rich proteins) and false negatives (e.g., metal-containing proteins).

## Methods Based on Inductively Coupled Plasma Mass Spectrometry (ICP-MS)

ICP-MS is a powerful metal analysis technique that is used as a standard technique in trace element analysis. The technique is based on the ionization of a sample by introducing it into an ICP, where it vaporizes and is broken down into atoms, of which many are ionized to form singly charged cations. Ions are subsequently transferred via an interface to a mass spectrometer. The interface is necessary to change the ion beam from the atmospheric pressure of the ICP to the high vacuum of the MS. Metals are identified based on their masses and isotopic distribution. The method is sensitive and has a large dynamic range for many metals and other elements. One inherent problem of ICP-MS is the occurrence of isobaric interferences originating from elements in the sample matrix or the ICP gas, e.g., $^{56}$Fe (m = 55.93494) and $^{40}$Ar$^{16}$O (m = 55.95729). High-resolution ICP-MS allows better separation of the different metal isotopes and prevents most isobaric interferences. ICP-MS has been used in quantitative proteomics by employing metal-coded affinity tags, which consist of three parts: (a) a metal chelate complex consisting of 1,4,7,10-tetraazacyclododecane-1,4,7,10-tetraacetic acid (DOTA) coordinating a lanthanide, (b) an affinity anchor for purification, and (c) a reactive group for the reaction with amino acids to label proteins (Ahrends et al. 2007). Below, two different strategies are presented for metalloproteomics using ICP-MS.

*2D Gel Electrophoresis – Laser Ablation ICP-MS*

Laser ablation ICP-MS (LA-ICP-MS) offers the possibility of directly analyzing metalloproteins following 1D or 2D-PAGE. This technique is based on the use of a focused laser beam to ablate part of the sample, which is transferred to the ICP using a continuous argon gas stream; the elemental ions are then analyzed by MS. Becker et al. (2004) used LA-ICP-MS to analyze the yeast mitochondrial proteome for phosphorus, sulfur, copper, zinc, and iron. Samples were separated by Blue Native PAGE in the first dimension and SDS-PAGE in the second. Two gels were produced in parallel: one analyzed for protein phosphorylation sites using MALDI-FTICR-MS; the other analyzed with LA-ICP-MS. This method offers primarily qualitative identification of metalloproteins and can provide element ratio, whereby the S content can be used as a measure of the protein amount.

LA-ICP-MS analysis of the same gel would require ICP-MS measurements of all parts of the gel, even those that do not contain any metals. Furthermore, during the process the gel is destroyed. However, ICP-MS has the advantage that it provides a multi-elemental analysis, and that nonmetal elements, such as sulfur, can be used to estimate the amount of protein.

LA-ICP-MS can be applied to a biological tissue directly and used to detect multiple different metals simultaneously. However, it has the disadvantage of being destructive to the biological sample and has a detection limit in the μM range for copper and zinc.

*2D Liquid Chromatography – ICP-MS*

A successful metalloproteomic workflow resulted in the finding that protein-folding location is used as a natural strategy to regulate metal ion binding in proteins of the cupin family in the cyanobacterium *Synechocystis* PCC 6803 (Tottey et al. 2008). The workflow was based on protein separation using 2D-LC and subsequent analysis of each fraction with ICP-MS for metals and

SDS-PAGE for proteins. The metal distribution is carefully aligned with the distribution of proteins after SDS-PAGE by using principal component analysis. The advantage of this method is that multiple different metals can be analyzed simultaneously and considerable flexibility in the separation is possible by changing LC techniques. The 2D-LC approach generates a large number of samples that have to be analyzed by ICP-MS and SDS-PAGE.

Cvetkovic et al. (2010) used a combination of 2D-LC, high-throughput tandem mass spectrometry, and ICP-MS to identify the metalloproteome of the thermophilic archaeon *Pyrococcus furiosus*. The organism was found to incorporate more metals in its proteins than anticipated, as Pb-, Mn-, Mo-, U-, and V-containing proteins were found. However, the incorporation of lead and uranium was found to be only substoichiometric; that is, only 0.01 U atom per ferritin (Pf0742) monomer (Cvetkovic et al. 2010). These data, together with a preliminary analysis of the metalloproteomes of *Escherichia coli* and *Sulfolobus solfataricus* by the same approach, led Cvetkovic et al. to conclude that the microbial metalloproteome is largely uncharacterized. The method employed by Cvetkovic et al. is laborious and does not appear to be suitable for the analysis of a large number of different biological samples (e.g., different microbial growth conditions). Multielement detection by ICP-MS is powerful, because it allows for the detection of metals that were not anticipated by the researcher. This method is a good starting point to explore the metalloproteome of a particular (micro-)organism.

**Methods Based on Radioactive Metal Isotopes**

Radioactive metal isotopes have great potential in metalloproteomics, as they offer superior sensitivity as well as the possibility of imaging metalloproteins and quantifying metal levels. Table 18.1 summarizes suitable radioactive isotopes for metalloproteomics based on their potential for imaging and relatively short half-life.

**Table 18.1** Metal radioisotopes with potential for metalloproteomics. The selection criteria are: $t_{1/2}$ between 2 and 100 hours; suitable $\beta^-$ abundance and energy.

| Radionuclide | Half-life time (hours) |
|---|---|
| $^{56}$Mn | 2.6 |
| $^{65}$Ni | 2.5 |
| $^{64}$Cu | 12.7 |
| $^{67}$Cu | 61.8 |
| $^{69}$Zn | 13.8 |
| $^{99}$Mo | 66.0 |
| $^{187}$W | 23.8 |

*Metal Isotope Native Radio Autography in Gel Electrophoresis (MIRAGE)*

MIRAGE is a metalloproteomics technique that involves four steps:

1. Labeling of target proteins with a radioisotope.
2. Separation of intact holoproteins using native isoelectric focusing, followed by Blue Native PAGE in the second dimension.
3. Spot visualization and quantification using autoradiography.
4. Protein identification by tandem mass spectrometry after in-gel trypsin digestion.

Step 1 can be achieved simply by growing a microorganism in a medium containing a radioactive metal isotope. The advantage of MIRAGE is that on a single 2D-PAGE gel, all proteins which contain a particular metal ion can be visualized (Figure 18.2). Furthermore by quantifying the beta emission from the radioisotopes, it is possible to obtain absolute quantities of the metal that is associated to a protein. Obtaining absolute quantities is challenging in conventional proteomic techniques, and the term quantitative proteomics nearly always refers to relative quantities. The main disadvantage of this technique is that one can detect only one type of metal at a time. This is especially interesting for researchers who are interested in a particular metal, rather than all types of metals at the same time. Protein identification by MS/MS typically results in several overlapping proteins for each metal-containing spot. Using the *E. coli* genome annotation, the proteins relevant to the metal under investigation can be selected.

MIRAGE has previously been used to determine the soluble Cu, Fe, and Zn proteome of *E. coli* and the Mo and W proteomes of *P. furiosus*. MIRAGE investigation of the soluble Cu proteome of *E. coli* showed that the multicopper oxidase CueO is the only detectable Cu protein. CueO is a multicopper oxidase responsible for the oxidation of $Cu^+$ to $Cu^{2+}$. Scavenging cytoplasmic free copper has been proposed as a possible physiological role of CueO (Sevcenco et al. 2009a). The soluble Fe proteome of *E. coli* was found to be dominated by just three different proteins: 90% of the Fe was associated with superoxide dismutase, ferritin, and bacterioferritin (Sevcenco et al. 2011). The Zn proteome of *E. coli* experiencing Zn stress was dominated by ZraP, a putative Zn storage protein (Sevcenco et al. 2011). MIRAGE investigation of the effect of molybdenum on the W proteome of *P. furiosus* revealed that the organism exhibits a strong preference for W over Mo incorporation in its enzymes, even when the intracellular concentration of molybdenum was higher than tungsten (Sevcenco et al. 2009b; Sevcenco et al. 2010).

The occurrence of numerous overlapping proteins in the spots following native-native 2D-PAGE can be resolved by improving the resolution of the native-native 2D-PAGE; for example, by using a more narrow pH range in the isoelectric focusing step or by employing pre-fractionation using other protein separation techniques. Quantitative data on the protein levels will provide

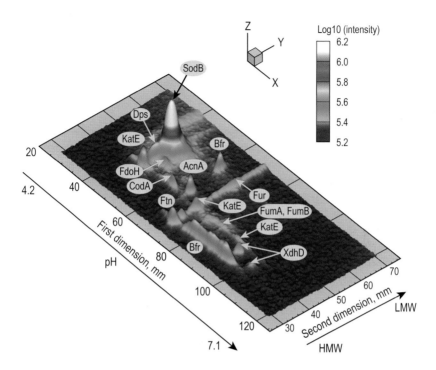

**Figure 18.2**   3D image of $^{59}$Fe–MIRAGE of *E. coli* soluble protein extract (575 µg protein) obtained from cells grown in 6 µM Fe (Sevcenco et al. 2012). AcnA: aconitase A; Bfr: bacterioferritin; CodA: cytosine deaminase; Dps: DNA-binding protein from starved cells; FdoH: formate dehydrogenase-O iron-sulfur cluster binding subunit; Ftn: ferritin; FumA: fumarase A; FumB: fumarase B; Fur: ferric uptake regulator; KatE: hydroperoxidase HPII; SodB: Fe superoxide dismutase; XdhD: xanthine dehydrogenase-like protein Mo and iron-sulfur cluster containing subunit. Reprinted with permission from John Wiley and Sons. Copyright © 1999–2014 John Wiley & Sons, Inc. All rights reserved.

valuable information on the metal/protein stoichiometry. At present, the absolute quantification of proteomes is difficult and laborious, although first studies into this area have recently appeared (Schmidt et al. 2011).

*2D-Denaturing, PAGE, Western Blotting, Phosphor Imaging*

Radioactive metal isotopes have been reported many times in the literature to identify and isolate metalloproteins. A relatively early approach to identify Zn-binding proteins in a comprehensive manner was published by Katayama et al. (2002). Proteins were separated using denaturing 2D-PAGE and, subsequently, the denatured proteins were transferred to a PVDF membrane using Western blotting. The resulting blot was incubated with a radioactive Zn isotope under non-denaturing conditions. The rationale behind this approach is that upon re-folding of the denatured proteins in the presence of zinc, the metal will be incorporated and the metalloproteins can be identified.

As this method is based on unfolding and refolding, there is a high risk of obtaining false positives as well as false negatives. Many of the Zn-containing proteins identified using MIRAGE were also found by Katayama et al. (2002), indicating that the method is apparently successful. This method does not pro-vide quantitative information on the (natural) distribution of zinc among the proteins in a biological sample.

**High-Throughput Colorimetric-Luminometric Metalloprotein Detection**

A very different approach has been published by Högbom et al. (2005) and involves an elegant combination of colorimetric and luminometric techniques to determine manganese, iron, cobalt, copper, and nickel or zinc. The proce-dure is a combination of two luminescence and one colorimetric assays. The protein sample (ca. 10 μg) was added to urea to denature the protein and release the metal ions. Subsequently luminol, sodium carbonate, and hydrogen perox-ide were added, and the first luminescence data were recorded. Metal ions are known to enhance the rate of the reaction of luminol with hydrogen peroxide under alkaline conditions. In the second step, 4-(2-pyridylazo)resorcinol (PAR) was added, and the second luminescence data were recorded. PAR is a metal ion chelator and forms colored complexes with various metal ions. After a two-hour incubation period and centrifugation step to release nitrogen gas bubbles resulting from the luminol reaction, the absorbance was measured at 492 nm. The combination of positive and negative responses on the three different as-says allows for the identification of the different metal ions (Figure 18.3).

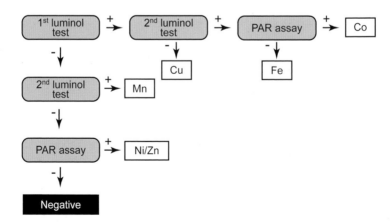

**Figure 18.3**   Schematic  workflow  of  the  luminometric/colorimetric  metallopro-teomics approach.

This method appeared to be powerful in the qualitative detection of metals in relatively pure protein samples, although it tolerates sub-stoichiometric levels of contaminating metals and can simultaneously measure copper and zinc or nickel. Since the identification of the metal ions in the colorimetric/ luminometric method relies on an ingenious combination of positive and negative results in the different assays, mixtures of metal ions will be difficult to analyze. It appears that this approach is most useful in cases where it is known that the sample contains relatively pure proteins and only one major metal is expected. An important advantage of this approach is that it can be implemented in existing high-throughput microplate-based platforms. The method was performed in a 384-well format and took three hours to complete, which, according to Högbom et al. (2005), makes it a true high-throughput method. The sensitivity of the method, however, is orders of magnitude lower than for most other techniques discussed here.

## Methods Based on Synchrotron Radiation X-Ray Absorption (XAS) and X-Ray Fluorescence (XRF)

XAS and XRF are based on the property that X-ray photons of a certain energy are able to expel electrons from the 1s electron shell around the nucleus. This hole is subsequently filled by another electron from a higher energy shell under the emission of a fluorescent X-ray photon. The fluorescence signals are highly characteristic of the type of metal. XAS and XRF have been used to structurally characterize metal sites in proteins in techniques such as EXAFS and XANES. SR-XRF has been used to obtain the distribution of certain metals in a single cell (McRae et al. 2009). In recent years, strategies have been developed to use XAS and XRF to perform metalloproteomics (Shi et al. 2005; Shi and Chance 2011). Spatial resolution of Synchrotron X-ray beams has improved to a resolution in the order of 0.1–1 μm with a penetration depth of approximately 1 mm. These metalloproteomic strategies involve performing high-throughput XAS on proteins produced in a structural genomics pipeline and detecting metalloproteins that have been separated using non-denaturing 1D or 2D gel electrophoresis using XRF or XAS.

High-throughput XAS to detect cobalt, nickel, copper, and zinc has been performed on recombinant proteins from *P. furiosus* produced in a structural genomics pipeline (Scott et al. 2005). This structural genomics pipeline involved the cloning, expression, and purification of ca. 2200 gene products from *P. furiosus*. Approximately 3 μl of 0.2–1.0 mM of each protein were required. In a similar approach, 654 proteins (100 μg each) from the New York Structural Genomics Research Consortium were analyzed for Mn, Fe, Co, Ni, Cu, and Zn content (Shi et al. 2005). Over 10% of the proteins were found to contain stoichiometric amounts of one of these metals. Scott et al. (2005) concluded that their method was approximately 95% accurate in predicting the stoichiometric metal content. When analyzing metalloproteins from such structural genomics pipelines, one must be careful as often his-tags and IMAC are used for high-throughput protein purification, and this may lead to improper metal incorporation or metal loss during purification (Jenney et al. 2005).

A different approach involves the use of XRF to directly scan proteins that have been separated on a non-denaturing electrophoresis gel (Native 2D-PAGE). This method was successfully applied to identify the metal composition of different isoforms of metalloproteins on a native 2D-PAGE (Ortega 2009). In principle, even information of the redox state and the chemical environment of the metal ion can be obtained (Kemner et al. 2005). A similar approach has been used in a metalloproteomic investigation of the response of *E. coli* to $Hg^{2+}$ (Gao et al. 2013). Proteins were separated using a conventional denaturing 2D-PAGE, after which differentially expressed proteins were identified using MS; Hg-containing proteins were found by scanning the gel using XRF. Apparently, Hg binding to these proteins was so tight that they were not disrupted by the extensive exposure of the protein to the denaturing agents (SDS and urea).

XAS and XRF are essentially noninvasive to the protein sample. These techniques, however, are only applicable to isolated pure proteins of high concentration. XAS provides more chemical information on the metal environment than any of the other techniques discussed in this chapter. The main disadvantage of the XRF- and XAS-based techniques is the requirement of a Synchrotron facility. In addition, although XRF is a very sensitive technique and allows the measurement of metals in small sample volumes, even within eukaryotic cells, the concentration of the metal required in the sample is relatively high (Ascone and Strange 2009).

## Computer-Based Metalloproteomics

Computer-based methods have already been used in several of the experimental strategies outlined above. Cvetkovic et al. (2010) used the Integrated Resource of Protein Domains and Functional Sites (InterPro database) to link the found metals to the proteins detected by MS. In the MIRAGE experiments, genome annotation was used to select the proteins relevant to the metal under investigation when a mixture of proteins was found to be present in a metal-containing spot (Sevcenco et al. 2011).

The wealth of genomic and protein structural information has not been overlooked by metalloproteomics researchers. The Metal MACiE database[1] provides structural and functional information on the metals involved in enzyme catalysis. Metal MACiE contains only metalloproteins with a known crystal structure and only a selected number of metal ions (Andreini et al. 2008). One typical example of this limitation is that there are no tungsten-containing

---

[1]  http://www.ebi.ac.uk/thornton-srv/databases/Metal_MACiE/home.html (accessed Dec. 2, 2014)

enzymes in the database, whereas in the Protein Data Bank there are at least four known tungsten enzyme crystal structures. More recently the MetalPDB database[2] has been constructed (Andreini et al. 2012). This database provides structural information about metal sites in proteins and is searchable by metal, by PDB entry, by enzyme or protein name, as well as by other identifiers and keywords. The information that can be retrieved from this database is predominantly structural. The user has to be aware that metal identities and coordination in crystal structures from proteins may contain errors: mismetallation may have occurred during protein production or crystallization, or the metal identity may not have been properly validated by structural biologists.

Several strategies to extract metalloproteomic information from such databases have been developed. One particularly comprehensive approach involves the following steps for one particular metal:

1. Interrogate literature and database resources to identify metalloproteins, transporters, cofactor biosynthesis proteins, and others (e.g., chaperones or regulatory proteins) and compile a set of proteins linked to one metal.
2. Perform BLAST searches of this set of proteins against sequenced genomes, identify homologs, and identify metal-using organisms and metal-containing proteins.
3. Analyze the data to construct metalloproteomes for a particular organism or group of organisms or identify the metalloproteome for a particular metal ion.

The search includes transporters, cofactor biosynthesis proteins, and regulatory proteins, most of which will not be metal containing. By using the strategy outlined above Zhang and Gladyshev (2009) have been able to investigate the metal usage by many different organisms.

Computer-based methods are interesting as they offer predictions that can be challenged experimentally. Furthermore, these methods offer an overview of metal usage in biology, based on our current knowledge. Their main drawback is that they are limited by our current knowledge and understanding of biological metal metabolisms. The strategies still require significant manual involvement and databases need to be curated. Unfortunately, two important metalloproteomics resources—Prosthetic centers and metal ions in protein active sites (PROMISE) and the Metalloprotein Database and Browser (MDB)—have recently been discontinued and no longer exist (Degtyarenko et al. 1998; Castagnetto et al. 2002). On the other hand, comprehensive genome, pathway, and protein databases like PROSITE and BioCyc are searchable for particular metals or metal-related biological functions (Caspi et al. 2010; Sigrist et al. 2012).

---

[2]  http://metalweb.cerm.unifi.it (accessed Dec. 2, 2014)

## Concluding Remarks

In a recent perspective article by Lothian et al. (2013), an integrative metalloproteomics strategy was envisioned, combining traditional proteomics and ICP-MS-based metalloproteomics on biological samples that have been enriched in particular stable isotopes for certain metals. In such a workflow, changes in protein level and metal content can be obtained, although no experimental data have yet been presented. Many of the methods presented in this chapter are comprehensive in nature. Some strategies are especially suitable for the systematic analysis of relatively pure recombinant proteins as produced in a structural genomics pipeline (e.g., SR-XRF and the high-throughput colorimetric/luminometric method). Other methods are suited to find and quantify metalloproteins that have been separated on a 2D-PAGE gel or by 2D-LC, such as methods based on LA-ICP-MS and MIRAGE. The first method allows for the detection of many metals simultaneously and requires analysis of large numbers of sample, whereas the second can only measure one (radioactive) metal isotope and provides a direct image of metal distribution and quantification of the metal levels in the different proteins. For the intracellular localization of metals in a single eukaryotic cell, SR-XRF appears to be the only amenable technology. For the multi-elemental imaging of a piece of tissue, LA-ICP-MS may well be the most suitable technique. For the identification and quantification of all proteins that contain a particular metal ion in any biological sample, MIRAGE is perhaps the optimal approach. Finally, in the near future, we can expect the interplay of computer-based and experimental strategies in metalloproteomics to advance the field significantly.

# 19

# Measuring Metals in Complex Biological Systems

Andreas Matusch, Ana-Maria Oros-Peusquens,
and J. Sabine Becker

## Abstract

This chapter presents a conceptual overview of techniques for element imaging in bio-logical specimens. Mass spectrometric techniques, particle and photon-induced X-ray emission techniques as well as X-ray and electron absorption techniques are described. In addition, it discusses frequent methodological issues common to elemental bioimag-ing in all of these techniques. These concern differential leaching of analyte species from distinct biological structures in contact with water and the use of reference pa-rameters correcting for nonhomogeneous material density and nonhomogeneous in-strument sensitivity. The use of 3D atlases of element concentrations for hypothesis generation is exemplified by manganese in the rat brain.

The data reported in this chapter were acquired from healthy tissue and illustrate the potential of measurement methods, which can have a major impact in clarifying the role of heavy metals in infectious disease. The examples described have been selected from among various applications of element imaging and may indirectly help infection biologists choose appropriate analytical strategies for their experiments.

## Overview of Methods for Element Imaging in Biological Tissue

Adapting element imaging to an analytical question involves a compromise between sensitivity and precision, on one hand, and spatial and possibly spec-tral resolution, on the other. The smallest detectable absolute amount of analyte determines the minimum volume of the smallest volume element (voxel).

Most of the methods discussed herein—laser ablation inductively coupled plasma mass spectrometry (LA-ICP-MS), scanning electron microscopy en-ergy dispersive X-ray analysis (SEM-EDX), and benchtop X-ray fluorescence (XRF)—are limited in spatial resolution and can be used to map infected or-gans or infected animals as a whole. They may help to determine quantita-tive element/metal balances in differentially affected zones or layers (e.g., in abscesses, granoluma, lymph nodes, affected gut segments) or in architectural subunits (e.g., liver lobule, nephron, or glandular unit).

When the topic of interest requires measurement of *in situ* element distribution in single bacteria in conjunction with that of its surroundings, including host cells, true microscopic techniques must be applied. A resolution of a few voxel per bacterium at 50 nm can be attained with nano secondary ion mass spectrometry (NanoSIMS) and, at a few synchrotron, XRF nanoimaging instruments, which recently have become operational. The only element-imaging techniques shown to provide structural details of bacteria are synchrotron X-ray absorption spectroscopy (XAS, 10–50 nm) and energy filtering transmission electron microscopy (EFTEM, 2–50 nm).

For the high-resolution techniques, laborious preparation of at least semithin (<2 μm), if not thin (<0.5 μm), sections through cryo-ultramicrotomy is necessary after high-pressure freezing to maintain original element distributions. Alternatively, the water in the sample can be sublimated and cryosubstituted by acetone in a freeze substitution apparatus, followed by infiltration/embedding by polyacrylate or polymetharylate resins (e.g., Lowicryl HM20™) and conventional ultra-microtomy.

## Techniques Involving Mass Spectrometry

*Laser Ablation Inductively Coupled Plasma Mass Spectrometry (LA-ICP-MS)*

For applications requiring absolute quantification of multiple elements, imaging by LA-ICP-MS is the method of choice. ICP-MS has an impressive dynamic range, reaching nine orders of magnitude in quadrupole and twelve orders of magnitude in the extended range configuration of sector field instruments. In a typical application of LA-quadrupole-ICP-MS for tissue imaging, we observed a range of $2 \cdot 10^7$ between the highest concentrations of the most abundant isotope $^{39}K$ and the lowest of all limits of detection determined for $^{208}Pb$. This is unparalleled among analytical methods and only comparable to the dynamic range of detection of radioactivity.

If we consider imaging techniques, the dynamic range of LA-ICP-MS is even superior to that involving radioactive detection. Furthermore, LA-ICP-MS can resolve very small sub ppm concentrations of one element in a matrix of highly concentrated (> 1000 ppm) elements of neighboring atomic number (Z) (Becker 2007). For polyisotopic elements, elemental mass spectrometry (LA-ICP-MS, SIMS) offers unique possibilities. For example, it can verify results by comparing the distribution images of several isotopes, such as $^{64}Zn$, $^{66}Zn$, and $^{67}Zn$. It can also perform stable isotope tracer studies using isotopically enriched preparations.

The principle of LA-ICP-MS is displayed in Figure 19.1 and explained in the legend. The x-length of one pixel is the product of the x-speed of the xyz stage and the acquisition time for one mass spectrum, which in turn is the sum

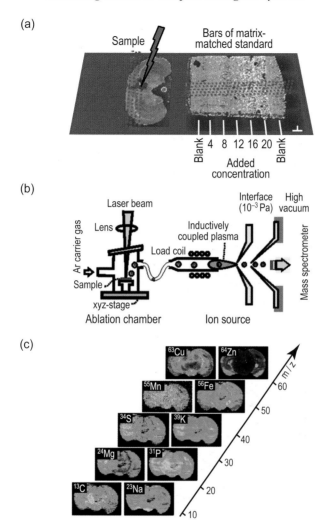

**Figure 19.1**    Principle of quantitative LA-ICP-MS bioimaging. (a) Native cryosections of sample and a stack of spiked homogenate standards are placed together in the ablation chamber, moved by the mobile xyz stage through the laser focus at fixed position and so ablated line by line. (b) The ablated material is transported as aerosol by about 1.1 l/min Ar or He/Ar into the inner of three concentric tubes of an ICP torch and crosses the argon plasma flame. The plasma acts as a secondary coil; the circulating currents therein are induced by the ~ 1500 W alternating voltage applied at radiofrequency to the four-winded primary (load) coil. In addition to the inner stream, the plasma is fed and regulated by an auxiliary Ar stream of about 0.7 l/min through the middle tube and cooled by the outer Ar stream of about 14 l/min. At about 7000 K, the material is atomized and ionized. Ions are accelerated and extracted into the mass analyzer where they are separated according to their m/z ratio. (c) For each pixel, a mass spectrum is obtained that contains ion intensities at the preselected m/z ratios. Adapted with permission from Matusch et al. (2012), copyright American Chemical Society.

of dwell times for the preselected m/z (e.g., 80 μm s$^{-1}$ × 0.1 s × 12 = 96 μm). The y-size of a pixel is the preselected distance between the centers of lines (e.g., 100 μm) which might be subdivided into the line width equalling the laser spot diameter (e.g., 70 μm) and a width of residual material between lines (e.g., 30 μm). When there is overlap (i.e., the spot size is larger than that of the pixel), this is termed oversampling. Due to a lack of appropriate calibration phantoms made of biological material, there is almost no formal determination of the spatial resolution of laser ablation in terms of full width at half maximum (FWHM). Pixel dimensions are considered equivalent with spatial resolution.

As a rule of thumb, spatial resolution will be in the range of the laser spot diameter. Commercial ablation systems, such as the NWR213 or the UP266, realistically allow resolutions down to 10 μm, although technically 5 μm is the smallest spot size that can be chosen. In 2013 the NWR-femto was launched, offering 1 μm spot size. Optimizing carrier gas flow, the particle composition of the ablated aerosol, transport efficiency by minimizing dead volume, and ion extraction efficiency of the mass spectrometer may leave some potential for further improvements. It should be kept in mind that longer scan times bring risks of hardware drift, plasma breakdown, or data overflow. From a practical point of view, scan times of 12 h can be used in an optimized setup without compromising data quality; however, the measurement time should not become substantially longer. Scanning an area of 1 cm$^2$ at 100 μm takes 2.8 h. Approximate realistic detection limits are 500 fg Cu and 50 fg Pt meaning 0.1 μg g$^{-1}$ and 0.01 μg g$^{-1}$ wet weight concentration, respectively, at 100 μm lateral resolution in a 30 μm native cryosection. The sensitivity of ICP-MS increases considerably with higher element order due to the lower first ionization energy and less noisy polyatomic interferences from biological matrix, argon, and residual traces of ambient air. We prefer that samples for LA-ICP-MS are placed onto Starfrost™ adhesive standard glass slides. Mounting onto coverslip glasses is an alternative, as these typically contain considerably lower element contamination than silicon and oxygen.

*Secondary Ion Mass Spectrometry (SIMS)*

In SIMS, a primary ion beam is shot onto the sample surface and launches (sputters) secondary atomic and molecular ions, which are then accelerated into mass analyzer and analyzed. Primary beams of $Au_n^+$ or $Bi_n^+$ clusters, $C_{60}^+$, $O_2^+$, or $O^-$ are used to create positively charged secondary ions, while $Cs^+$ or $SF_5^+$ are primarily used to produce negative secondary ions. The yield of secondary ions, and therefore the sensitivity, depends highly on (a) the first ionization energy, which is best for Li, Na, K, Rb, and Sr in positive ion mode, and on (b) the electron affinity (EA) in negative ion mode, which is best for Cl, Se, Br, F, Au, P, CN$^-$, CO$^-$, etc.; elements in between may be difficult to detect in some settings (Becker 2007). Due to the low penetration depth, this technique is highly sensitive to drying artifacts, whereby soluble compounds are transported to the surface forming a crust there, which makes it totally unsuitable to quantify elements present as mobile species (e.g., $K^+$ $Na^+$, $Li^+$, in part $Ca^{2+}$) in air-dried thicker sections. For meaningful SIMS measurements to reflect real element levels, a perfectly plane sample surface is provided by cryosubstituted resine-embedded ultramicrotome sections (discussed below). To allow higher primary ion currents or higher shoot frequency, with this higher penetration depth reaching 10 nm (dynamical mode), conductive support or coating is required (discussed further below). Otherwise, charge compensation through electron flooding makes the use of conventional glass slides possible.

In static SIMS mode, working with primary ion doses of $<10^{12}$ cm$^{-2}$, primary particles implanted into the sample and secondary particles sputtered away are almost in equilibrium providing secondary ions of low energy, narrow distribution of low initial velocities, and an information depth of about 5 atomic layers. In the dynamic SIMS mode, there is net removal of material of up to 10 nm in a single run and the possibility of depth profiling by multiple runs.

NanoSIMS, optimized for dynamic mode, provides high-spatial resolution down to about 50 nm in negative ion mode (see Figure 19.2) and 200 nm in

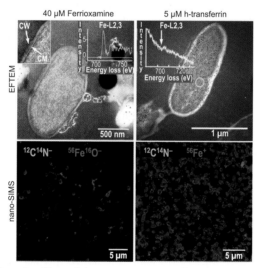

**Figure 19.2**  *Lactobacillus sakei* was grown on media supplemented with different iron sources (left and right column). Samples were high-pressure frozen, freeze-substituted with polyacryl embedding medium, and ultra-cut into 50 nM sections. Iron was imaged using EFTEM on a Zeiss CEM902; the 708 KeV energy edge corresponds to the characteristic L2,3 L-shell electron abstraction energy. Parallel electron energy loss spectra are inserted and 250 KeV energy loss (below the C K-edge) images are superimposed (upper images). Dynamic SIMS was acquired with a CAMECA NanoSIMS-50 ion microprobe equipped with a magnetic sector field analyzer, which is capable of detecting five secondary ion species simultaneously. Primary ion beams of about 6 pA Cs$^+$ were used to generate negative secondary ions and of O$^-$ to generate positive secondary ions. Pixel size was 390 nm $\times$ 117 nm. From Duhutrel et al. (2010); adapted with permission from the American Society for Microbiology.

positive ion mode. NanoSIMS uses a sector field analyzer equipped with up to seven collector detectors for highest sensitivity; this allows for continuously running the primary ion beam. Here about 5 ions reaching the detector are sufficient for detection, which requires sputtering 1000 Si atoms from the analytical volume.[1] Appendix 20.6 in Maret et al. (this volume) gives examples of sensitivities and limits of detections of NanoSIMS for the elements titanium through uranium. The use of time of flight (ToF) analyzers, better suited for static mode, requires pulses or shots of primary ion beams, and the ToF readout time limits lateral analysis speed. Suitable primary ions of lower energy (e.g., Au, $C_{60}$, or $Bi_{300}$ clusters) permit molecules that are larger than 1500 Da to be imaged. Spatial resolution is limited to about 0.5–5 µm, and can even go down to 100 nm in exceptional cases.

**Techniques Sensitive to Inner Electron Shell Transitions**

This group of quasi-nondestructive techniques employs focused X-ray photon, electron, proton, or particle beams of sufficient energy, which are scanned over the sample. Possible interactions between radiation and matter include absorption or inelastic scatter, which leads to specific ionization of an inner (K-, L-, M-) electron shell while lifting an electron by a discrete amount to a higher level. Here, the absorbed energy and, conversely, the energy loss of the incident particle ($\Delta W$) correspond to the potential difference of the shell electron (U), according to $U \cdot e = \Delta W$. Photons of the frequency $f$ are absorbed as entire quantum $h \cdot f = \Delta W + W_{kin}$ (where $W_{kin}$ represents the excess kinetic energy of ejected photoelectrons). For a given transition, the ionization energy is a function of $(Z-1)^2$, whereby $Z$ is the atomic number. This relationship was first observed and formulated for the XRF $K_{\alpha 1}$-lines, the energy of which is proportional to $(Z-1)^2$ (Moseley's Law).

*X-Ray and Electron Absorption Techniques*

Absorption spectra are not continuous but rather show element-specific edges. Spectra are measured using electron energy loss spectrometry (EELS) on transmission electron microscopy platforms that are equipped with a multisector field electron spectrometer at the sample stage, while working at a fixed acceleration voltage. XAS is available at some end stations of synchrotron sources, which allow incident X-ray energy to be fine-tuned. The element selective imaging modes thereof are termed energy filtering transmission electron microscopy (EFTEM) and scanning transmission X-ray microscopy (STXM), respectively. For fast imaging of a given element, the entire spectra does not need to be recorded per pixel; the difference or quotient of an absorption image is taken within an energy window (e.g., 40 eV width) above (i.e., at higher

---

[1]  http://www.cameca.com/literature/product-brochures.aspx (accessed December 4, 2014).

energy than) the absorption edge (post-edge), so that a background image can be generated from an extrapolation of one or several acquisitions below (i.e., at lower energy than) the absorption edge (pre-edge). To achieve high sensitivity in absorption techniques, a sharp absorption edge is required. The electron spectrometer of EFTEM is spatially resolving. Elements with full electron configurations (e.g., zinc, cadmium, and mercury) have particularly round edges, whereas elements with possible 2p → 3d transitions (potassium through nickel) and 3d → 4f transitions (tin through thulium) exhibit particularly sharp edges and eventually additional sharp "white" absorption lines. Normalizing to the spectrum integral can correct for sample thickness. Using EFTEM, single ferritin molecules of 8 nm diameter could be imaged at C, N, and O edges, and their Fe load of up to 4500 atoms was discriminated. In EFTEM, spatial resolutions of 2–50 nm were reached; in XAS, 10–50 nm.

In addition to measuring total element levels, XAS and EELS allow predictions to be made regarding the chemical environment of elements when acquired at high spectral resolution. Both techniques provide information on the electron environment, oxidation state, binding partners/ligands, and complex geometry. XAS even allows a classification of biomolecules and detects features of the C K-edge characteristic for proteins. The spectral range from 15 eV below to 150 eV above an absorption edge is termed near edge X-ray absorption fine structure (NEXAFS) and encompasses the range beyond extended X-ray absorption fine structure (EXAFS). In EELS, in addition to near edge and extended fine structure, the plasmon region of electron energy losses, ranging about 0–100 eV, provides additional speciation information. Obtaining spectra pixel per pixel is, however, time consuming and may be reserved for selected regions of interest. Another advantage of EFTEM is that filtering electrons with an energy loss of 250 eV, which is below the C K-edge at 284 eV, generates high-contrast structural elastic scatter images of unstained organic material suited for perfect superimposition with element images.

X-ray and electron absorption techniques allow the acquisition of high-quality structural images in the same session. XAS provides best structural contrast of hydrated samples in the "water" window: from above C K-edge at 284 eV to below the O K-edge at 543 eV.

*X-Ray Emission Techniques*

Once an electron shell has an inner electron (K-, L-, or M-) gap, this is filled by electrons from the outer shells. Two relevant processes control how the specific amount of excess energy can be released: (a) characteristic X-rays are emitted (this is termed X-ray fluorescence when excitation was by X-rays) or (b) outer shell electrons are ejected (this is termed Auger electron emission). The higher the atomic number $Z$, the lower the probability/quantum yield of Auger and the higher that of X-ray emission. The ratio for K-gaps is 50:50 for $Z = 38$

(strontium). X-ray emissions are typically detected in an angle of 45°–90° to the incident beam.

*Restrictions Related to the Interactions of Incident Beam and Matter*

The yield of X-ray emission per incident beam flux, termed the production cross section of characteristic X-ray emission, asymptotically decreases with $Z$ for particles while the photon-induced fluorescent X-ray production cross section increases with $Z$.

In addition to the characteristic element-specific discrete line spectrum, electron and particle beams produce a continuous spectrum of bremsstrahlung background. The production cross section of bremsstrahlung in the relevant range increases with energy for electrons, decreases with energy for protons and larger particles, and is proportional to $(z/m - Z/M)^2$ with $z/m$ and $Z/M$ corresponding to the charge to mass ratio of incident particle and target material, respectively. As $z/m$ is 1822 for electrons, 1 for protons and approximately ½ for other particles and matter, this explains that electrons produce considerably higher bremsstrahlung than do protons and particles. As the intensity spectrum of bremsstrahlung has its maximum close to the energy of the incident particle, the uppermost part of the spectrum cannot be exploited. Despite this, particle beams produce bremsstrahlung via secondary electrons which dominate and obscure the lower range of the energy spectrum.

In synchrotron XRF, elastic Raleigh scatter and inelastic Compton scatter produce a background spectrum which is continuous due to multiple scatter events and progressively increases toward the Compton peak (e.g., 8846 eV at 90° angle) closely below the Raleigh peak at the incident energy of, e.g., 9000 eV. Therefore, in XRF, the uppermost part of the spectrum from approximately 10% below the incident energy cannot be realistically exploited.

Any element is best detected at its Kα-line which is more intense than L- and these are more intense than M-lines, the respective fluorescence yield being about 40% and 0.6% for iron, 80% and 6% for cadmium (K and L) and 100%, 30%, and 2% for lead (K, L, M).

Given these prerequisites, it becomes clear that across atomic numbers and the periodic table there is a restricted window of highest sensitivity for each technique which can be shifted a bit by varying the energy of incident particles. Very light elements C–Si, because of the low fraction of X-ray versus Auger emissions, are best detected in absorption techniques, EFTEM and SXTM. Elements in the range between P–Fe are well suited for detection by electron induced X-ray emissions while the elements in the range between Mn–Mo (K-lines) and Hf–Pb (L-lines) are covered by 3 MeV PIXE. Finally XRF covers elements in the range between sodium to uranium.

*Restrictions Related to Detection*

For imaging purposes, X-ray emissions are recorded typically with energy-dispersive (EDX) detectors equipped with electron drift sensors which are fast but provide limited spectral energy resolution typically restricted to 120–140 eV at 5.9 KeV. Diffraction-based wavelength dispersive detectors, in turn, are considerably slower at excellent spectral resolution. At the entrance of most EDX detectors is a beryllium window which shields X-rays below ca. 1 KeV so that elements starting from about Na–Al are accessible at their K-lines. Detection below requires windowless detectors. Furthermore, the spectral range of X-ray optics and detectors is restricted in many settings; many synchrotron X-ray fluorescence end station instruments are optimized for a limited spectral range. Therefore, when the K-line energy of an element exceeds the available range, it has to be detected at its L-line and the heaviest elements even at their M-line. This leads to numerous spectral interferences with the major biological matrix elements, typical concentrations of which in animal tissue are 1500 µg g$^{-1}$ P, 800 µg g$^{-1}$ S, 900 µg g$^{-1}$ Cl, 2800 µg g$^{-1}$ K, 170 µg g$^{-1}$ Ca, 80 µg g$^{-1}$ Fe and, to a lower degree, 10 µg g$^{-1}$ Zn and 3 µg g$^{-1}$ Cu (Becker et al. 2010). Consequently the Co Kα is obscured by the Fe-Kβ1 and Sn-L and Sb-L disappear under the "mountain" of K- and Ca-K emission signal. Lastly, EDX detectors produce one type of artefact at 2·E caused by coinciding photons exciting the same electron in the electron drift sensor and another type of artefact caused by secondary XRF of the detector material when the captured X-ray energy is slightly over the respective absorption edge.

It becomes clear that spectral deconvolution is challenging in all X-ray emission techniques. Proper external calibration requires a checkerboard to cover the relevant combinatorial range instead of a standard stripe of dilutions of multielement standards. Spectral background and spectral interferences clearly limit the possibilities for quantification, even at synchrotron facilities, below those provided by LA-ICP-MS.

*Spatial Resolution and Additional Details*

The spatial resolution of X-ray emission techniques depends on the interaction volume of beam and sample, the area of which can be considerably larger than the beam spot size for electron and particle beams. Electron and particle beams, especially, penetrate deep into the sample as do harder X-rays; thus, thinner samples generally provide higher spatial resolution, but this comes at the expense of detection limits. The drop-shaped interaction volume of electron beams becomes higher with higher incident energy and reaches diameters of 5–10 µm in SEM-EDX of thick samples, thus practically limiting electron energy to about 25KeV. For proton and particle beams, the large part of the interaction volume occurs at higher depth, thus enabling spatial resolutions for protons (PIXE) down to 0.2–2 µm.

Benchtop XRF instruments provide beam diameters down to 10–25 µm. Since they are equipped with conventional X-ray tubes, the characteristic lines of anode material further restrict the number of elements accessible: a W-anode detection of copper and zinc is not possible because scatter from the W-L lines obscures the Cu-K signals. Depending on the analytical questions, anodes have to be changed: Cu, Rh, Mo, and W anodes are available. As these small X-ray tubes are typically operated at up to 50 KV, all elements can be measured at their K-lines. However, there is considerable background from scatter of the bremsstrahlung of the incident beam, and restricted beam intensity allows only for detection limits of about 20–100 µg g$^{-1}$ (see Figure 19.3).

At synchrotron facilities, monoenergetic highly focussed beams of sizes down to approximately 65 nm × 50 nm (ID22NI in Grenoble) are available with high photon fluxes (Kosior 2013). Furthermore, polarization of synchrotron X-rays allows considerably reduced background scatter at 90°. Therefore, synchrotron µXRF provides the highest sensitivity of all X-ray techniques. Commonly, the elastic Raleigh scatter around the incident energy is taken as reference, correcting for the sample thickness.

**Histochemical Techniques**

Prussian Blue staining for iron and Timm's autometallography for zinc after precipitation as zinc sulfide can be observed at light microscopic resolution (McRae et al. 2009). One considerable disadvantage of this technique is that there is often considerable heterogeneity of stain throughout a section, and calibration is challenging since sections are immersed into staining bathes and the washout from standards may likely be different from that of samples. The dynamic range of the detectable concentration is small. Depending on the precise

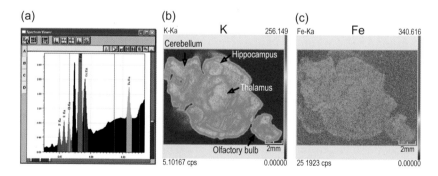

**Figure 19.3**   X-ray fluorescence image of a 150 µm horizontal section of a control mouse brain mounted onto Mylar obtained on a SEIKO SEA6000VX benchtop instrument. The scan duration was 4.8 h and pixel size was 30 µm: (a) shows the spectrum that was obtained during a prescan at a larger area on the sample (note the increasing background with increasing atomic number, $Z$); (b) K image; (c) Fe image.

redox conditions, the Prussian Blue method labels a poorly defined fraction of $Fe^{2+}$ and $Fe^{3+}$. Some washout of iron from the sample cannot be avoided. Thus the resulting signal does not reflect total iron but a quantity related to Fe activity. Histochemical techniques play a role for high-throughput/large-sample localization studies without need for precise quantification. Prussian Blue is routinely used to detect ultra-small superparamagnetic iron oxide nanoparticles *ex vivo* after MRI studies in living animals.

**Sample Preparation for Element Imaging**

One intrinsic challenge of microlocal analytical techniques is to maintain original concentrations and to avoid analyte washout. The best results are obtained when the slice thickness is adapted to the chosen lateral resolution. At a scale above 1 μm, for techniques such as LA-ICP-MS, histochemical techniques, and XRF and SEM-EDX at medium resolution, the use of native 10–50 μm thick cryosections was found to be appropriate. At a scale about 1 μm and below, (semi-)thin sections have to be produced by ultramicrotomy. To provide sufficient analytical volume for element detection and to allow stability to the incident beam, somewhat thicker sections are chosen (for EFTEM: 100–150 nm; for NanoSIMS: 0.75–1 μm) than is the case for ultrastructural imaging (down to 50–30 nm). To avoid tissue destruction and fissures during cutting, high-pressure freezing is paramount. Then there are two possible strategies to produce sections with a thickness going down to 50 nm. The sections obtained with cryo-ultramicrotomes have the advantage of being fully native and adduct-free but the practicability is limited, as they tend to break and spread fragments that risk contaminating the analytical instrument. An exception are tomography scanning electron microscopes, which do not image the section but the surface of the tissue block (block face) mounted on a cooled stage. Here an ultramicrotome is integrated to remove tissue layer by layer after being imaged (Gatan). Alternatively, in multibeam instruments a focused ion beam (FIB) typically originating from a liquid gallium gun and incident almost parallel to the layer surface is used to mill or polish away tissue layer by layer at approximately 5–50 nm thickness (Zeiss Auriga, Jeol JIB-4500 Multibeam) after SEM imaging (Kuo 2014). FIB can also be used for abrasion of material which is difficult to cut such as metal implants, bone or teeth.

The second strategy first cryosubstitutes water by acetone or by 10% acrolein in diethyl-ether in dedicated cryosubstitution instruments—a process which typically takes about one to three weeks. Thereafter it infiltrates/embeds the tissue by polymethyl-metacrylate (PMMA, Lowicryl HM20™) resin and finally produces conventional ultramicrotome sections.

For techniques using charged particle beams, the sample must be mounted onto a conductive substrate, grids for transmission techniques (EFTEM) or for other high-resolution techniques (NanoSIMS, SEM-EDX, PIXE), to be sputter-coated by 10–30 nm of carbon, lead, platinum, or gold. Glass slides or steel plates coated with gold or iron tin oxide are used with ToF analyzers which require high entrance voltage in SIMS and matrix-assisted laser desorption ionization (MALDI) ion sources. As in XRF, the incident X-rays penetrate the sample and support; XRF requires very thin plastic foils (e.g., polyethylenterephtalat 0.5–10 μm, Mylar™, Hostaphan™) to minimize background fluorescence from the support. XAS usually uses a sandwich of 0.5 μm thick $Si_3N_4$ windows for flat samples or very thin glass capillaries for biological samples such as bacteria in a hydrated environment.

## Differential Washout of Soluble Analytes during Fixation

A large part of the work performed in element imaging has been performed on formalin-fixed tissue sections due to simple reasons of availability. Immersion in water and aqueous formalin solution, however, leads to a washout of soluble species. This leaching is not necessarily uniform throughout biological compartments, because different elements and even species of a given element are highly differentially enriched throughout distinct structures. For instance, in highly specialized cerebral areas, soluble species of $Mn^{2+}$, $Cu^{2+}$, and $Zn^{2+}$ are stored in synaptic vesicles.

A first kinetic study detected evidence of Fe washout from spleen with a half life of ≈10 days (Figure 19.4a) (Chua-anusorn et al. 1997). Recently, Trunova et al. (2013) systematically studied the leaching of multiple elements from pieces of rat heart (Figure 19.4b) using ICP-MS.

Recently we froze one hemisphere of a rat brain at –80°C. The other half was immersed for 1 week in 4% buffered formalin to ensure complete fixation. Both halves were then cryocut and sections from similar levels were chosen for LA-ICP-MS. Element concentrations were averaged within a set of anatomically relevant regions of interest covering the slide entirely. The results are given in Figure 19.5 and Table 19.1.

The distribution of $Zn^{2+}$ undergoes a puzzling restructuring: from predominantly gray matter enrichment in native tissue to higher white matter concentration in fixed tissue.

Summarizing the results of our study: Cu, Zn, Mn, Na, K, Cl, and Ca measurements from fixed tissue are useless in most cases and do not allow any biological conclusions. Furthermore, the absolute concentrations of iron, phosphorus, and even carbon have to be interpreted with care. When formalin fixation is followed by immersion in 30% sucrose, which is common in immunohistochemistry, or dehydration in a series of increasing concentrations of alcohol for paraffin embedding, an even more considerable shrinkage of the tissue must be taken into account. This effect amounts to 15% in either direction and to 40% in volume (Boonstra et al. 1983). If referenced to the shrunken volume, the concentrations of elements would be 65% too high.

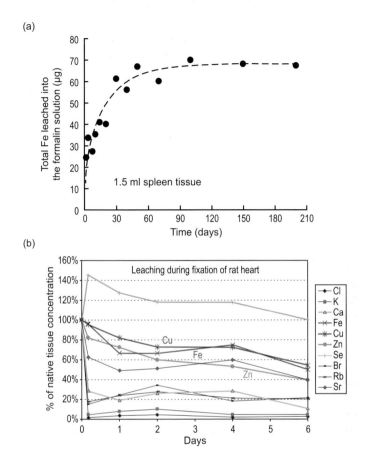

**Figure 19.4** Washout of elements during formalin fixation. (a) Iron was measured in the formalin solution where 1.5 ml of spleen tissue was immersed (Chua-anusorn et al. 1997; reprinted with permission from Elsevier). (b) Analogous pieces of approximately 60 mg of rat heart were measured by synchrotron-XRF either native or after different times of immersion in formalin solution (adapted from Trunova et al. 2013).

In conclusion, whenever possible, native cryosections should be used for element analysis. When fixation cannot be avoided, it is possible to precipitate zinc as ZnS by perfusion of the animal with a 1% $Na_2S$ solution (Moos 1993). When background from blood in organs, such as liver, may disturb measurements, a short perfusion by 0.9% saline should be undertaken, until a noticeable color change of the organ is detected, before removal, keeping in mind that the procedure might also lead to a washout of very mobile species.

*A. Matusch et al.*

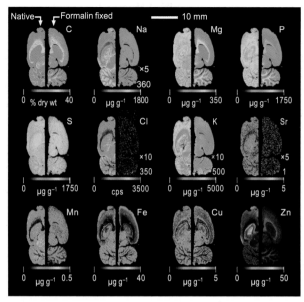

**Figure 19.5** LA-ICP-MS image of two horizontal cryosections of a native rat brain hemisphere (left) and a hemisphere that was immersed for 7 days in 4% buffered formalin solution (right). Sections were scanned with a laser spot diameter of 100 μm, residual space between lines of 60 μm, at an x-speed of 60 μm s$^{-1}$ and acquisition time per pixel of 1.4 s for 33 m/z making pixel dimension of 84 μm × 160 μm. Instrumentation was NWR213 coupled to Thermo X series 2, gas flows: sample 1.1 l/min auxiliary 0.8 l/min cooling 14 l/min Ar.

**Table 19.1** Differential washout of elements from rat brain after 7 days of formalin fixation. Average of changes obtained from two pairs of corresponding sections that were taken from native and formalin-fixed hemispheres imaged using LA-ICP-MS. Analysis of anatomically defined regions of interest.

| % Change | Entire section | Cortex | Corpus callosum | Preasu-biculum | CA3-hilus-pyr | Periven-tricular | Colliculus inferior |
|----------|--------|--------|--------|--------|--------|--------|--------|
| C | −14 | −5 | ref | | | | |
| Na | −87 | −85 | −78 | | | | |
| Mg | −22 | −30 | +8 | | | | |
| P | −34 | −36 | ref | | | | |
| S | −14 | −15 | ref | | | | |
| Cl | −98 | −98 | −98 | | | | |
| K | −90 | −91 | −86 | | | | |
| Mn | −20 | −25 | +155 | | | | −50 |
| Fe | −12 | −1 | −11 | | | | |
| Cu | −11 | −7 | +3 | −30 | | −54 | |
| Zn | −16 | −36 | +133 | −69 | −74 | | |
| Sr | −86 | −87 | −81 | | | | |

## Other Artifacts and Pitfalls in Element Imaging

When it comes to image treatment after acquisition, for any kind of image data, division operations (of the type voxel value of image A divided by voxel value of image B) are problematic because noise raises the risk of accentuating division by zero problems. Such problems arise especially at the edges and at uncovered space, where partial volume effects may accentuate. Therefore, generally, in image data treatment the divisor image is usually at least smoothed. In chemical instrumental imaging, it is highly problematic to use a per pixel reference, such as the Raleigh scatter per pixel in XRF, the total ion current in MALDI mass spectrometric imaging, or the $^{13}C^+$ ion intensity per pixel in LA-ICP-MS. A further problem is that these quantities correlate with the dry weight per area; however, the biologically relevant concentrations refer to the wet weight of tissue. The water content in fresh brain tissue is not homogeneous: cerebral white matter has 70% water content compared to cerebral gray matter, which has a water content of 80%. Therefore, it is more robust to select a per slice reference for data normalization, such as averaging the net Raleigh, net total ion current, or net $^{13}C^+$ signal across the section. The analogous normalization should be applied to the measurement of the slice with the element standards, which have a different thickness. The thickness variability of cryomicrotome slices was determined at a relative standard deviation of about 5% (Anthony et al. 1984), resulting in 7% for the pair of standard and sample.

## Preview of an Upcoming Element Atlas of the Rat Brain

Imaging the element distribution within a few slices already provides us with a glimpse of the anatomical variability. However, the brain is a highly heterogeneous structure; a complete description of its element distribution requires 3D analysis. Our goal has been to provide, for the first time, a reference for the variability of element distribution in the rat brain. To this end, we analyzed 31 horizontal native cryosections of a rat brain using LA-ICP mass spectrometric imaging. Each section was 30 μm thick, and the sections were spaced between 180 μm and 660 μm from each other. To ensure anatomical accuracy of the reconstruction, the rat was imaged *in vivo* by magnetic resonance imaging. Furthermore, we took macro-photographs of the tissue block before cutting each section. These so-called block face images show each undistorted plane; subsequent cutting and mounting onto a glass slide frequently caused shearing, local stretching, distortions, and even tissue defects. For an accurate concentration calibration over the entire volume, drift correction, and normalization throughout the stack, the frozen brain was embedded into a gel medium in which four 2 mm rods were placed. After the rods were removed, the holes were filled with 2 multielement-spiked tissue homogenates and 2 blank tissue

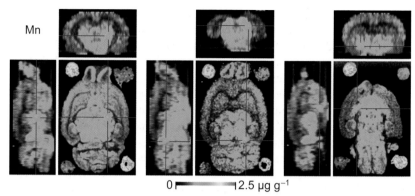

0 ▬▬▬▬ 2.5 µg g⁻¹

**Figure 19.6**   Element atlas of the rat brain obtained by LA-ICP-MS imaging. Example of navigation through the 3D data set of manganese using the orthogonal cross section viewer of Pmod 3.1 (Zurich, Switzerland). The blue cross hair gives the position of the respective two other planes and was centered on the right thalamus in the left panel, on the right colliculus inferior in the middle panel, and on the left ventral pallidum in the right panel. Given is unbiased wet weight concentration. The unbiased wet weight concentration is provided. Note that there are no concentration steps between sets of slices. The calibration points result from tissue homogenates blank containing 0.52 µg g⁻¹ manganese and spiked containing blank plus 1.11 µg g⁻¹ added (=1.63 µg g⁻¹) manganese.

homogenates. The brain and these four standard rods were cut together and the embedding gel was removed from the glass slides before LA-ICP-MS imaging.

Due to measurement time constraints, scan parameters varied slightly. This included spot sizes of 60 µm and 80 µm, residuals between lines 30 µm, x-scan speeds of 100 and 70 µm s⁻¹, acquisition times per pixel of 1.4 and 1.84 s, for 33 and 40 different m/z making pixel sizes of 140 µm × 90 µm and 129 µm × 110 µm, respectively.

We then combined the calibrated element concentration images obtained from the 31 slices into a three-dimensional data set. The 3D volume can be saved in various formats (e.g., ANALYZE, NIFTI, and INTERFILE) and navigated using different programs, as displayed for manganese in Figure 19.6. True 3D volumes of interest can be read out, and the data set can be compared to any other 3D rat brain data set for diverse correlations (Figure 19.6).

## Potential Application to Infections of the Central Nervous System

In view of the hypothesis supported by the study on liver abscesses of Corbin et al. (2008)—that manganese is a critical host factor for bacterial growth—it is tempting to compare the cerebral Mn distribution with predilection patterns known for bacterial infections. At a first glance, the colliculus inferior, marked by the crosshair in the middle image column of Figure 19.6, is the site of the highest Mn concentration, reaching 4 µg g⁻¹. By itself, the colliculus inferior as never been a characteristic site of infection, nor have other high-level Mn regions such as the thalamus, nucleus ruber, or nucleus oculomotorius accessorius. The localization of abscesses in the brain is more likely explained by continuity from adjacent structures (sinus, mastoid, etc.) or by emboli that get caught up at arterial bottlenecks.

Bacterial infections that take place in the central nervous system with a stereotypic characteristic distribution pattern are more the exception than the rule. These include basal menigoencephalitis, *Mycobacterium tuberculosis*, and listerial rhombencephalitis. At a second glance, there might be some congruencies of listerial rhomencephalitis, which has been reported to involve the thalamus and caudal portions of pons and medulla oblongata as well as Mn distribution. Indeed, inoculation experiments performed in 1966 determined the dose of *Listeria monocytogenes* leading to death in 50% (LD50) of mice after intraperitoneal injection. The LD50 was 7200 bacteria in controls, 31 bacteria in mice treated daily with 4 $\mu g \ g^{-1}$ per of intraperitoneal Mn, 6 bacteria under treatment with 4 $\mu g \ g^{-1}$ of $Fe^{2+}$, and 180 bacteria under treatment with 4 $\mu g \ g^{-1}$ of $Fe^{3+}$ per day (Sword 1966). We note that there are high overlaps of cerebral Fe and Mn distribution patterns, and only a minor fraction of tissular total iron is readily available as $Fe^{2+}$. Can the metalloarchitecture of the rat brain be transferred to the human? In our experience it can, but there are very few data on manganese, as it presents an analytical challenge. Inflammatory pathology with highly characteristic anatomical patterns (such as limbic encephalitis or diffuse perivenous encephalitis, which is also the pattern of multiple sclerosis) is paraneoplastic or postviral. Finally, there seems to be a link between Mn concentration and susceptibility to metronidazole encephalopathy (Lee et al. 2009). This example should illustrate that precise and quantitative anatomical localization can guide hypothesis generation in many cases.

## Acknowledgments

We thank Dr. Uwe Breuer (ZEA-3, Analytical Chemistry) as well as Brigitte Marshallsay and Dr. Astrid Rollenhagen (Institute of Neuroscience and Medicine, Forschungszentrum Jülich, Germany) for fruitful discussion of SIMS and electron microscopy, respectively. Figure 19.3 was compiled from the authors' data, and the contributing work of Dr. Nitzsche and Dr. Becker is gratefully acknowledged.

---

First column (top to bottom): Wolfgang Maret, Andreas Matusch, Richard Thompson, Andreas Matusch, Eric Skaar, Peter-Leon Hagedoorn, Joseph Caruso
Second column: Joseph Caruso, Christopher Contag, Eric Skaar, group discussion, David Giedroc, Christopher Contag, Eric Skaar
Third column: David Giedroc, Peter-Leon Hagedoorn, Joseph Caruso, Christopher Contag, Wolfgang Maret, Richard Thompson, Wolfgang Maret

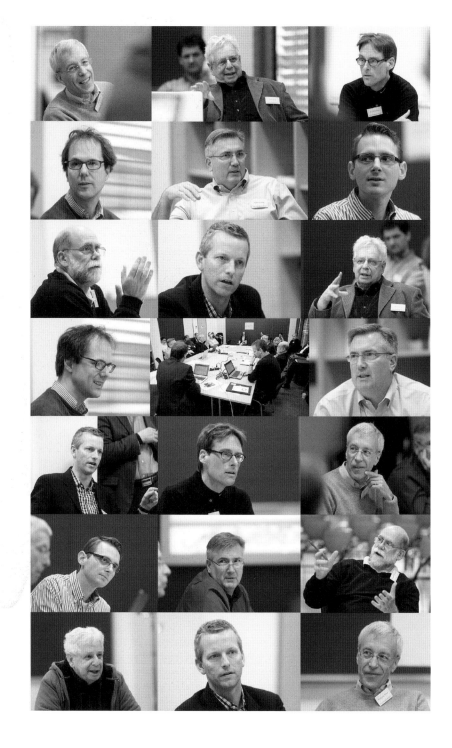

# 20

# Methods and Technologies for Studying Metals in Biological Systems

Wolfgang Maret, Joseph A. Caruso,
Christopher H. Contag, David P. Giedroc,
Peter-Leon Hagedoorn, Andreas Matusch,
Eric P. Skaar, and Richard B. Thompson

## Abstract

An extensive summary is provided on the methods and methodology available to analyze and image total metals in biological systems as well as to assess their speciation, in particular in metalloproteomes and as free metal ion concentrations. Discussion focuses on instrumental methods for analysis and separation and how they are complemented by genetic and bioinformatics approaches. The treatment of methods follows increased complexity and experimental challenges: from lysates and fluids, to cells and tissues, to living cells and animals, and finally to the prospects of applying extant technology to investigations in humans. Presently, method sensitivity is not sufficient for analysis of metals in the pathogen *in vivo*. Future analytical needs are presented to address metal ions in host–pathogen interactions for diagnosis and treatment of infectious disease. The material is presented in the context of both redistribution of metals in the host and known mechanisms of warfare to acquire the transition metal ions that are essential for growth and survival of either host or pathogen.

## Introduction

The struggle for metal between host and pathogen is a critical determinant to the clinical outcome of infection. Defining the importance of metals to infectious diseases requires the use of a host of techniques and focuses on measuring the levels of metal in both the host and pathogen. Measurement of metals is essential to understand their biology, particularly in the context of infectious disease. Measurement of metals in biological samples encompasses the total metal content, chemical speciation of metals, and additional information about distribution in biological space and time. For total metal content, inductively coupled plasma mass spectrometry (ICP-MS) is now the method of choice: it surpasses atomic absorption spectroscopy due to its multielement sensitivity, subpart per trillion detection levels, large dynamic range of up to nine orders of magnitude, and virtually no interference from the biological matrix for most elements. Whereas the traditional focus of analytical chemistry is the analysis of elements and molecules, present endeavors in systems biology aim at obtaining complete part lists and understanding the functions of all parts in the system. For metals, this is the metallome (i.e., the sum of all metal species).

Speciation science in metallobiology is primarily concerned with the functions of metals in proteins (metalloproteomics) and those that are not bound to proteins. For metalloproteomes, a combination of mass spectrometry for elemental and molecular analysis is employed: ICP-MS, electrospray mass spectrometry, and matrix-assisted laser desorption ionization mass spectrometry (MALDI-MS). Metalloproteomics requires techniques for protein separation, mostly chromatographic and electrophoretic, in combination with molecular mass spectrometry (hyphenated techniques).

A variety of imaging techniques can be used to achieve spatially resolved detection of total metal distribution (see section on Cells and Tissues). In contrast, the pool of nonprotein-bound metals, which is increasingly gaining attention due to its being "metabolically active," is addressed with fluorimetric techniques that have detection limits down to the zeptomolar range of concentrations; they even reach single molecule or single cell resolution with superresolution microscopy (see section on Fluorescence-Based Sensors That Measure Metal Ions in Cells).

Our understanding of the biology of metals in the context of infectious disease has been provided (and limited) by the various analytical tools. In this report, which is based on extensive discussions, our aim is (a) to provide an overview of the analytical techniques available for investigating the interaction of metals or metalloids ($Z \geq 22$) with both the microbe and host, (b) to specify needs for technological improvements, and (c) to identify emerging applications and analytical questions.

Another thematic axis of this report covers experimental paradigms, which span a wide range due to the large differences in size, reproductive speed, and experimental tractability of microbes and host animals. Microbes and cultured cells can be grown in media containing radioactive or stable isotope tracers; the total inventory of metal species can be identified and quantified by radioactivity detection or by the isotopic shift, respectively. In higher animals, tracer techniques allow application of uptake measurements and metal species turnover, but lack or bias the information on the total inventory of metals. To date, localization and speciation of total metals or the metallome in higher animals has been pursued only *ex vivo* in tissue sections or extracts of cells, tissues, or body fluids.

A third thematic axis involves transgenic constructs of metal sensors or reporter proteins from the cellular to the organismal level. Permanent or conditional knockouts of metal chaperones, transporters, chelators, or storage proteins elucidate the mechanism of metal-related host defense, but typically require the use of knockout mice. Fusions of fluorescent or luminescent proteins with metal-chelating proteins may report free metal ion[1] concentrations. Luminescent reporter proteins expressed under the control of promoters for genes of interest allow for the study of the regulation of metalloproteins or effector proteins responsive to metals and can provide an indication of the metal environment experienced by a pathogen during infection. Particular aspects pertaining to metal analysis in humans and reference values are discussed (see section on Reference Values).

ICP-MS has been established as the workhorse in nonradioactive metal speciation studies and, when coupled to a laser ablation (LA) instrument, imaging at the mesoscopic scale may be conducted. ICP-MS provides the lowest detection limits and the best sensitivities, highest concentration dynamic range, broad multiplex capability, and robustness toward matrix effects. Identification of metalloproteins after chromatographic or electrophoretic separation uses metal detection by ICP-MS (or autoradiography); for protein determination, tryptic digestion and high-resolution tandem mass spectrometry (MS[2]: fragmentation of a parent MS peak taken from the first MS spectrum) is used for peptide fragments to ideally obtain exact masses. Then the experimentally determined amino acid sequences of the peptides are compared with those organized in protein databases yielding acceptable or unacceptable probabilities of correct identifications. Unfortunately, protein databases lack many metalloproteins and contain numerous misassignments of metalloproteins (discussed further below).

A fourth thematic axis is introduced that addresses *in silico* approaches to metalloprotein function to predict and calculate the dynamics of metallomes for organisms, starting from their genome sequences. Existing or upcoming genome-wide expression studies utilizing real-time polymerase chain reaction are a valuable resource for identifying genes that encode metalloproteins, which are up- or downregulated in the host or microbe upon mutual contact and may mediate metal modulation of infectious disease.

---

[1] "Free" metal ions (also called mobile or exchangeable or labile): In aqueous solution most metal ions have other small molecules and ions bound, such as water or chloride. These weakly bound ligands typically exchange rapidly with other ligands, making the metal ion "bioavailable" to bind to other molecules and exert biological effects. In living cells and organisms, the molecules binding metals also include amino acids, proteins, and other macromolecules, and the binding may be relatively tight, such that the majority of the metal ions have other molecules tightly bound. These tight ligands exchange only slowly, which may furthermore prevent the metal ions from binding to other molecules, making them in effect unavailable.

In closing, we look at existing gaps and needs in technology. Upcoming methodological issues are discussed and analytical ways to study therapeutic or preventive interventions in the host–microbe interaction are analyzed, with a focus on further potential goals and applications.

## Lysates and Fluids

The most common analysis of metal content is performed on cellular lysate from either host or microbe cells, or on fluids removed from vertebrate hosts. Some methods allow a rough categorization of metal distribution over cellular compartments as well as over groups of chemical compounds or coordination environments. For acidic digestion of entire tissue or cell preparations, ICP-MS gives the total average metal content. Analysis of laser microdissected pieces of tissue or cell organelle fractions obtained by gradient ultracentrifugation provides information about cellular and subcellular localization. Metallic nanoparticles may, after enzymatic digestion and removal of organic and soluble matter, be separated by size through field-flow fractionation or microsieving. Soluble metal species may be separated by centrifugal ultrafiltration or dialysis at various molecular weight cutoffs.

A number of instrumental techniques allow for identification of the prevailing valence and/or chemical environment of metal atoms. Usually, they require a considerable amount of biological material. Two spectrographs have been instrumental in revealing coordination environments and valence states: extended X-ray absorption fine structure and X-ray absorption near edge structure. Both have been particularly useful in cases where other methods cannot be applied; however, these techniques require access to synchrotron radiation for work with biological material. Electron paramagnetic resonance spectroscopy (for use with all paramagnetic compounds with unpaired electrons: Ti, V, Cr, Mn, Fe, Co, Ni, Mo, Lanthanides, but not Zn) and Mössbauer spectroscopy (for Fe, Sn, Sb, Te) can detect the prevailing oxidation and spin state of metal atoms, the degree of coordinate covalency in metal-ligand bonds, electronegativity, and thus identity of donor atoms (O, N, or S) of ligands and the coordinative geometry (Pericone et al. 2003; Miao et al. 2008). Some metal nuclei also have a nuclear magnetic moment and spin suitable for nuclear magnetic resonance (NMR) spectroscopy such as [77]Se, [111]Cd, [113]Cd, [117]Sn, [119]Sn, and [183]W. New double spin resonance experiments performed on frozen whole cells allow for the direct detection of Mn(II)-orthophosphate complexes in bacteria and in yeast. These methods take advantage of the electron spin of Mn(II) coupled to naturally abundant NMR-active nuclei (e.g., [31]P) (McNaughton et al. 2010; Sharma et al. 2013).

Metalloproteomics of lysates (e.g., disrupted cells) and fluids (e.g., serum) can be performed using ICP-MS, MS$^2$, X-ray fluorescence (XRF), or radioactivity for metal analysis. To identify individual metalloproteins, separation is necessary using liquid chromatography or gel or capillary electrophoresis. Cross-linking proteins to membranes makes proteins resistant to digestion and hence precludes the use of $MS^2$ for protein identification.

## Sample Preparation

A critical parameter for the successful determination of metal levels in any sample is the quality of the sample preparation. In infection biology, this is complicated by safety concerns associated with working with pathogens and infected samples. When employing research instrumentation for clinical samples, contamination with infectious agents and radioactivity must be avoided and appropriate disinfection procedures must be implemented.

Cellular lysates can be prepared with or without detergent to investigate soluble and solubilized proteins, and they are used for proteomics investigations. The absence of detergents usually affords better resolution in separations. Redistribution of metals is an "endemic" problem in lysates. Thus the general disadvantage of using cell lysates for metalloproteomics is possible metal redistribution or loss as soon as the cells are broken. Readily exchangeable metals may be lost to some extent. Anaerobic treatment of the samples during the measurement may reduce the risk of oxidation of reduced cations and metal-coordinating sulfur (e.g., loss of iron from oxygen-sensitive Fe-S clusters). Currently used protocols for protein separations are not gentle enough to prevent metal loss, metal redistribution, or binding of adventitious metal ions. Another complicating factor is that only the most abundant proteins of a given metalloproteome can be investigated, as demonstrated by the seminal metalloproteomic studies of Robinson (Tottey et al. 2008) and Adams (Cvetkovic et al. 2010). One workaround is that immunoaffinity chromatography and immunoprecipitation can sometimes be used to remove highly abundant proteins from the lysate, thus gaining access to proteins in lower abundance (Kodali et al. 2012). The material removed from the bulk of the sample can then be investigated separately, either for metals or biological activity; in this way, an enrichment of less abundant proteins is possible.

These approaches, presented here for the analysis of cell lysates, can also be used for body fluids, since these samples are fully amenable to proteomics and metalloproteomics investigations. However, depending on the application, it may be similarly important to deplete these samples of the most abundant proteins (e.g., albumin in serum), given the limited dynamic range of molecule-specific mass spectrometry (5–6 orders of magnitude), so that less abundant proteins can be investigated.

## Protein Separation

The resolution in metalloproteomics can be dramatically improved through the use of protein separation techniques. Protein separation can be achieved by liquid chromatography (LC), two-dimensional polyacrylamide gel electrophoresis (2D-PAGE), or capillary electrophoresis (Kodali et al. 2012). The separation procedure has to be nondenaturing to avoid loss of the bound metal. Normal phase, but not reversed phase LC, can also be used to separate proteins in their native metal-bound state. 2D-PAGE offers the possibility of handling many different samples for metalloproteomic analysis. Full separation of proteins using LC may require up to six separate column steps (Cvetkovic et al. 2010), making it impractical for handling many different samples. In terms of the separation techniques, there is a trade-off between peak separation (resolution) and possible metal loss during the procedure. More separation steps improve protein resolution, which is necessary to assign a metal content unequivocally to a particular protein. However, it also leads to additional metal loss or redistribution. 2D-PAGE may be a useful approach to reach high-resolution separation in a single step. Following successful protein separation, samples are subjected to protein and/or metal identification using mass spectrometry technologies.

**In Gel Quantification of Metals**

An elegant alternative for direct quantification of up to two metals in biological samples is MIRAGE (metal isotope native radio autography in gel electrophoresis). MIRAGE involves the introduction, into the organism, of up to two metals as radioisotope tracers, and allows for full accounting of the amount of metal that is lost during the gel electrophoresis procedures. MIRAGE can detect over six orders of magnitude in concentration, which permits the simultaneous detection of low- and high-abundance proteins. For example, MIRAGE peaks that contain from 0.01 to up to 860 pmol zinc can be measured in the same gel (from a 450 µg protein *Escherichia coli* cell lysate) (Sevcenco et al. 2011). Despite this large dynamic range, only 20% of the Zn proteins predicted using bioinformatics resources were found. Failure to detect 80% of the Zn proteins may be due to (a) the detection limit of the methodology, (b) the fact that not all Zn proteins will be expressed at a particular growth condition, or (c) the reliability of the prediction itself.

Utilizing LA-ICP-MS on dried 2D polyacrylamide gels has the advantage of being capable of mapping more than two metals simultaneously; information on the stoichiometry can be obtained by measuring phosphorus and sulfur as references. However, a second analogous gel has to be prepared for spot picking. Incongruencies in the spot pattern of both gels may complicate correct spot assignment, and only small areas of interest can be mapped using LA-ICP-MS. Scanning an entire 86 mm × 68 mm polyacrylamide gel in a realistic time span of 15 h would allow for a resolution of only 300 µm. The major current limitation in metalloproteomics remains the ability to link the metal confidently to a particular protein. LC and 2D-PAGE still suffer from limited resolution of some proteins.

## Concomitant Metal and Protein Identification
## Using High-Resolution Mass Spectrometry

There is a clear need for a direct measurement of the metal bound to the protein via coordinate covalent bonds under native conditions. At present, this is only possible for high-affinity complexes coupled with relatively gentle ionization sources, e.g., electrospray ionization methods. Quantification of the percent iron occupancy of transferrin isolated from serum (del Castillo Busto et al. 2008) as well as Cd-thiolate (Chen et al. 2013), Cu(I)-thiolate (Banci et al. 2010), Zn-thiolate (Sutherland et al. 2012), and As(III)-thiolate (Ngu and Stillman 2006) complexes have all been detected using these methods. Very stable Cu(I)-coordination complexes can sometimes even be detected using MALDI methods (Chen et al. 2008). Although these investigations were conducted on purified proteins and not generally in crude cell lysates or fluids, the ongoing development of "top-down" proteomics approaches used to determine the exact masses and posttranslational modifications of proteins in crude lysates (Catherman et al. 2013), particularly in combination with a more conventional "bottom-up" tandem MS/MS proteomics workflow, may be used to detect specific metal complexes in proteins, as has recently been demonstrated for insulin-Pt adducts (Moreno-Gordaliza et al. 2009, 2010). The integration of top-down high-resolution mass spectrometry used to determine molecular formulas with bottom-up MS/MS peptide-based protein identification strategies has potential as both a discovery tool as well as a tool for the study of known proteins that are critical to the outcome of the host–pathogen interaction (Tombline et al. 2013).

Metalloproteomic analysis of membrane-bound proteins is possible but not well developed. 2D-PAGE combined with MIRAGE is compatible with membrane proteins, but mass spectrometric protein identification needs to be adjusted to handle more hydrophobic proteins (Fandino et al. 2005). Size exclusion chromatography (SEC) may also be used to separate from high- to low-molecular weight fractions, where a fraction is then further separated by another type of chromatography, such as reversed phase liquid chromatography (RPLC) or ion-pairing HPLC. Specific fractions may then be taken for LC-MS analysis. Determining the metalloproteome of a given single cell in one or a small number of experiments is not yet possible. In addition, with the exception of some proteins (e.g., ferritin and transferrin), few methods exist that allow for a determination of the native metallation state of a protein.

The identification of the respective protein from the peptide sequence of one or more diagnostic tryptic peptides, determined by $MS^n$, is an issue of deliberate database searches and appropriate organization and maintenance of these databases. Typically, $n$ refers to the number of times the mass spectrum is taken in one run of a particular sample; therefore, this would be the $MS^1$ run. If $n = 2$, the mass spectrum is taken from a peptide peak of $MS^1$, and if $n = 3$ it represents the mass spectrum taken from a peptide peak of $MS^2$, etc.

**Further Considerations for *Ex Vivo* Studies**

Additional experimental effort should be given to identifying individual metalloproteins and then determining the apoprotein versus holoprotein ratios. Masses of proteins are difficult to obtain, but high-resolution mass spectrometry is at hand (top down). For sample preparation, *in situ* tryptic digestion needs to be developed. Ion mobility mass spectrometry allows separating isobaric species that differ in drift time. Databases for *in vivo* masses of proteins are needed. No robust computational tool is available to calculate metal content from the total mass of the metalloprotein.

## Cells and Tissues

The ability to use specific approaches to image total metals and determine metalloprotein speciation state in more complex samples (e.g., cell specimens, sections of tissue sampled *ex vivo* or *post mortem*) depends on the type of sample. Development of methods that lower detection limits and provide better spatial resolution will be required to advance this field. In addition, specific strategies for sample preparation need to be considered. Of particular concern are the washout of soluble metal species during fixation or processing and the use of additives or other agents that react with metalloproteins, quench protein signals, or in the worst case may even introduce metal contamination. Whenever possible, snap-freezing of samples is generally recommended.

**Imaging Total Metal**

The extant methodology for imaging metals in biology has been reviewed comprehensively (McRae et al. 2009). The spatially resolved determination of total metals (imaging) is well within the realm of current technologies. An overview of current methods for imaging metals in biological systems is given in Appendices 20.1–20.4. Note that parameters given in these tables (e.g., spatial resolution, limit of detection, and speed) depend highly on the specific setup and application, and are thus solely intended for an initial orientation. It should be noted that all instrumental analytical techniques discussed here are, in general, time consuming, starting at 2 h per $cm^2$, and do not allow high throughput. For high throughput, one has to rely on histological stains for zinc and iron. Higher spatial resolution generally implies lower concentration sensitivity (as the absolute amount of analyte per smallest volume element is rather constant), a smaller field of view, and increased efforts in sample preparation. To analyze a higher number of elements or analytes quasi simultaneously (or a larger spectral range), more time is required or sensitivity may be compromised.

*LA-ICP-MS, Synchrotron μXRF, and Secondary*
*Ion Mass Spectrometry (SIMS)*

LA-ICP-MS is the technique of choice for quantitative multiplex imaging of almost all elements of the periodic table and their stable isotopes at the μg g$^{-1}$ level and below. The sample can be mounted onto a conventional glass slide and is ablated in its entire thickness. LA-ICP-MS is an established technique and is used in approximately twenty laboratories worldwide for biological imaging and in more than fifty for geological and archeological samples. At a spatial resolution of about 5 μm, this technique is at its practical limits; thus smaller cells and bacteria cannot be sufficiently resolved.

Here, analysis using synchrotron μXRF has the highest promise with respect to quantification, nano secondary ion mass spectrometry (NanoSIMS) provides spatial resolution down to 50 nm; electron microscope-based techniques can get down to 5 nm resolution but are not quantitative. For the analysis at the cell level, cultured cells and bacteria may be dried or frozen in total and sputtered with gold, carbon, platinum, or palladium for scanning electron microscopic techniques. For transmission techniques—applicable also for tissue—samples are high-pressure frozen and are either sectioned with an ultra-cryomicrotome or the water is cryosubstituted by a polyacrylmethacrylate resin, and the embedded tissue sectioned with a conventional ultramicrotome into 50–1000 nm thick sections. Samples for XRF have to be mounted onto plastic foil; any heavier support would introduce Raleigh and Compton scatter background. Samples for SIMS need to be mounted onto conductive substrates or conductively sputter-coated if a full analysis of speed and performance is desired. Nonconductive substrates necessitate charge compensation by an electron beam that limits frequency or current of the primary cation beam.

S-XRF and high-resolution NanoSIMS methods are now being used with increasing frequency to image algae, small organisms, and plant materials, particularly those from food crops, including rice (Meharg et al. 2008). Unfortunately, S-XRF is still limited in its availability, although it is increasingly being used. In addition, whole organisms can now be imaged at very high resolution with μXRF, a recent example of which is the water flea *Daphnia magna*, at 180 nm resolution (De Samber et al. 2013). Combining these two imaging modalities, while analyzing, for example, 10 μm sections in μXRF and neighboring 1 μm sections in SIMS with co-registration of the images, allows information to be obtained on the tissue distribution of metals with XRF (with μm, eventually, down to 100 nm resolution), followed by subcellular imaging of selected metals, isotopes, light elements, or polyatomic ions (phosphate, sulfate, cyanide) in smaller regions of interest with NanoSIMS (down to 50 nm resolution). Different leaf or mature crop sections have been imaged, as have been roots and bacteria. SIMS is predominantly a surface imaging methodology, whereas XRF penetrates the entire sample. Elements and matrices accessible by each technique are not identical (see Appendix 20.5). Especially in SIMS, sensitivities depend highly on the ionization energy of the analyte in positive ion mode and the electron affinity in negative ion mode, respectively. Abundant matrix elements, which have lower ionization energy or higher electron affinity, respectively, than the analyte, can reduce sensitivity considerably: examples include zinc oxide and cadmium. SIMS exhibits only modest sensitivities, and the Mn concentrations in biological samples are generally too low for SIMS detection. A recent study using this approach localized arsenic, zinc, and iron to vacuoles and copper and silicon to cell walls, respectively, in the nodes of rice plant stems (Moore et al. 2014). Localization and quantification of zinc in infected tissue may guide differential sampling of bacteria from high Zn and low Zn regions and increase understanding of resistance and adaptation mechanisms.

*Imaging Based on Particle Beam Platforms*

Imaging approaches based on particle beam (electron, proton, or focused ion) microscopy, particularly in combination with other light microscopy-based tools, have recently been employed to cryo-image single bacterial cells with 4 $nm^3$ tomographic resolution (Tocheva et al. 2013). Dramatic improvements with respect to the handling of native frozen hydrated samples were achieved by introducing cooled sample stages and using instruments that allowed for ablation and polishing of the sample surface with a focused ion beam ($Ne^+$ or $Ga^+$), and scanning the sample block face using a focused ion beam ($He^+$) or, in "cross beam" instruments, an electron beam. In both cases, backscattered electrons are detected to reconstruct an image. Several scanning electron microscopy platforms are equipped with energy-dispersive X-ray spectroscopy (EDX) detectors, and focused ion beam platforms can be similarly equipped to obtain surface element information at high resolution. EDX uses the element-specific characteristic X-rays emitted by the sample. As the available excited volume is higher in thick solid specimen than in thin sections, EDX is used in combination with scanning electron microscopy rather than with transmission electron microscopy. On the other hand, the larger interaction volume restricts spatial resolution. In contrast to XRF, where the photon-induced fluorescent X-ray production cross section (the yield per incident flux) increases with the atomic number, the particle-induced X-ray production cross section decreases with atomic number so that elements heavier than molybdenum are hardly accessible by particle-induced EDX techniques. The production of bremsstrahlung background is considerably lower for protons/particles compared to electrons, so that particle-induced X-ray emission allows lower detection limits and also imaging of Cu-Mo, which cannot be realized in electron beam EDX.

When co-registered with super-resolution light microscopy, specific proteins can be co-localized with specific subcellular assemblies (Tocheva et al. 2013). For tissue sections, transmission electron microscopy platforms equipped with an electron spectrometer to perform energy-filtering transmission electron microscopy and electron energy loss spectrometry are highly attractive as (a) the capability of imaging at the oxygen edge or below allows structural information (C, N, O) without counterstain, (b) elemental information can be obtained for elements (e.g., P, S, Si, Fe, and Cu), and (c) electron energy loss spectrometry provides speciation information about the coordination environment of the element of interest.

## Imaging Metal Uptake and Metal Species

A primary question in infection biology involves defining how microbial and host cells internalize and efflux metals during infection. The uptake and total level of metals can be measured using stable and radioactive isotopes (Appendix 20.5): discontinuously with the *ex vivo* techniques described here and in part continuously with the *in vivo* techniques described later.

Proteins can be identified with specific antibodies with very high sensitivity at nanomolar concentrations and co-localized with a particular metal(s). Accordingly, hundreds of antibodies developed for metalloproteins (e.g., cytochrome *c*, zinc finger protein 1, and ferritin) are commercially available. However, in most cases, no discrimination between apoprotein and metal-loaded protein is possible.

*Convergence of Elemental and Molecular Imaging,*
*Possibilities for* In Situ *Speciation*

Defining the suite of metalloproteins and their associated metals remains a significant challenge in biology. The integration of MALDI-MS and ICP-MS has significant potential for the identification of metalloproteins and metals in samples taken directly from tissues (Becker 2013). The current strategy is one of "guilt by association": MALDI-MS and LA-ICP-MS are performed to generate images of protein and metal localization within the sections (Corbin et al. 2008). Due to the destructive nature of these techniques, each method is applied to distinct sections, which are usually collected in parallel. This strategy has significant potential to identify proteins and metals that have characteristic distribution patterns. However, one obtains merely co-localization information. The definitive linking of the metal and protein remains a significant challenge.

Here expectations are directed toward high-resolution mass spectrometry to determine the exact mass of a protein of interest (Pedrero et al. 2012). One of these approaches is the coupling of an orbitrap instrument to a MALDI-imaging source. High-resolution mass spectrometry enables the identification or confirmation of the molecular formulas of compounds. As the absolute mass of each isotope differs from the nominal mass by some decimals—a feature caused by the mass defect, which is lowest for $^3$He and highest for $^{118}$Sn—it is possible, by simple combinatorics, to determine the sum formula of molecule ions and to predict metals therein. There might be more than one solution, however, and either the content of a high number of cysteines, glycines, aspartates, and phosphoserines (the amino acids with highest sum mass defect) or of a metal could make up the measured mass. The mass resolution of $\Delta m/m =$ 10,000 at m/z = 2,000 would allow for the correct assignment of copper to a peptide out of the mass range of about 2,000 Da in about 30% of cases—the result of easy simulations. Masses larger than 10,000 Da cannot be currently handled for theoretical reasons, as deisotoping procedures (deconvolution of C, N, O isotope patterns), which calculate the $^{12}$C-only monoisotopic mass from the number of different $^{13}$C isotopomer peaks on a background of thousands of peptides, are not feasible. Metal content has to be calculated manually from the total mass of the metalloprotein. A robust computational tool is needed urgently. Tryptic digestion, therefore, is paramount for the detection and assignment of larger proteins. Furthermore, it seems rather the exception than the rule that a metal ligand is preserved in a tryptic fragment in the gas phase, although cases have been described. Another possibility leading to suspicion of metal heteroelements in a molecular fragment ion of a peptide is the isotopic finger print (e.g., 69% $^{63}$Cu and 31% $^{65}$Cu), which can be further confirmed by measuring an analogous sample of an organism grown in the presence of an isotopically enriched tracer. For small molecules, desorption electrospray ionization may be of some interest.

An alternative approach, although limited in resolution, is spatially resolved micro-extraction from a series of spots on the tissue section using an automated pipette apparatus (liquid extraction surface analysis). In addition, local digestion using trypsin-loaded pipettes is possible. These extracts can then be treated, as described above (see discussion on Lysates and Fluids).

## Living Cells and Animals

New tools are being developed that will enable the investigation of metalloproteins as well as the speciation of metals and their relationship to infectious diseases in a nondestructive way in living cells, animals, and humans. Minimally, we can detect protein-bound metals and estimate nonprotein-bound ("free") metal ions and enumerate bacteria in cells and tissues. Through multiplexing we can begin to understand the distribution of metals in cells, tissues, and organs of intact living systems and evaluate the role of metals and metalloproteins in infection and disease progression. The imaging systems that can be used in these studies range from microscopes, for cellular and subcellular imaging, to macroscopes, for whole animal and whole human imaging.

These techniques employ energies across the electromagnetic spectrum and will together enable a greater understanding of metals in health and disease. The key to advancing this area of investigation is the development of molecular probes with a unique signature that can be detected both inside cells and outside of the body. Molecular probes that are targeted to specific subcellular locations and compartments are being developed. In each imaging approach, the signal-to-noise ratio determines the sensitivity and nature of what can be observed. Because of the difficulties in resolving pathogens from often abundant members of the existing microbiome in some tissues, as well as pathological changes in metal distribution among physiological metal ions which may also be relatively abundant, selective and sensitive probes and sensors will continually be required.

There is the possibility for *in vivo* tagging of proteins with specific inhibitors (or small molecules) or for introducing a tagged-fusion protein, thus allowing the protein to be assayed *in vivo*. Potentially, with sensors (such as fluorescence resonance energy transfer, FRET, sensors), it is possible to obtain information about the metal load of a protein. Probes that bind metal ions can be used. These can be low molecular weight probes, such as chelating fluorophores or proteins. Bioavailable zinc, for example, can be quantified in living cells with both temporal and spatial resolution using genetically encoded carbonic anhydrase (Bozym et al. 2008) or other genetically engineered proteins that sense metal ions in a FRET format[2] (Palmer et al. 2011; Qin et al. 2011; see below for further details). Aptamers could also be explored, as aptamer-based fluorescent biosensors have been developed for $Pb^{2+}$, $Hg^{2+}$ and hemin (Wang et al. 2011b). With proper control of experimental conditions, absolute measurement may be possible, but comparison of the different methods under the same experimental conditions across various protocols and sensors needs to be performed to advance this field. For approaches that rely on transcription and translation, such as green fluorescent protein reporters and gene fusions, there is a significant time delay (from 30 min to several hours) for the sensor to be transcribed and translated, and the fluorescent protein to "mature" into the active form. In addition, many of these reporter enzymes are oxygen dependent, limiting their value during oxygen limitation, such as might be encountered at certain sites of infection. Thus measurements can be done over hours, but time resolution in the realm of minutes can be a challenge, and other processes may limit the speed of response.

---

[2] FRET (fluorescence resonance energy transfer) is a versatile fluorescence technique. When one fluorescent compound ("the donor") has an emission whose wavelengths overlap the absorbance of a second fluorescent compound or moiety ("the acceptor") and the two are within 10 nm distance, energy can be transferred from the donor to the acceptor resulting in decreased donor emission and enhanced acceptor emission. The technique is frequently used in assays where the analyte causes a change in donor-acceptor distance due to a closer association of the two or a conformational change, resulting in increased FRET.

Some of the advances in this area include microscopic techniques for localizing probes that are introduced into cells: stimulated emission depletion (STED) laser fluorescence microscopy (Dyba and Hell 2002), reaching resolutions of $\lambda/23$, structured illumination microscopy, stochastic optical reconstruction microscopy (STORM), and photoactivated localization microscopy (PALM)[3] (Coltharp and Xiao 2012). Microscopic techniques can also be applied to larger living systems using fiberscopes that reach inside the body (e.g., CellVisio from Mauna Kea Technologies). Fiberscopes are being used for measurements of molecular probes in experimental animals. Although fiberscopes are used in humans, translating molecular probes for microbe and metal detection has been delayed pending regulatory approval by the FDA and other federal agencies.

## Fluorescence-Based Sensors That Measure Metal Ions in Cells

Metal ion determination or imaging of metal ion distribution with low molecular weight or protein fluorescent probes is frequently employed for calcium, copper, and zinc, and, to a lesser extent, iron. At present, corresponding sensor technology for manganese is not available. Research tools (e.g., heme sensors or peroxisomal fluorescence studies which measure whether or not catalase binds heme) seem to be within reach. Fluorescence-based sensors for metal ions have found wide utility in studies of metal ions in solution, isolated cells, and tissues. As yet, however, they have been of modest utility for *in vivo* experiments in mammalian model systems, which are frequently used in infectious disease studies. Since few metals are themselves appreciably fluorescent in aqueous solution, we define these sensors as consisting of molecules that recognize and bind (typically reversibly) to metal ions in solution; the binding reaction is accompanied by some change in fluorescence, which can be correlated with the presence or level of the ion. The fluorescence sensor approach has proven enormously powerful in understanding the biology of metals, largely because it can be applied to fluorescence microscopy of living cells for real time observation and mapping of concentrations and fluxes. By comparison, other analytical tools used to study metals often require (destructive) collection and processing of discrete samples that are inimical to living systems and which often lose spatial information.

The sensors can be usefully divided into small molecule (< 1000 Da) and macromolecule (> 1000 Da) sensors; most of the latter are proteins, with a few being peptides and polynucleotides (aptamers). Important *generic* advantages of these sensors include:

---

[3] PALM, STED, and STORM are fluorescence microscopy techniques which provide "super-resolution" of finer features (<80 nm) in the specimen than can be achieved by ordinary (diffraction-limited) optical microscopy ($\approx$ 300 nm).

- high-resolution imaging in cells and some tissues (to 200 nm with confocal fluorescence microscopy, and 50 nm with super-resolution microscopy methods like STED, PALM, and STORM),
- high sensitivity for the analyte (as low as zeptomolar),
- ease of use and flexibility,
- availability, mostly facile quantification, and
- modest cost.

Most of these sensors respond only to "rapidly exchangeable" metal ions in solution; that is, metal ions with weak ligands (water or chloride are typical) that exchange with other ligands in seconds or less. Fluorescence sensors are among the most powerful, widely used tools in the study of metallobiology, especially at the cellular level. They have provided insights into nonprotein-bound pools of metals in cells and hence have revealed new functions. In particular, for the spectroscopically "silent" Zn (and Ca) ions, they have made investigations of these metal ions possible.

*Sensor Characteristics*

Sensors have been described for scores of metals and some other elements; for brevity, we confine discussion to biological metal ions known to be of central interest with regard to infectious disease: iron, copper, and zinc. Sensors are also available for Ca, Mg, Na, K, $O_2$, NO, and $H^+$, as well as other xenobiotic heavy metals (discussed below). Furthermore, sensors have important properties that crucially affect their utility for virtually all experiments.

In biological systems, due to the complexity of biological environments, the most important attributes of metal sensors are *specificity* and *selectivity*. For example, one cannot reliably measure Zn ions at picomolar levels without being certain that other ions, such as calcium and magnesium, do not interfere when present at billionfold higher levels (specificity): the response needs to be only to the exchangeable metal ion (selectivity) and not to higher molecular weight complexes such as proteins. It is essential when molecule or macromolecule sensors are used to verify that selectivity and specificity are adequate for the measurement, particularly when quantitative results are desired beyond imaging spatial distribution or fluxes of the analyte. A recent example of these issues is shown in Figure 20.1 (Landero-Figueroa et al. 2013), where size exclusion chromatography together with fluorescence and ICP-MS detection was used to analyze a lysate of cells treated with a widely used fluorescent sensor for calcium, Fura Red AM™. Rather than responding solely to exchangeable $Ca^{2+}$ (shown as the rightmost Ca peak in blue), the chromatograms demonstrate that Fura Red AM™ also binds, not surprisingly (Grynkiewicz et al. 1985), to zinc and Cu(II) as small complexes (pink and green peaks on the right). Other metals can interfere, even if they do not induce a fluorescence change, merely by competing for the same binding site. Furthermore, the leftmost peaks on the

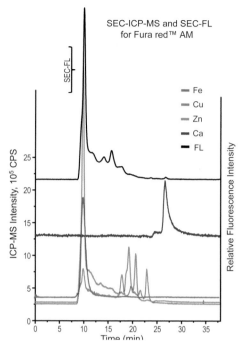

**Figure 20.1** Specificity and selectivity of Fura Red AM$^{TM}$ to Ca$^{2+}$ under conditions of classical *in vivo* cell imaging experiments. Macrophages were incubated with the dye, which was taken up into the cytoplasm. Then the release of Ca$^{2+}$ and eventually other cations from intracellular compartments (such as the endoplasmic reticulum) was stimulated by adding phorbol myristate acetate and/or ionomycin. Thereafter, cells were washed and lysed, and the lysate was injected into a size exclusion chromatography (SEC) column. SEC was run under conditions that preserved the metal-bound state. High molecular weight compounds elute first; low molecular weight compounds (e.g., free Ca$^{2+}$) last. Shown are SEC chromatograms with fluorescence detection (FL) and ICP-MS detection of iron, copper, zinc, and calcium. The Ca peak at 26 min must belong to free Ca$^{2+}$ and cannot be attributable to Fura Red Ca complexes, as no fluorescence is detected. None of the fluorescence signals can be attributed to Ca$^{2+}$ because calcium was not simultaneously detected. Therefore, Fura Red AM$^{TM}$ may detect other ions such as Zn$^{2+}$, but not Ca$^{2+}$. Modified after Landero-Figueroa et al. (2013), with permission of the Royal Society of Chemistry.

chromatograms, corresponding to high molecular weight species, demonstrate Fura Red's capability of binding to macromolecules, some of which also bind zinc, copper, or iron (red peaks), but evidently not calcium. These results illustrate the imperfect selectivity of Fura Red AM$^{TM}$, and the need for caution in interpreting results from all sensors.

The ease and reliability of *getting the sensor into the cell or tissue* is important: in intracellular measurements, macromolecule sensors must be expressed within the cell, microinjected, or conducted across the membrane by using protein transduction mechanisms (e.g., an attached peptide tag, such as TAT)

(Schwarze et al. 1999). By contrast, small molecule sensors that are nonpolar cross cell membranes readily, but they can also be easily washed out or "excreted" by multidrug resistance transporters. Small molecule sensors with iminodiacetate metal-binding moieties are often used as acetoxymethyl esters, which readily penetrate cells, but are trapped therein by esterases. Both types can be targeted to a degree to particular subcellular compartments (e.g., nuclei, mitochondria) or cell types.

*Dynamic range*

Dynamic range (i.e., the analyte concentration range that can be accurately measured) is an attribute that needs to be defined: plasma normal total $Zn^{2+}$ exhibits only a twofold range (Beers and Berkow 1999); other measurements may require a wider dynamic range. For typical reversible sensors that exhibit simple binding, the fractional occupancy of the binding site ($\Theta$) is proportional to the concentration of the metal [M], within the limits of $\Theta$ = 10–90%. This corresponds to an 80-fold concentration range of metal ion:

$$\Theta = \frac{[M]}{[M] + K_D},$$
(20.1)

where $K_D$ is the dissociation constant of the metal. Evidently the dynamic range is limited by the accuracy and precision with which small changes in $\Theta$ can be measured. In a few cases, fluorescence sensors can provide effective dynamic ranges of ten thousandfold or more (Szmacinski and Lakowicz 1993).

*Factors Biasing Fluorescence*

Two generic issues with fluorescence sensors involve *photodestruction* (bleaching) of the fluorescent moiety under prolonged illumination and the presence of interfering *background fluorescence* with comparable spectral properties. Photobleaching is strongly fluorophore dependent and can be reduced by choice of fluorophores or treatment with reagents, where these are feasible. Excessive background is usually a larger barrier to sensitivity of fluorescence determinations than one's ability to detect the target's fluorescence. In addition, for specimens thicker than 1 mm, *absorbance* and *scattering* can prohibitively reduce excitation and emission. The last three attributes are strongly wavelength dependent (Wolfbeis 1985; Cheong et al. 1990), so that in most tissues, typical ultraviolet and visibly excited fluorescent sensors are unusable at depths greater than 1 mm. Conversely, use of infrared fluorophores, which minimize background, absorbance, and scattering of specimens, permits visualization of the human lymphatic system *in vivo* at depths of centimeters (Marshall et al. 2010). To date, few metal sensors have been described with infrared fluorescence properties (Kiyose et al. 2006; Hirayama et al. 2012) or infrared 2-photon excitation (Thompson et al. 2000; Taki et al. 2004).

*Quantification*

Quantifying the metal is of central importance. Even under the most ideal circumstances, simple fluorescence intensity changes are almost unusable for quantification except *in vitro*. This arises from different local concentrations of the probe and bias of fluorescence through the above-mentioned effects. By comparison, the proportion of emission measured at two wavelengths (Grynkiewicz et al. 1985) that are sensitive to the analyte concentration in "wavelength ratiometric" probes has proved to be the most robust readout parameter. An often overlooked factor is the potential buffering effect on the metal ion concentration of the sensor itself, when it is present at high (micromolar and above) concentrations (Krezel and Maret 2006). To a large extent, lifetime- and anisotropy-based sensors also avoid these artifacts, but their use is less common due to instrument availability, despite their flexible implementation and imaging capacity. Whereas ill-suited for quantifying metals, simple intensity changes have proven very useful in identifying the presence, fluxes, and releases of metal ions (Frederickson et al. 1987; Burdette et al. 2001; Gee et al. 2002).

The *response time* of sensors is usually limited by the kinetics of the metal binding to the recognition site. Although the change in fluorescence properties of the sensor, once the ion is bound, is very fast (picoseconds), the time needed to respond to an increase in metal ion concentration is usually limited by the diffusion rate, speciation, and concentration of the metal ion; in addition, the time to equilibrate is controlled by the (concentration-independent) dissociation rate constant. Thus, at micromolar concentrations, a high-affinity site might respond in seconds, whereas at picomolar concentrations, equilibration might take hours. *In vivo*, we generally believe that catalysts facilitate equilibration of apoproteins (and apo-sensors) with low ambient metal ion concentrations.

*Types of Fluorescent Sensors*

Small molecule and macromolecule sensors exhibit important differences in their attributes which affect their utility in certain applications. Small molecule sensors are often available commercially, easy to use, and exhibit adequate sensitivity for some metal ions in some circumstances. Several examples have now been described with ratiometric or lifetime readout (Rolinski and Birch 1999; Chang et al. 2004; Kiyose et al. 2006). However, most sensors for zinc and Cu(II), described for use in biological matrices, utilize one of a few metal-binding motifs (Hirano et al. 2000; Burdette et al. 2001) because they exhibit adequate discrimination for zinc or Cu(II) against likely interfering metals, such as calcium and magnesium. When considering the use of metal sensors for a particular metal, it is important for the investigator to make certain that it is specific toward only that free metal, and selective to only the free metal at a low molecular weight range rather than across a range of higher molecular weights (Landero-Figueroa et al. 2013).

Macromolecule sensors typically exhibit high selectivity and sufficient sensitivity to determine ordinary Zn levels, even at the low levels present in mitochondria (Bozym et al. 2006; van Dongen et al. 2007; Qin et al. 2011). Most of these sensors are made by fusing genes for metal-binding proteins and domains to those for fluorescent proteins (Chalfie et al. 1994), and expressing the transfected gene in some suitable host. Among the important attributes of the macromolecules is that their sensitivity, selectivity, and also speed of response can all be modified and improved using basically the same process to produce a very similar molecule that typically behaves similarly. Thus, Zn sensors have been made with affinity varying over six orders of magnitude, thousandfold improvement in Cu(II) selectivity over Zn(II), and thousandfold improvement in metal equilibration kinetics, and thus response time (Fierke and Thompson 2001; Hurst et al. 2010). An important development is a macromolecule sensor for Cu(I) (Wegner et al. 2010), since this is doubtless the predominant intracellular form of copper present in metazoan cells.

*Current and Future Needs*

By comparison with ionic calcium, zinc, and copper, relatively few fluorescent sensors have been described for iron and manganese. Development of such sensors may be challenging, since $Fe^{2+}$ and $Mn^{2+}$ complexes are expected to be much less stable than $Cu^{2+}$ and $Zn^{2+}$, as reflected by their position in the Irving-Williams series (Irving and Williams 1948). These metals are suspected strongly of playing important roles in infectious disease and accompanying inflammatory responses (see Cavet et al. and Rehder et al., this volume). Recently, several groups have described novel fluorescence-based Fe sensors usable in living cells (Ma et al. 2006; Li et al. 2011; Au-Yeung et al. 2013). Whereas manganese generally plays fewer important roles in most organisms than iron (the Lyme disease pathogen Borrelia may be an exception; see Aguirre et al. 2013), the current modest understanding of Mn biochemistry would be dramatically enhanced by a sensor of appropriate sensitivity and selectivity, as has occurred with Ca sensors.

Fluorescent sensors could likely play a key part in elucidating the biology of xenobiotic and other toxic metal ions, as well as a role in infectious diseases. For instance, concern has arisen on the toxicity of "emerging elements" recently entering commerce (e.g., Ga, Pr, Nd, Te, Re, and Tl in addition to more established toxicants such as Pb, Hg, Cd, Co, Cr, U, As, and Ni). Sensors have been described for some of these elements in various forms, but most are poorly suited for biological applications due to limited selectivity and sensitivity as well as incompatibility with biological matrices.

In addition to imaging applications, fluorescence-based sensors have been incorporated into fiber optics (Peterson et al. 1980) to measure metal ions in remote (e.g., in the ocean; Zeng et al. 2003) and inaccessible *in vivo* samples (Zeng et al. 2005). Finally, work has begun to develop bioluminescence-based metal ion sensors; the elimination of the need for excitation is particularly desirable for *in vivo* imaging applications or austere applications, where an instrument would be inappropriate.

Fluorescence-based probes offer significant multiplexing capabilities, especially in small and transparent systems. As such, it may be possible to assess simultaneously the levels of metals, metalloproteins, and specific microbes in cells and relatively transparent organisms in real time. The development of microbe-specific molecular probes with fluorescent (Kong et al. 2010; Xie et al. 2012) or bioluminescent signatures, along with the advances discussed above for assessing metal levels, have begun to inform this field with a range of molecular probes for sensing and imaging of metal–pathogen and pathogen–host interactions in living systems. Furthermore, fluorescent proteins offer tremendous opportunities for sensing and imaging *in vivo* and these have been used to tag pathogens (see below) (Konjufca and Miller 2009; Melican and Richter-Dahlfors 2009; Coombes and Robey 2010) and further modified as elemental sensors for calcium (based on calmodulin proteins) (Miyawaki et al. 1997). Transcriptional reporters have been used to develop bacteria as biosensors of metals including iron (Cuero et al. 2012), and similar strategies could be developed for bacterial pathogens and metal sensors.

## Tools for Imaging or Assessing Metal–Microbe– Host Interactions in Living Animals

A range of instruments and technologies are available for imaging biological functions in living animals and humans (Helms et al. 2006), and many of these will help in understanding the influence of metals on infectious diseases. Although intrinsic signals from metals in tissues may be detectable in some cases, imaging of the low concentrations of metal and relatively small number of invading bacteria in living subjects will rely on the development and use of extrinsic tracers and molecular probes. Although some of the earliest papers in the field of molecular imaging were in the area of infectious disease (Contag et al. 1995; Piwnica-Worms et al. 2004), the majority of molecular probes developed to date have been designed for imaging changes in biology associated with malignant, cardiovascular, and neurological diseases. There have, however, been several recent advances in development of probes for infectious agents (Kong et al. 2010; Xie et al. 2012); the advances in probes for metal detection, mentioned above, may open up new opportunities for the study of the role of metals in infectious disease. Even with the current technologies, the total inventory of a metal is not accessible to *in vivo* measurement. Instead, the uptake of a given metal species in the chosen formulation via a particular path of delivery or some of the numerous effects of metals in an organism is measured. The colonization of an animal by a given microorganism, in turn, may well be quantified *in vivo* using specific probes or markers.

Some imaging modalities, largely based on optical methods, are ideally suited for small animal models of human biology and disease. There are also imaging modalities for rodents, which are essentially miniaturized versions of those used for humans and employ dedicated small animal scanners (discussed below). In many settings, no direct detection of metals will be possible; however, suitable, mostly genetically encoded reporter constructs can bring a wealth of new information to animal studies.

When using infected animals, heat shock or gamma inactivation is a way to erase infectivity. To protect the investigator, postexposure prophylactic treatment with antibiotics (amoxiclav after deep bites, even from healthy animals) should be considered and generously employed after inoculation with infectious material. Where applicable, vaccination should be considered.

*Bioluminescence Imaging*

In most cases, bioluminescence imaging requires genetic manipulation of the host or pathogen to express a protein-based bioluminescent probe (Contag et al. 1998). However, only a limited number of bioluminescence imaging strategies employ chemiluminescent or bioluminescent probes, which do not require genetic manipulation (Gross et al. 2009). In the vast majority of bioluminescence imaging studies, the bioluminescent probe is a modified luciferase enzyme that catalyzes a light-producing oxidation when chemical substrates (luciferin) are naturally present or supplied (Figure 20.2). The significant advantage of this approach is that the background levels are very low compared with fluorescence, and no exciting light needs to penetrate the specimen; this leads to extremely high signal-to-noise ratios and thus excellent sensitivity. Major limitations are that the signals are weak and not readily controlled; thus high-resolution images are difficult to obtain using tissues excised from these animals. Furthermore, as with all optical methods, detection of the signal is surface-weighted: the deeper the source of the signal, the less sensitive the detection. Therefore, signals from the surface are more readily detectable than those deeper in the tissue. This presents the greatest difficulty when there are both superficial and deep signals in the same subject, and the underlying

*W. Maret et al.*

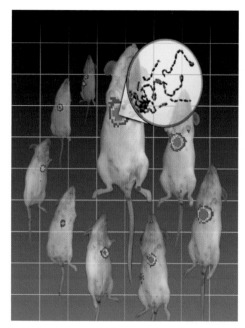

**Figure 20.2**  *In vivo* imaging of the bacterial pathogen, *Listeria monocytogenes*, which has been found to cause persistent infections in the gall bladder and exists in the gall bladder lumen as cell-free bacteria growing in chains. This image illustrates the persistence of the infection over time and the unusual nature of the bacterial growth in the gall bladder. Photos and layout by Jonathan Hardy and Christopher Contag, Stanford University.

signals are obscured by those at the surface. This is the case for all optically based imaging modalities.

*Fluorescence Imaging*

A wide range of genetically encoded reporters and fluorescent dyes can be used to image microbial pathogens *in vivo*, and there is an emerging set of fluorescent probes for similarly assessing levels of metals. As with all optical approaches, the ability to image fluorescence markers *in vivo* is dependent on wavelengths. In the case of fluorescence, both the wavelength of the excitation and emission light determine the level of detection: the longer the wavelength of light (i.e., redder), the better penetration can be achieved *in vivo*, with the optimal wavelengths lying between 800 and 1300 nm. A number of widely used dyes and reporters with emission between 600 and 800 nm are useful, although not necessarily optimal. High-resolution imaging is feasible with fluorescent reporters, and the tools that have been developed for fluorescent imaging of cells and tissues (i.e., confocal microscopy) can be used in living animals. This often requires exposing the tissues of interest surgically—a time-constrained procedure. Instrument miniaturization is ongoing. It increases the amount and type of information that can be obtained with fluorescent markers.

*Other Imaging Modalities*

A number of other modalities exist, based on optics or hybrid approaches, which have utility for work with mice and humans. These include optical coherence tomography, photoacoustic imaging where excitation is over a pulsed laser and detection over (ultrasound) microphones, and Raman spectroscopic imaging at tissue surfaces. Tomographs computed using XRF have been set up and allow for *in vivo* imaging of selected heavy elements (e.g., Au nanoparticles) that are well discriminated from other X-ray dense structures (e.g., bone). Since absorption of fluorescent X-rays by the surrounding tissue is an issue, X-rays should be sufficiently hard. Thus this technique is particularly suited for detecting heavy elements at their K-lines (Jones and Cho 2011).

*Labeled Pathogens*

Bacterial, fungal, parasitic, and viral pathogens have been labeled with both bioluminescent (Figure 20.3) and fluorescent genetic reporters, and imaged *in vivo*. Many of these labeled strains are broadly available for use in animal models, representing a wide range of pathogenic organisms. These can be tracked alone, as has been done in the vast majority of studies, or multiplexed in transgenic reporter mice (Kadurugamuwa et al. 2005).

There are a number of examples where reporter genes have been used to image the effects of metals on microbial gene transcription. *In vivo* bioluminescence has been used to monitor Fe-dependent gene expression in murine tissues infected with *Staphylococcus aureus* (Reniere and Skaar 2008) as well as to monitor heme-dependent gene expression in whole mice infected with *Bacillus anthracis* (Stauff and Skaar 2009). Green fluorescent proteins have also been used to monitor Zn-dependent gene expression *ex vivo* in lungs of mice infected with *Acinetobacter baumanii* (Hood et al. 2012).

*Transgenic Reporter Animals*

Animal models that are based on bioluminescence can be developed to enable imaging of the toxic effects of metals, as well as microbe-associated pathologies, using transcriptional reporters as transgenes in mice. A well-developed example of such a transgenic reporter mouse is one that uses the genetic promoter from heme oxygenase I to express the gene encoding a modified firefly luciferase (Zhang et al. 2001, 2002; Hajdena-Dawson et al. 2003; Malstrom et al. 2004; Su et al. 2006; Cao et al. 2008; Zhao et al. 2008). This reporter reveals patterns of transcription that are altered in response to heavy metal treatment (Figure 20.3) (Zhang et al. 2001; Malstrom et al. 2004).

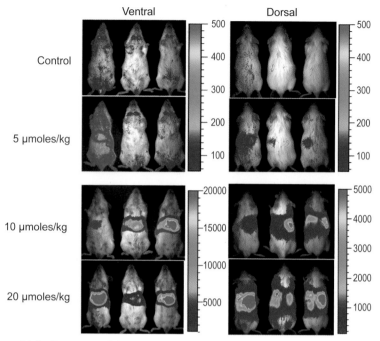

**Figure 20.3**   Response of the transcriptional reporter for heme oxygenase to various concentrations of cadmium chloride: signals that predominate from the liver (ventral) and kidney (dorsal). A transgene composed of the 15 kb heme oxygenase 1 promoter and the coding sequence of a modified firefly luciferase gene was introduced into mice by pronuclear injection. A selected transgene positive pup was selected, bred to wild-type, and subsequently bred to homozygosity to generate a line of mice called HO-luc. These animals were treated with cadmium chloride at the designated doses by intraperi-toneal injection and imaged using an ultrasensitive charged-coupled device camera in a light-tight box (called an IVIS system). After Zhang et al. (2001).

In the same way as luciferase, other reporter genes that code proteins sensitive to other imaging modalities can be expressed under the control of a promoter of interest. The highly specific thyroid iodide transporter works with the substrate $[^{123}I]$ or $[^{99m}Tc]O_4^-$ and single photon emission computed tomography (SPECT) or $[^{124}I]$ and positron emission tomography (PET). The Herpes simplex virus 1 thymidine kinase (HSV1-tk) works with different substrates labeled with $[^{123}I]$ for SPECT and $[^{18}F]$ or $[^{124}I]$ for PET.

## Tools for *In Vivo* Imaging and Assessing Metal Uptake, Metal Effects, and Microbes in Humans

To image humans, the methods or instruments derive largely from medical diagnostics. Still, there is a large range of molecular probes and tracers, used in experimental studies in mice and humans, available at single or select research centers. To date, however, they are not broadly used in routine clinical practice.

*Single Photon Emission Computed Tomography (SPECT)*

SPECT uses gamma emitter nuclides of suitable energy range (100–1000 KeV) as tracers. Typically, planar detector arrays acquire two-dimensional projection images using lamellar collimators for humans and the principle of the pin-hole camera, realized via multi-pinhole collimators for small-animal SPECT. While rotating one or several camera heads around the subject, projections from multiple angles are acquired. Using filtered back-projection or iterative reconstruction algorithms, three-dimensional data sets are calculated from the series of projections, termed sinograms. The spatial resolution of SPECT is limited by the diameter of the pinhole or the number and height of collimator plates, which in turn are inversely correlated with the yield of registered counts per radioactivity injected. The maximum radioactivity dose that can be applied is limited by radioprotection laws for humans (in Canada, 5 mSv; in Germany, 10 mSv and in exceptional circumstances, 20 mSv) as well as by the specific radioactivity of the tracer compound in mice, so as to avoid the saturation range with nonlinear binding or uptake, which is dependent on the assumed reversible or irreversible uptake kinetics. Practically, a resolution of 500 μm can be reached in mice and 5 mm in humans. The number of diagnostic SPECT radionuclides is, in practice, restricted to [$^{99m}$Tc] in [$^{99m}$Tc]chelates, [$^{123}$I] for labeling of small organics, [$^{111}$In] in DOTA[$^{111}$In], and [$^{147}$Gd] for the valida-tion of Gd MR probes (Appendix 20.6). Therefore, the role of SPECT is not in imaging metals but in probing effects via, for example, transgenic constructs. In contrast, PET nuclides have been produced for many metals of interest and are being used for bioimaging.

*Positron Emission Tomography (PET)*

PET acquires images of the spatial distribution of positron emitter nuclide trac-ers. After emission, the positron passes an average linear range according to its energy, which depends on the isotope (0.6 mm for $^{18}$F, $^{52}$Mn, $^{64}$Cu; 1.4 mm for $^{73}$Se) and theoretically limits the resolution of the image. After this distance, the positron collides with an electron from the surrounding material, and their mass is completely converted to energy, which leaves as two annihilation pho-tons of 512 keV emitted at roughly a 180° angle. PET cameras consist of rings of detectors. The readout passes an electronics, registering exclusively signals coincident within a window of 3–12 ns from any two detectors on either side of the object. It is thus possible to acquire data and generate three-dimensional images without collimator or optics. Registered coincidence events are grouped by the incident angle, re-binned into sinograms, and reconstructed as described for SPECT. Suitable and available positron emitter radioisotopes include the cyclotron nuclides [$^{18}$F], [$^{11}$C], [$^{15}$O], [$^{64}$Cu] as well as the generator nuclides [$^{68}$Ga], [$^{82}$Rb], which can be eluted as soluble daughter nuclide species from an insoluble, resin-bound mother nuclide.

One advantage of PET imaging is that a variety of chemical compounds can be labeled without changing their chemical identity. For a given dose of applied radioactivity, the sensitivity is considerably higher than for SPECT. This makes PET especially suitable for human studies. However, the constraints of scintillators and reconstruction further deteriorate resolution in modern scanners, allowing (at best) about 1.2 mm in small animals and 2.5 mm in humans. Nuclides that are not pure positron, but also gamma emitters (e.g., $^{52g}$Mn, $^{64}$Cu, and $^{62}$Zn) necessitate special correction algorithms to separate true from random coincidences, thus further deteriorating image quality.

*Magnetic Resonance Imaging (MRI)*

MRI was developed as an anatomic imaging tool. Today it allows plenty of high-frequency, magnetic gradient pulse sequences to be run, creating modalities sensible to innumerable features (e.g., optimized morphological contrast, water or fat content, mean interstitial liquid diffusion pathway, direction of fiber tracts, blood oxygen level, local perfusion, arteries, veins, and bone). Most of these use the magnetic resonance of hydrogen at about 42.6 MHz/Tesla. When optimized as "MR-microscopy," spatial resolutions down to 200 μm can be obtained.

Paramagnetic metal ions and ultrasmall superparamagnetic iron oxide particles can be used as MRI contrast agents because they reduce the T1 relaxation times of nearby protons. The oxidation state is important, as the metal ion has to be paramagnetic. For clinical use, Gd(III), Lu(III), and Eu(III) complexes are being developed for multimodal reporter molecules, incorporating fluorescence, MR contrast, and target-specific capabilities. Mn(II) is a strong contrast agent that has been used in animal studies (e.g., for retrograde axonal transport). In occasional nonlethal human Mn intoxications, manganese has been observed in the basal ganglia.

In addition to $^1$H resonance, some other nuclei can be imaged by MRI at their specific resonance frequency, thus necessitating a dedicated tuned coil. Unfortunately, a nuclear quadrupole momentum causes broadening of NMR peaks so that only some of the nuclei (i.e., with spin = ½) can be exploited. Commercially available $^{31}$P coils enable the study of abundant phosphates, such as ATP, ADP, and phosphocreatine. Several MRI work groups have established MRI for $^7$Li, $^{19}$F, $^{23}$Na. In addition, $^{19}$F MRI has been used to image antidepressants with trifluoromethyl groups in humans and may also be capable of imaging antibiotics with F$_3$C-groups, as well as chinolones with just one monofluor substituent. So far, $^{77}$Se, $^{111}$Cd, $^{113}$Cd, and $^{207}$Pb have only been used for analytical spectroscopy—not for imaging.

In addition to imaging nuclei at thermal equilibrium magnetic state, it is possible to hyperpolarize magnetically some nuclei ($^3$He, $^6$Li, $^{13}$C, $^{15}$N, $^{129}$Xe) with a half-life of this hyperpolarization in the range of hours. This allows preparations to be produced that can be applied to humans and used to label molecules covalently. The sensitivity of MRI for hyperpolarized nuclei is extremely high; for example, a dose of 10 mg hyperpolarized $^6$Li would be sufficient for acquiring meaningful images of a human adult. Recently Fura-2 $Ca^{2+}$ sensor molecules were labeled with $^{15}$N to produce a $Ca^{2+}$-sensitive NMR probe (Nonaka et al. 2013).

*Computed Tomography (CT)*

In this transmission X-ray imaging technique, an X-ray tube and a detector array, opposite, turn around the object, thus producing projections from multiple angles. These projections are reconstructed into three-dimensional image data sets. Gliding the object continuously through the gantry ring produces a spiral and enables continuous images of the whole body. The X-ray absorption is put out at the Houndsfield scale: 1000 is air and zero is water. This allows an absolute scanner-independent comparison. X-ray imaging is broadly used for anatomical orientation and co-registration with any chemical or functional imaging modality. Dual wavelength CT scanners perform the measurement at two different X-ray energies (e.g., 100 and 500 KeV). This allows bone density to be measured but adds no element information.

*Optical Imaging*

Optical coherence tomography is widely used in ophthalmology and is beginning to be used in gastroenterology for high-resolution imaging of tissue microstructure. Raman micro-imaging may be integrated into endoscopes, and photo-acoustic imaging obtains a role fueled by the development of photodynamic therapy using the selective uptake of fluorescent compounds into cancers.

Imaging systems for PET, SPECT, MRI, CT, some optical methods, and endoscopic and fiberoptic devices are available for small animals. Thus, similar imaging protocols used in mice could be translated to humans.

*Bioassays without Imaging Capacity*

Especially in gastroenterology, there are plenty of metabolic tests that measure the recovery in urine or exhaled air of test compounds or their metabolites. A series of organic compounds labeled with $^{13}$C provide an example whereby the concentration of $^{13}CO_2$ in exhaled air is the readout. $^{13}$C-urea serves to detect and eventually quantify urease, as this enzyme is exclusive to *Helicobacter pylori* in the stomach of patients with ulcers. In the Schilling Test, $^{57}$Co-labeled

cobalamin-intrinsic factor complex and [58]Co-labeled cobalamin are simultaneously applied orally and the recovery of [57]Co and [58]Co determined in urine. This
allows discrimination between deficient nutritional supply and malabsorption
of vitamin B12 in a single measurement, with an almost negligible radiation
dose (< 50 μSv). In an analogous way, suitable radionuclides of most transition
metals with very low radiotoxicity are available to study the oral bioavailability and disposition combined with the preexisting urine and plasma levels of
the most important species of the same metal in infected versus control persons
at baseline and during therapeutic interventions. For instance, [[54]Mn], [[51]Cr],
and [[75]Se] emit no β; [[66]Ni] and [[65]Zn] emit only very low energy β; and the
β exposure under [[59]Fe] and [[67]Cu] is very low due to the half-life of six and
nine weeks, respectively, and the extreme sensitivity of the method. The radionuclide species are highly concentrated in urine; samples can be counted over
24 h and longer, in contrast to *in vivo* imaging, where the acquisition time is
limited. It is also possible to place sensible gamma cameras with high spectral
resolution—assuring discrimination from background radioactivity—over organs of interest, such as liver or spleen for 0.5–3 h.

**Reference Values**

Whereas a few sources exist for total metal levels in human tissues (Linder
1991; Iyengar et al. 1997), data are fragmented, sometimes obtained with ob-
solete methods or sample collection, and typically obtained with low spatial
resolution (e.g., whole bone or brain). For nutrient metals in some bodily fluids, normal values have been published (Beers and Berkow 1999), and some
correlations between particular diseases and subject attributes (e.g., age, diet)
are known. There seems to be a general lack of reference texts and/or databases for metal ion concentrations in human tissues and body fluids. If available, data have not been obtained with the limits of detection of instruments
now available, and thus a new reference text/database is highly desirable. For
these studies, one needs fresh autopsies and snap-frozen samples. A normative
range in all tissues needs to be established. The technology to achieve this is
available because throughput is not hindered when ICP-MS is applied. In addition to total metals, studies on a database/text on metalloproteomics should
be encouraged; this information should lead to an atlas with the distribution of
elements and proteins in the body. Only when such values of healthy controls
have been established can data on infected tissue and fluids be interpreted.
Further stratification should include gender, age, race, and diet (i.e., nutritional
status). Variability needs to be established to interpret metal concentrations in
relation to the question of whether genetics predisposes to infectious diseases.
Such data could be further enhanced when considering toxicogenomics and
nutrigenomics.

## Database Development and Relevant Modeling Tools for Predictions about Metals in Biological Systems

Here we focus on state-of-the-art tools and approaches for predicting the number, structure, and functions of metalloproteins in either host or pathogen using bioinformatics. For clarification, we specify the term metalloprotein to be those proteins that have been verified to have the metal bound (holoform) at the time of analysis, as opposed to the apoform of the protein with the potential for metal binding. In addition, we refer to apoforms as putative metalloproteins and understand that these need to be experimentally verified.

Based on experimental data, homology searches have been performed to identify both metal-binding signatures and metal-binding domains. This approach allows for predictions to be made about the sizes of the metalloproteomes for zinc, copper, and iron (nonheme) for different organisms (Andreini et al. 2013), but data for the Mn metalloproteome are lacking. Given the challenges of assessing true metalloproteins, the databases for metalloproteins are, however, incomplete. The metalloprotein database from The Scripps Research Institute, now discontinued, and the MetalPDB (a database of metal sites in biological macromolecular structures; Andreini et al. 2013) are used as examples.

### Computational Approaches to Model the Metalloproteome

There has been a massive increase in the availability of whole genome sequences for a large number of organisms, including pathogens. In addition, significant advances have been made in the biochemistry of metalloprotein structure and function (Hsin et al. 2008a). In principal, these advances should allow for the development of approaches to query the protein sequence database to identify most, if not all, of the metalloproteins with the native "cognate" metal clearly indicated for a given organism. Despite significant advances (for a recent example, see Andreini et al. 2013), there remains, in practice, a paucity of data due to a number of limitations that we address as challenges for the future. One significant hurdle is that occasionally specific sequence signatures are not readily identifiable in the primary structural information. This is not an issue for canonical $Cys_2$-$His_2$ "zinc finger" proteins (Berg 1988), precisely because all four metal ligands are close to one another in the protein sequence and any multiple sequence alignment will readily pick this up. Predictions improve dramatically when the ligands which prepare the donor for metal binding are close in the sequence and significant gaps in the aligned sequences do not exist. Predictions of 2Fe-2S and 4Fe-4S clusters also seem to function quite well for the same reasons, with a low false positive rate. Cysteines are relatively rare amino acids in proteins, compared to other metal-coordinating amino acids (e.g., histidine, glutamate, or aspartate) and are therefore more conspicuous in amino acid sequence motifs. In contrast, many metalloproteins whose active sites employ ligands that are far apart in the primary structure are less predictable. This, coupled with the potential for an increased number of gaps in alignment that derive from insertions into metal-binding domains, makes the identification of metal-binding "sequence motifs" difficult.

The other major complication is that our knowledge of metalloprotein structure space remains limited relative to the anticipated large number of metalloproteins expected to be encoded by any genome; indeed, in mammalian cells, proteins harboring a metal cofactor are expected to comprise up to one-third of all proteins in the cell (Maret 2010). Briefly, we cannot model what we do not know. As a result, a significant increase in our collective knowledge of metalloproteins is required before we can fully exploit genome sequence databases. These advances will likely come from emerging metalloproteomics methodologies (Tottey et al. 2008), which will, over the longer term, improve our ability to identify new metalloproteins, and their cognate metal, simply by knowledge of the peptide sequence and perhaps three-dimensional structure.

Another complication is that if a metalloprotein sequence motif can be identified in a protein of interest, it is often not known with confidence what the cognate metal ion actually is. Many of the metalloproteins in the database predict the wrong metal binding, which in many cases is zinc, since zinc is a highly competitive metal (Braymer and Giedroc 2014). This observation is in accordance with the Irving-Williams series, in which Zn coordination complexes are among the most stable of the first-row divalent transition metal ions. In addition, certain proteins may not have a single "cognate" metal, but several, each of which is compatible with biological activity (Anjem et al. 2009; Anjem and Imlay 2012).

Finally, as the biological insights on metalloproteins continue to improve, efforts need to be maintained to ensure that sequence databases remain current and correctly annotated. Efforts in maintaining databases, such as the widely used Protein Databank, should consider the limitations in annotating metalloproteins and, if not in place, curators should be encouraged to provide the details of particular conditions that were used for purifying and crystallizing proteins designated as metalloproteins. This is critically important, as a subset of the annotations in the National Center for Biotechnology Information for metalloproteins may contain inaccuracies, and there needs to be a streamlined way in which new information, validated by and linked to specific publications, is continuously updated so that users extract the most accurate information. To make this maximally useful, query results from a "metalloproteome" search could be linked to human clinical data and disease outcomes. These approaches will increase the pace of discovery in this area. For example, databases that focus on a specific metal/organism/cell type/protein family could be developed utilizing known metal-binding domain information from one of the comprehensive databases (e.g., InterPro or UniProt), combined with protein sequence information produced by new genome sequencing projects. Examples of such databases are the PROsthetic centers and Metal Ions in protein active

SitEs database[4] (Degtyarenko et al. 1998), the Metalloprotein Database and Browser[5] (Castagnetto et al. 2002), and the Metal Sites in Proteins database[6] (Hsin et al. 2008b). Figure 20.4 illustrates another approach to the identification of Zn metalloproteins from *Histoplasma capsulatum, Hc,* a lung infecting fungus (Porollo and Daigle, pers. comm.). From the *Hc* genome (strain G217B), 11,220 proteins were predicted and used to generate a Mascot searchable proteomics database. *Hc* samples were fractionated using the Zn channel of SEC-ICP-MS. Proteins were identified from ICP-MS data and molecular MS[2] using Mascot with the custom proteomics database. These proteins were further fed to Blast2GO to narrow their list to zinc and metal-binding proteins only using sequence homology. This approach should be readily extendable to other metals within mammalian cells, such as macrophages, or for other microbial pathogens.

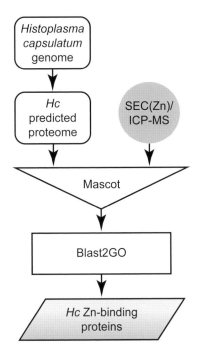

**Figure 20.4** Scheme for predicting Zn metalloproteins in *Histoplasma capsulatum* (*Hc*), a lung infecting pathogen.

---

4  http://metallo.scripps.edu/PROMISE/

5  https://lib.stanford.edu/metalloprotein-database-and-browser (accessed August 8, 2014)

6  http://mespeus.bch.ed.ac.uk/MESPEUS_10/

## Computational Modeling of Metal Speciation and Homeostasis

In addition to predicting the complexity and diversity of metalloproteomes, there is a need to further refine our understanding of metal speciation in small molecule (low molecular weight) ligands. Low molecular weight ligands can serve as buffers, metal chaperones, and sinks for metals. Together, the different species make up the metallome of a cell or organism. We have not yet identified, with certainty, the small molecules that buffer metal ions, although inorganic phosphates, glutathione, histidine, glutamate, and cysteine are candidates and likely play a significant role in metal biochemistry and the biology of the cell. That said, new double resonance electron spin resonance experiments carried out on frozen whole cells allow for the direct detection of Mn(II)-orthophosphate complexes in bacteria and in yeast. This method takes advantage of the electron spin of Mn(II) coupled to naturally abundant NMR-active nuclei, e.g., $^{31}P$ (McNaughton et al. 2010; Sharma et al. 2013). It is also possible to quantify uncomplexed iron in packed whole cell pellets (Pericone et al. 2003) and obtain insights into Fe-metalloprotein speciation in isolated organelles using a number of different approaches, including electron paramagnetic resonance and Mössbauer spectroscopies (Miao et al. 2008). Proteins and nucleic acids are also likely involved in buffering. These "pools" determine availability of metal ions, possibly "escorting" within and between host and pathogen.

Emerging evidence supports an intimate interaction between metals and microbes. Experimental evidence has been reported that metal ions redistribute in the host upon infection. Prime examples are the processes of nutritional immunity (moving Fe and Zn to tissues) and redistribution of zinc in macrophages (Corbin et al. 2008; Kehl-Fie et al. 2013; Vignesh et al. 2013a, b). Quantitative information on the rates and equilibria of the metal-binding capacity of these ligands and corresponding metal pools, as well as on metalloproteins in both host and pathogen, will be necessary for accurate computation and evaluation of metal competition within the microbial cell and between pathogen and resident microbial flora. Measurements of total metal concentrations at the sites of colonization and disease for a given invading organism would complement our understanding of pathogenesis and the role of individual metals. To model cellular and systemic metal redistribution, additional kinetic data, currently sparse, are needed. One caveat is that *in vivo* and *in vitro* kinetics of metal binding or metal exchange of metalloproteins are sometimes vastly different, consistent with the idea that small molecules may strongly influence metal trafficking *in vivo* (Bozym et al. 2008). Since modeling assists experimental designs, tools for effective modeling of the metallome are needed. Computational models can determine whether important participants in the system that have not yet been identified are missing. A number of emerging technologies, discussed above (see also Appendices 20.1–20.6)—including super resolution microscopy, SIMS, and high-resolution nano-XRF methods—allow direct observation of redistribution of total metal within single cells and small organisms (e.g., *D. magna*) (De Samber et al. 2013). Incorporation of these data will facilitate development of new algorithms and models for cellular and systemic metal homeostasis.

## Mining Genomic Databases to Identify New Players in Metal Metabolism Linked to the Susceptibility to Infectious Disease

With the advent of complete human genome sequences, appropriate tools exist for mining these databases for single nucleotide polymorphisms (SNPs) in genes coding metal-binding proteins that are associated with disease and host response. An excellent example is provided by metalloproteins involved in the nutritional immune response. In fact, polymorphisms in human hemoglobin represent the paradigm for how amino acid changes in a host metal-binding protein can impact susceptibility to infectious diseases. Increased resistance to malaria is observed in individuals who are heterozygous for the hemoglobin mutation that leads to sickle cell anemia (HbS) (Pishchany and Skaar 2012). In individuals who have a glutamine to valine substitution in a specific residue within the beta chain of hemoglobin, hemoglobin molecules aggregate within the erythrocytes, resulting in the sickling of red blood cells and severe anemia. Individuals who are heterozygous for the HbS mutation are not anemic and eliminate up to 90% of *Plasmodium* cells within their erythrocytes (Pishchany and Skaar 2012). Beyond simple associations, there is evidence that genetic mutations affect initiation and progression of infectious diseases. For example, *Acrodermatitis enteropathica* is a fatal disease where mutations in the Zn transporter Zip4 in the intestine lead to Zn deficiency that is linked to an increased risk for microbial infections. Knockout mouse models can be particularly useful in identifying new genes that are clearly linked to the susceptibility to microbial infection, as has been established for lipocalin 2 (Flo et al. 2004), calprotectin (Corbin et al. 2008), and others. Recently, SNPs in the gene that encodes the Fe transport protein ferroportin 1 have been found to influence the susceptibility to tuberculosis (Gemmati et al. 2012).

Metal-binding proteins that contribute to nutritional immunity are critical components of defense against infection. However, other than these few examples, the potential impact on susceptibility to infection of polymorphisms in genes encoding metal-sequestering proteins, such as lactoferrin, transferrin, calprotectin (S100A8/A9), and siderocalin, has not been evaluated in detail. In support of this link, aggressive periodontitis is associated with elevated levels of plasma calprotectin, and polymorphisms within S100A8 may influence the susceptibility and severity of aggressive periodontitis (Ren et al. 2009; Sun et al. 2011). In addition, polymorphisms within the transferrin gene have been linked to increased sensitivity to viral infections (Gehrke et al. 2003; Masaisa et al. 2012). These few examples lend support to the idea that sequence polymorphisms within metalloproteins may impact susceptibility to infection.

A publicly available comprehensive database on SNPs in the human genome is maintained and updated by the U.S. National Institutes of Health and the Human Genome Organisation. It is fully annotated as to origin and nature of sampled populations. In addition, the National Institute of Environmental Health Sciences maintains a separate database on genes and SNPs relevant to toxicity pathways, including metals. The U.S. Environmental Protection Agency maintains a database that links these toxicity pathways to known or proposed signaling pathways relevant to human diseases. These resources have the potential to be queried to identify SNPs that are associated with susceptibility to infection. One challenge for these analyses is access to human DNA samples from patients who have suffered from specific infections. Linking patient records from infected individuals to DNA samples has tremendous potential in uncovering gene polymorphisms that affect metalloproteins, metal metabolism, or control of metal homeostasis with impacting the susceptibility to infection.

## Future Directions and Challenges

Having discussed currently available methodologies to quantify and visualize metals ions at the host–pathogen interface—from lysates and fluid samples to single cells to tissues and whole animals—we now articulate future directions and technical challenges that need to be addressed to advance this field significantly.

### Studying Metals in the Microbe–Host Interaction

*LA-ICP-MS* does not have the resolution to study bacterial cells directly. Hence this technique is limited to the study of aspects of the host where granulomas, abscesses, affected segments, or layers can be investigated as well as functional units such as liver-lobuli, kidney-glomeruli and tubuli or lymphatic germ centers at different stages of infection. LA-ICP-MS has been applied to whole animal sections, an area that might be intensified in the future. Detection of microbes by, for example, fluorescence microscopic techniques in the same or an adjacent section allows superimposition and correlation of the images. There is still high potential for implementing the arsenal of image processing software established in the histological and MRI/PET imaging domain, such as co-registration, affine and elastic Z-stack registration, segmentation, and volume of interest readout tools in the domain of MS imaging.

*Whole body imaging* using PET, SPECT, and MRI offers the opportunity to image biological changes in humans; where there is a dire need for knowledge of metal distribution, location of pathogens, and the intersection of these biologies, it may be possible to conduct these human studies. The interest in directly imaging pathogens in relevant primate models and humans has led to the establishment of a biological safety level 4 imaging facility at the U.S. National Institutes of Health. Despite this, the interface with metals and infectious diseases is largely unexplored in the human host. The field suffers from the inability to measure metals in humans with the exception of some early work using radioactive tracers and body counters. For MRI there are possible tracers that can be injected, but imaging of endogenous metals cannot, in principle, be done. It is crucial that we clearly define the important questions that can or cannot be answered in animal models before embarking on programs to assess metal levels and infectious agents in humans. Although we like to be able to relate accumulation of toxic metals in lung or kidney to susceptibility to infection, the significant risks to the human subject and the difficult logistics of imaging of metal and infectious agents in humans may limit these studies to the scope of animal models or other model organisms. Even if there were a scientific rationale for these studies, there is no case/utility for human diagnosis at present. In summary, some methods exist, but there are no direct methods for studying metals in humans, and the utility of such methods, if and when developed, has not been clearly established.

**Clinical Opportunities, Diagnostics, and the Need for Miniaturization**

It should be borne in mind that some of the technologies described in this section have the potential to be developed into clinical tools as well as methods to answer research questions in human studies. Many examples of this are known: assays used in research to study liver and heart enzymes are now routinely used clinically to identify liver disease and heart attack. Clearly, developing a laboratory test into a clinical assay requires substantial refinement, and many research tools, such as two-dimensional gel electrophoresis or NMR spectrometers (except MRI), have attributes which make them difficult or impractical to use clinically. Nevertheless, some very sophisticated instruments and procedures, once exclusively the province of research laboratories, are now used clinically. Examples include tandem mass spectrometers for organic acid analysis of newborns, MALDI-TOF-MS of bacterial colonies for fingerprinting and identification, and short-lived radioisotopes for PET imaging. Some of the techniques described in this chapter (e.g., LA-ICP-MS, fluorescence biosensors, molecular imaging, and X-ray spectroscopy) have been used in animal studies and may potentially be used clinically. The requirement, of course, is that the analysis provides essential information accurately to the clinician in a timely manner, so as to enable the clinician to treat the patient successfully. We anticipate that better understanding of the biology of heavy metals in infectious disease will help identify opportunities to utilize these methods to improve diagnosis and treatment or prevent an infectious disease in the first place. The need for rapid diagnosis and identification of the pathogen in infectious disease at point of care is widely understood, not only because of prolonged disease—owing to the wrong antibiotic being initially employed in the absence of pathogen identification—but also the contribution to the development of resistant strains by this approach. The success of the Rapid Strep Test (measuring antibodies against the streptococcal antigen streptolysin) used widely in physician's offices is evidence of this. Other, mainly nucleic acid-based, methods are being developed for rapid pathogen identification. Clearly, the development of tools for imaging deep infections and for following their pathophysiology has the potential to contribute to the fight or avoidance of infectious disease.

An additional challenge is presented by the inability to bring large and expensive metal analysis equipment into the field where population studies are being conducted. An important class of instrument development that has potential application, particularly for field and epidemiological studies, is the development of miniaturized, low-cost, austere instruments and assays. Many of the techniques discussed herein generally require sophisticated instruments that are unusable outside the laboratory. Thus, the challenge is to identify which approaches, desirable for studies of epidemiology and individual exposure, can be adapted to simpler instrumentation. Instruments designed for person-portable field use without main power, air conditioning, low vibration, or trained operators require significant development, but are already appearing. Handheld XRF and laser-induced breakdown spectroscopy instruments are available today and can identify multiple elements in an alloy sample. However, can they perform well enough to address questions of interest? Miniaturized instruments ("lab on a chip") already exist for chromatographic, electrophoretic, and mass spectrometric separations. Similarly, the adaptation of fluorescence assays to inexpensive instruments has begun (e.g., Zinc-o-meter sensor, NeuroBioTex, Inc.), immunoassays are now commercially available and offer picogram sensitivity for macromolecule analytes (home pregnancy tests) without instrumentation, and Zn ion sensors with nanomolar sensitivity exist that require no instrumentation. The many needs potentially served by this technology have fueled its development and may well contribute to further studies.

**Additional Considerations for Animal Studies**

Most imaging studies image a single functional marker, and the majority overlay the data from this marker on some reference image. There is a need and a desire to begin to multiplex imaging studies, and this is possible for some imaging modalities. Three isotopes have been imaged by SPECT, two bioluminescent reporters have been used in one mouse and distinguished spectrally and biochemically, and a handful of fluorescent probes can be used—the number of which depends on tissue depth and detection method. To maximize the data that can be obtained from a single study subject (mouse or humans), one approach is to use multimodality approaches and image as many markers as possible.

The host–pathogen interaction has not been studied using the whole range of imaging techniques available in mice. An area in great need of further exploitation is bacterial reporter genes/sensors that are driven by metal-sensing transcription factors, such as Fur or Zur as a "barometer" for sensing the bacterial environment. Are the ecological niches in the host deprived of nutrient metals? There is an immediate and significant need for small molecules that sense iron and manganese. Transparent organisms, such as zebrafish, offer models to explore.

## Summary

The methodology for measuring total metals (and metalloids) in biological material has advanced significantly and relies primarily on ICP-MS with exquisite sensitivity, high dynamic range, and virtually no interference from biological matrices. In biology, metals are distributed and redistributed among a great number of species. Speciation analytics in biological time and space is a major challenge in the determination of biological function. One aspect of metals is their binding in metalloproteins. Here a combination of element- and molecule-specific techniques is employed, but determination of stoichiometries is rarely achieved. Addressing entire metalloproteomes is mostly out of reach with current techniques, in part because of the dynamics of biological systems and differences of orders of magnitude in concentrations. Another aspect concerns the state of metal ions that move in the cell and are bound to proteins only transiently. Here, fluorescence spectroscopy is the main technique. Additional approaches are quite indirect: one is the prediction of metal sites by bioinformatics, a method that *assumes* that the metal is indeed in its binding site; the other is the application of spectroscopic probes that *assume* that the same analyte is measured *in situ* or *in vivo* as *ex vivo*. Both approaches have enormous heuristic value but require further curation or validation.

Very bulky equipment is needed for most of the techniques described here. Thus future developments for field work will need to consider miniaturization. Major challenges for imaging remain, in terms of spatial and temporal resolution of the biological events that control the dynamics of metal redistribution during infection. At present, the methods for imaging metals in infectious agents have insufficient resolution in this regard.

There is great potential in harnessing the specificity and sensitivity of biological assays for monitoring metal ions.

**Appendix 20.1** Techniques to image total elements or tracer uptake at the *mesoscopic* scale.

| Technique | Spatial resolution | Time per 25 mm² | Detection limit, range | Remarks | Examples of Instruments |
|---|---|---|---|---|---|
| 1. LA-ICP-MS | 100 μm | 0.5 h | | | NWR213/260 |
| | 10 μm | 10 h | | | CetacLSX200 |
| | 2 μm | 25 h | | | NWR-Femto, Applied Spectra J100 |
| -single Q | | | Ti–Zn 25 fg >Rb 5 fg | ≈ 40 m/z per run | Bruker aurora, Thermo XSeries, Elan600/ NexION, Agilent7500ce, Thermo iCAP-Q |
| -triple Q | | | Improved for As, Se | only 1 m/z | Agilent 8800 |
| -sector field | | | < 1 fg for >Rb | typically < 10 m/z | Element 2 /XR |
| 2. bXRF | 50 μm | 1 h | | | Zeiss iMOXS[a] |
| | 25 μm | 2 h | 1–5 pg; 20–100 μg g⁻¹ | | EDAX Orbis, Bruker Tornado |
| | 10 μm | 4 h | | | Hitachi EA8000 HoribaXGT5000 |
| 3. MALDI-hr-MS | 5–50 μm | 2 h | < 1 fmol | m/z < 4000 m/z < 10,000 | LTQ-Orbitrap Bruker solariX-MI |
| 4. Autoradiography | ≈ 100 μm (β-range) | < 7 d exposure | 1 fmol, e.g., ≈ 50 fg Fe | | FujifilmBAS PerkinElmerTyphoon |
| 5. SEM-EDX/ EPMA | 5–20 μm | ≈ 2 h | 0.1–1 mg g⁻¹, 10 ag | Hook et al. (1985) | TEI, Bruker, EDAX, XMaxN |
| 6. INAA | > 300 μm | < 7 d exposure | 1 pg B 100 pg Se | | Research reactors |
| 7. LIBS | 100 μm | Quite fast | 1–100 μg g⁻¹ | | Applied spectra |
| 8. SECM | 20 μm | | | | Individual setup |

[a] A 50 KeV microfocus X-ray source that can be mounted to SEM platforms using preexistent EDX detectors

**Explanation:**

1. LA-ICP-MS offers high sensitivity throughout the periodic table, accurate quantitative measurements, highest dynamical range, and matrix independence. 10 cm × 10 cm ablation chamber standard; Li–U accessible, Cr, As, Se, Sb, Hg challenging; at some m/z isobaric interferences, collision/reaction cell improves some m/z at the expense of others. Triple Q is an option for dedicated As and Se imaging but lacks an internal standard. Sector field analyzers offer the highest sensitivity and separation, and unequivocal identification of many isobaric interferences.

2. Benchtop XRF scanners use, e.g., 50 KeV X-ray tubes and polychromatic excitation, and have a background of scattered bremsstrahlung and characteristic peaks from the anode material (Cu, Rh, Mo, W available), and a spectrum of accessible elements with gaps: P, S, K, Fe (Na–Mo; Sn–Tb, Ho, W–U). It is easy to handle, requires no laborious tuning, has no consumables, and some instruments offer a simultaneous X-ray transmission imaging mode.

3. MALDI high-resolution MS with Orbitrap (m/Δm 60 000 at m/z 400) or ion cyclotron resonance (m/Δm 650 000 at m/z 400) analyzers permit detection of small molecules, small proteins, tryptic fragments of larger proteins, metallo-organic compounds, etc. Isobaric ions of different sum formula can be separated upon absolute mass. Exceptionally tightly bound metal ligands can be identified due to the mass defect of the complex or through isotopic shift experiments.

4. The spatial resolution of autoradiography depends on the range of β emitted by the radionuclides (e.g., 600 µm for $^{64}$Cu; cf. Appendix 20.5) and is limited to about 100 µm due to geometrical issues for low-energy particles with a range below the slice thickness (e.g., $^3$H β⁻ or Auger e⁻). Highest resolution is obtained when sections are dipped into photoemulsion; highest throughput is assured with single-use X-ray films or washable storage foils. Only uptake measurements are possible, not more than two available radionuclides.

5. In EPMA an EDX detector analyzes the characteristic X-ray spectrum emitted at the site of incident electrons. Energy resolution of detectors is about 100–140 eV at 5 KeV (Kuo 2014). Interaction volume of droplet shape lies below the sample surface and depends on the energy difference of incident electrons and emitted characteristic X-rays and the density of matrix material. To keep the interaction volume low, only limited electron energies (~20 KeV) are used, thus restricting the range of elements accessible. Bremsstrahlung background.

6. In INAA, the sample is exposed to neutron radiation. The analyte is transmuted into a radionuclide. The analyte is transmuted into a radionuclide through, e.g., (n, γ) or (n, p) reactions. Detection is by auto-radiography. α, β, γ after irradiation; α also during irradiation. Only stable isotopes with sufficient interaction cross section and appropriate product radioisotopes are accessible. 0.1 µg g⁻¹ of B were detected; large numbers of slices can be processed in parallel (Stone et al. 1987).

7. LIBS after per pixel pulsed laser induction of a plasma (atomization and ionization of the sample). Within a delay of 10 µs a characteristic optical emission spectrum is recorded; typical laser wavelength 532 nm; typical spectral range 190–1040 nm; 5 × 5 cm² scanning area. Differential volatility of analytes, spectral interferences; relatively cheap; no or minor sample preparation; field applications.

8. Scanning electrochemical microscopy (SECM) measures per pixel currents through a conductive tip clamped at the specific redox potential of a compound of interest. While the tip is scanned over the sample, selected small organic molecules are accessible. Bacterial pyocyanine or $H_2O_2$ and micro-local redox conditions were imaged (Liu et al. 2011).

**Appendix 20.2** Imaging of total elements and tracer uptake at the *microscopic* scale.

| Technique | Spatial resolution | Time per 25 mm² | Detection limit, range | Remarks | Examples of Instruments |
|---|---|---|---|---|---|
| 1. S-μXRF | 50 nm –20 μm | 9 h at 20 μm | 1 ag, μg g⁻¹ range | | ESRF, DESY, NSLS, SSRF |
| 2. PIXE | 0.2–2 μm | | 1–10 μg g⁻¹ | | Selected sites |
| 3. ToF-SIMS | 250 nm 0.2 nm depth | 4 h[b] | 500 atoms Mn 900 atoms Fe 50 atoms Ga [c] | m/z range ca. 1–1000 | IonToF, Cameca, PHI physical electronics NanoToF |
| NanoSIMS | 50 nm (–)[a] 200 nm (+) 10 nm depth | 19 h[b] | 75 atoms Mn 140 atoms Fe 8 atoms Ga [c] | 5–7 m/z | Cameca |
| 4. Histochemistry | 300 nm | 1–2h[d] | 5 μg g⁻¹ | Fe, Cu, Zn | Any light microscope |

[a] 50 nm resolution can be reached in negative and 200 nm in positive ion modus.

[b] for 2500 μm²

[c] 1% of sputtered Si matrix is assumed to be ionized

[d] Staining may take 1–2 h plus the exposition time for Zn

**Explanation:**

1. S-μXRF: Irradiation with monoenergetic, polarized microfocused X-rays; detection of fluorescent K, L lines by fast EDX. Available energy range and resolution given by instrumentation at an end station can limit the spectrum of accessible elements (Ducic et al. 2013). Sensitivity at a given line (K, L, M) increases with Z as the photon-induced fluorescent X-ray production cross section increases. Background of multiple elastic (Raleigh) and inelastic (Compton) scatter events and by escape and coincidence peaks. A 50 nm beam of 17 or 29 KeV at EH2-ID22NI at ESRF in Grenoble; a 350 nm beam of 2–9 KeV at ID21. Here 4 h were required to scan 2500 μm². ID21-D at Argonne: 200 nm and 6.5–20 KeV. The range of elements that can be detected at the K-line is restricted: 9 KeV ≤Cu; 17 KeV ≤Zr; 20KeV ≤Mo; 29 KeV ≤Sn. Abundant matrix elements obscure large parts of the spectrum and a series of L- and M- lines. Further facilities: NSLS-II-X27A at Brookhaven; Diamond Source, UK I18; LNLS Campinas; SSRF Shanghai.

2. PIXE, occasionally coupled with spectroscopy of Rutherford backscattered and transmitted (STIM) particles: 2–4 MeV protons are typically used. The particle-induced characteristic X-ray production cross section decreases with higher Z. Bremsstrahlung of protons is considerably lower than of electrons, proportional to $(z/m·Z/M)^2/E$; $z/m$, $Z/M$ incident and target element atomic number/mass. Secondary electrons account for bremsstrahlung at the lower part of the spectrum.

3. A focused primary ion beam sputters material from the sample surface of which about 1% are secondarily ionized and extracted into a mass analyzer. Elements and polyatomic ions with low ionization energy in positive ion mode or with high electron affinity in negative ion mode can be measured. Relative sensitivity factors are extremely element, modus, and matrix dependent. Analytes with higher ionization energy are suppressed, e.g., by Na and K matrix in biological samples in positive ion mode. NanoSIMS is optimized for highest transmission of 5–7 preselected m/z while ToF-SIMS allows acquisition of complete spectra per pixel, measuring elements and small molecules simultaneously.

4. Zn autometallography requires precipitation of Zn as ZnS, by perfusion with $Na_2S$. Sections are immersed in a photoemulsion, where ZnS catalyzes reduction of $Ag^+$ to Ag. Prussian Blue staining for Fe, classical, or as Perl-DAB is used, e.g., to detect Fe nanoparticles, including ultrasmall super-paramagnetic iron oxide particles. Dithiooxamide forms a green complex with $Cu^{2+}$.

**Appendix 20.3** Imaging of total elements at the *electron microscopic* scale.

| Technique | Spatial resolution | Time (h/10 $\mu m^2$) | Detection limit, range | Remarks | Examples of Instruments |
|---|---|---|---|---|---|
| 1. EFTEM | 2–50 nm | 1–5 min | 1000 atoms Fe in 8 nm diameter, 0.1 ag | | Zeiss Libra120 Jeol JEM3200FS FEI Tecnai TF30 |
| 2. TEM-EDX | 100 nm | probing | 1 mg $g^{-1}$, 10 ag | | Bruker, EDAX, Oxford Instruments |
| 3. SAM | 10 nm | | 1000 $\mu g$ $g^{-1}$ | 6 nm depth | Jeol 9510F, PHI710 |
| 4. (N)EXAFS-STXM | 10–50 nm | slow | 1–0.1 ag > 1000 $\mu g$ $g^{-1}$ | Pecher et al. (2003) | Beamlines (e.g., SSRL-SLAC 6-2c) |

**Explanation:**

1. EFTEM/EELS use an electron spectrometer after the specimen to analyze electrons inelastically scattered due to inner electron shell ionizations; energy losses correspond to specific potential differences. Element-specific images can be obtained by subtracting an image obtained slightly behind an absorption edge from background images obtained in front of an absorption edge (all with, e.g., 40 eV energy window). Typically used are transitions from more outer shells than it is the case for XRF. For example, for P the L2,3 in the range 120–155 eV was used whereas in XRF the $K\alpha 1$ at 2014 eV is used. The energy resolution is about 1 eV and the electron energy loss range accessible, e.g., 3.5 KeV in the Libra120. The local thickness of the sample can be measured from the ratio of zero loss peak and entire spectrum integrals. Sections of 100–150 nm are ideal (Hook et al. 1985). In EELS mode, 100–1000 spectra per second and some speciation information can be obtained. A high contrast between low-level and high-level regions is necessary and imaging of concentrations is possible, rather than the detection of deposits.

2. In TEM-EDX, the interaction volume is usually smaller than in SEM-EDX; thus at better spatial resolution, LODs are higher. A probing of structures of interest (not imaging) is possible. TEM-EDX may complement EFTEM by analysis of, e.g., zinc and perhaps calcium in the speciation of crystals and inclusions.

3. Scanning Auger electron microanalysis records Auger electrons emitted by a sample area exited by an electron beam and is particularly suited for material science, not biological samples. Light elements < Ge in conductive samples preferentially accessible. Measurement of insulator samples with charge compensation via $Ar^+$ ion gun. Imaging and spectrum mode; information on the chemical environment and lattice provided; huge matrix effects.

4. Near edge X-ray absorption fine structure scanning transmission X-ray microscopy (or XANES): spectral range 0.1–2.0 KeV, typically 150 eV around the absorption edge. The spectrum at 150 eV–800 eV above the absorption edge is termed extended X-ray absorption fine structure (EXAFS). Energy resolution of wavelength dispersive detectors (e.g., $E/\Delta E > 3000$) is suited for hydrated samples, e.g., bacterial biofilms, enrichment of Mn, Fe, Ni in the silicate-rich sheaths of filamentous bacteria, redox mechanisms of $Fe^{2+}$ oxidizing bacteria, bacterial magnetosomes, $Mn^{2+}$ oxidation in Pseudomonas were studied. Element images

are generated by subtracting pre- from post-edge images. Classification of organic compounds into, e.g., proteins is possible. Studies of organic coatings on metal particles. At some end stations, combined XRF and NEXAFS are possible (Hook et al. 1985). Imaging at preselected energy windows or per pixel acquisition of entire spectra. Sample thickness <300 nm, otherwise absorption saturation, photoreduction of $Cu^{2+}$ by high photon fluxes, artificial deposition of carbon. Speciation information of metals and organics.

**Appendix 20.4** Imaging uptake and effects of metals *in vivo*.

| Technique | Spatial resolution | Detection limit | Examples of Instruments |
|---|---|---|---|
| 1. PET | 1.3 mm [$^{18}$F], [$^{64}$Cu]<br>2 mm [$^{11}$C]<br>2.5 mm [$^{68}$Ga]<br>5.3 mm [$^{76}$Br] | 10 fmol | Small animal PET/SPECT/CT[a]<br>Siemens CTI Inveon<br>MILabs VECTor[+]<br>Bruker Albira |
| 2. SPECT | 5 mm humans<br>0.3 mm small animals | 50 fmol | Small animals: MILabs U-SPECT[a]<br>SciVis NanoSPECT<br>TriFoil Triumph II |
| 3. Luminescence, fluorescence imaging | 20 μm in microscopic mode | 0.5 pmol | Bruker In Vivo MS FX Pro<br>Perkin Elmer IVIS200<br>TriFoil FLECT |
| 4. MRI:<br>contrast<br>X-nuclei | <br>100 μm<br>1–2 mm | <br>50 pmol | <br>small animals[a]<br>Bruker BioSpin<br>Trifoil LabPET/MR |

[a] For humans, PET, SPECT, and MRI scanners are available from Philips, Siemens, General Electric, and Hitachi, usually at 1.2; 1.5; 3 and 7T

**Explanation:**

1. Coincidence detection allows imaging without collimator and thus 1/3 of decays can be exploited for image acquisition, rendering PET extremely sensitive. Beyond standard nuclides [$^{11}$C], [$^{15}$O], [$^{18}$F], suitable PET radionuclides of most elements are available at few cyclotron centers. A large variety of covalently labeled compounds has been established. The spatial resolution is influenced by the mean range of $\beta^+$.

2. As SPECT requires pinhole or lamellar collimators, a compromise of sensitivity and spatial resolution must be taken. The radioactivity dose to humans is restricted by radiation protection and to mice by the mass of cold compound (tracer criterion). Mostly used with covalently labeled compounds; not many metals established.

3. Luminescent/fluorescent probes are only established for a few metals (e.g., Ca$^{2+}$ and Zn$^{2+}$). Transgenic constructs allow studies of gene expression and biomarkers. The 2D mode is mostly applied; several instruments are combined with planar X-ray imaging. Sufficient tissue optical transmission is obtained in the range 600–900 nm. Fluorescence emission computed tomography enables full 3D scans.

4. $^1H$ resonance is primarily used for bioimaging. A large variety of high-frequency sequences and gradient pulses has been established to yield various tissue contrasts, structural and functional information. $^1H$ and $^{31}P$ spectroscopy allow speciation of abundant small molecules in, e.g., 5 mm voxels. T2* and $R_{2p}$ measured during adiabatic pulses reflect, in part, native Fe distribution. Paramagnetic species shorten T1 relaxation time and act as contrast agents, especially for Mn, Eu, Gd, and Tb. Ultrasmall superparamagnetic iron oxide particles shorten T2. A few other paramagnetic nuclei without quadrupole moment are suitable for MRI (e.g., $^7Li$, $^{13}C$, $^{19}F$, $^{23}Na$). Compounds of some nuclei (e.g., $^3He$, $^{13}C$, $^{129}Xe$) can by hyperpolarized and applied as very strong contrast agents.

**Note:** Of the techniques mentioned in Appendices 20.1–20.4, only LA-ICP-MS and autoradiography are quantitative over large concentration dynamical ranges. SIMS allows only reliable quantification of isotope ratios. In all X-ray emission techniques, scatter and spectral interferences from the matrix limit absolute quantification; in the particle-induced techniques there is background from bremsstrahlung. Sample supports are glass slides in LA-ICP-MS, MALDI-hr-MS, LIBS, SECM, autoradiography, INAA, and histochemical techniques; plastic foil for bXRF and S-µXRF; copper grids or carbon plates and sputter coating with C, Pd, Pt, or Au for EPMA, PIXE, EFTEM, NanoSIMS; $Si_3N_4$ plates for NEXAFS-STXM.

**Appendix 20.5** Nuclides for biomedical tracing and imaging purposes (jointly authored with Syed M. Qaim, INM-5 Nuclear Chemistry, Forschungszentrum Jülich, Germany). Applications include clinical routine (*CR*), studies in humans (*sH*), studies in small animals (*sA*), *in vitro* studies (*iV*), future studies (*f*), and *hC*, historical clinical.

| Nuclide[a] | Production/Mother[a, b] | Emitted particles (energy: MeV for $\beta$, KeV for $\gamma$)[a] | Half-life | Examples of applications |
|---|---|---|---|---|
| *1. SPECT*: clinical,[c] all (Qaim 2012, 2013) | | | | |
| $^{67}$Ga | $^{68}$Zn (p, 2n) | $\varepsilon$, $\gamma$ 93, 185, 300 | 3.3 d | [$^{67}$Ga]$^{3+}$ imaging of subacute inflammatory foci and tumors. Uptake as Fe$^{3+}$ mimetic via transferrin, leukocyte lactoferrin and bacterial siderophores *CR*; [$^{67}$Ga]trastuzumab in mice, *sA*. |
| $^{99m}$Tc | $^{99}$Mo, gn, 2.8 d fission product | IT, $\gamma$ 141 | 6.0 h | [$^{99m}$Tc]O$_4^-$ as analog for I$^-$. [$^{99m}$Tc]TRODAT D$_2$-receptor ligand, *CR*. |
| $^{123}$I | $^{124}$Xe (p, 2n)$^{123}$Cs → $^{123}$Xe, 2.1 h $^{124}$Xe (p, pn)$^{123}$Xe | $\varepsilon$, $\gamma$ 159 | 13.2 h | [$^{123}$I]FP-CIT, DAT ligand, *CR*; [$^{123}$I]MIBG, noradrenergic marker, *CR*; I$^-$ channel expressed by a reporter gene (Niu et al. 2005), *sA*. |
| $^{111}$In | $^{112}$Cd (p, 2n) | $\varepsilon$, $\gamma$ 173, 247 | 2.8 d | [$^{111}$In]DOTA-TOC, somatostatin analog, carcinoid tumors, *CR*; [$^{111}$In]albumin for cerebrospinal fluid tracing, *CR*; labeling proteins, antibodies, *sH*, bacteria, *f*. |
| *2. SPECT*: experimental (Qaim 2012, 2013) | | | | |
| $^{147}$Gd | $^{144}$Sm ($\alpha$, n) (Denzler et al. 1997) | $\varepsilon$, $\gamma$ 229, 396, 929 | 38.1 h | Production established, development, validation, and dosimetry of Gd-labeled contrast agents for MRI, theranostics, *f*. |
| $^{213}$Bi | $^{225}$Ac gn, 3$\alpha$ | $\beta^-$ 1.4, $\alpha$ 5.9, $\gamma$ 440 | 46 min | Antibody conjugates, anticancer; SPECT, MIRAGE, *f*. |
| *3. PET*: clinical,[c] all (Qaim 2012, 2013) | | | | |
| $^{11}$C | $^{14}$N (p, $\alpha$) | $\beta^+$ 1.0; mr = 1.0 mm | 20.4 min | Labeling of any organic compound, *CR*. |
| $^{13}$N | $^{16}$O (p, $\alpha$) | $\beta^+$ 1.2; mr = 1.3 mm | 10.0 min | [$^{13}$N]NH$_3$, myocardial perfusion imaging, *CR*. |
| $^{15}$O | $^{14}$N (d, n) | $\beta^+$ 1.7; mr = 2.0 mm | 2.0 min | [$^{15}$O]H$_2$O, [$^{15}$O]CO$_2$, [$^{15}$O]CO for basal metabolic studies, *CR*. |

**Appendix 20.5 (continued)**

| Nuclide[a] | Production/Mother[a, b] | Emitted particles (energy: MeV for β, KeV for γ)[a] | Half-life | Examples of applications |
|---|---|---|---|---|
| $^{18}$F | $^{18}$O (p, n) | β+ 0.6; mr = 0.6 mm | 109.8 min | Labeling of organic compounds, e.g. [$^{18}$F]FDG as glucose analog with cellular trapping kinetics; [$^{18}$F]– for bone imaging, CR. |
| $^{68}$Ga | $^{68}$Ge gn, 271 d; $^{nat}$Ga (p, xn)$^{68}$Ge | β+ 1.9, γ 1077; mr = 2.2 mm | 67.6 h | [$^{68}$Ga]DOTA as label for peptides somatostatin, CR; proteins, antibodies –anti CD20 = Ibritumomab, ZEVALIN, CR. |
| $^{82g}$Rb | $^{82}$Sr gn 25.3 d; $^{85}$Rb (p, 4n)$^{82}$Sr | β+ 0.8, γ 776, 554, 619; mr = 4.3 mm | 6.3 h | [$^{82}$Rb]+ as analog of K+, imaging of myocardial infarct, CR. |

4. *PET*: experimental (Qaim 2011, 2013)

| Nuclide | Production/Mother | Emitted particles | Half-life | Examples of applications |
|---|---|---|---|---|
| $^{45}$Ti | $^{45}$Sc (p, n) | β+ 1.0, γ (720) | 3.1 h | Ti(OH)$_3$+ uptake and distribution in rats, label of transferrin (Vavere and Welch 2005). |
| $^{51}$Mn | $^{50}$Cr (d, n) | β+ 2.2, γ (749) | 46 min | $^{51}$Cr daughter, animal only. |
| $^{52g}$Mn | $^{nat}$Cr (p, xn) | ε, β+ 0.6, γ 1434, 936, 744 | 5.6 d | Bioavailability sH, PET i.v.; icv biodistribution sA (Davidson and Ward 1988; Davidsson et al. 1988; Topping et al. 2013). |
| $^{52m}$Mn | $^{52}$Fe gn | β+ 2.6, γ 1434, 378 | 21 min | Myocard perfusion tracer (Buck et al. 1996) sA. |
| $^{52}$Fe | $^{55}$Mn (p, 4n) | β+ 0.8, γ 169 | 8.3 h | $^{52m}$Mn daughter, uptake of $^{52}$Fe into human tumors (Roelcke et al. 1996) sH. |
| $^{55}$Co | $^{58}$Ni (p, α) | β+ 1.5, γ 931, 477, 1409 | 17.5 h | Uptake analog to Ca$^{2+}$ into ischemic cerebral tissue (De Reuck et al. 2004) sH. |
| $^{61}$Cu | $^{61}$Ni (p, n) | β+ 1.2, γ 283, 656, 67, 1186 | 3.1 h | Cu-ATSM for hypoxia imaging (Fujibayashi et al. 1997) sH. |
| $^{64}$Cu[c] | $^{64}$Ni (p, n) | ε, β– 0.6, β+ 0.9, γ (1346) | 12.7 h | Labeling of proteins, antibodies, e.g. [$^{64}$Cu]DOTA-trastuzumab CR, organic complexes, Au nanoparticles; Cu disposition in models of Wilson disease (Bahde et al. 2012) sA; inoculation of mice with $^{64}$Cu-PTSM labeled bacteria (Herzog et al. 1993); monitoring of Wilson disease $^{64}$CuCl$_2$ (Wesch et al. 1980) CR. |

**Appendix 20.5 (continued)**

| Nuclide[a] | Production/Mother[a,b] | Emitted particles (energy: MeV for $\beta$, KeV for $\gamma$)[a] (Qaim 2011, 2013) | Half-life | Examples of applications |
|---|---|---|---|---|
| **4.** *PET*: experimental (continued) (Qaim 2011, 2013) | | | | |
| $^{62}$Zn | $^{63}$Cu (p, 2n) | $\varepsilon$, $\beta^+$ 0.7, $\gamma$ 597, 548, 508 → $^{62}$Cu | 9.1 h | Uptake in bovine hereditary Zn deficiency vs. controls, $\gamma$-probe positioned over the liver (Bauer et al. 1992). |
| $^{72}$As | $^{72}$Se gn, or $^{nat}$Ge (p, xn) | $\beta^+$ 2.5, 3.5, $\gamma$ 834, 630 | 25.9 h | Covalent labeling of polymers with thiol groups (Herth et al. 2010). |
| $^{73g}$Se | $^{75}$As (p, 3n) | $\beta^+$ 1.3, 1.7, $\gamma$ 361, 67 | 7.1 h | Labeling of amines with tissue pH selective uptake *sA* (Plenevaux et al. 1990). |
| $^{76}$Br | $^{76}$Se (p, n) / $^{75}$As ($^3$He, 2n) | $\beta^+$ 3.4, 3.9, $\gamma$ 559, 657,1857 | 16 h | Label of organics, proteins, and oligonucleotides, [$^{76}$Br]BrdU as proliferation marker. |
| $^{86g}$Y[c] | $^{86}$Sr (p, n) | $\varepsilon$, $\beta^+$ 1.2, 1.5, $\gamma$ 1077, 628, 1153 | 14.7 h | Dosimetry for therapeutic $^{90}$Y complexes (Rosch et al. 1996) *sH*, peptides and antibodies (Koi et al. 2014) *sA*. |
| $^{89}$Zr[c] | $^{89}$Y (p, n) | $\varepsilon$, $\beta^+$ 0.9 | 3.3 d | Labeling of antibodies, e.g. bevacizumab (Gaykema et al. 2013) *sH*. |
| $^{94m}$Tc | $^{94}$Mo (p, n) | $\varepsilon$, $\beta^+$ 0.8, $\gamma$ 871, 703, 850 | 4.9 h | Use of Tc-chelators established for SPECT in PET, e.g. [$^{94m}$Tc] sestamibi *sH* (Stone et al. 1994). |
| $^{124}$I[c] | $^{124}$Te (p, n) | $\varepsilon$, $\beta^+$ 2.1,$\gamma$ 603, 1691, 723 | 4.2 d | Labeling of DNA analogs IUdR (Blasberg et al. 2000) and antibodies, cf. [$^{123}$I]. |
| **5.** *In vivo assays*[d] (IAEA 2003; Qaim 2011, 2012) | | | | |
| $^{48}$V | $^{50}$Cr (d, α) | $\varepsilon$, $\beta^+$ 0.7, $\gamma$ 984, 1312, 944 | 16.0 d | Uptake and distribution of VO$^{2+}$ antidiabetics, VOSO$_4$ vs. BEOV (Setyawati et al. 1998) *sA*. |
| $^{51}$Cr[c] | $^{50}$Cr (n, $\gamma$) / **$^{55}$Mn** (p, α) | $\varepsilon$, $\gamma$ 320 | 16.0 d | Labeling of blood cells, *CR*, accurate renal glomerular filtration rate [$^{51}$Cr]EDTA pretransplant (Macias et al. 2013), very mild radiator, *CR*. |
| $^{54}$Mn[c] | $^{56}$Fe (d, α) | $\varepsilon$, $\gamma$ 835 | 312 d | Bioavailability (Davidson and Ward 1988; Davidsson et al. 1988; Topping et al. 2013) mild radiator *sH*. |

**Appendix 20.5 (continued)**

| Nuclide[a, b] | Production/Mother[a, b] | Emitted particles (energy: MeV for $\beta$, KeV for $\gamma$)[a] | Half-life | Examples of applications |
|---|---|---|---|---|
| $^{55}$Fe[c] | $^{55}$Mn (p, n) | $\varepsilon$, no $\gamma$ | 2.73 y | Mild radiator. |
| $^{59}$Fe[c] | $^{58}$Fe (n, $\gamma$) | $\beta^-$ 0.5, 1.6, $\gamma$ 1099, 1292 | 44.5 d | Diagnosis of haemochromatosis *hC*, MIRAGE label bacterial Fe-proteome (Sevcenco et al. 2011). |
| $^{57}$Co[c] | $^{56}$Fe (d, n) | $\varepsilon$, $\gamma$ 122,136,14 | 271.8 d | Schilling-Test, double labeling of Intrinsic factor Cobalamin Complex and Cobalamin alone, *CR*. |
| $^{58}$Co[c] | $^{57}$Fe (d, n) | $\varepsilon$, $\beta^+$ 0.5, $\gamma$ 811 | 70.9 d | Labeling bacterial cuprophores, *f*. |
| $^{67}$Cu | $^{67}$Zn (n, p), $^{68}$Zn (p, 2p) | $\beta^-$ 0.14, $\gamma$ 185, 93, 91 | 2.6 d | [$^{67}$Cu]radioimmunotherapy (O'Donnell et al. 1999). |
| $^{65}$Zn[c] | $^{65}$Cu (d, 2n) | $\varepsilon$, $\beta^+$ 0.3, $\gamma$ 1115 | 244.3 d | $^{65}$Zn uptake studies in cultured cells, bioavailability studies. |
| $^{69m}$Zn | $^{68}$Zn (n, $\gamma$) | IT, $\gamma$ 439 → $^{69g}$Zn, $\beta^-$ 0.9 | 13.8 h | MIRAGE, label of bacterial Zn-proteome (Sevcenco et al. 2011). |
| $^{74}$As | $^{74}$Ge (d, 2n) | $\beta^-$ 1.4, $\beta^+$ 0.9, 1.5, $\gamma$ 596, 635 | 17.8 d | Toxicokinetics and metabolism in rabbits (De Kimpe et al. 1999). |
| $^{75}$Se | **$^{75}$As** (p, n), $^{74}$Se (n, $\gamma$) | $\varepsilon$, $\gamma$ 265, 136, 280, 121, 401 | 119.6 d | Large parts of the biochemistry of organo-Se compounds was unravelled with $^{75}$Se (Behne et al. 1994); [$^{75}$Se]HCAT test, *CR*. |
| $^{88}$Y | $^{88}$Sr (p, n) | $\varepsilon$, $\gamma$ 1836, 898 | 106.6 d | cf. $^{86g}$Y. |
| $^{99}$Mo | $^{235}$U fission product | $\beta^-$ 1.2, $\gamma$ 740, 182, 778 | 66 h | MIRAGE label of bacterial Mo-proteome (Sevcenco et al. 2011). |
| $^{110m}$Ag | $^{110}$Pd (d, 2n) | $\beta^-$ 0.5, $\gamma$ 658, 885 | 250 d | Label of Ag nanoparticles (Al-Sid-Cheikh et al. 2013), biodistribution. |
| $^{109}$Cd | $^{nat}$Ag (p, n) | $\varepsilon$ no $\gamma$ | 463 d | Biodistribution in insect larvae (Inza et al. 2001). |
| $^{117m}$Sn | $^{116}$Cd ($\alpha$, 3n) | $\gamma$ 159, e$^-$ | 13.6 d | Biodistribution in rats (Hurst et al. 1986). |
| $^{187}$W | $^{186}$W (n, $\gamma$) | $\beta^-$ 0.6, 1.3 $\gamma$ 686, 480, 72 | 23.7 d | MIRAGE label of bacterial W-proteome (Sevcenco et al. 2011). |
| $^{198g}$**Au** | **$^{197}$Au** (n, $\gamma$) | $\beta^-$ 1.0, 1.4, $\gamma$ 412 | 2.7 d | Distribution of Au cytostatics (Akerman et al. 2013), $^{198}$Au colloid for liver imaging *hC*. |
| $^{203}$Hg | $^{202}$Hg (n, $\gamma$) | $\beta^-$ 0.2, $\gamma$ 279 | 46.6 d | Biodistribution in insect larvae, historical use for renal studies. |
| $^{203}$Pb | $^{205}$Tl (p, 3n) | $\varepsilon$, $\gamma$ 279, 401 | 52 h | Labeling of antibodies. |

**Appendix 20.5 (continued)**

| Nuclide[a] | Production/Mother[a, b] | Emitted particles (energy: MeV for β, KeV for γ)[a] | Half-life | Examples of applications |
|---|---|---|---|---|
| 6. *Frequent therapeutic radionuclides, may be used for MIRAGE* | | | | |
| 90Y | 90Sr gn, 28.6 a fission product | β⁻ 2.3, γ (2186) | 64 h | Antibody conjugates, mr = 8.8 mm. |
| 103Pd | **103Rh** (p, n) | ε, γ (357) | 17.0 d | Radionuclide, brachytherapy seeds. |
| 131I | 130Te (n, γ)131Te 25 min | β⁻ 0.6, 0.8, γ 364, 637, 284 | 8.0 d | Thyroid cancer, thyroid ablation *CR*, mr = 2.0 mm. |
| 153Sm | 152Sm (n, γ) | β⁻ 0.7, 0.8, γ 103, 70 | 46.3 h | Intra-articular 153Sm EDTMP, mr = 3.8 mm. |
| 166Ho | 165Ho (n, γ) | β⁻ 1.9, γ 81 e⁻ | 26.8 h | Microembolization of liver metastases. |
| 169Er | 168Er (n, γ) | β⁻ 0.3, γ (110) | 9.4 d | Intra-articular. |
| 177Lu | 176Yb (n, γ)177Yb 1.9 h or 176Yb (d, n) | β⁻ 0.5, γ 208, 113 | 6.7 d | Antibody conjugates, anticancer, mr = 0.16 mm. |
| 186Re | 186W (p, n) | β⁻ 1.1, ε, γ 137 | 3.7 d | Intra-articular, 186Re HEDP for palliation of bone metastases, mr = 8.7 mm. |
| 188Re | 188W Gen. 69d | β⁻ 2.1, γ 155, 633 | 17.0 h | 188Re HEDP for palliation of bone metastases. |
| 223Ra | 226Ra (n, γ)227Ra → 227Ac → 227Th | α5.6, 5.7, γ 269, 154, 324 | 11.4 d | Bone metastases, i.v. application RaCl₂, *CR*. |
| 7. *Upcoming therapeutic radionuclides* | | | | |
| 140Nd | natCe (³He, xn) | ε, no γ | 3.4 d | PET detection via daughter 140Pr, 3.4 min. |
| 193mPt | 192Os (α, 3n) | γ (136), e⁻ | 4.3 d | Biodistribution of Pt cytostatics, dosimetry on target site *sH* |
| 195mPt | 192Os (α, n) | γ 99, 130, e⁻ | 4.0 d | (Sathekge et al. 2013). |
| 197Hg | **197Au** (d, 2n) | ε, γ 77, 191 e⁻ | 2.7 d | Methyl mercury production in lakes and seas (Koron et al. 2012). |

a    Nuclides: β⁺, positron emission; β⁻, β⁻ decay; c, commercially available; d, deuteron; e⁻, emission of conversion electrons; ε, electron capture from K- or L-shell, when the K- or L-shell gap is filled the excess energy leaves by K- or L-characteristic X-ray or Auger electron emissions; gn, generator nuclide with half life of parent; IT, internal transition; MIRAGE, metal isotope native radioautography in gel electrophoresis; mr, mean range of emitted particles in water, b    determines the spatial resolution of PET; n, neutron; p, proton; SeHCAT, 23-seleno-25-homo-tauro-cholic acid used for bile absorption test. Mono-isotopic elements are set in boldface.

   The most common radionuclide production route is shown (producing minimal long-lived by-products at acceptable product yields) with low- to medium-energy p- or d-particle beams available in standard cyclotrons. The production of some nuclides (e.g. $^{51}$Mn, $^{52}$Fe, $^{73}$Se, $^{83}$Sr) requires higher beam energies available on intermediate energy cyclotrons (Qaim 2012).

c    Low suitability of $^{62}$Zn for PET because of $\gamma$ in the window of 512 KeV annihilation and $^{62}$Cu daughter emitting 2.9 MeV $\beta^+$, T½ = 9.7 min

d    In vivo assays: before going into PET/SPECT, cell-assays and ex vivo biodistributions may be conducted with a batch of species of interest of a longer-lived nuclide of the same element, classical is e.g. establishing iodinated compounds first with $^{125}$I (T½ = 59 d) before labeling with $^{123}$I (T½ = 13 h) for SPECT.

## Explanation:

Typically, reactor nuclides produced by (n, $\gamma$) cannot be obtained carrier-free and thus are of limited suitability for in vivo tracing of specific saturable biological processes at sub nM concentrations. Nonetheless, using carrier-added nuclide MIRAGE studies, toxicological studies, labeling of particles, and studies of trapping processes, e.g., irreversible deposition in bone are feasible and were reported. Upcoming uses of radionuclides in the context of metals and microbes may include:

- [$^{11}$C] and [$^{18}$F]labeling of metallophores, antibiotics and virustatics
- [$^{68}$Ga]$^{3+}$ in ADEM and dose-finding studies to establish Ga$^{3+}$ against Pseudomonas aeruginosa
- [$^{52g}$Mn]$^{2+}$ distribution studies in abscess, calprotectin knockout vs. wildtype
- differential uptake and availability of Fe$^{2+}$, Fe$^{3+}$ species, free or heme/ferritin bound in bacteria
- [$^{64}$Cu]$^{2+}$ in Yersinia enterocolitica infections to understand pathophysiology and extent of altered Cu disposition via Ybt bacterial chelator/cuprophorin
- [$^{72}$As] polymer microspheres with reactive group for labeling proteins
- [$^{73}$Se ], [$^{75}$Se] for viral mutagenesis studies as a function of the offer of Se-methionine
- [$^{124}$I] for imaging gene expression using Na iodide symporter (NIS) as reporter gene [18]
- [$^{51}$Cr]O$_4$]$^{2-}$ uptake studies into bacteria in the host
- [$^{54}$Mn] uptake into P. aeruginosa, with or without Zn$^{2+}$
- disposition of [$^{54}$Mn] in the calprotectin knockout mouse vs. wildtype
- [$^{59}$Fe] labeled siderocalin/lipocalin;
- uptake studies for controlled release Fe supplement formulations transdermal/wafer
- [$^{57}$Co]/[$^{58}$Co] for identification of the true MRP1 substrate in intestinal mucosa
- disposition of [$^{65}$Zn] in the calprotectin knockout mouse vs. wildtype
- pathobiochemistry of [$^{65}$Zn] in pneumococcal infection, effect of Zn substitution
- [$^{74}$As] for identification of arsenated proteins in T-cells mechanisms for deteriorated immunity
- [$^{109}$Cd ] for elucidating the fate of CdSe nanoparticles in vivo
- [$^{117m}$Sn] for elucidating the fate of organo-tin compounds in vivo
- [$^{203}$Hg] for toxicokinetics of diverse Hg compounds.

**Appendix 20.6** Techniques of imaging elements in biological systems, suitably listed by element. (a) LA–ICP-MS, SIMS, radionuclide techniques, and MRI; (b) X–ray emission techniques, EFTEM and EPR. Native composition with preserved Na, Mg, Cl, K, Ca, Fe, Zn, and Cu was assumed. Atomic number (Z), limits of detection (LODs), instrumental neutron activation analysis (INAA), electron paramagnetic resonance (EPR). Some techniques are scored: +++ very good; ++ good; + sufficient; – low; – – very low or impossible to detect; –/+ possible/not possible. Because their full electron configurations have smooth electron absorption edges, Zn and Cd, e.g., are not suited for EFTEM, no electron paramagnetic resonance, and thus cannot realistically be seen in SIMS negative ion mode as atomic ions. Furthermore, there is no stable Zn isotope with a spin of 1/2 yielding sufficiently exploitable nuclear magnetic resonance signals, no suitable SPECT nuclide, a poorly suited PET nuclide, and instrumental neutron activation analysis is possible because interaction cross section and activation product are suitable. No entry means no data, but principally possible. Symbols of monoisotopic elements are set in boldface.

| (a) | | LA–ICP-MS | | SIMS | | | | Radionuclide techniques | | | | MRI |
|---|---|---|---|---|---|---|---|---|---|---|---|---|
| Z | | Score | LOD $\mu g\ g^{-1}$ (1,2) | Pos. ion mode[10] | Neg. ion mode[10] | Ion species used for bioimaging | LOD $\mu g\ g^{-1}$ [11] | INAA | Auto-radiography | PET[15] | SPECT[15] | Contrast or resonance[16] |
| 22 | Ti | ++ | $0.1^{(3)}$ | +++ | – – | | 1 | – | ++ | ++ | – | – |
| 23 | V | ++ | $0.07^{(3)}$ | +++ | – – | | 2 | – | ++ | – | – | – |
| 24 | Cr | + | $0.7^{(3)}$ | +++ | – – | | 2 | + | ++ | – | – | – |
| 25 | **Mn** | +++ | $0.1^{(3)}$ | ++ | | $MnO^-$ | 3 | – | ++ | + | – | ++ |
| 26 | Fe | ++ | $0.9^{(3)}$ $0.24^{(4)}$ | ++ | | $Fe^+, FeO^-$ | $7^{(12)}$ | + | ++ | ++ | – | – |
| 27 | **Co** | ++ | $0.01^{(3)}$ | + | – | | 65 | + | ++ | + | – | – |
| 28 | Ni | ++ | $0.2^{(3)}$ | + | – | | 20 | –/+ | | – | – | – |
| 29 | Cu | ++ | $0.3^{(3,4)}$ | + | – | | 44 | – | ++ | +++ | – | – |
| 30 | Zn | ++ | $0.3^{(3,4)}$ | – | – – | $ZnO^-$ | $1222^{(12)}$ | + | ++ | + | – | – |
| 31 | Ga | ++ | $0.1^{(5)}$ | +++ | – – | | 0.5 | – | + | +++ | + | – |
| 32 | Ge | +++ | $0.01^{(5)}$ | + | + | | 90 | – | + | – | – | – |
| 33 | **As** | ++ | $0.1^{(6)}$ | – | | $AsO^+, As^-$ $AsO^-$ | $2600^{(12)}$ $6^{(13)}$ | + | + | +++ | – | – |

| (a) | | LA–ICP–MS | | SIMS | | | | Radionuclide techniques | | | | MRI |
|---|---|---|---|---|---|---|---|---|---|---|---|---|
| Z | | Score | LOD $\mu g\,g^{-1}$ [1,2] | Pos. ion mode[10] | Neg. ion mode[10] | Ion species used for bioimaging | LOD $\mu g\,g^{-1}$ [11] | INAA | Auto-radiography | PET[15] | SPECT[15] | Contrast or resonance[16] |
| 34 | Se | + | 0.2[5] | – – | +++ | $^{80}Se^-$ | 820[12] 40[13] | + | + | ++ | – | $^{77}Se$ |
| 37 | Rb | +++ | 0.2[3] | +++ | – – | | 1 | + | – | + | – | – |
| 38 | Sr | +++ | 0.1[3] | +++ | – – | $Sr^+$ | 2 | + | + | – | – | – |
| 39 | Y | +++ | 0.02[5] | +++ | – – | | 3 | – | ++ | ++ | – | – |
| 40 | Zr | ++ | 0.1[7] | +++ | – – | | 8 | + | + | ++ | – | – |
| 41 | Nb | +++ | 0.02[5] | +++ | – – | | 19 | – | + | – | – | – |
| 42 | Mo | ++ | 0.1[3] | ++ | – – | | $^{26}7$ | – | ++ | – | – | – |
| 44 | Ru | +++ | | + | – | | 73 | – | – | – | – | – |
| 45 | Rh | +++ | | ++ | | | 58 | – | – | – | – | – |
| 46 | Pd | +++ | | + | – – | | 309 | – | ++ | – | – | – |
| 47 | Ag | ++ | 0.04[5] | + | + | | 90 | + | + | – | – | – |
| 48 | Cd | +++ | 0.05[5] | – | – – | | 1900 | –/+ | ++ | – | – | $^{111}Cd, ^{113}Cd$ |
| 49 | In | +++ | 0.01[5] | +++ | – – | | 4 | – | + | – | + | – |
| 50 | Sn | ++ | 0.5[7] | ++ | + | | 74 | – | ++ | – | – | $^{117}Sn, ^{119}Sn$ |
| 51 | Sb | ++ | 0.1[5] | – | – | | 51 | + | – | – | – | – |
| 52 | Te | +++ | | – | +++ | | $^{21}/1059$ | – | – | – | – | $^{123}Te, ^{125}Te$ |
| 55 | Cs | +++ | 0.04[5] | +++ | – – | | 0.2 | + | ++ | – | – | – |
| 56 | Ba | +++ | 0.3[7] | +++ | – – | $Ba^+$ | 4 | + | – | – | – | – |
| 57 | La | +++ | 0.06[8] | +++ | – – | | 8 | + | – | – | – | – |
| 58 | Ce | +++ | 0.08[8] | +++ | – – | | 7 | + | – | – | – | – |

**Appendix 20.6a (continued)**

| (a) | | LA–ICP-MS | | SIMS | | | | Radionuclide techniques | | | | MRI |
|---|---|---|---|---|---|---|---|---|---|---|---|---|
| Z | | Score | LOD μg g⁻¹ (1, 2) | Pos. ion mode[10] | Neg. ion mode[10] | Ion species used for bioimaging | LOD μg g⁻¹ (11) | INAA | Auto-radiography | PET[15] | SPECT[15] | Contrast or resonance[16] |
| 59 | **Pr** | +++ | 0.04[8] | +++ | – – | | 5 | – | – | – | – | |
| 60 | Nd | +++ | 0.16[8] | +++ | – – | | 1 | + | – | – | – | |
| 62 | Sm | +++ | 0.09[8] | +++ | – – | | 7 | + | + | – | + | |
| 63 | Eu | +++ | 0.08[8] | +++ | – – | | 5 | + | – | – | – | +++ |
| 64 | Gd | +++ | 0.10[8] | +++ | – – | | 9 | + | + | – | + | +++ |
| 65 | **Tb** | +++ | 0.06[8] | +++ | – – | | 7 | + | – | – | – | ++ |
| 66 | Dy | +++ | 0.10[8] | +++ | – – | | 7 | – | – | – | – | |
| 67 | **Ho** | +++ | 0.07[8] | +++ | – – | | 8 | – | – | – | + | |
| 68 | Er | +++ | 0.15[8] | +++ | – – | | 5 | – | + | – | – | |
| 69 | **Tm** | +++ | 0.07[8] | +++ | – – | | 10 | + | – | – | – | |
| 70 | Yb | +++ | 0.17[8] | +++ | – – | | 8 | + | – | – | – | ¹⁷¹Yb |
| 71 | Lu | +++ | 0.03[8] | +++ | – – | | 11 | + | + | – | + | |
| 72 | Hf | +++ | 0.1[6] | ++ | – – | | 210 | + | – | – | – | – |
| 73 | Ta | +++ | 0.01[5] | + | – – | | 75 | + | – | – | – | – |
| 74 | W | +++ | 0.04[5] | + | – – | | 153 | + | ++ | – | – | – |
| 75 | Re | +++ | 0.04[5] | – – | – – | | 31 | – | + | – | + | – |
| 76 | Os | +++ | 0.04[5] | – | – | | 142 | – | – | – | – | – |
| 77 | Ir | +++ | 0.04[5] | – | + | | 320 | + | – | – | – | – |

(a)

| Z | | LA–ICP–MS | | SIMS | | | | Radionuclide techniques | | | | MRI |
|---|---|---|---|---|---|---|---|---|---|---|---|---|
| | | Score | LOD µg g⁻¹ [1,2] | Pos. ion mode[10] | Neg. ion mode[10] | Ion species used for bioimaging | LOD µg g⁻¹ [11] | INAA | Auto-radiography | PET[15] | SPECT[15] | Contrast or resonance[16] |
| 78 | Pt | +++ | 0.04[9] | – – | ++ | Pt⁻ | 85 | –/+ | + | – | – | $^{195}$Pt |
| 79 | **Au** | +++ | 0.04[5] | – – | +++ | Au⁻ | 41 | + | + | – | – | – |
| 80 | Hg | + | 1[3] | – – | – – | | 555 | – | + | – – | – | $^{199}$Hg |
| 81 | Tl | +++ | 0.04[5] | +++ | – – | | 1 | – | + | – | + | – |
| 82 | Pb | +++ | 0.0005[3] | + | – – | | 34 | – | ++ | – | – | $^{207}$Pb |
| 83 | **Bi** | +++ | 0.04[5] | + | – | | 360 | – | + | – | + | – |
| 88 | Ra | +++ | | ++ | – – | | | – | + | – | – | – |
| 90 | **Th** | +++ | 0.04[5] | +++ | – – | | 10 | – | – | – | – | – |
| 92 | U | +++ | 0.001[3] | +++ | – – | | 8 | + | – | – | – | – |
| 94 | Pu | +++ | | ++ | – – | | | + | – | – | – | – |

**Appendix 20.6 (b)**

| (b) | | Basic data | | | X-ray emission techniques | | | | | Absorption | |
| | | | | | Photon-induced (XRF) | | | | Particle-induced | | |
| | | | | | Synchrotron | | | | | | |
| Z | | Electron configuration ground state | Characteristic X-ray energy $K_{\alpha 1}$, KeV | Characteristic X-ray energy $L_{\alpha 1}$, KeV | Argonne, ID21-D (6.5–20 KeV)[13] | ESRF BL21 (2–9 KeV)[13] | bXRF[14] 50 KeV, Rh anode | EM-EDX (–20 KeV)[14] | PIXE (–30 KeV, 1–4 MeV Protons)[14] | EF–TEM / ESI | EPR[17] |
|---|---|---|---|---|---|---|---|---|---|---|---|
| 14 | Si | $3p^2$ | 1.7 | – | ++ | ++ | + | + | (+) | ++ | – |
| 15 | P | $3p^3$ | 2.0 | – | ++ | ++ | + | + | (+) | ++ | – |
| 16 | S | $3p^4$ | 2.3 | – | ++ | ++ | + | + | (+) | ++ | – |
| 17 | Cl | $3p^5$ | 2.6 | – | ++ | ++ | (+) | + | (+) | ++ | – |
| 19 | K | $3p^6, 4s^1$ | 3.3 | – | ++ | ++ | + | + | (+) | ++ | – |
| 20 | Ca | $3p^6, 4s^2$ | 3.7 | 0.34 | ++ | ++ | + | + | (+) | ++ | – |
| 22 | Ti | $3d^2, 4s^2$ | 4.5 | 0.45 | ++ | ++ | + | + | (+) | ++ | + |
| 23 | V | $3d^3, 4s^2$ | 4.9 | 0.51 | ++ | ++ | + | + | (+) | ++ | + |
| 24 | Cr | $3d^5, 4s^1$ | 5.4 | 0.57 | ++ | ++ | + | + | (+) | ++ | + |
| 25 | Mn | $3d^5, 4s^2$ | 5.9 | 0.64 | ++ | ++ | + | + | + | ++ | + |
| 26 | Fe | $3d^6, 4s^2$ | 6.4 | 0.71 | +++ | +++ | + | ++ | + | ++ | + |
| 27 | Co | $3d^7, 4s^2$ | 6.9 | 0.78 | – | – | – | – | – | ++ | + |
| 28 | Ni | $3d^8, 4s^2$ | 7.5 | 0.85 | ++ | ++ | + | + | + | ++ | + |
| 29 | Cu | $3d^{10}, 4s^1$ | 8.0 | 0.93 | +++ | ++ | + | + | ++ | + | + |
| 30 | Zn | full | 8.6 | 1.0 | +++ | +/– | + | + | ++ | – | – |
| 31 | Ga | $4p^1$ | 9.3 | 1.1 | ++ | – | + | + | ++ | – | – |
| 32 | Ge | $4p^2$ | 9.9 | 1.2 | ++ | + | + | + | ++ | – | – |
| 33 | As | $4p^3$ | 10.5 | 1.3 | ++ | – | + | + | ++ | – | – |

| (b) | | Basic data | | | X-ray emission techniques | | | | | Absorption | |
|---|---|---|---|---|---|---|---|---|---|---|---|
| | | | | | Photon-induced (XRF) | | | Particle-induced | | | |
| | | | | | Synchrotron | | | | | | |
| Z | | Electron configuration ground state | Characteristic X-ray energy $K_{\alpha 1}$, KeV | Characteristic X-ray energy $L_{\alpha 1}$, KeV | Argonne, ID21-D (6.5–20 KeV)[13] | ESRF BL21 (2–9 KeV)[13] | bXRF[14] 50 KeV, Rh anode | EM-EDX (~20 KeV)[14] | PIXE (~30 KeV, 1–4 MeV Protons)[14] | EF-TEM / ESI | EPR[17] |
| 34 | Se | $4p^4$ | 11.2 | 1.4 | ++ | + | + | + | ++ | – | – |
| 37 | Rb | $4d^0, 5s^1$ | 13.4 | 1.7 | ++ | – | + | + | ++ | + | – |
| 38 | Sr | $4d^0, 5s^2$ | 14.2 | 1.8 | ++ | – | – | + | ++ | – | – |
| 39 | Y | $4d^1, 5s^2$ | 15.0 | 1.9 | ++ | – | + | + | + | – | – |
| 40 | Zr | $4d^2, 5s^2$ | 15.8 | 2.0 | ++ | – | + | + | + | – | + |
| 41 | Nb | $4d^4, 5s^1$ | 16.6 | 2.2 | ++ | – | + | + | + | – | – |
| 42 | Mo | $4d^5, 5s^1$ | 17.5 | 2.3 | ++ | – | + | + | + | – | + |
| 44 | Ru | $4d^7, 5s^1$ | 19.3 | 2.6 | – | – | – | + | + | – | + |
| 45 | Rh | $4d^8, 5s^1$ | 20.2 | 2.7 | – | – | – | + | + | – | + |
| 46 | Pd | $4d^{10}, 5s^0$ | 21.2 | 2.8 | ++ | + | – | – | + | – | + |
| 47 | Ag | $4d^{10}, 5s^1$ | 22.1 | 3.0 | ++ | ++ | – | – | + | – | – |
| 48 | Cd | full | 23.2 | 3.1 | ++ | ++ | – | – | – | – | – |
| 49 | In | $4f^0, 5p^1$ | 24.2 | 3.3 | – | – | – | – | – | – | – |
| 50 | Sn | $4f^0, 5p^2$ | 25.3 | 3.4 | – | – | + | – | – | + | – |
| 51 | Sb | $4f^0, 5p^3$ | 26.4 | 3.6 | – | – | + | – | – | + | + |
| 52 | Te | $4f^0, 5p^4$ | 27.5 | 3.8 | – | – | + | – | + | + | – |
| 55 | Cs | $4f^0, 5p^6, 6s^1$ | 31.0 | 4.3 | ++ | ++ | + | – | – | + | – |
| 56 | Ba | $4f^0, 5p^6, 6s^2$ | 32.2 | 4.5 | ++ | ++ | + | – | – | + | – |

**Appendix 20.6 (b) (continued)**

| (b) | | | Basic data | | | X-ray emission techniques | | | | | Absorption | |
| --- | --- | --- | --- | --- | --- | --- | --- | --- | --- | --- | --- | --- |
| | | | | | | Photon-induced (XRF) | | | Particle-induced | | | |
| | | | | | | Synchrotron | | | | | | |
| Z | | Electron configuration ground state | Characteristic X-ray energy $K_{\alpha 1}$, KeV | Characteristic X-ray energy $L_{\alpha 1}$, KeV | | Argonne, ID21-D (6.5–20 KeV)[13] | ESRF BL21 (2–9 KeV)[13] | bXRF[14] 50 KeV, Rh anode | EM-EDX (~20 KeV)[14] | PIXE (~30 KeV, 1–4 MeV Protons)[14] | EF–TEM / ESI | EPR[17] |
| 57 | La | $4f^0, 5d^1, 6s^2$ | 33.4 | 4.7 | | ++ | ++ | ++ | – | – | + | + |
| 58 | Ce | $4f^2, 5d^0, 6s^2$ | 34.7 | 4.8 | | ++ | ++ | ++ | – | – | + | + |
| 59 | Pr | $4f^3, 5d^0, 6s^2$ | 36.0 | 5.0 | | ++ | ++ | ++ | – | – | + | + |
| 60 | Nd | $4f^4, 5d^0, 6s^2$ | 37.4 | 5.2 | | ++ | ++ | ++ | – | – | + | + |
| 62 | Sm | $4f^6, 5d^0, 6s^2$ | 40.1 | 5.6 | | ++ | ++ | ++ | – | – | + | + |
| 63 | Eu | $4f^7, 5d^0, 6s^2$ | 41.5 | 5.8 | | + | + | ++ | – | – | + | + |
| 64 | Gd | $4f^7, 5d^1, 6s^2$ | 43.0 | 6.1 | | + | + | ++ | – | – | + | + |
| 65 | Tb | $4f^9, 5d^0, 6s^2$ | 44.5 | 6.3 | | – | – | ++ | – | – | + | + |
| 66 | Dy | $4f^{10}, 5d^0, 6s^2$ | 46.0 | 6.5 | | – | – | – | – | – | + | + |
| 67 | Ho | $4f^{11}, 5d^0, 6s^2$ | 47.5 | 6.7 | | ++ | ++ | ++ | – | – | + | + |
| 68 | Er | $4f^{12}, 5d^0, 6s^2$ | 49.1 | 6.9 | | ++ | – | – | – | – | + | + |
| 69 | Tm | $4f^{13}, 5d^0, 6s^2$ | 50.7 | 7.2 | | ++ | – | – | – | – | + | + |
| 70 | Yb | $4f^{14}, 5d^0, 6s^2$ | 52.4 | 7.4 | | ++ | + | + | – | – | (+) | + |
| 71 | Lu | $4f^{14}, 5d^1, 6s^2$ | 54.1 | 7.7 | | ++ | + | + | – | – | – | + |
| 72 | Hf | $5d^2, 6s^2$ | 55.8 | 7.9 | | – | – | – | – | – | – | – |
| 73 | Ta | $5d^3, 6s^2$ | 57.5 | 8.1 | | – | – | – | – | – | – | – |
| 74 | W | $5d^4, 6s^2$ | 59.3 | 8.4 | | ++ | – | + | – | +/– | – | + |

| (b) | | Basic data | | | X-ray emission techniques | | | | | Absorption | |
| | | | | | Photon-induced (XRF) | | | Particle-induced | | | |
| | | | | | Synchrotron | | | | | | |
| Z | Electron configuration ground state | Characteristic X-ray energy $K_{α1}$, KeV | Characteristic X-ray energy $L_{α1}$, KeV | | Argonne, ID21-D (6.5–20 KeV)[13] | ESRF BL21 (2–9 KeV)[13] | bXRF[14] 50 KeV, Rh anode | EM-EDX (~20 KeV)[14] | PIXE (~30 KeV, 1–4 MeV Protons)[14] | EF–TEM / ESI | EPR[17] |
|---|---|---|---|---|---|---|---|---|---|---|---|
| 75 | Re | $5d^5, 6s^2$ | 61.1 | 8.7 | – | – | + | – | – | – | + |
| 76 | Os | $5d^6, 6s^2$ | 63.0 | 8.9 | – | – | + | – | – | – – | + |
| 77 | Ir | $5d^7, 6s^2$ | 64.9 | 9.2 | ++ | – | + | – | +/– | – | + |
| 78 | Pt | $5d^9, 6s^1$ | 66.8 | 9.4 | ++ | ++ | + | – | +/– | – | + |
| 79 | Au | $5d^{10}, 6s^1$ | 68.8 | 9.7 | ++ | ++ | + | – | +/– | – | – |
| 80 | Hg | full | 70.8 | 10.0 | ++ | ++ | + | – | +/– | – | – |
| 81 | Tl | $6p^1$ | 72.9 | 10.3 | ++ | – – | + | – | +/– | – | – |
| 82 | Pb | $6p^2$ | 75.0 | 10.6 | ++ | – – | + | – | +/– | – – | + |
| 83 | Bi | $6p^3$ | 77.1 | 10.8 | ++ | ++ | + | – | +/– | – | – |
| 88 | Ra | $6d^0, 7s^1$ | 88.5 | 12.3 | ++ | – | + | – | +/– | – | + |
| 90 | Th | $6d^2, 7s^2$ | 95.9 | 13.0 | ++ | ++ | + | – | +/– | – | + |
| 92 | U | $5f^3, 6d^1, 7s^2$ | 98.4 | 13.6 | ++ | – | + | – | +/– | – – – | + |
| 94 | Pu | $5f^6, 6d^0, 7s^2$ | 103.8 | 14.3 | ++ | – | – | – | +/– | – – | + |

1 Limits of detection (LODs) data for LA-ICP-MS in biological tissue were only available for some elements (black text). LODs obtained in glass were available for almost all elements (gray text) and showed high congruency with bio-LOD as LA-ICP-MS is considerable less matrix-dependent than SIMS. Cr, Se, and to some degree Fe are problematic due to the interferences ($^{52}Cr/^{40}Ar^{12}C$, $^{53}Cr/^{40}Ar^{13}C$, $^{56}Fe/^{40}Ar^{16}O$, $^{78}Se/^{38}Ar^{40}Ar$, $^{80}Se/^{40}Ar_2$) and may require the use of a collision/reaction cell for decomposition of interfering polyatomic species or a sector-field instrument for resolution. In addition, As, Se, Ag, and Sb may be challenging due to their high ionization potentials (Becker 2007).

2 All LODs were calculated for full ablation of a pixel of 50 μm × 50 μm × 50 μm (in line scan mode x-feed × spotsize) of dried cryosections cut at a wet thickness of 30 μm and thus refer to wet weight. Multiplication with the factor 75 fg ($\mu g\ g^{-1}$) gives absolute LODs.

3   Newly calculated data published in Sussulini et al. (2012).

4   Data adapted from Lear et al. (2012).

5   Data adapted from Jenner and O'Neill (2012), determined on an Agilent 7500S quadrupole instrument.

6   Data adapted from Stadlbauer et al. (2007).

7   Data adapted from Trejos et al. (2013).

8   Data adapted from Dressler et al. (2007).

9   Data adapted from Moreno-Gordaliza et al. (2011).

10  Element sensitivity was classified according to the relative sensitivity factors determined in a silicium matrix (Wilson 1995) on CAMECA sector field instruments using 4 KeV O$^-$/8 KeV O$_2^+$ or 14.5 KeV Cs$^+$ into the following categories:

    −    impossible/ bad sensitivity, $2 \times 10^{23} < RSF < 2 \times 10^{24}$ cm$^{-3}$
    − −  impossible / very bad sensitivity, $2 \times 10^{24}$ cm$^{-3}$ < RSF
    +    possible / sufficient sensitivity, $3 \times 10^{22} < RSF < 2 \times 10^{23}$ cm$^{-3}$
    ++   good sensitivity, $10^{22} < RSF < 3 \times 10^{22}$ cm$^{-3}$
    +++  excellent sensitivity, RSF $< 10^{22}$ cm$^{-3}$

    No comprehensive relative sensitive factor (RSF) data were available for biological tissue. Here and under otherwise different conditions (primary ions, incident angle, mass analyzer), RSF for a given element may vary, but these data may give an overall orientation. In biological tissue, a series of elements can best be detected as monoxide ion species.

11  Numbers in black were calculated from RSF in graphite assuming 1% ionization of ablated material and 6 atoms in the detector as detection threshold, numbers in gray were calculated from RSF in silicium given by Wilson (1995). LOD wet weight was calculated for full sputtering of 200 nm × 200 nm × 10 nm dry material corresponding to 200 nm × 200 nm × 50 nm wet material. Multiplication by $2 \times 10^{-21}$ g ($\mu$g g$^{-1}$) gives absolute detection limits, multiplication by 1200 ($\mu$g g$^{-1}$ × atomic weight) gives the number of atoms.

12  LODs are given for the monoatomic ions; LODs of biatomic ions, such as ZnO$^-$ may be considerably lower.

13  Data adapted from Moore et al. (2010).

14  Spectral background from a typical native biological matrix containing 1500 $\mu$g g$^{-1}$ P, 800 $\mu$g g$^{-1}$ S, 900 $\mu$g g$^{-1}$ Cl, 2800 $\mu$g g$^{-1}$ K 170 $\mu$g g$^{-1}$ Ca, 80 $\mu$g g$^{-1}$ Fe, 10 $\mu$g g$^{-1}$ Zn, 3 $\mu$g g$^{-1}$ Cu was assumed for all X-ray emission techniques. Sensitivity for an element depends on whether (a) the energy range offered in a given configuration of X-ray optics and detector permits detection at its K lines, which are most sensitive, or (b) it has to be detected at L or M lines. These are generally less intense and risk to be completely overlain by dispersed K signals of matrix elements. Different examples are presented. The other limiting factor is the energy resolution of the X-ray detector which is typically 120−140 eV in fast energy dispersive detectors used for bioimaging at synchrotron end stations as well as on electron or particle beam platforms.

15  Some PET and SPECT nuclides are only available with comparatively short half-lives so that only a short uptake phase can be studied before more specific mechanisms of disposition come into play (e.g., $^{55}$Co$^{2+}$ behaved as Ca$^{2+}$ analog and $^{82}$Rb$^+$ or $^{201}$Tl$^+$ as K$^+$ analog).

16  Those nuclei with exploitable NMR (spin ±½, without signal broadening by quadrupole moment) are given with the mass number; elements acting as contrast agent which shorten $^1$H signal T1 or T2 relaxation time are indicated by +++.

17  An EPR signal can be obtained from compounds or states containing unpaired (radical) electrons and be paramagnetic or ferromagnetic. Thus the presence of an EPR signal depends on the species/compound—some Cu(II) species display EPR but not Cu(I)—and only species most relevant for biological matter were taken into consideration (e.g., not metallic K, Ca but K$^+$ and Ca$^{2+}$). Especially species or ions with incomplete 3d, 4d, 5d, 4f or 5f shells may present EPR. Most appropriately (solutions of) pure isolated compounds may be studied and characterized by EPR. EPR can contribute valuable information on speciation/coordination environment, e.g., Mn$^{2+}$ complexed by appropriate ligands at low temperature shows a six-line hyperfine splitting of the EPR signal while free Mn$^{2+}$ shows a similar signal without fine structure.

# List of Acronyms

| | |
|---|---|
| ABC | ATP-binding cassette |
| ADP | adenosine diphosphate |
| AI | adequate intake |
| ATP | adenosine triphosphate |
| BFR | bacterioferritin |
| bXRF | benchtop XRF |
| cGMP | cyclic guanosine monophosphate |
| CHA | carbonated hydroxyapatite |
| CQ | chloroquine |
| CsoR | Cu-sensitive operon repressor |
| CT | computed tomography |
| CTP | choline phosphate cytidylyltransferase |
| CTZ | clotrimazole |
| DcytB | duodenal cytochrome B |
| DMT1 | divalent metal transporter 1 |
| Dps | DNA-binding protein from starved cells |
| DRI | dietary reference intake |
| EAR | estimated average requirement |
| EDX | energy-dispersive X-ray spectroscopy |
| EELS | electron energy loss spectrometry |
| Efb | extracellular fibrinogen-binding |
| EFTEM | energy filtering transmission electron microscopy |
| Ent | enterobactin |
| EPMA | electron probe micro analysis |
| ES-MS | electrospray mass spectrometry |
| EXAFS | extended X-ray absorption fine structure |
| FQ | ferroquine |
| FRET | fluorescence resonance energy transfer |
| GM-CSF | granulocyte macrophage colony stimulating factor |
| GTP | guanosine-5'-triphosphate |
| HAMP | hepcidin-encoding gene |
| HIF-1 | hypoxia inducible factor-1 |
| HmbR | heme/hemoglobin receptor |
| HO-1 | heme oxygenase-1 |
| iAsV | inorganic arsenate |
| iAsIII | inorganic arsenite |
| ICP-MS | inductively coupled plasma mass spectrometry |
| IMAC | immobilized metal ion affinity chromatography |
| IFN | interferon |
| IL | interleukin |
| iNOS | inducible nitric oxide synthase |
| IRE | iron-responsive element |
| IRP | iron regulatory proten |
| KO | knockout |
| KTZ | ketoconazole |

| | |
|---|---|
| LA-ICP-MS | laser ablation inductively coupled plasma mass spectrometry |
| LC | liquid chromatography |
| LC-ESI-MS | liquid chromatography–electrospray ionization–mass spectrometry |
| Lcn2 | lipocalin 2 |
| Lf | lactoferrin |
| LIBS | laser-inseduced breakdown spectroscopy |
| LOD | limits of detection |
| LPS | lipopolysaccharide |
| MALDI-MS | matrix-assisted laser desorption ionization mass spectrometry |
| MctB | mycobacterial Cu transport protein B |
| MFP | membrane fusion protein |
| MIRAGE | metal isotope native radioautography in gel electrophesis |
| MRI | magnetic resonance imaging |
| MRP | multidrug resistance protein |
| MS | mass spectrometry |
| $MS^2$ | tandem mass spectroscopy |
| NAD | nicotine adenine dinucleotide |
| NanoSIMS | nano secondary ion mass spectrometry |
| NEAT | near iron transporter |
| (N)EXAFS-STXM | near edge X-ray absorption fine structure scanning transmission X-ray microscopy |
| NGAL | neutrophil gelatinase-associated lipocalin |
| NHANES | National Health and Nutrition Examination Survey |
| NK cell | natural killer cell |
| NMR | nuclear magnetic resonance |
| NOS | nitric oxide synthases |
| NRAMP | natural resistance-associated macrophage protein |
| NTD | neglected tropic disease |
| OMF | outer membrane factor |
| PALM | photoactivated localization microscopy |
| PDTC | pyridine-2,6-bis(thiocarboxylic acid) |
| PET | positron emission tomography |
| PLGA | polylactic-co-glycolic acid |
| RDA | recommended dietary allowance |
| RDI | recommended daily intake or reference daily intake |
| RicR | regulated-in Cu repressor |
| RND | resistance-nodulation-cell division |
| RPLC | reverse phase liquid chromatography |
| Sbi | staphylococcal immunoglobulin G-binding protein |
| SDS-PAGE | sodium dodecyl sulfate–polyacrylamide gel electrophoresis |
| SEC | size exclusion chromatography |
| SEM-EDX | scanning electron microscopy energy dispersive X-ray analysis |
| SIMS | secondary ion mass spectrometry |
| S-μXRF | synchrotron micro X-ray fluorescence |
| SOD | superoxide dismutase |
| SNP | single nucleotide polymorphism |
| SpA | protein A |

| SPECT | single photon emission computed tomography |
| SPION | superparamagnetic iron oxide nanoparticles |
| SR-XRF | synchrotron radiation X-ray fluorescence |
| STED | stimulated emission depletion (laser fluorescence microscopy) |
| STIM | scanning transmission ion microscopy |
| STORM | stochastic optical reconstruction microscopy |
| STXM | scanning transmission X-ray microscopy |
| 2D-PAGE | two-dimensional polyacrylamide gel electrophoresis |
| TCA | tricarboxylic acide |
| TEM | transmission electron microscopy |
| Tf | transferrin |
| TfR | transferring receptor |
| Th | thymus helper |
| TLR-4 | Toll-like receptor 4 |
| TNF | tumor necrosis factor |
| ToF | time-of-flight |
| TTP | tri-tolyl phosphate |
| UIL | upper intake level |
| UPEC | uropathogenic *E. coli* |
| XRF | X-ray fluorescence |
| XRM | X-ray fluorescence microprobe |
| Ybt | yersiniabactin |

# Bibliography

Note: Numbers in square brackets denote the chapter in which an entry is cited.

Abergel, R. J., M. C. Clifton, J. C. Pizarro, et al. 2008. The Siderocalin/Enterobactin Interaction: A Link between Mammalian Immunity and Bacterial Iron Transport. *J. Am. Chem. Soc.* **130**:11524–11534. [3]

Abramovich, M., A. Miller, H. Yang, and J. K. Friel. 2011. Molybdenum Content of Canadian and U.S. Infant Formulas. *Biol. Trace Elem. Res.* **143**:844–853. [11]

Abu-Kwaik, Y., and D. Bumann. 2013. Microbial Quest for Food *in Vivo*: "Nutritional Virulence" as an Emerging Paradigm. *Cell. Microbiol.* **15**:882–890. [1]

Achard, M. E., S. L. Stafford, N. J. Bokil, et al. 2012. Copper Redistribution in Murine Macrophages in Response to *Salmonella* Infection. *Biochem. J.* **444**:51–57. [7]

Ackland, M. L., and A. Michalczyk. 2006. Zinc Deficiency and Its Inherited Disorders: A Review. *Genes Nutr.* **1**:41–49. [7]

Adamzik, M., T. Hamburger, F. Petrat, et al. 2012. Free Hemoglobin Concentration in Severe Sepsis: Methods of Measurement and Prediction of Outcome. *Crit. Care* **16**:R125. [13]

Adlard, P. A., R. A. Cherny, D. I. Finkelstein, et al. 2008. Rapid Restoration of Cognition in Alzheimer's Transgenic Mice with 8-Hydroxy Quinoline Analogs Is Associated with Decreased Interstitial Aβ. *Neuron* **59**:43–55. [6]

Afridi, H. I., T. G. Kazi, N. Kazi, et al. 2008. Evaluation of Status of Toxic Metals in Biological Samples of Diabetes Mellitus Patients. *Diabetes Res. Clin. Pract.* **80**:280–288. [12]

Afridi, H. I., T. G. Kazi, F. N. Talpur, et al. 2014. Evaluation of Chromium and Manganese in Biological Samples (Scalp Hair, Blood and Urine) of Tuberculosis and Diarrhea Male Human Immunodeficiency Virus Patients. *Clin. Lab.* **60**:1333–1341. [11]

Aggett, P. J. 1991. The Assessment of Zinc Status: A Personal View. *Proc. Nutr. Soc.* **50**:9–17. [17]

Aguiar, A. C., E. M. Rocha, N. B. Souza, T. C. Franca, and A. U. Krettli. 2012. New Approaches in Antimalarial Drug Discovery and Development: A Review. *Mem. Inst. Oswaldo Cruz* **107**:831–845. [10]

Aguirre, J. D., H. M. Clark, M. McIlvin, et al. 2013. A Manganese-Rich Environment Supports Superoxide Dismutase Activity in a Lyme Disease Pathogen, *Borrelia burgdorferi*. *J. Biol. Chem.* **288**:8468–8478. [20]

Ahmed, M. F., S. A. J. Shamsuddin, S. G. Mahmud, et al. 2005. Risk Assessment of Arsenic Mitigation Options (RAAMO). Arsenic Policy Support Unit (APSU), Ministry of Local Government, Rural Development and Cooperatives, Government of Bangladesh, Dhaka. http://www.buet.ac.bd/itn/pages/apsudocs/rammo_full_document.pdf. (accessed April 15, 2013). [17]

Ahokas, R. A., P. V. Dilts, Jr., and E. B. LaHaye. 1980. Cadmium-Induced Fetal Growth Retardation: Protective Effect of Excess Dietary Zinc. *Am. J. Obstet. Gynecol.* **136**:216–221. [8]

Ahrends, R., S. Pieper, A. Kuhn, et al. 2007. A Metal-Coded Affinity Tag Approach to Quantitative Proteomics. *Mol. Cell. Proteomics* **6**:1907–1916. [18]

*Bibliography*

Akerman, M. P., O. Q. Munro, M. Mongane, et al. 2013. Biodistribution (as Determined by the Radiolabelled Equivalent) of a Gold(III) Bis(Pyrrolide-Imine) Schiff Base Complex: A Potential Chemotherapeutic. *J. Labelled Comp. Radiopharm.* **56**:530–535. [20]

Akesson, A., M. Berglund, A. Schutz, et al. 2002. Cadmium Exposure in Pregnancy and Lactation in Relation to Iron Status. *Am. J. Public Health* **92**:284–287. [11]

Akhtar, S. 2013. Zinc Status in South Asian Populations: An Update. *J. Health Popul. Nutr.* **31**:139–149. [7]

Al Bayati, M. A., O. G. Raabe, and S. V. Teague. 1992. Effect of Inhaled Dimethylselenide in Fisher 344 Male Rat. *J. Toxicol. Environ. Health* **37**:549–557. [14]

Alessio, E. 2011. Bioinorganic Medicinal Chemistry. Weinheim: Wiley-VCH. [10]

Alisjahbana, B., E. Sahiratmadja, E. J. Nelwan, et al. 2007. The Effect of Type 2 Diabetes Mellitus on the Presentation and Treatment Response of Pulmonary Tuberculosis. *Clin. Infect. Dis.* **45**:428–435. [12]

Allard, K. A., J. Dao, P. Sanjeevaiah, et al. 2009. Purification of Legiobactin and the Importance of This Siderophore in Lung Infection by *Legionella pneumophila.* *Infect. Immun.* **77**:2887–2895. [3]

Allen, L. H. 2002. Iron Supplements: Scientific Issues Concerning Efficacy and Implications for Research and Programs. *J. Nutr.* **132**:813S–819S. [8]

Al-Sid-Cheikh, M., C. Rouleau, and E. Pelletier. 2013. Tissue Distribution and Kinetics of Dissolved and Nanoparticulate Silver in Iceland Scallop (*Chlamys islandica*). *Mar. Environ. Res.* **86**:21–28. [20]

Altuvia, S., M. Almiron, G. Huisman, R. Kolter, and G. Storz. 1994. The *Dps* Promoter Is Activated by OxyR During Growth and by IHF and Sigma S in Stationary Phase. *Mol. Microbiol.* **13**:265–272. [5]

Amar, S., Q. Zhou, Y. Shaik-Dasthagirisaheb, and S. Leeman. 2007. Diet-Induced Obesity in Mice Causes Changes in Immune Responses and Bone Loss Manifested by Bacterial Challenge. *PNAS* **104**:20466–20471. [12]

An, Y. H., and R. J. Friedman. 1998. Concise Review of Mechanisms of Bacterial Adhesion to Biomaterial Surfaces. *J. Biomed. Mater. Res.* **43**:338–348. [16]

Anaya, D. A., and E. P. Dellinger. 2006. The Obese Surgical Patient: A Susceptible Host for Infection. *Surg. Infect.* **7**:473–480. [12]

Anbar, A. D. 2008. Elements and Evolution. *Science* **322**:1481–1483. [5]

Anderson, J. E., M. M. Hobbs, G. D. Biswas, and P. F. Sparling. 2003. Opposing Selective Forces for Expression of the Gonococcal Lactoferrin Receptor. *Mol. Microbiol.* **48**:1325–1337. [2]

Anderson, R. A. 1995. Chromium and Parenteral Nutrition. *Nutrition* **11**:83–86. [8]

———. 1997. Nutritional Factors Influencing the Glucose/Insulin System: Chromium. *J. Am. Coll. Nutr.* **16**:404–410. [8]

Ando, N., E. J. Brignole, C. M. Zimanyi, et al. 2011. Structural Interconversions Modulate Activity of *Escherichia coli* Ribonucleotide Reductase. *PNAS* **108**:21046–21051. [4]

Andreini, C., L. Banci, I. Bertini, and A. Rosato. 2006a. Counting the Zinc-Proteins Encoded in the Human Genome. *J. Proteome Res.* **5**:196–201. [12]

———. 2006b. Zinc through the Three Domains of Life. *J. Proteome Res.* **5**:3173–3178. [5]

Andreini, C., I. Bertini, and G. Cavallaro. 2011. Minimal Functional Sites Allow a Classification of Zinc Sites in Proteins. *PLoS One* **6**:e26325. [4]

Andreini, C., I. Bertini, G. Cavallaro, G. L. Holliday, and J. M. Thornton. 2008. Metal Ions in Biological Catalysis: From Enzyme Databases to General Principles. *J. Biol. Chem.* **13**:1205–1218. [4, 18]

————. 2009. Metal-Macie: A Database of Metals Involved in Biological Catalysis. *Bioinformatics* **25**:2088–2089. [4]

Andreini, C., G. Cavallaro, S. Lorenzini, and A. Rosato. 2012. MetalPDB: A Database of Metal Sites in Biological Mactromolecular Structures. *Nucl. Acids Res.* **41**:D312–D319. [18]

————. 2013. MetalPDB: A Database of Metal Sites in Biological Macromolecular Structures. *Nucl. Acids Res.* **41**:D312–319. [20]

Andrew, J. P., M. Korbas, G. N. George, and J. Gailer. 2007. Reversed-Phase High-Performance Liquid Chromatographic Separation of Inorganic Mercury and Methylmercury Driven by Their Different Coordination Chemistry Towards Thiols. *J. Chromatogr. A* **1156**:331–339. [14]

Andrews, N. C. 1999. Disorders of Iron Metabolism. *N. Engl. J. Med.* **341**:1986–1995. [8]

Andrews, S. C. 2010. The Ferritin-Like Superfamily: Evolution of the Biological Iron Storeman from a Rubrerythrin-Like Ancestor. *Biochim. Biophys. Acta* **1800**:691–705. [4]

Anjem, A., and J. A. Imlay. 2012. Mononuclear Iron Enzymes Are Primary Targets of Hydrogen Peroxide Stress. *J. Biol. Chem.* **287**:15544–15556. [4, 5, 7, 20]

Anjem, A., S. Varghese, and J. A. Imlay. 2009. Manganese Import Is a Key Element of the OxyR Response to Hydrogen Peroxide in *Escherichia coli. Mol. Microbiol.* **72**:844–858. [5, 20]

Anna, K., R. Biyyani, C. Veluru, and K. Mullen. 2009. Is Obesity a Risk Factor for Anemia? *Am. J. Gastroenterol.* **104**:S114. [12]

Anthony, A., G. J. Colurso, T. M. Bocan, and J. A. Doebler. 1984. Interferometric Analysis of Intrasection and Intersection Thickness Variability Associated with Cryostat Microtomy. *Histochem. J.* **16**:61–70. [19]

Anton, A., C. Große, J. Reißmann, T. Pribyl, and D. H. Nies. 1999. CzcD Is a Heavy Metal Ion Transporter Involved in Regulation of Heavy Metal Resistance in *Ralstonia* sp. Strain CH34. *J. Bacteriol.* **181**:6876–6881. [4]

Apostoli, P., and S. Catalani. 2011. Metal Ions Affecting Reproduction and Development. *Met. Ions. Life Sci.* **8**:263–303. [8]

Appia-Ayme, C., A. Hall, E. Patrick, et al. 2012. Zrap Is a Periplasmic Molecular Chaperone and a Repressor of the Zinc-Responsive Two-Component Regulator Zrasr. *Biochem. J.* **442**:85–93. [5]

Archibald, F. 1983. *Lactobacillus plantarum*, an Organism Not Requiring Iron. *FEMS Microbiology Letters* **19**:29–32. [5]

Archibald, F., and I. Fridovich. 1981. Manganese and Defenses against Oxygen Toxicity in *Lactobacillus plantarum. J. Bacteriol.* **145**:442–451. [5]

Arguello, J. M., D. Raimunda, and T. Padilla-Benavides. 2013. Mechanisms of Copper Homeostasis in Bacteria. *Front. Cell. Infect. Microbiol.* **3**:73. [4, 5]

Arita, A., and M. Costa. 2009. Epigenetics in Metal Carcinogenesis: Nickel, Arsenic, Chromium and Cadmium. *Metallomics* **1**:222–228. [17]

Arnich, N., V. Sirot, G. Riviere, et al. 2012. Dietary Exposure to Trace Elements and Health Risk Assessment in the 2nd French Total Diet Study. *Food Chem. Toxicol.* **50**:2432–2449. [11]

Arrieta, M. C., and B. B. Finlay. 2012. The Commensal Microbiota Drives Immune Homeostasis. *Front. Immunol.* **3**:33. [7]

Arsenault, J. E., P. J. Havel, D. López de Romaña, et al. 2007. Longitudinal Measures of Circulating Leptin and Ghrelin Concentrations Are Associated with the Growth of Young Peruvian Children but Are Not Affected by Zinc Supplementation. *Am. J. Clin. Nutr.* **86**:1111–1119. [12]

Arslan, E., H. Atilgan, and I. Yavasoglu. 2009. The Prevalence of *Helicobacter pylori* in Obese Subjects. *Eur. J. Int. Med.* **20**:695–697. [12]

Aschner, J. L., and M. Aschner. 2005. Nutritional Aspects of Manganese Homeostasis. *Mol. Aspects Med.* **26**:353–362. [17]

Aschner, M., K. M. Erikson, E. H. Hernandez, and R. Tjalkens. 2009. Manganese and Its Role in Parkinson's Disease: From Transport to Neuropathology. *Neuromol. Med.* **11**:252–266. [13]

Aschner, M., and M. Gannon. 1994. Manganese (Mn) Transport across the Rat Blood-Brain Barrier: Saturable and Transferrin-Dependent Transport Mechanisms. *Brain Res. Bull.* **33**:345–349. [3, 13]

Ascone, I., and R. Strange. 2009. Biological X-Ray Absorption Spectroscopy and Metalloproteomics. *J. Synchrotron Rad.* **16**:413–421. [18]

Asmuss, M., L. H. Mullenders, and A. Hartwig. 2000. Interference by Toxic Metal Compounds with Isolated Zinc Finger DNA Repair Proteins. *Toxicol. Lett.* **112**–**113**:227–231. [11]

Ausk, K. J., and G. N. Ioannou. 2008. Is Obesity Associated with Anemia of Chronic Disease? A Population-Based Study. *Obesity* **16**:2356–2361. [12]

Autenrieth, I., K. Hantke, and J. Heesemann. 1991. Immunosuppression of the Host and Delivery of Iron to the Pathogen: A Possible Dual Role of Siderophores in the Pathogenesis of Microbial Infections. *Med. Microbiol. Immunol.* **180**:135–141. [3]

Autenrieth, I. B., E. Bohn, J. H. Ewald, and J. Heesemann. 1995. Deferoxamine B but Not Deferoxamine G1 Inhibits Cytokine Production in Murine Bone Marrow Macrophages. *J. Infect. Dis.* **172**:490–496. [3]

Au-Yeung, H. Y., J. Chan, T. Chantarojsiri, and C. J. Chan. 2013. Molecular Imaging of Labile Iron(II) Pools in Living Cells with a Turn-on Fluorescent Probe. *J. Am. Chem. Soc.* **135**:15165–15173. [20]

Ayres, J. S., and D. S. Schneider. 2009. The Role of Anorexia in Resistance and Tolerance to Infections in *Drosophila*. *PLoS Biol.* **7**:e1000150. [17]

———. 2012. Tolerance of Infections. *Annu. Rev. Immunol.* **30**:271–294. [1, 17]

Bachman, M. A., S. Lenio, L. Schmidt, J. E. Oyler, and J. N. Weiser. 2012. Interaction of Lipocalin 2, Transferrin, and Siderophores Determines the Replicative Niche of *Klebsiella pneumoniae* During Pneumonia. *MBio* **3**:e00224–00211. [3, 7]

Bachman, M. A., V. L. Miller, and J. N. Weiser. 2009. Mucosal Lipocalin 2 Has Pro-Inflammatory and Iron-Sequestering Effects in Response to Bacterial Enterobactin. *PLoS Pathog.* **5**:e1000622. [3]

Bachman, M. A., J. E. Oyler, S. H. Burns, et al. 2011. *Klebsiella pneumoniae* Yersiniabactin Promotes Respiratory Tract Infection through Evasion of Lipocalin 2. *Infect. Immun.* **79**:3309–3316. [3, 7]

Backhed, F., J. K. Manchester, C. F. Semenkovich, and J. I. Gordon. 2007. Mechanisms Underlying the Resistance to Diet-Induced Obesity in Germ-Free Mice. *PNAS* **104**:979–984. [12]

Bahde, R., S. Kapoor, K. K. Bhargava, et al. 2012. PET with [64]Cu-Histidine for Noninvasive Diagnosis of Biliary Copper Excretion in Long-Evans Cinnamon Rat Model of Wilson Disease. *J. Nucl. Med.* **53**:961–968. [20]

Baillie, J. K. 2014. Targeting the Host Immune Response to Fight Infection. *Science* **344**:807–808. [1]

Baiocco, P., A. Ilari, P. Ceci, et al. 2011. Inhibitory Effect of Silver Nanoparticles on Trypanothione Reductase Activity and Leishmania Infantum Proliferation. *ACS Med. Chem. Lett.* **2**:230–233. [10]

Baker-Austin, C., M. S. Wright, R. Stepanauskas, and J. V. McArthur. 2006. Co-Selection of Antibiotic and Metal Resistance. *Trends Microbiol.* **14**:176–182. [4, 17]

Balazs, D. J., K. Triandafillu, P. Wood, et al. 2004. Inhibition of Bacterial Adhesion on PVC Endotracheal Tubes by RF-Oxygen Glow Discharge, Sodium Hydroxide and Silver Nitrate Treatments. *Biomaterials* **25**:2139–2151. [16]

Baltaci, A. K., R. Mogulkoc, and I. Halifeoglu. 2005. Effects of Zinc Deficiency and Supplementation on Plasma Leptin Levels in Rats. *Biol. Trace Elem. Res.* **104**:41–46. [12]

Baltes, N., I. Hennig-Pauka, and G. F. Gerlach. 2002. Both Transferrin Binding Proteins Are Virulence Factors in *Actinobacillus pleuropneumoniae* Serotype 7 Infection. *FEMS Microbiol. Lett.* **209**:283–287. [2]

Banci, L. 2013. Metallomics and the Cell, vol. 12. Metal Ions in Life Sciences. New York: Springer. [4]

Banci, L., I. Bertini, S. Ciofi-Baffoni, et al. 2010. Affinity Gradients Drive Copper to Cellular Destinations. *Nature* **465**:645–648. [20]

Banerjee, R., and S. W. Ragsdale. 2003. The Many Faces of Vitamin B12: Catalysis by Cobalamin-Dependent Enzymes. *Annu. Rev. Biochem.* **72**:209–247. [2, 8]

Banerjee, S., A. K. Nandyala, P. Raviprasad, N. Ahmed, and S. E. Hasnain. 2007. Iron-Dependent RNA-Binding Activity of *Mycobacterium tuberculosis* Aconitase. *J. Bacteriol.* **189**:4046–4052. [5]

Bao, G., M. C. Clifton, T. M. Hoette, et al. 2010a. Iron Traffics in Circulation Bound to a Siderocalin (NGAL)-Catechol Complex. *Nat. Chem. Biol.* **6**:602–609. [3]

Bao, S., M. J. Liu, B. Lee, et al. 2010b. Zinc Modulates the Innate Immune Response *in Vivo* to Polymicrobial Sepsis through Regulation of NFκB. *Am. J. Physiol. Lung Cell. Mol. Physiol.* **298**:L744–754. [12]

Baqui, A. H., R. E. Black, S. El Arifeen, et al. 2002. Effect of Zinc Supplementation Started During Diarrhea on Morbidity and Mortality in Bangladeshi Children: Community Randomised Trial. *Br. Med. J.* **325**:1059. [13]

Baran, E. J. 2004. Trace Elements Supplementation: Recent Advances and Perspectives. *Mini Rev. Med. Chem.* **4**:1–9. [8]

Barba-Gutierrez, Y., B. Adenso-Diaz, and M. Hop. 2008. An Analysis of Some Environmental Consequences of European Electrical and Electronic Waste Regulations. *Res. Conserv. Recycl.* **52**:481–495. [15]

Barceloux, D. G. 1999. Cobalt. *J. Toxicol. Clin. Toxicol.* **37**:201–206. [8]

Basaki, M., M. Saeb, S. Nazifi, and H. A. Shamsaei. 2012. Zinc, Copper, Iron, and Chromium Concentrations in Young Patients with Type 2 Diabetes Mellitus. *Biol. Trace Elem. Res.* **148**:161–164. [12]

Basnet, S., M. Mathisen, and T. A. Strand. 2014. Oral Zinc and Common Childhood Infections: An Update. *J. Trace Elem. Med. Biol.* doi: 10.1016/j.jtemb.2014.1005.1006. [Epub ahead of print]. [8]

Bauer, R., E. Brummerstedt, M. Jensen, H. Mejborn, and M. Smith. 1992. Reduced Rate of Uptake of Zinc Ions in a Calf Affected with the Lethal Syndrome A46 Relative to Clinically Normal Calves Using Whole Body Radio-Isotope Scanning of 62Zn. *APMIS* **100**:347–352. [20]

Baum, M. K., A. Campa, S. Lai, et al. 2013. Effect of Micronutrient Supplementation on Disease Progression in Asymptomatic, Antiretroviral-Naive, HIV-Infected Adults in Botswana: A Randomized Clinical Trial. *JAMA* **310**:2154–2163. [11]

Baum, M. K., S. Lai, S. Sales, J. B. Page, and A. Campa. 2010. Randomized, Controlled Clinical Trial of Zinc Supplementation to Prevent Immunological Failure in HIV-Infected Adults. *Clin. Infect. Dis.* **50**:1653–1660. [8]

Bayram, E., Y. Topcu, P. Karakaya, et al. 2013. Molybdenum Cofactor Deficiency: Review of 12 Cases (MoCD and Review). *Eur. J. Paediatr. Neurol.* **17**:1–6. [8]

Beard, S. J., R. Hashim, G. Wu, et al. 2000. Evidence for the Transport of Zinc(II) Ions via the Pit Inorganic Phosphate Transport System in *Escherichia coli. FEMS Microbiol. Lett.* **184**:231–235. [5]

Beasley, F. C., C. L. Marolda, J. Cheung, S. Buac, and D. E. Heinrichs. 2011. *Staphylococcus aureus* Transporters Hts, Sir, and Sst Capture Iron Liberated from Human Transferrin by Staphyloferrin a, Staphyloferrin B, and Catecholamine Stress Hormones, Respectively, and Contribute to Virulence. *Infect. Immun.* **79**:2345–2355. [2]

Beck, M. A., P. C. Kolbeck, Q. Shi, et al. 1994. Increased Virulence of a Human Enterovirus (Coxsackievirus B3) in Selenium-Deficient Mice. *J. Infect. Dis.* **170**:351–357. [17]

Beck, M. A., O. A. Levander, and J. Handy. 2003. Selenium Deficiency and Viral Infection. *J. Nutr.* **133**:1463S–1467S. [13]

Becker, J. S. 2007. Inorganic Mass Spectrometry: Principles and Applications. Chichester: John Wiley and Sons. [19, 20]

———. 2013. Imaging of Metals in Biological Tissue by Laser Ablation Inductively Coupled Plasma Mass Spectrometry (LA-ICP-MS): State of the Art and Future Developments. *J. Mass Spectrom.* **48**:255–268. [20]

Becker, J. S., U. Breuer, H. F. Hsieh, et al. 2010. Bioimaging of Metals and Biomolecules in Mouse Heart by Laser Ablation Inductively Coupled Plasma Mass Spectrometry and Secondary Ion Mass Spectrometry. *Anal. Chem.* **82**:9528–9533. [19]

Becker, J. S., M. Zoriy, U. Krause-Buchholz, et al. 2004. In-Gel Screening of Phosphorus and Copper, Zinc and Iron in Proteins of Yeast Mitochondria by LA-ICP-MS and Identification of Phosphorylated Protein Structures by MALDI-FT-ICR-MS after Seperation with Two-Dimentional Gel-Electrophoresis. *J. Anal. At. Spectrom.* **19**:1236–1243. [18]

Bednorz, C., S. Guenther, K. Oelgeschläger, et al. 2013. Feeding the Probiotic *Enterococcus faecium* Strain NCIMB 10415 to Piglets Specifically Reduces the Number of *Escherichia coli* Pathotypes Adherent to the Gut Mucosa. *Appl. Environ. Microbiol.* **79**:7896–7904. [17]

Beers, M. H., and R. Berkow, eds. 1999. The Merck Manual of Diagnosis and Therapy. Whitehouse Station, NJ: Merck Research Laboratories. [20]

Behne, D., C. Weiss-Nowak, M. Kalcklosch, et al. 1994. Application of Nuclear Analytical Methods in the Investigation and Identification of New Selenoproteins. *Biol. Trace Elem. Res.* **43-45**:287–297. [20]

Beisel, W. R. 1998. Metabolic Response of the Host to Infections. In: Textbook of Pediatric Infectious Disease, ed. R. D. Feigin and J. D. Cherry, pp. 54–56. Philadelphia: W. B. Saunders. [17]

Belbraouet, S., H. Biaudet, A. Tébi, et al. 2007. Serum Zinc and Copper Status in Hospitalized vs. Healthy Elderly Subjects. *J. Am. Coll. Nutr.* **26**:650–654. [8]

Belcher, J. D., C. Chen, J. Nguyen, et al. 2014. Heme Triggers TLR4 Signaling Leading to Endothelial Cell Activation and Vaso-Occlusion in Murine Sickle Cell Disease. *Blood* **123**:377–390. [13]

Belmonte, N., O. Rivera, and J. Herkovits. 1989. Zinc Protection against Cadmium Effects of Preimplantation Mice Embryos. *Bull. Environ. Contam. Toxicol.* **45**:107–110. [14]

Ben-Bassat, A., K. Bauer, S. Y. Chang, et al. 1987. Processing of the Initiation Methionine from Proteins: Properties of the *Escherichia coli* Methionine Aminopeptidase and Its Gene Structure. *J. Bacteriol.* **169**:751–757. [4]

Bengmark, S. 2013. Gut Microbiota, Immune Development and Function. *Pharmacol. Res.* **69**:87–113. [17]

Benítez, J., I. Correia, L. Becco, et al. 2013. Searching for Vanadium-Based Prospective Agents against *Trypanosoma cruzi*: Oxidovanadium(IV) Compounds with Phenanthroline Derivatives as Ligands. *Z. Anorg. Allg. Chem.* **639**:1417–1425. [10]

Berg, J. M. 1988. Proposed Structure for the Zinc-Binding Domains from Transcription Factor IIIA and Related Proteins. *PNAS* **85**:99–102. [20]

Berglund, M., A. Akesson, B. Nermell, and M. Vahter. 1994. Intestinal Absorption of Dietary Cadmium in Women Depends on Body Iron Stores and Fiber Intake. *Environ. Health Perspect.* **102**:1058–1066. [11]

Berhane, K., M. Widersten, A. Engstrom, J. W. Kozarich, and B. Mannervik. 1994. Detoxication of Base Propenals and Other Unsaturated Aldehyde Products of Radical Reactions and Lipid Peroxidation by Human Glutathione Transferases. *PNAS* **91**:1480–1484. [17]

Berni, C. R., V. Buccigrossi, and A. Passariello. 2011. Mechanisms of Action of Zinc in Acute Diarrhea. *Curr. Opin. Gastroenterol.* **27**:8–12. [8]

Bhargava, P., and R. Singh. 2012. Developments in Diagnosis and Antileishmanial Drugs. Article Id 626838. *Interdiscip. Perspect. Infect. Dis.* http://www.hindawi.com/journals/ipid/2012/626838/. (accessed Sept. 30, 2014). [10]

Bhutta, Z. A., R. A. Salam, and J. K. Das. 2013. Meeting the Challenges of Micronutrient Malnutrition in the Developing World. *Br. Med. Bull.* **106**:7–17. [7]

Bierer, B. E., and D. G. Nathan. 1990. The Effect of Desferrithiocin, an Oral Iron Chelator, on T-Cell Function. *Blood* **76**:2052–2059. [3]

Biot, C., W. Castro, C. Y. Botté, and M. Navarro. 2012. The Therapeutic Potential of Metal-Based Antimalarial Agents: Implications for the Mechanism of Action. *Dalton Trans.* **41**:6335–6349. [10, 13]

Birner, R., S. A. Kone, N. Linacre, and D. Resnick. 2007. Biofortified Foods and Crops in West Africa: Mali and Burkina Faso. *AgBioForum* **10**:192–200. [17]

Bishayi, B., and M. Sengupta. 2006. Synergism in Immunotoxicological Effects Due to Repeated Combined Administration of Arsenic and Lead in Mice. *Int. Immunopharmacol.* **6**:454–464. [17]

Bjermo, H., S. Sand, C. Nalsen, et al. 2013. Lead, Mercury, and Cadmium in Blood and Their Relation to Diet among Swedish Adults. *Food Chem. Toxicol.* **57**:161–169. [11]

Bjornsdottir, S., M. Gottfredsson, A. S. Thorisdottir, et al. 2005. Risk Factors for Acute Cellulitis of the Lower Limb: A Prospective Case-Control Study. *Clin. Infect. Dis.* **41**:1416–1422. [12]

Black, R. E., H. A. Lindsay, Z. A. Bhutta, et al. 2008. Maternal and Child Undernutrition: Global and Regional Exposures and Health Consequences. *Lancet* **371**:243–260. [17]

Black, R. E., C. G. Victora, S. P. Walker, et al. 2013. Maternal and Child Undernutrition and Overweight in Low-Income and Middle-Income Countries. *Lancet* **382**:427–451. [8]

Blackwell, J. M., T. Goswami, C. A. Evans, et al. 2001. SLC11A1 (Formerly NRAMP1) and Disease Resistance. *Cell. Microbiol.* **3**:773–874. [6, 9, 13]

Blanusa, M., N. Ivicic, and V. Simeon. 1990. Lead, Iron, Copper, Zinc and Ash in Deciduous Teeth in Relation to Age and Distance from a Lead Smelter. *Bull. Environ. Contam. Toxicol.* **50**:724–729. [17]

Blasberg, R. G., U. Roelcke, R. Weinreich, et al. 2000. Imaging Brain Tumor Proliferative Activity with [124I]Iododeoxyuridine. *Cancer Res.* **60**:624–635. [20]

Bloom, M. S., E. F. Fitzgerald, K. Kim, I. Neamtiu, and E. S. Gurzau. 2010. Spontaneous Pregnancy Loss in Humans and Exposure to Arsenic in Drinking Water. *Int. J. Hyg. Environ. Health* **213**:401–413. [8]

Boden, G., X. Chen, J. Ruiz, G. D. van Rossum, and S. Turco. 1996. Effects of Vanadyl Sulfate on Carbohydrate and Lipid Metabolism in Patients with Non-Insulin-Dependent Diabetes Mellitus. *Metabolism* **45**:1130–1135. [11]

Bodwell, J. E., J. A. Gosse, A. P. Nomikos, and J. W. Hamilton. 2006. Arsenic Disruption of Steroid Receptor Gene Activation: Complex Dose-Response Effects Are Shared by Several Steroid Receptors. *Chem. Res. Toxicol.* **19**:1619–1629. [12]

Boelaert, J. R., S. J. Vandecasteele, R. Appelberg, and V. R. Gordeuk. 2007. The Effect of the Host's Iron Status on Tuberculosis. *J. Infect. Dis.* **195**:1745–1753. [6]

Bogaert, D., A. van Belkum, M. Sluijter, et al. 2004. Colonisation by *Streptococcus pneumoniae* and *Staphylococcus aureus* in Healthy Children. *Lancet* **363**:1871–1872. [3]

Boonstra, H., J. W. Oosterhuis, A. M. Oosterhuis, and G. J. Fleuren. 1983. Cervical Tissue Shrinkage by Formaldehyde Fixation, Paraffin Wax Embedding, Section Cutting and Mounting. *Virchows Arch. A. Pathol. Anat. Histopathol.* **402**:195–201. [19]

Boosz, B., C. Davis, and D. Malamud. 1983. Comparison of Saliva- and Zn-Mediated Bacterial Aggregation. *J. Dent. Res.* **62A**:226. [17]

Bornhorst, J., S. Meyer, T. Weber, et al. 2013. Molecular Mechanisms of Mn-Induced Neurotoxicity: Rons Generation, Genotoxicity, and DNA-Damage Response. *Mol. Nutr. Food Res.* **57**:1255–1269. [17]

Borresen, E. C., and E. P. Ryan. 2014. Rice Bran: A Food Ingredient with Global Public Health Opportunity. In: Wheat and Rice in Disease Prevention and Health, ed. R. R. Watson et al., pp. 301–310. Oxford: Elsevier. [17]

Botella, H., P. Peyron, F. Levillain, et al. 2011. Mycobacterial $P_1$-Type ATPases Mediate Resistance to Zinc Poisoning in Human Macrophages. *Cell Host Microbe* **10**:248–259. [7]

Botella, H., G. Stadthagen, G. Lugo-Villarino, C. de Chastellier, and O. Neyrolles. 2012. Metallobiology of Host–Pathogen Interactions: An Intoxicating New Insight. *Trends Microbiol.* **20**:106–112. [3, 9]

Bou-Abdallah, F., H. Yang, A. Awomolo, et al. 2014. Functionality of the Three-Site Ferroxidase Center of *Escherichia coli* Bacterial Ferritin (EcFtnA). *Biochemistry* **53**:483–495. [4]

Bouchard, M., F. Laforest, L. Vandelac, D. Bellinger, and D. Mergler. 2007. Hair Manganese and Hyperactive Behaviors: Pilot Study of School-Age Children Exposed through Tap Water. *Environ. Health Perspect.* **115**:122–127. [11]

Bouchard, M. F., S. Sauve, B. Barbeau, et al. 2011. Intellectual Impairment in School-Age Children Exposed to Manganese from Drinking Water. *Environ. Health Perspect.* **119**:138–143. [11]

Bouis, H. E. 2003. Micronutrient Fortification of Plants through Plant Breeding: Can It Improve Nutrition in Man at Low Cost? *Proc. Nutr. Soc.* **62**:403–411. [17]

Bouis, H. E., E. Boy-Gallego, and J. V. Meenakshi. 2012. Micronutrient Malnutrition: Prevalence, Consequences, and Interventions. In: Fertilizing Crops to Improve Human Health: A Scientific Review, vol. 1, Food and Nutrition Security, pp. 29–64. Norcross, GA: International Plant Nutrition Institute. [17]

Bowman, A. B., G. F. Kwakye, E. H. Hernandez, and M. Aschner. 2011. Role of Manganese in Neurodegenerative Diseases. *J. Trace Elem. Med. Biol.* **25**:25:191–203. [13]

Bowman, S. A., and B. T. Vinyard. 2004. Fast Food Consumption of U.S. Adults: Impact on Energy and Nutrient Intakes and Overweight Status. *J. Am. Coll. Nutr.* **23**:163–168. [17]

Bozym, R., T. K. Hurst, N. Westerberg, et al. 2008. Determination of Zinc Using Carbonic Anhydrase-Based Fluorescence Biosensors. *Methods Enzymol.* **450**:287–309. [20]

Bozym, R. A., R. B. Thompson, A. K. Stoddard, and C. A. Fierke. 2006. Measuring Picomolar Intracellular Exchangeable Zinc in PC-12 Cells Using a Ratiometric Fluorescence Biosensor. *ACS Chem. Biol.* **1**:103–111. [20]

Bradsher, K. 2010. After China's Rare Earth Embargo, a New Calculus. *New York Times*. Oct. 29, 2010. [15]

Brandel, J., N. Humbert, M. Elhabiri, et al. 2012. Pyochelin, a Siderophore of *Pseudomonas aeruginosa*: Physicochemical Characterization of the Iron(III), Copper(II) and Zinc(II) Complexes. *Dalton Trans.* **41**:2820–2834. [2]

Braud, A., V. Geoffroy, F. Hoegy, G. L. Mislin, and I. J. Schalk. 2010. Presence of the Siderophores Pyoverdine and Pyochelin in the Extracellular Medium Reduces Toxic Metal Accumulation in *Pseudomonas aeruginosa* and Increases Bacterial Metal Tolerance. *Environ. Microbiol. Rep.* **2**:419–425. [4]

Braydich-Stolle, L., S. Hussain, J. J. Schlager, and M. C. Hofmann. 2005. In Vitro Cytotoxicity of Nanoparticles in Mammalian Germline Stem Cells. *Toxicol. Sci.* **88**:412–419. [16]

Brayman, T. G., and R. P. Hausinger. 1996. Purification, Characterization, and Functional Analysis of a Truncated *Klebsiella aerogenes* Uree Urease Accessory Protein Lacking the Histidine-Rich Carboxyl Terminus. *J. Bacteriol.* **178**:5410–5416. [4]

Braymer, J. J., and D. P. Giedroc. 2014. Recent Developments in Copper and Zinc Homeostasis in Bacterial Pathogens. *Curr. Opin. Chem. Biol.* **19**:59–66. [20]

Brennan, R. F., and M. D. A. Bolland. 2006. Residual Values of Soil-Applied Zinc Fertilizer for Early Vegetative Growth of Six Crop Species. *Aust. J. Exp. Agr.* **46**:1341–1347. [17]

Brickman, T. J., and S. K. Armstrong. 2009. Temporal Signaling and Differential Expression of *Bordetella* Iron Transport Systems: The Role of Ferrimones and Positive Regulators. *Biometals* **22**:33–41. [7]

Brickman, T. J., T. Hanawa, M. T. Anderson, R. J. Suhadolc, and S. K. Armstrong. 2008. Differential Expression of *Bordetella pertussis* Iron Transport System Genes During Infection. *Mol. Microbiol.* **70**:3–14. [3]

Brickman, T. J., and M. A. McIntosh. 1992. Overexpression and Purification of Ferric Enterobactin Esterase from *Escherichia coli*. Demonstration of Enzymatic Hydrolysis of Enterobactin and Its Iron Complex. *J. Biol. Chem.* **267**:12350–12355. [5]

Brita, T. M., A. S. Karel, and R. J. Colin. 2006. Mechanisms of Chronic Water Borne Zn Toxicity in Daphniamagna. *Aquat. Toxicol.* **77**:393–401. [16]

Britigan, B. E., G. T. Rasmussen, and C. D. Cox. 1994. *Pseudomonas* Siderophore Pyochelin Enhances Neutrophil-Mediated Endothelial Cell Injury. *Am. J. Physiol.* **266**:L192–L198. [3]

———. 1997. Augmentation of Oxidant Injury to Human Pulmonary Epithelial Cells by the *Pseudomonas aeruginosa* Siderophore Pyochelin. *Infect. Immun.* **65**:1071–1076. [3]

Britigan, B. E., G. T. Rasmussen, O. Olakanmi, and C. D. Cox. 2000. Iron Acquisition from *Pseudomonas aeruginosa* Siderophores by Human Phagocytes: An Additional Mechanism of Host Defense through Iron Sequestration? *Infect. Immun.* **68**:1271–1275. [3]

Brocklehurst, K. R., J. L. Hobman, B. Lawley, et al. 1999. ZntR Is a Zn(II)-Responsive MerR-Like Transcriptional Regulator of *zntA* in *Escherichia coli. Mol. Microbiol.* **31**:893–902. [5]

Brooks, W. A., M. Santosham, A. Naheed, et al. 2005. Effect of Weekly Zinc Supplements on Incidence of Pneumonia and Diarrhoea in Children Younger Than 2 Years in an Urban, Low-Income Population in Bangladesh: Randomised Controlled Trial. *Lancet* **366**:999–1004. [3]

Brown, K. H., J. M. Peerson, S. K. Baker, and S. Y. Hess. 2009. Preventive Zinc Supplementation among Infants, Preschoolers, and Older Prepubertal Children. *Food Nutr. Bull.* **30**:S12–S44. [13]

Bruins, M. R., S. Kapil, and F. W. Oehme. 2000. Microbial Resistance to Metals in the Environment. *Ecotoxicol. Environ. Saf.* **45**:198–207. [4]

Brunst, K. J., Y. K. Leung, P. H. Ryan, et al. 2013. Forkhead Box Protein 3 (FOXP3) Hypermethylation Is Associated with Diesel Exhaust Exposure and Risk for Childhood Asthma. *J. Allergy Clin. Immunol.* **131**:592–594. [17]

Buchman, A. L. 2012. Manganese. In: Modern Nutrition in Health and Disease, ed. A. C. Ross et al., pp. 238–243, vol. 11. Philadelphia: Wolters Kluwer Health/Lippincott Williams & Wilkins. [8]

Buck, A., N. Nguyen, C. Burger, et al. 1996. Quantitative Evaluation of Manganese-52m as a Myocardial Perfusion Tracer in Pigs Using Positron Emission Tomography. *Eur. J. Nucl. Med.* **23**:1619–1627. [20]

Buckling, A., F. Harrison, M. Vos, et al. 2007. Siderophore-Mediated Cooperation and Virulence in *Pseudomonas aeruginosa. FEMS Microbiol. Ecol.* **62**:135–141. [3]

Buck Louis, G. M., and R. Sundaram. 2012. Exposome: Time for Transformative Research. *Stat. Med.* **31**:2569–2575. [17]

Buffie, C. G., and E. G. Pamer. 2013. Microbiota-Mediated Colonization Resistance against Intestinal Pathogens. *Nat. Rev. Immunol.* **13**:790–801. [7]

Bumgardner, J. D., P. Adatrow, W. O. Haggard, and P. A. Norowski. 2011. Emerging Antibacterial Biomaterial Strategies for the Prevention of Peri-Implant Inflammatory Diseases. *Int. J. Oral Maxillofac. Implants* **26**:553–560. [16]

Burdette, S. C., G. K. Walkup, B. Spingler, R. Y. Tsien, and S. J. Lippard. 2001. Fluorescent Sensors for $Zn^{2+}$ Based on a Fluorescein Platform: Synthesis, Properties and Intracellular Distribution. *J. Am. Chem. Soc.* **123**:7831–7841. [20]

Burguera, E., Z. Romero, M. Burguera, et al. 2002. Determination of Some Cationic Species in Temporary Teeth. *J. Trace Elem. Med. Biol.* **16**:103–112. [17]

Butterman, W. C., and J. F. Carlin, Jr. 2004. Mineral Commodity Profiles: Antimony. Open-File Report 03-019. U.S. Department of the Interior, U.S. Geological Survey. http://pubs.usgs.gov/of/2003/of03-019/of03-019.pdf. (accessed Oct. 10, 2014). [15]

Cabrera, A., E. Alonzo, E. Sauble, et al. 2008. Copper Binding Components of Blood Plasma and Organs, and Their Responses to Influx of Large Doses of (65)Cu, in the Mouse. *Biometals* 21:525–543. [8]

Cakmak, I., H. Wolfgang, W. H. Pfeiffer, and B. McClafferty. 2010. Biofortification of Durum Wheat with Zinc and Iron. *Cereal Chem.* 87:10–20. [17]

Calvano, S. E., W. Xiao, D. R. Richards, et al. 2005. A Network-Based Analysis of Systemic Inflammation in Humans. *Nature* 437:1032–1037. [12]

Campanale, M., E. Nucera, V. Ojetti, et al. 2014. Nickel Free-Diet Enhances the *Helicobacter pylori* Eradication Rate: A Pilot Study. *Dig. Dis. Sci.* 59:1851–1855. [11]

Cani, P. D., J. Amar, and M. A. Iglesias. 2007. Metabolic Endotoxemia Initiates Obesity and Insulin Resistance. *Diabetes* 56:1761–1772. [12]

Cannata, J. B., and J. L. Domingo. 1989. Aluminum Toxicity in Mammals: A Minireview. *Vet. Hum. Toxicol.* 31:577–583. [8]

Cao, D., P. A. Bromberg, and J. M. Samet. 2007. Cox-2 Expression Induced by Diesel Particles Involves Chromatin Modification and Degradation of Hdac1. *Am. J. Respir. Cell Mol. Biol.* 37:232–239. [17]

Cao, Y. A., A. J. Wagers, H. Karsunky, et al. 2008. Heme Oxygenase-1 Deficiency Leads to Disrupted Response to Acute Stress in Stem Cells and Progenitors. *Blood* 112:4494–4502. [20]

Carlton, B. D., M. B. Beneke, and G. L. Fisher. 1982. Assessment of the Teratogenicity of Ammonium Vanadate Using Syrian Golden Hamsters. *Environ. Res.* 29:256–262. [8]

Carrondo, M. A. 2003. Ferritins, Iron Uptake and Storage from the Bacterioferritin Viewpoint. *EMBO J.* 22:1959–1968. [4]

Cartron, M. L., S. Maddocks, P. Gillingham, and S. C. Andrews. 2006. Feo: Transport of Ferrous Iron into Bacteria. *Biometals* 19:143–157. [5]

Caruso, T. J., C. G. Prober, and J. M. Gwaltney, Jr. 2007. Treatment of Naturally Acquired Common Colds with Zinc: A Structured Review. *Clin. Infect. Dis.* 45:569–574. [8]

Caspi, R., T. Altman, J. M. Dale, et al. 2010. The MetaCyc Database of Metabolic Pathways and Enzymes and the BioCyc Collection of Pathway/Genome Databases. *Nucl. Acids Res.* 38:D473–D479. [18]

Cassat, J. E., and E. P. Skaar. 2013. Iron in Infection and Immunity. *Cell Host Microbe* 13:509–519. [7, 9]

Castagnetto, J. M., S. W. Hennessy, V. A. Roberts, et al. 2002. MDB: The Metalloprotein Database and Browser at the Scripps Research Institute. *Nucl. Acids Res.* 30:379–382. [4, 18, 20]

Castro-Gonzalez, M. I., and M. Mendez-Armenta. 2008. Heavy Metals: Implications Associated to Fish Consumption. *Environ. Toxicol. Pharmacol.* 26:263–271. [8]

Catherman, A. D., K. R. Durbin, D. R. Ahlf, et al. 2013. Large-Scale Top-Down Proteomics of the Human Proteome: Membrane Proteins, Mitochondria, and Senescence. *Mol. Cell. Proteomics* 12:3465–3473. [20]

Catling, D. C., and M. W. Claire. 2005. How Earth's Atmosphere Evolved to an Oxic State: A Status Report. *Earth Planetary Sci. Lett.* 237:1–20. [4]

Caulfield, L. E., and R. E. Black. 2004. Zinc Deficiency. In: Comparative Quantification of Health Risks Global and Regional Burden of Disease Attributable to Selected Major, ed. M. Ezzati et al. Geneva: WHO. [17]

Cavaco, L. M., M. Hasman, M. Stegger, et al. 2010. Cloning and Occurrence of czrC, a Gene Conferring Cadmium and Zinc Resistance in Methicillin-Resistant *Staphylococcus aureus* CC398 Isolates. *Antimicrob. Agents Chemother.* 54:3605–3608. [17]

Cavan, K. R., R. S. Gibson, C. F. Grazioso, et al. 1993. Growth and Body Composition of Periurban Guatemalan Children in Relation to Zinc Status: A Longitudinal Zinc Intervention Trial. *Am. J. Clin. Nutr.* **57**:344–352. [12]

Cefalu, W. T., J. Rood, P. Pinsonat, and J. Qin. 2010. Characterization of the Metabolic and Physiologic Response to Chromium Supplementation in Subjects with Type 2 Diabetes Mellitus. *Metabol. Clin. Exp.* **59**:755–762. [13]

Cellier, M. F. 2012. NRAMP: From Sequence to Structure and Mechanism of Divalent Metal Import. *Curr. Top. Membr.* **69**:249–293. [17]

Cellier, M. F., P. Courville, and C. Campion. 2007. NRAMP1 Phagocyte Intracellular Metal Withdrawal Defense. *Microbes Infect.* **9**:1662–1670. [7]

Chai, S. C., W.-L. Wang, and Q.-Z. Ye. 2008. Fe(II) Is the Native Cofactor for *Escherichia coli* Methionine Aminopeptidase. *J. Biol. Chem.* **283**:26879–26885. [4]

Chakraborti, D., M. K. Sengupta, M. M. Rahman, et al. 2004. Groundwater Arsenic Contamination and Its Health Effects in the Ganga-Meghna-Brahmaputra Plain. *J. Environ. Monit.* **6**:74N–83N. [8]

Chalfie, M., D. Prasher, and W. Ward. 1994. GFP as Expression Probe. *Science* **263**:802–805. [20]

Chambers, E. C., S. Heshka, D. Gallagher, et al. 2006. Serum Iron and Body Fat Distribution in a Multiethnic Cohort of Adults Living in New York City. *J. Am. Diet. Assoc.* **106**:680–684. [12]

Chan, Y. R., J. S. Liu, D. A. Pociask, et al. 2009. Lipocalin 2 Is Required for Pulmonary Host Defense against Klebsiella Infection. *J. Immunol.* **182**:4947–4956. [3]

Chancerel, P., C. E. M. Meskers, C. Hageluken, and V. S. Rotter. 2009. Assessment of Precious Metal Flows During Preprocessing of Waste Electrical and Electronic Equipment. *J. Indus. Ecol.* **13**:791–810. [15]

Chang, C. J., J. Jaworski, E. M. Nolan, M. Sheng, and S. J. Lippard. 2004. A Tautomeric Zinc Sensor for Ratiometric Fluorescence Imaging: Application to Nitric Oxide-Induced Release of Intracellular Zinc. *PNAS* **101**:1129–1134. [20]

Chang, L. W., ed. 1996. Toxicology of Metals, vol. 1. Boca Raton: CRC Press. [15]

Chang, L. W., P. R. Wade, J. G. Pounds, and K. R. Reuhl. 1980. Prenatal and Neonatal Toxicology and Pathology of Heavy Metals. *Adv. Pharmacol. Chemother.* **17**:195–231. [8]

Chang, S. Y., E. C. McGary, and S. Chang. 1989. Methionine Aminopeptidase Gene of *Escherichia coli* Is Essential for Cell Growth. *J. Bacteriol.* **171**:4071–4072. [4]

Changela, A., K. Chen, Y. Xue, et al. 2003. Molecular Basis of Metal-Ion Selectivity and Zeptomolar Sensitivity by Cuer. *Science* **301**:1383–1387. [4, 5]

Chao, Y., M. Makale, P. P. Karmali, et al. 2012. Recognition of Dextran-Superparamagnetic Iron Oxide Nanoparticle Conjugates (Feridex) via Macrophage Scavenger Receptor Charged Domains. *Bioconjugate Chem.* **23**:1003–1009. [17]

Chasapis, C. T., A. C. Loutsidou, C. A. Spiliopoulou, and M. E. Stefanidou. 2012. Zinc and Human Health: An Update. *Arch. Toxicol.* **86**:521–534. [13]

Chaturvedi, K. S., C. S. Hung, J. R. Crowley, A. E. Stapleton, and J. P. Henderson. 2012. The Siderophore Yersiniabactin Binds Copper to Protect Pathogens During Infection. *Nat. Chem. Biol.* **8**:731–736. [2–4]

Checconi, P., R. Sgarbanti, I. Celestino, et al. 2013. The Environmental Pollutant Cadmium Promotes Influenza Virus Replication in MDCK Cells by Altering Their Redox State. *Int. J. Mol. Sci.* **14**:4148–4162. [11]

Chen, H., J. N. Seiber, and M. Hotze. 2014. ACS Select on Nanotechnology in Food and Agriculture: A Perspective on Implications and Applications. *J. Agric. Food Chem.* **62**:1209–1212. [17]

Chen, J. 2012. An Original Discovery: Selenium Deficiency and Keshan Disease (an Endemic Heart Disease). *Asia Pac. J. Clin. Nutr.* **21**:320. [6]

Chen, M., P. Lin, V. Cheng, and W. Lin. 1996. Zinc Supplementation Aggravates Body Fat Accumulation in Genetically Obese Mice and Dietary Obese Mice. *Biol. Trace Elem. Res.* **34**:176–185. [12]

Chen, S. H., W. K. Russell, and D. H. Russell. 2013. Combining Chemical Labeling, Bottom-up and Top-Down Ion-Mobility Mass Spectrometry to Identify Metal-Binding Sites of Partially Metalated Metallothionein. *Anal. Chem.* **85**:3229–3237. [20]

Chen, X., H. Hua, K. Balamurugan, et al. 2008. Copper Sensing Function of Drosophila Metal-Responsive Transcription Factor-1 Is Mediated by a Tetranuclear Cu(I) Cluster. *Nucl. Acids Res.* **36**:3128–3138. [20]

Cheng, N., R. He, J. Tian, P. P. Ye, and R. D. Ye. 2008. Cutting Edge: TLR2 Is a Functional Receptor for Acute-Phase Serum Amyloid A. *J. Immunol.* **181**:22–26. [12]

Cheong, W. F., S. A. Prahl, and A. J. Welch. 1990. A Review of the Optical Properties of Biological Tissues. *IEEE J. Quantum Electronics* **26**:2166–2185. [20]

Cherny, R. A., C. S. Atwood, M. E. Xilinas, et al. 2001. Treatment with a Copper-Zinc Chelator Markedly and Rapidly Inhibits B-Amyloid Accumulation in Alzheimer's Disease Transgenic Mice. *Neuron* **30**:665–676. [6]

Cheung, R. C., J. H. Wong, and T. B. Ng. 2012. Immobilized Metal Ion Affinity Chromatography: A Review on Its Applications. *Appl. Microbiol. Biotechnol.* **96**:1411–1420. [18]

Chifman, J., K. Kniss, P. Neupane, et al. 2012. The Core Control System of Intracellular Iron Homeostasis: A Mathematical Model. *J. Theor. Biol.* **300**:91–99. [17]

Chivers, P. T., and R. T. Sauer. 2002. Nikr Repressor: High-Affinity Nickel Binding to the C-Terminal Domain Regulates Binding to Operator DNA. *Chem. Biol.* **9**:1141–1148. [4]

Choi, E. Y., E. C. Kim, H. M. Oh, et al. 2004. Iron Chelator Triggers Inflammatory Signals in Human Intestinal Epithelial Cells: Involvement of P38 and Extracellular Signal-Regulated Kinase Signaling Pathways. *J. Immunol.* **172**:7069–7077. [3]

Chong, E. W., T. Y. Wong, A. J. Kreis, J. A. Simpson, and R. H. Guymer. 2007. Dietary Antioxidants and Primary Prevention of Age Related Macular Degeneration: Systematic Review and Meta-Analysis. *Br. Med. J.* **335**:755. [8]

Christensen, B. C., and C. J. Marsit. 2011. Epigenomics in Environmental Health. *Front. Genet.* **2**:84. [17]

Chua-anusorn, W., J. Webb, D. J. Macey, P. Pootrakul, and T. G. St. Pierre. 1997. The Effect of Histological Processing on the Form of Iron in Iron-Loaded Human Tissues. *Biochim. Biophys. Acta* **1360**:255–261. [19]

Citiulo, F., I. D. Jacobsen, P. Miramon, et al. 2012. *Candida albicans* Scavenges Host Zinc via Pra1 During Endothelial Invasion. *PLoS Pathog.* **8**:e1002777. [7]

Clark, N. A., K. Teschke, K. Rideout, and R. Copes. 2007. Trace Element Levels in Adults from the West Coast of Canada and Associations with Age, Gender, Diet, Activities, and Levels of Other Trace Elements. *Chemosphere* **70**:155–164. [11]

Clarkson, T. W. 1997. The Toxicology of Mercury. *Crit. Rev. Clin. Lab. Sci.* **34**:369–403. [14]

Clarkson, T. W., and L. Magos. 2006. The Toxicology of Mercury and Its Chemical Compounds. *Crit. Rev. Toxicol.* **36**:609–662. [8]

Cobrado, L., A. Silva-Dias, M. M. Azevedo, C. Pina-Vaz, and A. G. Rodrigues. 2013. *In Vivo* Antibiofilm Effect of Cerium, Chitosan and Hamamelitannin against Usual Agents of Catheter-Related Bloodstream Infections. *J. Antimicrob. Chemother.* **68**:126–130. [17]

Cocho, J. A., J. F. Escanero, and J. M. González de Buitrago. 1998. Elementos Traza: Aspectos Bioquímicos, Analíticos y Clínicos. Barcelona: Sociedad Española de Bioquímica Clínica y Patología Molecular. [14]

Coffman, T. J., C. D. Cox, B. L. Edeker, and B. E. Britigan. 1990. Possible Role of Bacterial Siderophores in Inflammation. Iron Bound to the *Pseudomonas* Siderophore Pyochelin Can Function as a Hydroxyl Radical Catalyst. *J. Clin. Invest.* **86**:1030–1037. [3]

Cogswell, M. E., I. Parvanta, L. Ickes, R. Yip, and G. M. Brittenham. 2003. Iron Supplementation During Pregnancy, Anemia, and Birth Weight: A Randomized Controlled Trial. *Am. J. Clin. Nutr.* **78**:773–781. [8]

Cole, S. P. C. 2014. Targeting Multidrug Resistance Protein 1 (MRP1, ABCC1): Past, Present, and Future. *Annu. Rev. Pharmacol. Toxicol.* **54**:95–117. [2]

Collins, J. F., J. R. Prohaska, and M. D. Knutson. 2010. Metabolic Crossroads of Iron and Copper. *Nutr. Rev.* **68**:133–147. [2]

Coltharp, C., and J. Xiao. 2012. Superresolution Microscopy for Microbiology. *Cell. Microbiol.* **14**:1808–1818. [20]

Combs, G. F., Jr. 2001. Selenium in Global Food Systems. *Br. J. Nutr.* **85**:517–547. [11]

Compan, I., and D. Touati. 1993. Interaction of Six Global Transcription Regulators in Expression of Manganese Superoxide Dismutase in *Escherichia coli* K-12. *J. Bacteriol.* **175**:1687–1696. [5, 7]

Contag, C. H., P. R. Contag, J. I. Mullins, et al. 1995. Photonic Detection of Bacterial Pathogens in Living Hosts. *Mol. Microbiol.* **18**:593–603. [20]

Contag, P. R., I. N. Olomu, D. K. Stevenson, and C. H. Contag. 1998. Bioluminescent Indicators in Living Mammals. *Nat. Med.* **4**:245–247. [20]

Cooke, G. M., H. Tryphonas, O. Pulido, et al. 2004. Oral (Gavage), *in Utero* and Postnatal Exposure of Sprague-Dawley Rats to Low Doses of Tributyltin Chloride. Part 1: Toxicology, Histopathology and Clinical Chemistry. *Food Chem. Toxicol.* **42**:211–220. [12]

Coombes, J. L., and E. A. Robey. 2010. Dynamic Imaging of Host–Pathogen Interactions *in Vivo*. *Nat. Rev. Immunol.* **10**:353–364. [20]

Coombs, G. F. 2000. Food System-Based Approaches to Improving Micronutrient Nutrition: The Case for Selenium. *Biofactors* **12**:39–43. [17]

Cooper, C. E. 1999. Nitric Oxide and Iron Proteins. *Biochim. Biophys. Acta* **1411**:290–309. [13]

Corbett, J. V. 1995. Accidental Poisoning with Iron Supplements. *Am. J. Matern. Child Nurs.* **20**:234. [8]

Corbin, B. D., E. H. Seeley, A. Raab, et al. 2008. Metal Chelation and Inhibition of Bacterial Growth in Tissue Abscesses. *Science* **319**:962–965. [3, 11, 13, 19, 20]

Cornelis, P., and J. Dingemans. 2013. *Pseudomonas aeruginosa* Adapts Its Iron Uptake Strategies in Function of the Type of Infections. *Front. Cell. Infect. Microbiol.* **3**:75. [7]

Correnti, C., V. Richardson, A. K. Sia, et al. 2012. Siderocalin/Lcn2/NGAL/24p3 Does Not Drive Apoptosis through Gentisic Acid Mediated Iron Withdrawal in Hematopoietic Cell Lines. *PLoS One* **7**:e43696. [3]

Correnti, C., and R. K. Strong. 2012. Mammalian Siderophores, Siderophore-Binding Lipocalins, and the Labile Iron Pool. *J. Biol. Chem.* **287**:13524–13531. [3]

Cotruvo, J. A., Jr., and J. Stubbe. 2011. *Escherichia coli* Class Ib Ribonucleotide Reductase Contains a Dimanganese(III)-Tyrosyl Radical Cofactor *in Vivo*. *Biochemistry* **50**:1672–1681. [5, 7]

————. 2012. Metallation and Mismetallation of Iron and Manganese Proteins *in Vitro* and *in Vivo*: The Class I Ribonucleotide Reductases as a Case Study. *Metallomics* **4**:1020–1036. [4]

Cotton, J. A., J. K. Beatty, and A. G. Buret. 2011. Host Parasite Interactions and Pathophysiology in Giardia Infections. *Int. J. Parasitol.* **41**:925–933. [11]

Counago, R. M., M. P. Ween, S. L. Begg, et al. 2013. Imperfect Coordination Chemistry Facilitates Metal Ion Release in the Psa Permease. *Nat. Chem. Biol.* **10**:35–41. [7]

Cowan, J. A. 2002. Structural and Catalytic Chemistry of Magnesium-Dependent Enzymes. *Biometals* **15**:225–235. [4]

Craig, M., and J. M. Slauch. 2009. Phagocytic Superoxide Specifically Damages an Extracytoplasmic Target to Inhibit or Kill *Salmonella*. *PLoS One* **4**:e4975. [7]

Crichton, R. R., and J. P. Declercq. 2010. X-Ray Structures of Ferritins and Related Proteins. *Biochim. Biophys. Acta* **1800**:706–718. [4]

Critchfield, J. W., and C. L. Keen. 1992. Manganese+2 Exhibits Dynamic Binding to Multiple Ligands in Human Plasma. *Metab. Clin. Exp.* **41**:1087–1092. [3]

Crouch, M.-L. V., M. Castor, J. E. Karlinsey, T. Kalhorn, and F. C. Fang. 2008. Biosynthesis and Iroc-Dependent Export of the Siderophore Salmochelin Are Essential for Virulence of *Salmonella enterica* serovar *Typhimurium*. *Mol. Microbiol.* **67**:971–983. [3]

Crownover, B. K., and C. J. Covey. 2013. Hereditary Hemochromatosis. *Am. Fam. Physician* **87**:183–190. [8]

Cuero, R., J. Lilly, and D. S. McKay. 2012. Constructed Molecular Sensor to Enhance Metal Detection by Bacterial Ribosomal Switch-Ion Channel Protein Interaction. *J. Biotechnol.* **158**:1–7. [20]

Cummins, L. M., and E. T. Kimura. 1971. Safety Evaluation of Selenium Sulfide Antidandruff Shampoos. *Toxicol. Appl. Pharmacol.* **20**:89–96. [14]

Cunningham-Rundles, S., D. F. McNeeley, and A. Moon. 2005. Mechanisms of Nutrient Modulation of the Immune Response. *J. Allergy Clin. Immunol.* **115**:1119–1128. [12]

Cvetkovic, A., A. L. Menon, M. P. Thorgersen, et al. 2010. Microbial Metalloproteomes Are Largely Uncharacterized. *Nature* **466**:779–782. [18, 20]

Daley, B., A. T. Doherty, B. Fairman, and C. P. Case. 2004. Wear Debris from Hip or Knee Replacements Causes Chromosomal Damage in Human Cells in Tissue Culture. *J. Bone Joint Surg. Br.* **86**:598–606. [16]

Daly, M. J., E. K. Gaidamakova, V. Y. Matrosova, et al. 2004. Accumulation of Mn(II) in *Deinococcus radiodurans* Facilitates Gamma-Radiation Resistance. *Science* **306**:1025–1028. [5]

Damo, S. M., T. E. Kehl-Fie, N. Sugitani, et al. 2013. Molecular Basis for Manganese Sequestration by Calprotectin and Roles in the Innate Immune Response to Invading Bacterial Pathogens. *PNAS* **110**:3841–3846. [9]

Dardenne, M., and J.-M. Pleau. 1994. Interactions between Zinc and Thymulin. *Met. Based Drugs* **1**:233–239. [13]

Darnton-Hill, I., I. Darnton-Hill, and R. Nalubola. 2002. Fortification Strategies to Meet Micronutrient Needs: Successes and Failures. *Proc. Nutr. Soc.* **61**:231–241. [11]

Dart, A. M., J. L. Martin, and S. Kay. 2002. Association between Past Infection with *Chlamydia pneumoniae* and Body Mass Index, Low-Density Lipoprotein Particle Size and Fasting Insulin. *Int. J. Obes. Relat. Metab. Disord.* **26**:464–468. [12]

Daston, G. P. 1982. Toxic Effects of Cadmium on the Developing Rat Lung. II. Glycogen and Phospholipid Metabolism. *J. Toxicol. Environ. Health* **9**:51–61. [8]

Dave, M., P. D. Higgins, S. Middha, and K. P. Rioux. 2012. The Human Gut Microbiome: Current Knowledge, Challenges, and Future Directions. *Transl. Res.* **160**:246–257. [17]

Davey, J. C., J. E. Bodwell, J. A. Gosse, and J. W. Hamilton. 2007. Arsenic as an Endocrine Disruptor: Effects of Arsenic on Estrogen Receptor-Mediated Gene Expression *in Vivo* and in Cell Culture. *Toxicol. Sci.* **98**:75–86. [12]

Davidson, D. L., and N. I. Ward. 1988. Abnormal Aluminium, Cobalt, Manganese, Strontium and Zinc Concentrations in Untreated Epilepsy. *Epilepsy Res.* **2**:323–330. [20]

Davidson, S. M., and M. R. Duchen. 2012. Imaging Mitochondrial Calcium Signalling with Fluorescent Probes and Single or Two Photon Confocal Microscopy. *Methods Mol. Biol.* **810**:219–234. [7]

Davidsson, L., A. Cederblad, E. Hagebo, B. Lonnerdal, and B. Sandstrom. 1988. Intrinsic and Extrinsic Labeling for Studies of Manganese Absorption in Humans. *J. Nutri.* **118**:1517–1521. [20]

Davidsson, L., B. Lönnerdal, B. Sandström, C. Kunz, and C. L. Keen. 1989. Identification of Transferrin as the Major Plasma Carrier Protein for Manganese Introduced Orally or Intravenously or after *in Vitro* Addition in the Rat. *J. Nutri.* **119**:1461–1464. [3]

Davies, S., H. J. McLaren, A. Hunnisett, and M. Howard. 1997. Age-Related Decreases in Chromium Levels in 51,665 Hair, Sweat, and Serum Samples from 40,872 Patients: Implications for the Prevention of Cardiovascular Disease and Type II Diabetes Mellitus. *Metabolism* **46**:469–473. [8]

Day, F. A., A. E. Funk, and F. O. Brady. 1984. *In Vivo* and *ex Vivo* Displacement of Zinc from Metallothionein by Cadmium and by Mercury. *Chem. Biol. Interactions* **50**:159–174. [14]

de Almeida, A., L. Bruno, J. Oliveira, et al. 2013. Emerging Protein Targets for Metal-Based Pharmaceutical Agents: An Update. *Coord. Chem. Rev.* **257**:2689–2704. [10]

de Almeida, M. P., and S. A. C. Carabineiro. 2013. The Role of Nanogold in Human Tropical Diseases: Research, Detection and Therapy. *Gold Bull.* **46**:65–79. [10]

De Domenico, I., D. McVey Ward, and J. Kaplan. 2008. Regulation of Iron Acquisition and Storage: Consequences for Iron-Linked Disorders. *Nat. Rev. Mol. Cell Biol.* **9**:72–81. [2]

Degtyarenko, K. N., A. C. T. North, D. N. Perkins, and J. B. C. Findlay. 1998. PROMISE: A Database of Information on Prosthetic Centers and Metal Ions in Protein Active Sites. *Nucl. Acids Res.* **26**:376–381. [18, 20]

De Kimpe, J., R. Cornelis, L. Mees, R. Vanholder, and G. Verhoeven. 1999. [74]As-Arsenate Metabolism in Flemish Giant Rabbits with Renal Insufficiency. *J. Trace Elem. Med. Biol.* **13**:7–14. [20]

del Castillo Busto, M. E., M. Montes-Bayon, J. Bettmer, and A. Sanz-Medel. 2008. Stable Isotope Labelling and FPLC-ICP-SFMS for the Accurate Determination of Clinical Iron Status Parameters in Human Serum. *Analyst* **133**:379–384. [20]

Denkhaus, E., and K. Salnikow. 2002. Nickel Essentiality, Toxicity, and Carcinogenicity. *Crit. Rev. Oncol. Hematol.* **42**:35–56. [8]

Denzler, F. O., N. A. Lebedev, A. F. Novgorodov, F. Rosch, and S. M. Qaim. 1997. Production and Radiochemical Separation of Gd-147. *Appl. Radiat. Isot.* **48**:319–326. [20]

Deretic, V., and B. Levine. 2009. Autophagy, Immunity, and Microbial Adaptations. *Cell Host Microbe* **5**:527–549. [17]

Bibliography

De Reuck, J., K. Paemeleire, P. Santens, K. Strijckmans, and I. Lemahieu. 2004. Cobalt-55 Positron Emission Tomography in Symptomatic Atherosclerotic Carotid Artery Disease: Borderzone versus Territorial Infarcts. *Clin. Neurol. Neurosurg.* **106**:77–81. [20]

Deriu, E., J. Z. Liu, M. Pezeshki, et al. 2013. Probiotic Bacteria Reduce *Salmonella typhimurium* Intestinal Colonization by Competing for Iron. *Cell Host Microbe* **14**:26–37. [3]

De Samber, B., K. A. De Schamphelaere, C. R. Janssen, et al. 2013. Hard X-Ray Nanoprobe Investigations of the Subtissue Metal Distributions within *Daphnia magna*. *Anal. Bioanal. Chem.* **405**:6061–6068. [20]

Devireddy, L. R., C. Gazin, X. Zhu, and M. R. Green. 2005. A Cell-Surface Receptor for Lipocalin 24p3 Selectively Mediates Apoptosis and Iron Uptake. *Cell* **123**:1293–1305. [3]

Devirgiliis, C., C. Murgia, G. Danscher, and G. Perozzi. 2004. Exchangeable Zinc Ions Transiently Accumulate in a Vesicular Compartment in the Yeast *Saccharomyces cerevisiae*. *Biochem. Biophys. Res. Commun.* **323**:58–64. [7]

Dhurandhar, N. V. 2011. A Framework for Identification of Infections That Contribute to Human Obesity. *Lancet Infect. Dis.* **11**:963–969. [12]

Diamond, G. L., P. E. Goodrum, S. P. Felter, and W. L. Ruoff. 1998. Gastrointestinal Absorption of Metals. *Drug Chem. Toxicol.* **21**:223–251. [17]

Diaz-Ochoda, V. E., S. Jellbauer, S. Klaus, and M. Raffatellu. 2014. Transition Metal Ions at the Crossroads of Mucosal Immunity and Microbial Pathogenesis. *Front. Cell Infect. Microbiol.* **4**:1–10. [13]

Diaz-Villasenor, A., A. L. Burns, M. Hiriart, M. E. Cebrian, and P. Ostrosky-Wegman. 2007. Arsenic-Induced Alteration in the Expression of Genes Related to Type 2 Diabetes Mellitus. *Toxicol. Appl. Pharmacol.* **225**:123–133. [12]

Di Bella, S., E. Grilli, M. A. Cataldo, and N. Petrosillo. 2010. Selenium Deficiency and HIV Infection. *Infect. Dis. Rep.* **2**:e18. [8]

Dietert, R. R. 2009. Developmental Immunotoxicology: Focus on Health Risks. *Chem. Res. Toxicol.* **22**:17–23. [1]

Di Martino, G., M. G. Matera, B. De Martino, et al. 1993. Relationship between Zinc and Obesity. *J. Med.* **24**:177–183. [12]

Dinelli, M. I. S., and M. I. Moraes-Pinto. 2008. Seroconvertion to Hepatitis B Vaccine after Weight Reduction in Obese Non-Responder. *Rev. Inst. Med. Trop. S. Paulo* **50**:129–130. [12]

Ding, C., R. A. Festa, Y. L. Chen, et al. 2013. *Cryptococcus neoformans* Copper Detoxification Machinery Is Critical for Fungal Virulence. *Cell Host Microbe* **13**:265–276. [7, 13]

Ding, C., J. Yin, E. M. Tovar, et al. 2011. The Copper Regulon of the Human Fungal Pathogen *Cryptococcus neoformans* H99. *Mol. Microbiol.* **81**:1560–1576. [7]

DiSilvestro, R. A. 2000. Zinc in Relation to Diabetes and Oxidative Disease. *J. Nutr.* **130**:S1509–S1511. [12]

Dodani, S. C., D. W. Domaille, C. I. Nam, et al. 2011. Calcium-Dependent Copper Redistributions in Neuronal Cells Revealed by a Fluorescent Copper Sensor and X-Ray Fluorescence Microscopy. *PNAS* **108**:5980–5985. [7]

Domingo, J. L. 1994. Metal-Induced Developmental Toxicity in Mammals: A Review. *J. Toxicol. Environ. Health* **42**:123–141. [8]

———. 2002. Vanadium and Tungsten Derivatives as Antidiabetic Agents: A Review of Their Toxic Effects. *Biol. Trace Elem. Res.* **88**:97–112. [11]

Domingo, J. L., M. Gomez, J. M. Llobet, and J. Corbella. 1991. Influence of Some Dietary Constituents on Aluminum Absorption and Retention in Rats. *Kidney Int.* **39**:598–601. [8]

Donati, R. M., M. M. McLaughlin, E. A. Levri, A. R. Berman, and L. R. Stromberg. 1969. The Response of Iron Metabolism to the Microbial Flora: Studies on Germfree Mice. *Proc. Soc. Exp. Biol. Med.* **130**:920–922. [7]

Dongarra, G., D. Varrica, E. Tamburo, and D. D'Andrea. 2012. Trace Elements in Scalp Hair of Children Living in Differing Environmental Contexts in Sicily (Italy). *Environ. Toxicol. Pharmacol.* **34**:160–169. [11]

Douillet, C., J. Currier, J. Saunders, et al. 2013. Methylated Trivalent Arsenicals Are Potent Inhibitors of Glucose Stimulated Insulin Secretion by Murine Pancreatic Islets. *Toxicol. Appl. Pharmacol.* **267**:11–15. [12]

Drakesmith, H., and A. Prentice. 2008. Viral Infection and Iron Metabolism. *Nat. Rev. Microbiol.* **6**:541–552. [6]

Drennan, C. L., S. Huang, J. T. Drummond, R. G. Matthews, and M. L. Lidwig. 1994. How a Protein Binds B12: A 3.0 a X-Ray Structure of B12-Binding Domains of Methionine Synthase. *Science* **266**:1669–1674. [4]

Dressler, V. L., D. Pozebon, A. Matusch, and J. S. Becker. 2007. Micronebulization for Trace Analysis of Lanthanides in Small Biological Specimens by ICP-MS. *Int. J. Mass Spectrom.* **266**:25–33. [20]

Ducic, T., E. Barski, M. Salome, et al. 2013. X-Ray Fluorescence Analysis of Iron and Manganese Distribution in Primary Dopaminergic Neurons. *J. Neurochem.* **124**:250–261. [20]

Duhutrel, P., C. Bordat, T. D. Wu, et al. 2010. Iron Sources Used by the Nonpathogenic Lactic Acid Bacterium *Lactobacillus sakei* as Revealed by Electron Energy Loss Spectroscopy and Secondary-Ion Mass Spectrometry. *Appl. Environ. Microbiol.* **76**:560–565. [19]

Dupont, C. L., A. Butcher, R. E. Valas, P. E. Boume, and G. Caetano-Anolles. 2010. History of Biological Metal Utilization Inferred through Phylogenomic Analysis of Protein Structures. *PNAS* **107**:10567–10572. [5]

Dupont, C. L., S. Yang, B. Palenik, and P. E. Bourne. 2006. Modern Proteomes Contain Putative Imprints of Ancient Shifts in Trace Metal Geochemistry. *PNAS* **103**:17822–17827. [5]

Durmus, N. G., E. N. Taylor, K. M. Kummer, and T. J. Webster. 2013. Enhanced Efficacy of Superparamagnetic Iron Oxide Nanoparticles against Antibiotic-Resistant Biofilms in the Presence of Metabolites. *Adv. Mater.* **25**:5706–5713. [16]

Dyba, M., and S. W. Hell. 2002. Focal Spots of Size Lambda/23 Open up Far-Field Florescence Microscopy at 33 nm Axial Resolution. *Phys. Rev. Lett.* **88**:163901. [20]

Eaton, K. A., C. L. Brooks, D. R. Morgan, and S. Krakowka. 1991. Essential Role of Urease in Pathogenesis of Gastritis Induced by *Helicobacter pylori* in Gnotobiotic Piglets. *Infect. Immun.* **59**:2470–2475. [4]

Eckhert, C. D. 2012. Trace Elements. In: Modern Nutrition in Health and Disease, ed. A. C. Ross et al., pp. 246–257, vol. 11. Philadelphia: Wolters Kluwer Health/ Lippincott Williams & Wilkins. [8]

Eddins, D., A. Petro, N. Pollard, J. H. Freedman, and E. D. Levin. 2008. Mercury-Induced Cognitive Impairment in Metallothionein-1/2 Null Mice. *Neurotoxicol. Teratol.* **30**:88–95. [12]

EFSA Panel on FEC. 2011. Scientific Opinion on the Safety Evaluation of the Substance, Silver Zeolite a (Silver Zinc Sodium Ammonium Alumino Silicate), Silver Content 2–5%, for Use in Food Contact Materials. *EFSA Journal* **9**:1999–2011. [17]

————. 2012. Scientific Opinion on the Safety Evaluation of the Substance, Titanium Nitride, Nanoparticles, for Use in Food Contact Materials. *EFSA Journal* **10**:2641–2649. [17]

Ekici, S., H. Yang, H. G. Koch, and F. Daldal. 2012. Novel Transporter Required for Biogenesis of Cbb3-Type Cytochrome C Oxidase in *Rhodobacter capsulatus*. *MBio* **3**:e00293–00211. [4]

Eliakim, A., C. Swindt, F. Zaldivar, P. Casali, and D. M. Cooper. 2006. Reduced Tetanus Antibody Titers in Overweight Children. *Autoimmunity* **39**:137–141. [12]

Ellis, J. K., T. J. Athersuch, L. D. Thomas, et al. 2012. Metabolic Profiling Detects Early Effects of Environmental and Lifestyle Exposure to Cadmium in a Human Population. *BMC Med.* **10**:61. [11]

Elreedy, S., N. Krieger, P. B. Ryan, et al. 1999. Relations between Individual and Neighborhood-Based Measures of Socioeconomic Position and Bone Lead Concentrations among Community-Exposed Men: The Normative Aging Study. *Am. J. Epidemiol.* **150**:129–141. [11]

Evans, G. W., and E. Kantrowitz. 2002. Socioeconomic Status and Health: The Potential Role of Environmental Risk Exposure. *Annu. Rev. Public Health* **23**:303–331. [11]

Everson da Silva, L., P. Teixeira de Sousa, Jr., E. Nunes Maciel, et al. 2010. *In Vitro* Antiprotozoal Evaluation of Zinc and Copper Complexes Based on Sulphonamides Containing 8-Aminoquinoline Ligands. *Lett. Drug Des. Discov.* **7**:679–685. [10]

Eze, J. I., M. C. Okeke, A. A. Ngene, J. N. Omeje, and F. O. Abonyi. 2013. Effects of Dietary Selenium Supplementation on Parasitemia, Anemia and Serum Proteins of *Trypanosoma brucei* Infected Rats. *Exp. Parasitol.* **135**:331–336. [13]

Fahrni, C. J. 2007. Biological Applications of X-Ray Fluorescence Microscopy: Exploring the Subcellular Topography and Speciation of Transition Metals. *Curr. Opin. Chem. Biol.* **11**:121–127. [7]

Failla, M. L. 2003. Trace Elements and Host Defense: Recent Advances and Continuing Challenges. *J. Nutri.* **133**:1443S–1447S. [1]

Falagas, M. E., and M. Kompoti. 2006. Obesity and Infection. *Lancet Infect. Dis.* **6**:438–446. [12]

Faller, P. 2012. Copper in Alzheimer Disease: Too Much, Too Little, or Misplaced? *Free Radic. Biol. Med.* **52**:747–748. [6]

Fandino, A. S., I. Rais, M. Vollmer, et al. 2005. LC-Nanospray-MS/MS Analysis of Hydrophobic Proteins from Membrane Protein Complexes Isolated by Blue-Native Electrophoresis. *J. Mass Spectrometry* **40**:1223–1231. [20]

Farrell, N. 2002. Biomedical Uses and Application of Inorganic Chemistry Overview. *Coord. Chem. Rev.* **232**:1. [10]

Farrugia, M. A., L. Macomber, and R. P. Hausinger. 2013. Biosynthesis of the Urease Metallocenter. *J. Biol. Chem.* **288**:13178–13185. [4, 5]

Ferdousi, S., and A. R. Mia. 2012. Serum Levels of Copper and Zinc in Newly Diagnosed Type-2 Diabetic Subjects. *Mymensingh Med. J.* **21**:475–478. [12]

Fernández-Real, J. M., M. J. Ferri, J. Vendrell, and W. Ricart. 2007. Burden of Infection and Fat Mass in Healthy Middle-Aged Men. *Obesity* **15**:245–252. [12]

Fernández-Sánchez, A., E. Madrigal-Santillán, M. Bautista, et al. 2011. Inflammation: Oxidative Stress and Obesity. *Int. J. Mol. Sci.* **12(5)**: 3117–3132. [7]

Ferreira, A., J. Balla, V. Jeney, G. Balla, and M. P. Soares. 2008. A Central Role for Free Heme in the Pathogenesis of Severe Malaria: The Missing Link? *J. Mol. Med.* **86**:1097–1111. [13]

*Bibliography*

Fetherston, J. D., O. Kirillina, A. G. Bobrov, J. T. Paulley, and R. D. Perry. 2010. The Yersiniabactin Transport System Is Critical for the Pathogenesis of Bubonic and Pneumonic Plague. *Infect. Immun.* **78**:2045–2052. [3, 7]

Fetherston, J. D., I. Mier, Jr., H. Truszczynska, and R. D. Perry. 2012. The Yfe and Feo Transporters Are Involved in Microaerobic Growth and the Virulence of *Yersinia pestis* in Bubonic Plague. *Infect. Immun.* **80**:3880–3891. [3, 7]

Fiehn, O., J. Kopka, P. Dörmann, et al. 2000. Metabolite Profiling for Plant Functional Genomics. *Nat. Biotechnol.* **18**:1157. [14]

Fierke, C. A., and R. B. Thompson. 2001. Fluorescence-Based Biosensing of Zinc Using Carbonic Anhydrase. *Biometals* **14**:205–222. [20]

Filipov, N. M., and C. A. Dodd. 2011. Role of Glial Cells in Manganese Neurotoxicity. *J. Appl. Toxicol.* **32**:310–317. [13]

Fillat, M. F. 2014. The Fur (Ferric Uptake Regulator) Superfamily: Diversity and Versatility of Key Transcriptional Regulators. *Arch. Biochem. Biophys.* **546**:41–52. [4]

Finley, J. W., J. G. Penland, R. E. Pettit, and C. D. Davis. 2003. Dietary Manganese Intake and Type of Lipid Do Not Affect Clinical or Neuropsychological Measures in Healthy Young Women. *J. Nutr.* **133**:2849–2856. [13]

Fischbach, M. A., H. Lin, Z. L., et al. 2006. The Pathogen-Associated iroA Gene Cluster Mediates Bacterial Evasion of Lipocalin 2. *PNAS* **103**:16502–16507. [3]

Fischer, W. C., and R. E. Black. 2004. Zinc and the Risk for Infectious Disease. *Annu. Rev. Nutr.* **24**:255–275. [8]

Fleury, C., A. Petit, F. Mwale, et al. 2006. Effect of Cobalt and Chromium Ions on Human MG-63 Osteoblasts *in Vitro*: Morphology, Cytotoxicity, and Oxidative Stress. *Biomaterials* **27**:3351–3360. [16]

Flo, T. H., K. D. Smith, S. Sato, et al. 2004. Lipocalin 2 Mediates an Innate Immune Response to Bacterial Infection by Sequestrating Iron. *Nature* **432**:917–921. [2, 3, 6, 7, 9, 13, 20]

Foote, J. W., and H. T. Delves. 1984. Albumin Bound and A$_2$-Macroglobulin Bound Zinc Concentrations in the Sera of Healthy Adults. *J. Clin. Pathol.* **37**:1050–1054. [3]

Forbes, J. M., M. T. Coughlan, and M. E. Cooper. 2008. Oxidative Stress as a Major Culprit in Kidney Disease in Diabetes. *Diabetes* **57**:1446–1454. [12]

Forbes, J. R., and P. Gros. 2001. Divalent-Metal Transport by NRAMP Proteins at the Interface of Host-Pathogen Interactions. *Trends Microbiol.* **9**:397–403. [9, 13]

Fortes, G. B., L. S. Alves, R. de Oliveira, et al. 2012. Heme Induces Programmed Necrosis on Macrophages through Autocrine TNF and ROS Production. *Blood* **119**:2368–2375. [13]

Fortin, A., L. Abel, J. L. Casanova, and P. Gros. 2007. Host Genetics of Mycobacterial Diseases in Mice and Men: Forward Genetic Studies of BCG-osis and Tuberculosis. *Annu. Rev. Hum. Genet.* **8**:163–192. [12]

Fraga, C. G. 2005. Relevance, Essentiality and Toxicity of Trace Elements in Human Health. *Mol. Aspects Med.* **26**:235–244. [17]

Franck, F., S. M. Kelly, and W. Ben. 2004. Silver Nanoparticles and Polymeric Medical Devices: A New Approach to Prevention of Infection? *J. Antimicrob. Chemother.* **54**:1019–1024. [16]

Franke, S., G. Grass, C. Rensing, and D. H. Nies. 2003. Molecular Analysis of the Copper-Transporting Efflux System CusCFBA of *Escherichia coli. J. Bacteriol.* **185**:3804–3812. [5]

Frawley, E. R., M.-L. V. Crouch, L. K. Bingham-Ramos, et al. 2013. Iron and Citrate Export by a Major Facilitator Superfamily Pump Regulates Metabolism and Stress Resistance in *Salmonella typhimurium. PNAS* **110**:12054–12059. [5]

Frederickson, C. J., E. J. Kasarskis, D. Ringo, and C. J. Frederickson. 1987. A Quinoline Fluorescence Method for Visualizing and Assaying Histochemically Reactive Zinc (Bouton Zinc) in the Brain. *J. Neurosci. Meth.* **20**:91–103. [20]

Friedman, D. B., D. L. Stauff, G. Pishchany, et al. 2006. *Staphylococcus aureus* Redirects Central Metabolism to Increase Iron Availability. *PLoS Pathog.* **2**:e87. [4]

Frisk, P., P. Darnerud, G. Friman, J. Blomberg, and N.-G. Ilbäck. 2007. Sequential Trace Element Changes in Serum and Blood During a Common Viral Infection in Mice. *J. Trace Elem. Med. Biol.* **21**:29–36. [17]

Frisk, P., Y. Molin, and N.-G. Ilbäck. 2008. Tissue Uptake of Mercury Is Changed During the Course of a Common Viral Infection in Mice. *Environ. Res.* **106**:178–184. [17]

Fritsche, G., M. Nairz, S. J. Libby, F. C. Fang, and G. Weiss. 2012. SLC11A1 (NRAMP1) Impairs Growth of *Salmonella enterica* serovar *Typhimurium* in Macrophages via Stimulation of Lipocalin-2 Expression. *J. Leukoc. Biol.* **92**:353–359. [9, 13]

Fujibayashi, Y., H. Taniuchi, Y. Yonekura, et al. 1997. Copper-62-ATSM: A New Hypoxia Imaging Agent with High Membrane Permeability and Low Redox Potential. *J. Nucl. Med.* **38**:1155–1160. [20]

Furukawa, K., and K. Tonomura. 1972. Metallic Mercury-Releasing Enzyme in Mercury-Resistant *Pseudomonas*. *Agric. Biol. Chem.* **36**:217–226. [4]

Furukawa, S., T. Fujita, M. Shimabukuro, et al. 2004. Increased Oxidative Stress in Obesity and Its Impact on Metabolic Syndrome. *J. Clin. Invest.* **114**:1752–1761. [12]

Gaggelli, E., H. Kozlowski, D. Valensin, and G. Valensin. 2006. Copper Homeostasis and Neurodegenerative Disorders (Alzheimer's, Prion, and Parkinson's Diseases and Amyotrophic Lateral Sclerosis). *Chem. Rev.* **106**:1995–2044. [16]

Gajski, G., Z. Jelčić, V. Oreščanin, et al. 2014. Physico-Chemical Characterization and the *in Vitro* Genotoxicity of Medical Implants Metal Alloy (TiAlV and CoCrMo) and Polyethylene Particles in Human Lymphocytes. *Biochim. Biophys. Acta* **1840**:565–576. [16]

Gale, T. F. 1973. The Interaction of Mercury with Cadmium and Zinc in Mammalian Embryonic Development. *Environ. Res.* **6**:95–105. [14]

Galhardi, C. M., Y. S. Diniz, L. A. Faine, et al. 2004. Toxicity of Copper Intake: Lipid Profile, Oxidative Stress and Susceptibility to Renal Dysfunction. *Food Chem. Toxicol.* **42**:2053–2060. [12]

Galsfeld, A., E. Guedon, J. D. Helmann, and R. G. Brennan. 2003. Structure of the Manganese-Bound Manganese Transport Regulator of *Bacillus subtilis*. *Nat. Struct. Biol.* **10**:652–657. [5]

Gambino, D., and L. Otero. 2012. Perspectives on What Ruthenium-Based Compounds Could Offer in the Development of Potential Antiparasitic Drugs. *Inorganica Chim. Acta* **393**:103–114. [10]

Ganz, T. 2009. Iron in Innate Immunity: Starve the Invaders. *Curr. Opin. Immunol.* **21**:63–67. [3, 9]

Gao, Y., X. Peng, J. Zhang, et al. 2013. Cellular Response of *E. coli* Upon $H^{2+}$ Exposure: A Case Study of Advanced Nuclear Analytical Approach to Metalloproteomics. *Metallomics* **5**:913–919. [18]

García, O. P., K. Z. Long, and J. L. Rosado. 2009. Impact of Micronutrient Deficiencies on Obesity. *Nutr. Rev.* **67**:559–572. [12]

García-Barrera, T., J. L. Gómez-Ariza, M. González-Fernández, et al. 2012. Biological Responses Related to Agonistic, Antagonistic and Synergistic Interactions of Chemical Species. *Anal. Bioanal. Chem.* **403**:2237–2253. [14]

Gaykema, S. B., A. H. Brouwers, M. N. L.-d. Hooge, et al. 2013. [89]Zr-Bevacizumab PET Imaging in Primary Breast Cancer. *J. Nucl. Med.* **54**:1014–1018. [20]

Gee, K. R., Z. L. Zhou, D. Ton-That, S. L. Sensi, and J. H. Weiss. 2002. Measuring Zinc in Living Cells: A New Generation of Sensitive and Selective Fluorescent Probes. *Cell Calcium* **31**:245–251. [20]

Gehrke, S. G., W. Stremmel, I. Mathes, et al. 2003. Hemochromatosis and Transferrin Receptor Gene Polymorphisms in Chronic Hepatitis C: Impact on Iron Status, Liver Injury and HCV Genotype. *J. Molec. Med.* **81**:780–787. [20]

Gemmati, D., G. Zeri, E. Orioli, et al. 2012. Polymorphisms in the Genes Coding for Iron Binding and Transporting Proteins Are Associated with Disability, Severity, and Early Progression in Multiple Sclerosis. *BMC Med. Genet.* **13**:70. [20]

Gergely, V., K. M. Kubachka, S. Mounicou, P. Fodor, and J. A. Caruso. 2006. Selenium Speciation in *Agaricus bisporus* and *Lentinula edodes* Mushroom Proteins Using Multi-Dimensional Chromatography Coupled to Inductively Coupled Plasma Mass Spectrometry. *J. Chromatogr. A* **1101**:94–102. [14]

Ghazali, A. R., F. Kamarulzaman, C. D. Normah, et al. 2013. Levels of Metallic Elements and Their Potential Relationships to Cognitive Function among Elderly from Federal Land Development Authority (FELDA) Settlement in Selangor Malaysia. *Biol. Trace Elem. Res.* **153**:16–21. [8]

Ghio, A. J. 2014. Particle Exposures and Infections. *Infection* **42**:459–467. [17]

Gibson, R. S. 1994. Content and Bioavailability of Trace Elements in Vegetarian Diets. *Am. J. Clin. Nutr.* **59**:1223S–1232S. [11]

Gielda, L. M., and V. J. DiRita. 2012. Zinc Competition among the Intestinal Microbiota. *MBio* **3**:e00171–00112. [3, 7]

González-Fernández, M., T. García-Barrera, J. Jurado, et al. 2008. Integrated Application of Transcriptomics, Proteomics and Metallomics in Environmental Issues. *Pure Appl. Chem.* **80**:2609–2626. [14]

Gonzalez-Guerrero, M., and J. M. Arguello. 2008. Mechanism of Cu[+]-Transporting ATPases:Soluble Cu[+] Chaperones Directly Transfer Cu[+] to Transmembrane Transport Sites. *PNAS* **105**:5992–5997. [5]

Gonzalez-Guerrero, M., D. Raimunda, X. Cheng, and J. M. Argüello. 2010. Distinct Functional Roles of Homologous Cu[+] Efflux ATPases in *Pseudomonas aeruginosa*. *Mol. Microbiol.* **78**:1246–1258. [4, 5]

Gordeuk, V. R., A. Caleffi, E. Corradini, et al. 2003. Iron Overload in Africans and African-Americans and a Common Mutation in the Scl40a1 (Ferroportin 1) Gene. *Blood Cells Mol. Dis.* **31**:299–304. [9, 13]

Govindaraj, M., P. Kannan, and P. Arunachalam. 2011. Implication of Micronutrients in Agriculture and Health with Special Reference to Iron and Zinc. *Int. J. Agricul. Manage. Develop.* **1**:207–220. [17]

Goyette, J., and C. Geczy. 2011. Inflammation Associated S100 Proteins: New Mechanisms That Regulate Function. *Amino Acids* **41**:821–842. [13]

Gozzelino, R., B. B. Andrade, R. Larsen, et al. 2012. Metabolic Adaptation to Tissue Iron Overload Confers Tolerance to Malaria. *Cell Host Microbe* **12**:693–704. [9, 13, 17]

Gozzelino, R., V. Jeney, and M. P. Soares. 2010. Mechanisms of Cell Protection by Heme Oxygenase-1. *Annu. Rev. Pharmacol. Toxicol.* **50**:323–354. [13]

Gozzelino, R., and M. P. Soares. 2014. Coupling Heme and Iron Metabolism via Ferritin H Chain. *Antioxid. Redox Signal.* **20**:1754–1769. [13]

Graham, A. I., S. Hunt, S. L. Stokes, et al. 2009. Severe Zinc Depletion of *Escherichia coli*: Roles for High Affinity Zinc Binding by Zint, Zinc Transport and Zinc-Independent Proteins. *J. Biol. Chem.* **284**:18377–18389. [5]

Graham, R. D., M. Marija Knez, and R. M. Welch. 2012. How Much Nutritional Iron Deficiency in Humans Globally Is Due to an Underlying Zinc Deficiency? *Adv. Agronomy* **115**:1–29. [1, 6, 17]

Granchi, D., E. Cenni, G. Ciapetti, et al. 1998. Cell Death Induced by Metal Ions: Necrosis or Apoptosis? *J. Mater. Sci. Mater. Med.* **9**:31–37. [16]

Granchi, D., E. Cenni, D. Tigani, et al. 2008. Sensitivity to Implant Materials in Patients with Total Knee Arthroplasties. *Biomaterials* **29**:1494–1500. [16]

Grass, G., B. Fan, B. P. Rosen, et al. 2001. Zitb (Ybgr), a Member of the Cation Diffusion Facilitator Family, Is an Additional Zinc Transporter in *Escherichia coli*. *J. Bacteriol.* **183**:4664–4667. [5]

Grass, G., S. Franke, N. Taudte, et al. 2005a. The Metal Permease Zupt from *Escherichia coli* Is a Transporter with a Broad Substrate Spectrum. *J. Bacteriol.* **187**:1604–1611. [5]

Grass, G., M. Otto, B. Fricke, et al. 2005b. FieF (YiiP) from *Escherichia coli* Mediates Decreased Cellular Accumulation of Iron and Relieves Iron Stress. *Arch. Microbiol.* **183**:9–18. [5]

Grass, G., and C. Rensing. 2001. CueO Is a Multi-Copper Oxidase That Confers Copper Tolerance in *Escherichia coli*. *Biochem. Biophys. Res. Commun.* **286**:902–908. [5]

Grass, G., M. D. Wong, B. P. Rosen, R. L. Smith, and C. Rensing. 2002. Zupt Is a Zn(II) Uptake System in *Escherichia coli*. *J. Bacteriol.* **184**:864–866. [5]

Griffin, A. S., S. A. West, and A. Buckling. 2004. Cooperation and Competition in Pathogenic Bacteria. *Nature* **430**:1024–1027. [3]

Gross, S., S. T. Gammon, B. L. Moss, et al. 2009. Bioluminescence Imaging of Myeloperoxidase Activity *in Vivo. Nat. Med.* **15**:455–461. [20]

Gruber, K., E. Rosenkranz, M. Maywald, B. Plümäkers, and L. Rink. 2013. Zinc Deficiency Adversely Influences Interleukin-4 and Interleukin-6 Signaling. *J. Biol. Regul. Homeost. Agents* **27**:661–671. [13]

Grüneberg, R. N. 1969. Relationship of Infecting Urinary Organism to the Faecal Flora in Patients with Symptomatic Urinary Infection. *Lancet* **2**:766–778. [4]

Grynkiewicz, G., M. Poenie, and R. Y. Tsien. 1985. A New Generation of Calcium Indicators with Greatly Improved Fluorescence Properties. *J. Biol. Chem.* **260**:3440–3450. [20]

Gu, M., and J. A. Imlay. 2013. Superoxide Poisons Mononuclear Iron Enzymes by Causing Mismetallation. *Mol. Microbiol.* **89**:123–134. [5]

Guan, Y., P. An, Z. Zhang, et al. 2013. Screening Identifies the Chinese Medicinal Plant Caulis Spatholobi as an Effective Hamp Expression Inhibitor. *J. Nutr.* **143**:1061–1066. [6]

Guerrero-Romero, F., and M. Rodriguez-Moran. 2006. Hypomagnesemia, Oxidative Stress, Inflammation, and Metabolic Syndrome. *Diabetes Metab. Res. Rev.* **22**:471–476. [12]

Gundacker, C., S. Frohlich, K. Graf-Rohrmeister, et al. 2010. Perinatal Lead and Mercury Exposure in Austria. *Sci. Total Environ.* **408**:5744–5749. [11]

Gunther, M. R., P. M. Hanna, R. P. Mason, and M. S. Cohen. 1995. Hydroxyl Radical Formation from Cuprous Ion and Hydrogen Peroxide: A Spin-Trapping Study. *Arch. Biochem. Biophys.* **316**:515–522. [5]

Guo, F., X. Guo, A. Xie, Y. L. Lou, and Y. Wang. 2011. The Suppressive Effects of Lanthanum on the Production of Inflammatory Mediators in Mice Challenged by LPS. *Biol. Trace Elem. Res.* **142**:693–703. [17]

Guo, Z., and P. J. Sadler. 1999. Metals in Medicine. *Angew. Chem. Int. Ed.* **38**:1512–1531. [10]

Gupta, A., K. Matsui, J. F. Lo, and S. Silver. 1999. Molecular Basis for Resistance to Silver Cations in *Salmonella*. *Nat. Med.* **5**:183–188. [4]

Gutierrez-Barranquero, J. A., A. de Vicente, V. J. Carrion, G. W. Sundin, and F. M. Cazorla. 2013. Recruitment and Rearrangement of Three Different Genetic Determinants into a Conjugative Plasmid Increase Copper Resistance in *Pseudomonas syringae*. *Appl. Environ. Microbiol.* **79**:1028–1033. [7]

Haase, H. 2013. An Element of Life: Competition for Zinc in Host-Pathogen Interaction. *Immunity* **39**:623–624. [8, 13]

Haase, H., E. Mocchegiani, and L. Rink. 2006. Correlation between Zinc Status and Immune Function in the Elderly. *Biogerontology* **7**:421–428. [8]

Haase, H., S. Overbeck, and L. Rink. 2008. Zinc Supplementation for the Treatment or Prevention of Disease: Current Status and Future Perspectives. *Exp. Gerontol.* **43**:394–408. [1]

Haase, H., and L. Rink. 2009. Functional Significance of Zinc-Related Signaling Pathways in Immune Cells. *Annu. Rev. Nutr.* **29**:133–152. [8, 13]

———. 2013. Zinc Signals and Immune Function. *Biofactors* **40**:27–40. [8]

———. 2014. The Multiple Impacts of Zinc on Immune Function. *Metallomics* **6**:1175–1180. [13, 17]

Hagan, E. C., and H. L. T. Mobley. 2009. Haem Acquisition Is Facilitated by a Novel Receptor Hma and Required by Urapathogenic *Escherichia coli* for Kidney Infection. *Mol. Microbiol.* **71**:79–91. [5]

Hajdena-Dawson, M., W. Zhang, P. R. Contag, et al. 2003. Effects of Metalloporphyrins on Heme Oxygenase-1 Transcription: Correlative Cell Culture Assays Guide *in Vivo* Imaging. *Mol. Imaging* **2**:138–149. [20]

Hallab, N. J., and J. J. Jacobs. 2009. Biologic Effects of Implant Debris. *Bull. NYU Hosp. Jt. Dis.* **67**:182–188. [16]

Halliwell, B., and J. M. Gutteridge. 1984. Oxygen Toxicity, Oxygen Radicals, Transition Metals and Disease. *Biochem. J.* **219**:1–14. [8]

Halwani, M., B. Yebio, Z. E. Suntres, et al. 2008. Co-Encapsulation of Gallium with Gentamicin in Liposomes Enhances Antimicrobial Activity of Gentamicin against *Pseudomonas aeruginosa*. *J. Antimicrob. Chemother.* **62**:1291–1297. [7]

Hamza, I., J. Prohaska, and J. D. Gitlin. 2003. Essential Role for Atox1 in the Copper-Mediated Intracellular Trafficking of the Menkes ATPase. *PNAS* **100**:1215–1220. [8]

Hantke, K. 2001. Iron and Metal Regulation in Bacteria. *Curr. Opin. Microbiol.* **4**:172–177. [5]

Harthill, M. 2011. Review: Micronutrient Selenium Deficiency Influences Evolution of Some Viral Infectious Diseases. *Biol. Trace Elem. Res.* **143**:1325–1336. [8]

Hattori, M., N. Iwase, N. Furuya, et al. 2009. $Mg^{2+}$-Dependent Gating of Bacterial Mgte Channel Underlies $Mg^{2+}$ Homeostasis. *EMBO J.* **28**:3602–3612. [5]

Haxel, G. B., J. B. Hedrick, and G. J. Orris. 2002. Rare Earth Elements: Critical Resources for High Technology. Usgs Fact Sheet 087-02, U.S. Geological Survey. http://pubs.usgs.gov/fs/2002/fs087-02/fs087-02.pdf. (accessed Oct. 10, 2014). [15]

He, G., E. I. Pearce, and C. H. Sissons. 2002. Inhibitory Effect of ZnCl(2) on Glycolysis in Human Oral Microbes. *Arch. Oral Biol.* **47**:117–129. [17]

Hegde, V., and N. V. Dhurandhard. 2013. Microbes and Obesity: Interrelationship between Infection, Adipose Tissue and the Immune System. *Clin. Microbiol. Infect.* **19**:314–320. [12]

Heitman, J., T. R. Kozel, J. Kwon-Chung, J. R. Perfect, and A. Casadevall, eds. 2011. *Cryptococcus*: From Human Pathogen to Model Yeast. Washington, D.C.: ASM Press. [7]

Helge, J. W., B. Stallknecht, B. K. Pedersen, et al. 2003. The Effect of Graded Exercise on Il-6 Release and Glucose Uptake in Human Skeletal Muscle. *J. Physiol.* **546**:299–305. [11]

Helms, M. W., B. H. Brandt, and C. H. Contag. 2006. Options for Visualizing Metastatic Disease in the Living Body. *Contrib. Microbiol.* **13**:209–231. [20]

Helmstaedt, K., S. Krappmann, and G. H. Braus. 2001. Allosteric Regulation of Catalytic Activity: *Escherichia coli* Aspartate Transcarbamoylase versus Yeast Chorismate Mutase. *Microbiol. Mol. Biol. Rev.* **65**:404–421. [5]

Henderson, J. P., J. R. Crowley, J. S. Pinkner, et al. 2009. Quantitative Metabolomics Reveals an Epigenetic Blueprint for Iron Acquisition in Uropathogenic *Escherichia coli*. *PLoS Pathog.* **5**:e1000305. [3]

Hensley, M. P., T. S. Gunasekera, J. A. Easton, et al. 2012. Characterization of Zn(II)-Responsive Ribosomal Proteins Ykgm and L31 in *E. coli*. *J. Inorg. Biochem.* **111**:164–172. [5]

Hernandez-Sanchez, A., P. Tejada-Gonzalez, and M. Arteta-Jimenez. 2013. Aluminium in Parenteral Nutrition: A Systematic Review. *Eur. J. Clin. Nutr.* **67**:230–238. [8]

Herth, M. M., M. Barz, M. Jahn, R. Zentel, and F. Rosch. 2010. $^{72/74}$As-Labeling of HPMA Based Polymers for Long-Term *in Vivo* PET Imaging. *Bioorg. Med. Chem. Lett.* **20**:5454–5458. [20]

Herwaldt, L. A., J. J. Cullen, P. French, et al. 2004. Preoperative Risk Factors for Nasal Carriage of *Staphylococcus aureus*. *Infect. Control Hosp. Epidemiol.* **25**:481–484. [12]

Herzog, H., F. Rosch, G. Stocklin, et al. 1993. Measurement of Pharmacokinetics of Yttrium-86 Radiopharmaceuticals with PET and Radiation Dose Calculation of Analogous Yttrium-90 Radiotherapeutics. *J. Nucl. Med.* **34**:2222–2226. [20]

Hesham, M. S., A. B. Edariah, and M. Norhayati. 2004. Intestinal Parasitic Infections and Micronutrient Deficiency: A Review. *Med. J. Malaysia* **59**:284–293. [11]

Hetrick, E. M., and M. H. Schoenfisch. 2006. Reducing Implant-Related Infections: Active Release Strategies. *Chem. Soc. Rev.* **35**:780–789. [16]

Hileti, D., P. Panayiotidis, and A. V. Hoffbrand. 1995. Iron Chelators Induce Apoptosis in Proliferating Cells. *Br. J. Haematol.* **89**:181–187. [3]

Hill, K. E., S. Wu, A. K. Motley, et al. 2012. Production of Selenoprotein P (Sepp1) by Hepatocytes Is Central to Selenium Homeostasis. *J. Biol. Chem.* **287**:40414–40424. [8]

Hirano, T., K. Kikuchi, Y. Urano, T. Higuchi, and T. Nagano. 2000. Highly Zinc-Selective Fluorescent Sensor Molecules Suitable for Biological Applications. *J. Am. Chem. Soc.* **122**:12399–12400. [20]

Hirayama, T., G. C. Van de Bittner, L. W. Gray, S. Lutsenko, and C. J. Chang. 2012. Near-Infrared Fluorescent Sensor for *in Vivo* Copper Imaging in a Murine Wilson Disease Model. *PNAS* **109**:2228–2233. [20]

Ho, E., C. Courtemanche, and B. N. Ames. 2003. Zinc Deficiency Induces Oxidative DNA Damage and Increases P53 Expression in Human Lung Fibroblasts. *J. Nutr.* **133**:2543–2548. [12]

Ho, S. M., A. Johnson, P. Tarapore, et al. 2012. Environmental Epigenetics and Its Implication on Disease Risk and Health Outcomes. *ILAR J.* **53**:289–305. [17]

Hoffman, A. E., M. DeStefano, C. Shoen, et al. 2013. Co(II) and Cu(II) Pyrophosphate Complexes Have Selectivity and Potency against Mycobacteria Including *Mycobacterium tuberculosis. Eur. J. Med. Chem.* **70**:589–593. [11]

Högbom, M., U. B. Ericsson, R. Lam, et al. 2005. A High Throughput Method for the Detection of Metalloproteins on a Microgram Scale. *Mol. Cell. Proteomics* **4**:827–834. [18]

Hohle, T. H., and M. R. O'Brian. 2012. Manganese Is Required for Oxidative Metabolism in Unstressed *Bradyrhizobium japonicum* Cells. *Mol. Microbiol.* **84**:766–777. [5, 7]

Holt, D., and M. Webb. 1986. The Toxicity and Teratogenicity of Mercuric Mercury in the Pregnant Rat. *Arch. Toxicol.* **58**:243–248. [8]

Hood, M. I., B. L. Mortensen, J. L. Moore, et al. 2012. Identification of an *Acinetobacter baumannii* Zinc Acquisition System that Facilitates Resistance to Calprotectin-Mediated Zinc Sequestration. *PLoS Pathog.* **8**:e1003068. [20]

Hood, M. I., and E. P. Skaar. 2012. Nutritional Immunity: Transition Metals at the Pathogen-Host Interface. *Nat. Rev. Microbiol.* **10**:525–537. [2, 3, 7, 9]

Hook, G. R., J. M. Hosseini, and R. J. Elin. 1985. Analytical Approaches for Biomedical Elemental Analysis. *J. Am. Coll. Nutr.* **4**:599–612. [20]

Hsin, J., A. Arkhipov, Y. Yin, J. E. Stone, and K. Schulten. 2008a. Using VMD: An Introductory Tutorial. *Curr. Protoc. Bioinform.* **5**:5.7. [20]

Hsin, K., Y. Sheng, M. M. Harding, P. Taylor, and M. D. Walkinshaw. 2008b. MESPEUS: A Database of the Geometry of Metal Sites in Proteins. *J. Appl. Cryst.* **41**:963–968. [20]

Hsu, A., D. M. Aronoff, J. Phipps, D. Goel, and P. Mancuso. 2007. Leptin Improves Pulmonary Bacterial Clearance and Survival in ob/ob Mice During Pneumococcal Pneumonia. *Clin. Exp. Immunol.* **150**:332–339. [12]

Hu, H., M. Rabinowitz, and D. Smith. 1998. Bone Lead as a Biological Marker in Epidemiologic Studies of Chronic Toxicity: Conceptual Paradigms. *Environ. Health Perspect.* **106**:1–8. [12]

Hu, H., W. Zhang, Y. Qiao, et al. 2012. Antibacterial Activity and Increased Bone Marrow Stem Cell Functions of Zn-Incorporated $TiO_2$ Coatings on Titanium. *Acta Biomater.* **8**:904–915. [16]

Hua, Y., S. Clark, J. Ren, and N. Sreejayan. 2012. Molecular Mechanisms of Chromium in Alleviating Insulin Resistance. *J. Nutr. Biochem.* **23**:313–319. [8]

Huang, C. F., Y. W. Chen, C. Y. Yang, et al. 2011. Arsenic and Diabetes: Current Perspectives. *Kaohsiung J. Med. Sci.* **27**:402–410. [12]

Huang, H. L., Y. Y. Chang, J. H. Weng, et al. 2012a. Anti-Bacterial Performance of Zirconia Coatings on Titanium Implants. *Thin Solid Films* **528**:151–156. [16]

Huang, L., Y. Y. Yu, C. P. Kirschke, E. R. Gertz, and K. K. Lloyd. 2007. Znt7 (Slc30a7)-Deficient Mice Display Reduced Body Zinc Status and Body Fat Accumulation. *J. Biol. Chem.* **282**:37053–37063. [12]

Huang, X. F., and P. Arvan. 1995. Intracellular Transport of Proinsulin in Pancreatic Beta-Cells. Structural Maturation Probed by Disulfide Accessibility. *J. Biol. Chem.* **270**:20417–20423 [12]

Huang, Z., A. H. Rose, and P. R. Hoffmann. 2012b. The Role of Selenium in Inflammation and Immunity: From Molecular Mechanisms to Therapeutic Opportunities. *Antioxid. Redox Signal.* **16**:705–743. [13]

Hunt, J. R., S. K. Gallagher, and L. K. Johnson. 1994. Effect of Ascorbic Acid on Apparent Iron Absorption by Women with Low Iron Stores. *Am. J. Clin. Nutr.* **59**:1381–1385. [8]

Hurrell, R. F. 1997. Preventing Iron Deficiency through Food Fortification. *Nutr. Rev.* **55**:210–222. [8]

Hurst, L. C., M. A. Badalamente, Z. H. Oster, H. L. Atkins, and D. Weissberg. 1986. Incorporation of a New Radioactive Compound, 4+Sn-117m DTPA, into Normal and Burred Rat Femurs. *Clin. Orthop. Relat. Res.* **206**:290–294. [20]

Hurst, T. K., D. Wang, R. B. Thompson, and C. A. Fierke. 2010. Carbonic Anhydrase II-Based Metal Ion Sensing: Advances and New Perspectives. *Biochim. Biophys. Acta* **1804**:393–403. [20]

Huttunen, R., and J. Syrjanen. 2013. Obesity and the Risk and Outcome of Infection. *Int. J. Obes.* **37**:333–340. [12]

Hvidberg, V., C. Jacobsen, R. K. Strong, et al. 2005. The Endocytic Receptor Megalin Binds the Iron Transporting Neutrophil-Gelatinase-Associated Lipocalin with High Affinity and Mediates Its Cellular Uptake. *FEBS Lett.* **579**:773–777. [3]

IAEA. 2003. Manual for Reactor Produced Radioisotopes. Vienna, Austria: IAEA. [20]

Ibrahim, F., T. Halttunen, R. Tahvonen, and S. Salminen. 2006. Probiotic Bacteria as Potential Detoxification Tools: Assessing Their Heavy Metal Binding Isotherms. *Can. J. Microbiol.* **52**:877– 885. [17]

Ibs, K. H., and L. Rink. 2003. Zinc-Altered Immune Function. *J. Nutr.* **133**:1452S–1456S. [11]

Ikeda, J., A. Janakiraman, D. G. Kehres, M. E. Maguire, and J. M. Slauch. 2005. Transcriptional Regulation of *SitABCD* of *Salmonella enterica* serovar *Typhimurium* by MntR and Fur. *J. Bacteriol.* **187**:912–922. [5]

Ikejima, S., S. Sasaki, H. Sashinami, et al. 2005. Impairment of Host Resistance to Listeria monocytogenes Infection in Liver of db/db and ob/ob Mice. *Diabetes* **54**:182–189. [12]

Ilari, A., P. Ceci, D. Ferrari, G. Rossi, and E. Chiancone. 2002. Iron Incorporation into *E. coli* Dps Gives Rise to a Ferritin-Like Microcrystalline Core. *J. Biol. Chem.* **277**:37619–37623. [5]

Ilbäck, N. G., G. Benyamin, U. Lindh, J. Fohlman, and G. Friman. 2003. Trace Element Changes in the Pancreas During Viral Infection in Mice. *Pancreas* **26**:190–196. [17]

Ilbäck, N. G., P. Frisk, N. Mohamed, et al. 2007. Virus Induces Metal-Binding Proteins and Changed Trace Element Balance in the Brain During the Course of a Common Human Infection (Coxsackievirus B3) in Mice. *Sci. Total Environ.* **381**:88–98. [17]

Ilbäck, N. G., A. W. Glynn, L. Wikberg, E. Netzel, and U. Lindh. 2004. Metallothionein Is Induced and Trace Element Balance Changed in Target Organs of a Common Viral Infection. *Toxicology* **199**:241–250. [17]

Imlay, J. A. 2013. The Molecular Mechanisms and Physiological Consequences of Oxidative Stress: Lessons from a Model Bacterium. *Nat. Rev. Microbiol.* **11**:443–454. [5]

Imlay, J. A., and S. Linn. 1988. DNA Damage and Oxygen Radical Toxicity. *Science* **240**:1302–1309. [5]

Inadera, H. 2006. The Immune System as a Target for Environmental Chemicals: Xenoestrogens and Other Compounds. *Toxicol. Lett.* **164**:191–206. [1]

Iniguez, E., A. Sánchez, M. A. Vasquez, et al. 2013. Metal–Drug Synergy: New Ruthenium(II) Complexes of Ketoconazole Are Highly Active against *Leishmania major* and *Trypanosoma cruzi* and Nontoxic to Human or Murine Normal Cells. *J. Inorg. Biochem.* **18**:779–790. [10]

434                                    *Bibliography*

Inza, B., C. Rouleau, H. Tjalve, et al. 2001. Fine-Scale Tissue Distribution of Cadmium, Inorganic Mercury, and Methylmercury in Nymphs of the Burrowing Mayfly *Hexagenia rigida* Studied by Whole-Body Autoradiography. *Environ. Res.* **85**:265–271. [20]

Iranpour, R., A. Zandian, M. Mohammadizadeh, et al. 2009. Comparison of Maternal and Umbilical Cord Blood Selenium Levels in Term and Preterm Infants. *Zhongguo Dang Dai Er. Ke. Za Zhi* **11**:513–516. [8]

Irreverre, F., S. H. Mudd, W. D. Heizer, and L. Laster. 1967. Sulfite oxidase deficiency: studies of a patient with mental retardation, dislocated ocular lenses, and abnormal urinary excretion of S-sulfo-L-cysteine, sulfite, and thiosulfate. *Biochem. Med.* **1**:187–217. [8]

Irving, H., and R. J. P. Williams. 1948. Order of Stability of Metal Complexes. *Nature* **162**:746–747. [5, 20]

Iyengar, V. G., K. S. Subramanian, and J. R. W. Woittiez. 1997. Element Analysis of Biological Samples Principles and Practice. New York: CRC Press. [20]

Jabado, N., A. Jankowski, S. Dougaparsad, et al. 2000. Natural Resistance to Intracellular Infections: Natural Resistance-Associated Macrophage Protein 1 (NRAMP1) Functions as a pH-Dependent Manganese Transporter at the Phagosomal Membrane. *J. Exp. Med.* **192**:1237–1248. [7]

Jacobi, C. A., S. Gregor, A. Rakin, and J. Heesemann. 2001. Expression Analysis of the Yersiniabactin Receptor Gene *fyuA* and the Heme Receptor *hemR* of *Yersinia enterocolitica in Vitro* and *in Vivo* Using the Reporter Genes for Green Fluorescent Protein and Luciferase. *Infect. Immun.* **69**:7772–7782. [7]

Jacquamet, L., D. Aberdam, A. Adrait, et al. 1998. X-Ray Absorption Spectroscopy of a New Zinc Site in the Fur Protein from *Escherichia coli*. *Biochemistry* **37**:2564–2571. [4]

Jang, S., and J. A. Imlay. 2007. Micromolar Intracellular Hydrogen Peroxide Disrupts Metabolism by Damaging Iron-Sulfur Enzymes. *J. Biol. Chem.* **282**:929–937. [5]

Jansen, J., W. Karges, and L. Rink. 2009. Zinc and Diabetes: Clinical Links and Molecular Mechanisms. *J. Nutr. Biochem.* **20**:399–417. [11]

Jarup, L., and A. Akesson. 2009. Current Status of Cadmium as an Environmental Health Problem. *Toxicol. Appl. Pharmacol.* **238**:201–208. [11]

Jedrychowski, W., U. Maugeri, E. Flak, E. Mroz, and I. Bianchi. 1998. Predisposition to Acute Respiratory Infections among Overweight Preadolescent Children: An Epidemiologic Study in Poland. *Public Health* **112**:189–195. [12]

Jeejeebhoy, K. N., R. C. Chu, E. B. Marliss, G. R. Greenberg, and A. Bruce-Robertson. 1977. Chromium Deficiency, Glucose Intolerance, and Neuropathy Reversed by Chromium Supplementation, in a Patient Receiving Long-Term Total Parenteral Nutrition. *Am. J. Clin. Nutr.* **30**:531–538. [8]

Jenner, F. E., and H. S. O'Neill. 2012. Analysis of 60 Elements in 616 Ocean Floor Basaltic Glasses. *Geochem. Geophys. Geosys.* **13**:Q02005. [20]

Jenney, F. E., P. S. Brereton, M. Izumi, et al. 2005. High-Throughput Production of *Pyrococcus furiosus* Proteins: Considerations for Metalloproteins. *J. Synchrotron Rad.* **12**:8–12. [18]

Jensen, L. T., and V. C. Culotta. 2005. Activation of CuZn Superoxide Dismutases from *Caenorhabditis elegans* Does Not Require the Copper Chaperone Ccs. *J. Biol. Chem.* **280**:41373–41379. [7]

Jia, Y., S. R. Tang, R. G. Wang, et al. 2010. Effects of Elevated $CO_2$ on Growth, Photosynthesis, Elemental Composition, Antioxidant Level, and Phytochelatin Concentration in *Lolium mutiforum* and *Lolium perenne* under Cd Stress. *J. Hazard Materials* **180**:384–394. [17]

Johnson, A. R., J. J. Milner, and L. Makowski. 2012. The Inflammation Highway: Metabolism Accelerates Inflammatory Traffic in Obesity. *Immunol Rev.* **249(1)**: 218–238. [12]

Johnson, D. C., D. R. Dean, A. D. Smith, and M. K. Johnson. 2005a. Structure, Function, and Formation of Biological Iron-Sulfur Clusters. *Annu. Rev. Biochem.* **74**:247–281. [4]

Johnson, D. R., J. C. O'Connor, R. Dantzer, and G. G. Freund. 2005b. Inhibition of Vagally Mediated Immune-to-Brain Signaling by Vanadyl Sulfate Speeds Recovery from Sickness. *PNAS* **102**:15184–15189. [8]

Jomova, K., and M. Valko. 2011. Advances in Metal-Induced Oxidative Stress and Human Disease. *Toxicology* **283**:65–87. [1, 8, 12]

Jones, B. L., and S. H. Cho. 2011. The Feasibility of Polychromatic Cone-Beam X-Ray Fluorescence Computed Tomography (XFCT) Imaging of Gold Nanoparticle-Loaded Objects: A Monte Carlo Study. *Phys. Med. Biol.* **56**:3719–3730. [20]

Jones, C., S. A. Badger, M. Hoper, et al. 2013. Hepatic Cytokine Response Can Be Modulated Using the Kupffer Cell Blocker Gadolinium Chloride in Obstructive Jaundice. *Int. J. Surg.* **11**:46–51. [17]

Jubber, A. 2004. Respiratory Complications of Obesity. *Int. J. Clin. Pract.* **58**:573–580. [12]

Kadurugamuwa, J. L., K. Modi, O. Coquoz, et al. 2005. Reduction of Astrogliosis by Early Treatment of Pneumococcal Meningitis Measured by Simultaneous Imaging, *in Vivo*, of the Pathogen and Host Response. *Infect. Immun.* **73**:7836–7843. [20]

Kalogeropoulos, N., S. Karavoltsos, A. Sakellari, et al. 2012. Heavy Metals in Raw, Fried and Grilled Mediterranean Finfish and Shellfish. *Food. Chem. Toxicol.* **50**:3702–2708. [11]

Kaluarachchi, H., K. C. Chan Chung, and D. B. Zamble. 2010. Microbial Nickel Proteins. *Nat. Prod. Rep.* **27**:681–694. [7]

Kaluarachchi, H., J. W. Zhang, and D. B. Zamble. 2011. *Escherichia coli* SlyD, More Than a Ni(II) Reservoir. *Biochemistry* **50**:10761–10763. [4]

Kambe, T., B. P. Weaver, and G. K. Andrews. 2008. The Genetics of Essential Metal Homeostasis During Development. *Genesis* **46**:214–228. [8]

Kamen, M. D., and T. Horio. 1970. Bacterial Cytochromes: I. Structural Aspects. *Annu. Rev. Biochem.* **39**:673–700. [4]

Kanda, T., T. Takahashi, S. Kudo, et al. 2004. Leptin Deficiency Enhances Myocardial Necrosis and Lethality in a Murine Model of Viral Myocarditis. *Life Sci.* **75**:1435–1447. [12]

Kaneko, Y., M. Thoendel, O. Olakanmi, B. E. Britigan, and P. K. Singh. 2007. The Transition Metal Gallium Disrupts *Pseudomonas aeruginosa* Iron Metabolism and Has Antimicrobial and Antibiofilm Activity. *J. Clin. Invest.* **117**:877–888. [3]

Karjala, Z., D. Neal, and J. Rohrer. 2011. Association between HSV1 Seropositivity and Obesity: Data from the National Health and Nutritional Examination Survey, 2007–2008. *PLoS One* **6**:e19092. [12]

Karlsson, E. A., and M. A. Beck. 2010. The Burden of Obesity on Infectious Disease. *Exp. Biol. Med.* **235**:1412–1424. [12]

Karlsson, H. L., P. Cronholm, J. Gustafsson, and L. Möller. 2008. Copper Oxide Nanoparticles Are Highly Toxic: A Comparison between Metal Oxide Nanoparticles and Carbon Nanotubes. *Chem. Res. Toxicol.* **21**:1726–1732. [16]

Karppelin, M., T. Siljander, J. Vuopio-Varkila, et al. 2010. Factors Predisposing to Acute and Recurrent Bacterial Non-Necrotizing Cellulitis in Hospitalized Patients: A Prospective Case-Control Study. *Clin. Microbiol. Infect.* **16**:729–734. [12]

Katayama, A., A. Tsujii, A. Wada, T. Nishino, and A. Ishihama. 2002. Systematic Search for Zinc-Binding Proteins in *Escherichia coli*. *Eur. J. Biochem.* **269**:2403–2413. [18]

Katona, P., and J. Katona-Apte. 2008. The Interaction between Nutrition and Infection. *Clin. Infect. Dis.* **46**:1582–1588. [8]

Keaney, J. F., Jr., M. G. Larson, R. S. Vasan, et al. 2003. Obesity and Systemic Oxidative Stress: Clinical Correlates of Oxidative Stress in the Framingham Study. *Arterioscler. Thromb. Vasc. Biol.* **23**:434–439. [12]

Keen, C. L., J. Y. Uriu-Hare, S. N. Hawk, et al. 1998. Effect of Copper Deficiency on Prenatal Development and Pregnancy Outcome. *Am. J. Clin. Nutr.* **67**:1003S–1011S. [8]

Kehl-Fie, T. E., and E. P. Skaar. 2010. Nutritional Immunity Beyond Iron: A Role for Manganese and Zinc. *Curr. Opin. Chem. Biol.* **14**:218–224. [3, 7]

Kehl-Fie, T. E., Y. Zhang, J. L. Moore, et al. 2013. MntABC and MntH Contribute to Systemic *Staphylococcus aureus* Infection by Competing with Calprotectin for Nutrient Manganese. *Infect. Immun.* **81**:3395–3405. [11, 20]

Kehres, D. G., A. Janakiraman, J. M. Slauch, and M. E. Maguire. 2002a. Regulation of *Salmonella enterica* serovar *Typhimurium mntH* Transcription by $H_2O_2$, $Fe^{2+}$, and $Mn^{2+}$. *J. Bacteriol.* **184**:3151–3158. [5]

———. 2002b. SitABCD Is the Alkaline $Mn^{(2+)}$ Transporter of *Salmonella enterica* serovar *Typhimurium*. *J. Bacteriol.* **184**:3159–3166. [5]

Kehres, D. G., M. L. Zaharik, B. B. Finlay, and M. E. Maguire. 2000. The NRAMP Proteins of *Salmonella typhimurium* and *Escherichia coli* Are Selective Manganese Transporters Involved in the Response to Reactive Oxygen. *Mol. Microbiol.* **36**:1085–1100. [5]

Kemna, E., P. Pickkers, E. Nemeth, H. van der Hoeven, and D. Swinkels. 2005. Time-Course Analysis of Hepcidin, Serum Iron, and Plasma Cytokine Levels in Humans Injected with LPS. *Blood* **106**:1864–1866. [9]

Kemner, K. M., S. D. Kelly, E. J. O'Loughlin, et al. 2005. XRF and XAFS Analysis of Electrophoretically Isolated Nondenatured Proteins. *Phys. Scr.* **T115**:940–942. [18]

Kenyon, E. M., L. M. Del Razo, and M. F. Hughes. 2005. Tissue Distribution and Urinary Excretion of Inorganic Arsenic and Its Methylated Metabolites in Mice Following Acute Oral Administration of Arsenate. *Toxicol. Sci.* **85**:468–475. [8]

Keyer, K., A. S. Gort, and J. A. Imlay. 1995. Superoxide and the Production of Oxidative DNA Damage. *J. Bacteriol.* **177**:6782–6790. [5]

Khor, C. C., and M. L. Hibberd. 2012. Host-Pathogen Interactions Revealed by Human Genome-Wide Surveys. *Trends Genet.* **28**:233–243. [17]

Khosravi, A. D., F. Ahmadi, S. Salmanzadeh, A. Dashtbozorg, and E. A. Montazeri. 2009. Study of Bacteria Isolated from Orthopedic Implant Infections and Their Antimicrobial Susceptibility Pattern. *Res. J. Microbiol.* **4**:158–163. [16]

Kile, M. L., E. G. Rodrigues, M. Mazumdar, et al. 2014. A Prospective Cohort Study of the Association between Drinking Water Arsenic Exposure and Self-Reported Maternal Health Symptoms During Pregnancy in Bangladesh. *Environ. Health* **13**:29. [11]

Kim, B. E., T. Nevitt, and D. J. Thiele. 2008. Mechanisms for Copper Acquisition, Distribution and Regulation. *Nat. Chem. Biol.* **4**:176–185. [2]

Kim, D. K., J. H. Jeong, J. M. Lee, et al. 2014. Inverse Agonist of Estrogen-Related Receptor Gamma Controls *Salmonella typhimurium* Infection by Modulating Host Iron Homeostasis. *Nat. Med.* **20**:419–424. [11]

Kim, H. W., U. S. Ha, J. C. Woo, et al. 2012. Preventive Effect of Selenium on Chronic Bacterial Prostatitis. *J. Infect. Chemother.* **18**:30–34. [13]

Kim, R., H. Hu, A. Rotnitzky, D. Bellinger, and H. Needleman. 1995. A Longitudinal Study of Chronic Lead Exposure and Physical Growth in Boston Children. *Environ. Health Perspect.* **103**:952–957. [12]

Kim, S., and H. Kang. 2011. Effects of Elevated $CO_2$ and Pb on Phytoextraction and Enzyme Activity. *Water Air Soil Pollut.* **219**:365–375. [17]

Kimber, I., and D. A. Basketter. 1996. Contact Hypersensitivity to Metals. In: Toxicology of Metals, ed. L. W. Chang, vol. 1. Boca Raton: CRC Press. [15]

Kinnamon, K. E., E. A. Steck, and D. S. Rane. 1979. Activity of Antitumor Drugs against African Trypanosomes. *Antimicrob. Agents Chemother.* **15**:157–160. [10]

Kirchner, S., T. Kieu, C. Chow, S. Casey, and B. Blumberg. 2010. Prenatal Exposure to the Environmental Obesogen Tributyltin Predisposes Multipotent Stem Cells to Become Adipocytes. *Mol. Endocrinol.* **24**:526–539. [12]

Kirsten, A., M. Herzberg, A. Voigt, et al. 2011. Contributions of Five Secondary Metal Uptake Systems to Metal Homeostasis of *Cupriavidus metallidurans* CH34. *J. Bacteriol.* **193**:4652–4663. [5]

Kittleson, J. T., I. R. Loftin, A. C. Hausrath, et al. 2006. Periplasmic Metal-Resistance Protein CusF Exhibits High Affinity and Specificity for Both Cui and Agi. *Biochemistry* **45**:11096–11102. [5]

Kiyose, K., H. Kojima, Y. Urano, and T. Nagano. 2006. Development of a Ratiometric Fluorescent Zinc Ion Probe in Near-Infrared Region, Based on Tricarbocyanine Chromophore. *J. Am. Chem. Soc.* **128**:6548–6549. [20]

Knapp, C. W., S. M. McCluskey, B. K. Singh, et al. 2011. Antibiotic Resistance Gene Abundances Correlate with Metal and Geochemical Conditions in Archived Scottish Soils. *PLoS One* **6**:e27300. [4]

Knoell, D. L., M. W. Julian, S. Bao, et al. 2009. Zinc Deficiency Increases Organ Damage and Mortality in a Murine Model of Polymicrobial Sepsis. *Crit. Care Med.* **37**:1380–1388. [12]

Knoell, D. L., and M. J. Liu. 2010. Impact of Zinc Metabolism on Innate Immune Function in the Setting of Sepsis. *Int. J. Vitam. Nutr. Res.* **80**:271–277. [3]

Kobayashi, M., and S. Shimizu. 1999. Cobalt Proteins. *Eur. J. Biochem.* **261**:1–9. [4]

Kobayashi, Y., Y. Ogra, K. Ishiwata, et al. 2002. Selenosugars Are Key and Urinary Metabolites for Selenium Excretion within the Required to Low-Toxic Range. *PNAS* **99**:15932–15936. [8]

Kodali, P., J. Landero-Figueroa, K. R. Chitta, J. A. Caruso, and A. Opeolu. 2012. Detection of Metalloproteins and Metal Levels in Blood Plasma of Stroke Patients by Metallomics Mass Spectrometry Methods. *Metallomics* **4**:1077–1087. [20]

Koenig, S. M. 2001. Pulmonary Complications of Obesity. *Am. J. Med. Sci.* **321**:249–279. [12]

Kohanski, M. A., D. J. Dwyer, B. Hayete, C. A. Lawrence, and J. J. Collins. 2007. A Common Mechanism of Cellular Death Induced by Bactericidal Antibiotics. *Cell* **130**:797–810. [3]

Koi, L., R. Bergmann, K. Bruchner, et al. 2014. Radiolabeled Anti-EGFR-Antibody Improves Local Tumor Control after External Beam Radiotherapy and Offers Theragnostic Potential. *Radiother. Oncol.* **110**:362–369. [20]

Koller, L. D. 1975. Methylmercury: Effect on Oncogenic and Nononcogenic Viruses in Mice. *Am. J. Vet. Res.* **36**:1501–1504. [17]

Komolova, M., S. L. Bourque, K. Nakatsu, and M. A. Adams. 2008. Sedentariness and Increased Visceral Adiposity in Adult Perinatally Iron-Deficient Rats. *Int. J. Obes.* **32**:1441–1444. [12]

Kondilis-Mangum, H. D., and P. A. Wade. 2013. Epigenetics and the Adaptive Immune Response. *Mol. Aspects Med.* **34**:813–825. [17]

Kong, Y., H. Yao, H. Ren, et al. 2010. Imaging Tuberculosis with Endogenous Beta-Lactamase Reporter Enzyme Fluorescence in Live Mice. *PNAS* **107**:12239–12244. [20]

Konjufca, V., and M. J. Miller. 2009. Two-Photon Microscopy of Host-Pathogen Interactions: Acquiring a Dynamic Picture of Infection *in Vivo*. *Cell. Microbiol.* **11**:551–559. [20]

Koron, N., A. Bratkic, S. Ribeiro Guevara, M. Vahcic, and M. Horvat. 2012. Mercury Methylation and Reduction Potentials in Marine Water: An Improved Methodology Using $^{197}$Hg Radiotracer. *Appl. Radiat. Isot.* **70**:46–50. [20]

Kosior, E. 2013. Combined Phase and X-Ray Fluorescence Imaging at the Sub-Cellular Level. PhD thesis, European Synchrotron Radiation Facility, Université de Grenoble, Grenoble. [19]

Kovtunovych, G., M. A. Eckhaus, M. C. Ghosh, H. Ollivierre-Wilson, and T. A. Rouault. 2010. Dysfunction of the Heme Recycling System in Heme Oxygenase 1-Deficient Mice: Effects on Macrophage Viability and Tissue Iron Distribution. *Blood* **116**:6054–6062. [13]

Kowalewski, B., J. Poppe, U. Demmer, et al. 2012. Nature's Polyoxometalate Chemistry: X-Ray Structure of the Mo Storage Protein Loaded with Discrete Polynuclear Mo-O Clusters. *J. Am. Chem. Soc.* **134**:9768–9774. [4]

Kowolenko, M., L. Tracy, and D. Lawrence. 1991. Early Effects of Lead on Bone Marrow Cell Responsiveness in Mice Challenged with Listeria monocytogenes. *Fundam. Appl. Toxicol.* **17**:75–82. [17]

Kozlovsky, A. S., P. B. Moser, S. Reiser, and R. A. Anderson. 1986. Effects of Diets High in Simple Sugars on Urinary Chromium Losses. *Metabolism* **35**:515–518. [8]

Kozyraki, R., and O. Cases. 2013. Vitamin B12 Absorption: Mammalian Physiology and Acquired and Inherited Disorders. *Biochimie* **95**:1002–1007. [2]

Krewski, D., R. A. Yokel, E. Nieboer, et al. 2007. Human Health Risk Assessment for Aluminium, Aluminium Oxide, and Aluminium Hydroxide. *J. Toxicol. Environ. Health B Crit. Rev.* **10(Suppl 1)**:1–269. [8]

Krewulak, K. D., and H. J. Vogel. 2008. Structural Biology of Bacterial Iron Uptake. *Biochim. Biophys. Acta* **1778**:1781–1804. [2]

Krezel, A., and W. Maret. 2006. Zinc-Buffering Capacity of a Eukaryotic Cell at Physiological pZn. *J. Biol. Inorg. Chem.* **11**:1049–1062. [20]

Krishna, S. S., I. Majumdar, and N. V. Grishin. 2003. Structural Classification of Zinc Fingers: Survey and Summary. *Nucl. Acids Res.* **31**:532–550. [4]

Krishnakumar, R., M. Craig, J. A. Imlay, and J. M. Slauch. 2004. Differences in Enzymatic Properties Allow SodCI but Not SodCII to Contribute to Virulence in *Salmonella enterica* serovar *Typhimurium* Strain 14028. *J. Bacteriol.* **186**:5230–5238. [5]

Kronstad, J. W., G. Hu, and W. H. Jung. 2013. An Encapsulation of Iron Homeostasis and Virulence in *Cryptococcus neoformans*. *Trends Microbiol.* **21**:457–465. [7]

Kucharzewski, M., J. Braziewicz, U. Majewska, and S. Gozdz. 2002. Concentration of Selenium in the Whole Blood and the Thyroid Tissue of Patients with Various Thyroid Diseases. *Biol. Trace Elem. Res.* **88**:25–30. [8]

Kuo, C. C., K. Moon, K. A. Thayer, and A. Navas-Acien. 2013. Environmental Chemicals and Type 2 Diabetes: An Updated Systematic Review of the Epidemiologic Evidence. *Curr. Diab. Rep.* **13**:831–849. [12]

Kuo, J., ed. 2014. Electron Microscopy, Methods and Protocols (3rd edition). Methods in Molecular Biology, vol. 1117. J. M. Walker, series ed. Hatfield, UK: Humana Press. [19, 20]

Lag, M., D. Rodionov, J. Ovrevik, et al. 2010. Cadmium-Induced Inflammatory Responses in Cells Relevant for Lung Toxicity: Expression and Release of Cytokines in Fibroblasts, Epithelial Cells and Macrophages. *Toxicol. Lett.* **193**:252–260. [11]

Lamberti, L. M., C. L. Fischer Walker, K. Y. Chan, W.-J. Jian, and R. E. Black. 2013. Oral Zinc Supplementation for the Treatment of Acute Diarrhea in Children: A Systematic Review and Meta-Analysis. *Nutrients* **5**:4715–4740. [13]

Landero-Figueroa, J., K. Subramanian Vignesh, G. S. Deepe, Jr., and J. A. Caruso. 2013. Selectivity and Specificity of Small Molecule Fluorescent Dyes/Probes Used for the Detection of $Zn^{2+}$ and $Ca^{2+}$ in Cells. *Metallomics* **6**:301–315. [20]

Larmas, M. 1993. Plaque-Mediated Diseases: Basic and Clinical Studies Using the Value of Saliva Monitoring. *Ann. NY Acad. Sci.* **694**:253–264. [17]

Larsen, R., Z. Gouveia, M. P. Soares, and R. Gozzelino. 2012. Heme Cytotoxicity and the Pathogenesis of Immune-Mediated Inflammatory Diseases. *Front. Pharmacol.* **3**:77. [13]

Larsen, R., R. Gozzelino, V. Jeney, et al. 2010. A Central Role for Free Heme in the Pathogenesis of Severe Sepsis. *Sci. Transl. Med.* **2**:51ra71. [13, 17]

Lauwerys, R., and D. Lison. 1994. Health Risks Associated with Cobalt Exposure: An Overview. *Sci. Total Environ.* **150**:1–6. [8]

Lawlor, M. S., C. O'Connor, and V. L. Miller. 2007. Yersiniabactin Is a Virulence Factor for *Klebsiella pneumoniae* During Pulmonary Infection. *Infect. Immun.* **75**:1463–1472. [3]

Leach, L. H., J. C. Morris, and T. A. Lewis. 2007. The Role of the Siderophore Pyridine-2,6-Bis (Thiocarboxylic Acid) (PDTC) in Zinc Utilization by *Pseudomonas putida* DSM 3601. *Biometals* **20**:717–726. [4]

Lear, J., D. J. Hare, F. Fryer, et al. 2012. High-Resolution Elemental Bioimaging of Ca, Mn, Fe, Co, Cu, and Zn Employing LA-ICP-MS and Hydrogen Reaction Gas. *Anal. Chem.* **84**:6707–6714. [20]

Leasure, L., A. Giddabasappa, S. Chaney, et al. 2008. Low-Level Human Equivalent Gestational Lead Exposure Produces Sex-Specific Motor and Coordination Abnormalities and Late-Onset Obesity in Year-Old Mice. *Environ. Health Perspect.* **116**:355–361. [12]

Le Brun, N. E., A. Crow, M. E. Murphy, A. G. Mauk, and G. R. Moore. 2010. Iron Core Mineralisation in Prokaryotic Ferritins. *Biochim. Biophys. Acta* **1800**:732–744. [4]

Lechardeur, D., B. Cesselin, U. Liebl, et al. 2012. Discovery of Intracellular Heme-Binding Protein HrtR, Which Controls Heme Efflux by the Conserved HrtB-HrtA Transporter in *Lactococcus lactis*. *J. Biol. Chem.* **287**:4752–4758. [4]

Lecube, A., A. Carrera, E. Losada, et al. 2006. Iron Deficiency in Obese Postmenopausal Women. *Obesity* **14**:1724–1730. [12]

Lee, H. J., S. C. Choi, E. Y. Choi, et al. 2005. Iron Chelator Induces MIP-A/CCL20 in Human Intestinal Epithelial Cells: Implication for Triggering Mucosal Adaptive Immunity. *Exp. Mol. Med.* **37**:297–310. [3]

Lee, J. W., C. K. Lee, C. S. Moon, et al. 2012. Korea National Survey for Environmental Pollutants in the Human Body 2008: Heavy Metals in the Blood or Urine of the Korean Population. *Int. J. Hyg. Environ. Health* **215**:449–457. [11]

Lee, S., S. H. Cha, S. Y. Lee, and C. J. Song. 2009. Reversible Inferior Colliculus Lesion in Metronidazole-Induced Encephalopathy: Magnetic Resonance Findings on Diffusion-Weighted and Fluid Attenuated Inversion Recovery Imaging. *J. Comput. Assist. Tomogr.* **33**:305–308. [19]

Lee, S., J. K. Yu, K. Park, et al. 2010. Phylogenetic Groups and Virulence Factors in Pathogenic and Commensal Strains of *Escherichia coli* and Their Association with blaCTX-M. *Ann. Clin. Lab. Sci.* **40**:361–367. [4]

Lee-Lewis, H., and D. M. Anderson. 2010. Absence of Inflammation and Pneumonia During Infection with Nonpigmented *Yersinia pestis* Reveals a New Role for the *pgm* Locus in Pathogenesis. *Infect. Immun.* **78**:220–230. [3, 7]

Lei, L., X. Chang, G. Rentschler, et al. 2012. A Polymorphism in Metallothionein 1a (MT1A) Is Associated with Cadmium-Related Excretion of Urinary Beta 2-Microglobulin. *Toxicol. Appl. Pharmacol.* **265**:373–379. [17]

Leitch, J. M., P. J. Yick, and V. C. Culotta. 2009. The Right to Choose: Multiple Pathways for Activating Copper,Zinc Superoxide Dismutase. *J. Biol. Chem.* **284**:24679–24683. [5]

Levina, A., R. Codd, and P. A. Lay. 2009. Chromium in Cancer and Dietary Supplements. *Biol. Magn. Reson.* **28**:551–579. [13]

Lewin, A., G. R. Moore, and N. E. Le Brun. 2005. Formation of Protein-Coated Iron Minerals. *Dalton Trans.* **22**:3597–3610. [4]

Li, B., J. Y. Sun, L. Z. Han, et al. 2010a. Phylogenetic Groups and Pathogenicity Island Markers in Fecal *Escherichia coli* Isolates from Asymptomatic Humans in China. *Appl. Environ. Microbiol.* **76**:6698–6700. [4]

Li, P., L. Fang, H. Zhou, et al. 2011. A New Ratiometric Fluorescent Probe for Detection of $Fe^{2+}$ with High Sensitivity and Its Intracellular Imaging Applications. *Chemistry* **17**:10520–10523. [20]

Li, Y., Q. Zhang, R. Wang, et al. 2012. Temperature Changes the Dynamics of Trace Element Accumulation in *Solanum tuberosum* L. *Clim. Change* **112**:655–672. [17]

Li, Z. Y., S. R. Tang, X. F. Deng, R. G. Wang, and Z. G. Song. 2010b. Contrasting Effects of Elevated $CO_2$ on Cu and Cd Uptake by Different Rice Varieties Grown on Contaminated Soils with Two Levels of Metals: Implication for Phytoextraction and Food Safety. *J. Hazard Materials* **177**:352–361. [17]

Lichten, L. A., and R. J. Cousins. 2009. Mammalian Zinc Transporters: Nutritional and Physiologic Regulation. *Annu. Rev. Nutr.* **29**:153–176. [2, 7, 13]

Lim, K. H., L. J. Riddell, C. A. Nowson, A. O. Booth, and E. A. Szymlek-Gay. 2013. Iron and Zinc Nutrition in the Economically-Developed World: A Review. *Nutrients* **5**:3184–3211. [7]

Lim, S. S., T. Vos, A. D. Flaxman, et al. 2012. A Comparative Risk Assessment of Burden of Disease and Injury Attributable to 67 Risk Factors and Risk Factor Clusters in 21 Regions, 1990–2010: A Systematic Analysis for the Global Burden of Disease Study 2010. *Lancet* **380**:2224–2260. [17]

Lim, T. H., T. Sargent, III, and N. Kusubov. 1983. Kinetics of Trace Element Chromium(III) in the Human Body. *Am. J. Physiol.* **244**:R445–R454. [8]

Lin, S., Q. Shi, F. B. Nix, et al. 2002. A Novel S-Adenosyl-L-Methionine:Arsenic(III) Methyltransferase from Rat Liver Cytosol. *J. Biol. Chem.* **277**:10795–10803. [8]

Linder, M. C. 1991. Biochemistry of Copper. New York: Plenum. [20]

Lindgren, A., B. R. Danielsson, L. Dencker, and M. Vahter. 1984. Embryotoxicity of Arsenite and Arsenate: Distribution in Pregnant Mice and Monkeys and Effects on Embryonic Cells *in Vitro*. *Acta Pharmacol.Toxicol.* **54**:311–320. [8]

Liochev, S. I., and I. Fridovich. 1994. The Role of $O_2^-$ in the Production of HO: *In Vitro* and *in Vivo*. *Free Radic. Biol. Med.* **16**:29–33. [5]

Lippard, S. J., and J. M. Berg. 1994. Principles of Bioinorganic Chemistry. Mill Valley, CA: University Science Books. [14]

Lisher, J. P., and D. P. Giedroc. 2013. Manganese Acquisition and Homeostasis at the Host-Pathogen Interface. *Front. Cell. Infect. Microbiol.* **3**:91. [4]

Liu, J., M. Ballaney, U. Al-alem, et al. 2008 Combined Inhaled Diesel Exhaust Particles and Allergen Exposure Alter Methylation of T Helper Genes and IgE Production *in Vivo*. *Toxicol. Sci.* **102**:76–81. [17]

Liu, J. Z., S. Jellbauer, A. J. Poe, et al. 2012. Zinc Sequestration by the Neutrophil Protein Calprotectin Enhances *Salmonella* Growth in the Inflamed Gut. *Cell Host Microbe* **11**:227–239. [7, 9, 13]

Liu, M.-J., B. Bao, E. R. Bolin, et al. 2013. Zinc Deficiency Augments Leptin Production and Exacerbates Macrophage Infiltration into Adipose Tissue in Mice Fed a High-Fat Diet. *J. Nutr.* **143**:1036–1045. [12]

Liu, M.-J., S. Bao, J. R. Napolitano, et al. 2014. Zinc Regulates the Acute Phase Response and Serum Amyloid A Production in Response to Sepsis Through JAK-STAT3 Signaling. *PLoS ONE* **9(4)**:e94934. [12]

Liu, X., J. A. Buffington, and R. B. Tjalkens. 2005. NF-κB-Dependent Production of Nitric Oxide by Astrocytes Mediates Apoptosis in Differentiated PC12 Neurons Following Exposure to Manganese and Cytokines. *Brain Res. Mol. Brain Res.* **141**:39–47. [13]

Liu, X., M. M. Ramsey, X. Chen, et al. 2011. Real-Time Mapping of a Hydrogen Peroxide Concentration Profile across a Polymicrobial Bacterial Biofilm Using Scanning Electrochemical Microscopy. *PNAS* **108**:2668–2673. [20]

Liu, X. B., M. Tanaka, and Y. Matsui. 2006. Generation Amount Prediction and Material Flow Analysis of Electronic Wastes: A Case Study in Beijing, China. *Waste Manag. Res.* **24**:434–445. [15]

Liu, Y., and J. A. Imlay. 2013. Cell Death from Antibiotics without the Involvement of Reactive Oxygen Species. *Science* **339**:1210–1213. [3]

Liuzzi, J. P., L. A. Lichten, S. Rivera, et al. 2005. Interleukin-6 Regulates the Zinc Transporter Zip14 in Liver and Contributes to the Hypozincemia of the Acute-Phase Response. *PNAS* **103**:6843–6848. [3]

Lizarazo-Jaimes, E. H., R. L. Monte-Neto, P. G. Reis, et al. 2012. Improved Antileishmanial Activity of Dppz through Complexation with Antimony(III) and Bismuth(III): Investigation of the Role of the Metal. *Molecules* **17**:12622–12635. [10]

Ljung, K., B. Palm, M. Grandér, and M. Vahter. 2011. High Concentrations of Essential and Toxic Elements in Infant Formula and Infant Foods: A Matter of Concern. *Food Chem.* **127**:943–951. [17]

Lobinski, R., J. S. Becker, H. Haraguchi, and B. Sarkar. 2010. Metallomics: Guidelines for Terminology and Critical Evaluation of Analytical Chemistry Approaches (IUPAC Technical Report). *Pure Appl. Chem.* **82**:493–504. [14]

Loferski, P. J. 2011. 2010 Minerals Yearbook; Platinum-Group Metals. Usgs Mineral Resources Program. http://minerals.usgs.gov/minerals/pubs/commodity/platinum/myb1-2010-plati.pdf (accessed Oct. 10, 2014). [15]

Loiseau, L., C. Gerez, M. Bekker, et al. 2007. ErpA, an Iron Sulfur (Fe S) Protein of the a-Type Essential for Respiratory Metabolism in *Escherichia coli*. *PNAS* **104**:13626–13631. [5]

Lokuge, K. M., W. Smith, B. Caldwell, K. Dear, and A. H. Milton. 2004. The Effect of Arsenic Mitigation Interventions on Disease Burden in Bangladesh. *Environ. Health Perspect.* **112**:1172–1177. [17]

Lönnerdal, B., C. L. Keen, and L. S. Hurley. 1985. Manganese Binding Proteins in Human and Cow's Milk. *Am. J. Clin. Nutr.* **41**:550–559. [3]

Lothian, A., D. J. Hare, R. Grimm, et al. 2013. Metalloproteomics: Principles, Challenges, and Applications to Neurodegeneration. *Front. Aging Neurosci.* **5**:35. [18]

Lu, C. C., N. Matsumoto, and S. Iijima. 1979. Teratogenic Effects of Nickel Chloride on Embryonic Mice and Its Transfer to Embryonic Mice. *Teratology* **19**:137–142. [8]

Lu, J., A. J. Stewart, P. J. Sadler, T. J. Pinheiro, and C. A. Blindauer. 2008. Albumin as a Zinc Carrier: Properties of Its High-Affinity Zinc-Binding Site. *Biochem. Soc. Trans.* **36**:1317–1321. [2]

Lu, K., P. H. Cable, R. P. Abo, et al. 2013. Gut Microbiome Perturbations Induced by Bacterial Infection Affect Arsenic Biotransformation. *Chem. Res. Toxicol.* **26**:1893–1903. [17]

Lu, M., J. Chai, and D. Fu. 2009. Structural Basis for Autoregulation of the Zinc Transporter YiiP. *Nat. Struct. Mol. Biol.* **16**:1063–1068. [5]

Ludwiczek, S., E. Aigner, I. Theurl, and G. Weiss. 2003. Cytokine-Mediated Regulation of Iron Transport in Human Monocytic Cells. *Blood* **101**:4148–4154. [9]

Lukaski, H. C., W. W. Bolonchuk, W. A. Siders, and D. B. Milne. 1996. Chromium Supplementation and Resistance Training: Effects on Body Composition, Strength, and Trace Element Status of Men. *Am. J. Clin. Nutr.* **63**:954–965. [8]

Lynch, R. J. M. 2011. Zinc in the Mouth, Its Interactions with Dental Enamel and Possible. *Int. Dental J.* **61(Suppl. 3)**:46–54. [17]

Lyons, G., and I. Cakmak. 2012. Agronomic Biofortification of Food Crops with Micronutrients. In: Fertilizing Crops to Improve Human Health: A Scientific Review, vol. 1, Food and Nutrition Security, pp. 97–122. Norcross, GA: International Plant Nutrition Institute. [17]

Lyons, M. J., I. M. Faust, R. B. Hemmes, et al. 1982. A Virally Induced Obesity Syndrome in Mice. *Science* **216**:82–85. [12]

Ma, Y., H. de Groot, Z. Liu, R. C. Hider, and F. Petrat. 2006. Chelation and Determination of Labile Iron in Primary Hepatocytes by Pyridinone Fluorescent Probes. *Biochem. J.* **395**:49–55. [20]

Ma, Z., M. J. Faulkner, and J. D. Helmann. 2012. Origins of the Specificity and Cross-Talk in Metal Ion Sensing by *Bacillus subtilis* Fur. *Mol. Microbiol.* **86**:1144–1155. [5]

Ma, Z., S. E. Gabriel, and J. D. Helmann. 2011. Sequential Binding and Sensing of Zn(II) by *Bacillus subtilis* Zur. *Nucl. Acids Res.* **39**:9130–9138. [5]

Ma, Z., F. E. Jacobsen, and D. P. Giedroc. 2009. Coordination Chemistry of Bacterial Metal Transport and Sensing. *Chem. Rev.* **109**:4644–4681. [5]

Macara, I. G., T. G. Hoy, and P. M. Harrison. 1973. The Formation of Ferritin from Apoferritin: Inhibition and Metal Ion-Binding Studies. *Biochem. J.* **135**:785–789. [3]

Macias, L. B., M. S. Poblet, R. I. Jerez, et al. 2013. Study of Renal Function in Living Kidney Donors: Estimated or Measured Glomerular Filtration. *Transplant. Proc.* **45**:3612–3615. [20]

Macomber, L., and J. A. Imlay. 2009. The Iron-Sulfur Clusters of Dehydratases Are Primary Intracellular Targets of Copper Toxicity. *PNAS* **106**:8344–8349. [5]

Macomber, L., C. Rensing, and J. A. Imlay. 2007. Intracellular Copper Does Not Catalyze the Formation of Oxidative DNA Damage in *Escherichia coli*. *J. Bacteriol.* **189**:1616–1626. [5]

Madejczyk, M. S., and N. Ballatori. 2012. The Iron Transporter Ferroportin Can Also Function as a Manganese Exporter. *Biochim. Biophys. Acta* **1818**:651–657. [2]

Madiwale, T., and E. Liebelt. 2006. Iron: Not a Benign Therapeutic Drug. *Curr. Opin. Pediatr.* **18**:174–179. [8]

Madureira, J., C. I. Ramos, M. Marques, et al. 2013. Nonclassic Metallointercalators with Dipyridophenazine: DNA Interaction Studies and Leishmanicidal Activity. *Inorg. Chem.* **52**:8881–8894. [10]

Magnuson, B. A., T. S. Jonaitis, and J. W. Card. 2011. A Brief Review of the Occurrence, Use, and Safety of Food-Related Nanomaterials. *J. Food Sci.* **76**:R126–133. [17]

Makita, Y., M. Omura, A. Tanaka, and C. Kiyohara. 2005. Effects of Concurrent Exposure to Tributyltin and 1,1-Dichloro-2,2 Bis (P-Chlorophenyl) Ethylene (P,P'-DDE) Onimmature Male Wistar Rats. *Basic Clin. Pharmacol. Toxicol.* **97**:364–368. [12]

Makui, H., E. Roig, S. T. Cole, et al. 2000. Identification of the *Escherichia coli* K-12 NRAMP Orthologue (MntH) as a Selective Divalent Metal Ion Transporter. *Mol. Microbiol.* **35**:1065–1078. [5]

Malstrom, S. E., D. Jekic-McMullen, L. Sambucetti, et al. 2004. *In Vivo* Bioluminescent Monitoring of Chemical Toxicity Using Heme Oxygenase-Luciferase Transgenic Mice. *Toxicol. Appl. Pharmacol.* **200**:219–228. [20]

Mancuso, P. 2013. Obesity and Respiratory Infections: Does Excess Adiposity Weigh Down Host Defense? *Pulm. Pharmacol. Ther.* **26**:412–419. [12]

Mancuso, P., A. Gottschalk, S. M. Phare, et al. 2002. Leptin-Deficient Mice Exhibit Impaired Host Defense in Gram-Negative Pneumonia. *J. Immunol.* **168**:4018–4024. [12]

Mantzoros, C. S., A. S. Prasad, F. W. Beck, et al. 1998. Zinc May Regulate Serum Leptin Concentrations in Humans. *J. Am. Coll. Nutr.* **17**:270–275. [12]

Marcellini, F., C. Giuli, R. Papa, et al. 2006. Zinc Status, Psychological and Nutritional Assessment in Old People Recruited in Five European Countries: Zincage Study. *Biogerontology* **7**:339–345. [11]

Marco, M. L., and S. Tachon. 2013. Environmental Factors Influencing the Efficacy of Probiotic Bacteria. *Curr. Opin. Biotechnol.* **24**:207–213. [17]

Maret, W. 2010. Metalloproteomics, Metalloproteomes, and the Annotation of Metalloproteins. *Metallomics* **2**:117–125. [4, 14, 20]

———. 2012. New Perspectives of Zinc Coordination Environments in Proteins. *J. Inorg. Biochem.* **111**:110–116. [8]

———. 2013. Zinc and the Zinc Proteome. In: Metallomics and the Cell, ed. L. Banci, pp. 479–501, Metal Ions in Life Sciences, vol. 12. Amsterdam: Springer. [2]

Maret, W., and M. Copsey. 2012. Metallomics: Whence and Whither. *Metallomics* **4**:1017–1019. [14]

Maret, W., and H. H. Sandstead. 2006. Zinc Requirements and the Risks and Benefits of Zinc Supplementation. *J. Trace Elem. Med. Biol.* **20**:3–18. [8]

Mariani, E., F. Mangialasche, F. T. Feliziani, et al. 2008. Effects of Zinc Supplementation on Antioxidant Enzyme Activities in Healthy Old Subjects. *Exp. Gerontol.* **43**:445–451. [11]

Marks, R. 1993. Stained Glass in England During the Middle Ages. London: Routledge. [15]

Marri, P. R., M. Paniscus, N. J. Weyand, et al. 2010. Genome Sequencing Reveals Widespread Virulence Gene Exchange among Human *Neisseria* Species. *PLoS One* **5**:e11835. [2, 7]

Marshall, M. V., J. C. Rasmussen, I.-C. Tan, et al. 2010. Near-Infrared Fluorescence Imaging in Humans with Indocyanine Green: A Review and Update. *Open Surg. Oncol. J.* **2**:12–25. [20]

Marti, A., A. Marcos, and J. A. Martinez. 2010. Obesity and Immune Function Relationships. *Obes. Rev.* **2**:131–140. [12]

Marti-Cid, R., A. Bocio, J. M. Llobet, and J. L. Domingo. 2007. Intake of Chemical Contaminants through Fish and Seafood Consumption by Children of Catalonia, Spain: Health Risks. *Food Chem. Toxicol.* **45**:1968–1974. [11]

Martin, J. E., and J. A. Imlay. 2011. The Alternative Aerobic Ribonucleotide Reductase of *Escherichia coli*, NrdEF, Is a Manganese-Dependent Enzyme That Enables Cell Replication During Periods of Iron Starvation. *Mol. Microbiol.* **80**:319–334. [4, 5]

Martínez, A., T. Carreon, E. Iniguez, et al. 2012. Searching for New Chemotherapies for Tropical Diseases: Ruthenium-Clotrimazole Complexes Display High *in Vitro* Activity against *Leishmania major* and *Trypanosoma cruzi* and Low Toxicity Towards Normal Mammalian Cells. *J. Med. Chem.* **55**:3867–3877. [10]

Martinez, J. L. 2009. Environmental Pollution by Antibiotics and by Antibiotic Resistance Determinants. *Environ. Pollut.* **157**:2893–2902. [17]

Masaisa, F., J. B. Gahutu, J. Mukiibi, J. Delanghe, and J. Philippé. 2012. Transferrin Polymorphism and Opportunistic Infections in HIV-Infected Women in Rwanda. *Acta Haematol.* **128**:100–106. [20]

Masharani, U., C. Gjerde, S. McCoy, et al. 2012. Chromium Supplementation in Non-Obese Non-Diabetic Subjects Is Associated with a Decline in Insulin Sensitivity. *BMC Endocr. Disord.* **12**:31. [8]

Masse, E., C. K. Vanderpool, and S. Gottesman. 2005. Effect of RyhB Small RNA on Global Iron Use in *Escherichia coli*. *J. Bacteriol.* **187**:6962–6971. [5, 7]

Mathema, V., B. Thakuri, and M. Sillanpää. 2011. Bacterial Mer Operon-Mediated Detoxification of Mercurial Compounds: A Short Review. *Arch. Microbiol.* **193**:837–844. [4]

Matsuzawa-Nagata, N., T. Takamura, H. Ando, et al. 2008. Increased Oxidative Stress Precedes the Onset of High-Fat Diet-Induced Insulin Resistance and Obesity. *Metabolism* **57**:1071–1077. [12]

Matusch, A., L. S. Fenn, C. Depboylu, et al. 2012. Combined Elemental and Biomolecular Mass Spectrometry Imaging for Probing the Inventory of Tissue at a Micrometer Scale. *Anal. Chem.* **84**:3170–3178. [19]

Maull, E. A., H. Ahsan, J. Edwards, and et al. 2012. Evaluation of the Association between Arsenic and Diabetes: A National Toxicology Program Workshop Review. *Environ. Health Perspect.* **120**:1658–1670. [12]

Mayer, D. R., W. Kosmus, H. Pogglitsch, D. Mayer, and W. Beyer. 1993. Essential Trace Elements in Humans: Serum Arsenic Concentrations in Hemodialysis Patients in Comparison to Healthy Controls. *Biol. Trace Elem. Res.* **37**:27–38. [8]

McClelland, E. E., and J. M. Smith. 2011. Gender Specific Differences in the Immune Response to Infection. *Arch. Immunol. Ther. Exp.* **59**:203–213. [17]

McClung, J. P., and J. P. Karl. 2009. Iron Deficiency and Obesity: The Contribution of Inflammation and Diminished Iron Absorption. *Nutr. Rev.* **67**:100–104. [12]

McDevitt, C. A., A. D. Ogunniyi, E. Valkov, et al. 2011. A Molecular Mechanism for Bacterial Susceptibility to Zinc. *PLoS Pathog.* **7**:e1002357. [3, 7]

McKelvey, W., R. C. Gwynn, N. Jeffery, et al. 2007. A Biomonitoring Study of Lead, Cadmium, and Mercury in the Blood of New York City Adults. *Environ. Health Perspect.* **115**:1435–1441. [11]

McNaughton, R. L., A. R. Reddi, M. H. Clement, et al. 2010. Probing *in Vivo* $Mn^{2+}$ Speciation and Oxidative Stress Resistance in Yeast Cells with Electron-Nuclear Double Resonance Spectroscopy. *PNAS* **107**:15335–15339. [20]

McRae, R., P. Bagchi, S. Sumalekshmy, and C. J. Fahrni. 2009. *In Situ* Imaging of Metals in Cells and Tissues. *Chem. Rev.* **109**:4780–4827. [18–20]

Mealman, T. D., N. J. Blackburn, and M. M. McEvoy. 2012. Metal Export by CusCFBA, the Periplasmic Cu(I)/Ag(I) Transport System of *Escherichia coli. Curr. Top. Membr.* **69**:163–196. [4]

Medzhitov, R., D. S. Schneider, and M. P. Soares. 2012. Disease Tolerance as a Defense Strategy. *Science* **335**:936–941. [1, 10, 13, 17]

Meeker, J. D., M. G. Rossano, B. Protas, et al. 2008. Cadmium, Lead, and Other Metals in Relation to Semen Quality: Human Evidence for Molybdenum as a Male Reproductive Toxicant. *Environ. Health Perspect.* **116**:1473–1479. [11]

Meharg, A. A., E. Lombi, P. N. Williams, et al. 2008. Speciation and Localization of Arsenic in White and Brown Rice Grains. *Environ. Sci. Technol.* **42**:1051–1057. [20]

Melican, K., and A. Richter-Dahlfors. 2009. Real-Time Live Imaging to Study Bacterial Infections *in Vivo. Curr. Opin. Microbiol.* **12**:31–36. [20]

Mencacci, A., E. Cenci, J. R. Boelaert, et al. 1997. Iron Overload Alters Innate and T Helper Cell Responses to *Candida albicans* in Mice. *J. Infect. Dis.* **175**:1467–1476. [9, 13]

Mendel, R. R., and F. Bittner. 2006. Cell Biology of Molybdenum. *Biochim. Biophys. Acta* **1763**:621–635. [8]

Mendel, R. R., and T. Kruse. 2012. Cell Biology of Molybdenum in Plants and Humans. *Biochim. Biophys. Acta* **1823**:1568–1579. [2]

Merrill, M. L., and L. S. Birnbaum. 2011. Childhood Obesity and Environmental Chemicals. *Mt. Sinai J. Med.* **78**:22–48. [12]

Mertz, W. 1993. Chromium in Human Nutrition. *J. Nutr.* **123**:626–633. [13]

Merza, M., P. Farnia, S. Anoosheh, et al. 2009. The NRAMP1, VDR and TNF-Alpha Gene Polymorphisms in Iranian Tuberculosis Patients: The Study on Host Susceptibility. *Braz. J. Infect. Dis.* **13**:252–256. [17]

Meyer, J., M. R. Stohle, and M. J. Stablein. 1981. Correlation of Changes in Capillary Supply and Epithelial Dimensions in the Hyperplastic Buccal Mucosa of Zinc-Deficient Rats. *J. Oral Biol.* **10**:49–59. [17]

Miao, R., M. Martinho, J. G. Morales, et al. 2008. EPR and Mossbauer Spectroscopy of Intact Mitochondria Isolated from Yah1p-Depleted *Saccharomyces cerevisiae. Biochemistry* **47**:9888–9899. [20]

Michalak, I., M. Mikulewicz, K. Chojnacka, et al. 2012. Exposure to Nickel by Hair Mineral Analysis. *Environ. Toxicol. Pharmacol.* **34**:727–734. [11]

Michalke, B., S. Halbach, and V. Nischwitz. 2007. Speciation and Toxicological Relevance of Manganese in Humans. *J. Environ. Monit.* **9**:650–656. [2, 11]

Miethke, M., J. Hou, and M. A. Marahiel. 2011. The Siderophore-Interacting Protein yqjH Acts as a Ferric Reductase in Different Iron Assimilation Pathways of *Escherichia coli. Biochemistry* **50**:10951–10964. [5]

Mijnendonckx, K., N. Leys, J. Mahillon, S. Silver, and R. Van Houdt. 2013. Antimicrobial Silver: Uses, Toxicity and Potential for Resistance. *Biometals* **26**:609–621. [7]

Miller, G. W., and D. P. Jones. 2014. The Nature of Nurture: Refining the Definition of the Exposome. *Toxicol. Sci.* **138**:1–2. [17]

Miller, L. H., H. C. Ackerman, X. Z. Su, and T. E. Wellems. 2013. Malaria Biology and Disease Pathogenesis: Insights for New Treatments. *Nat. Med.* **19**:156–167. [13]

Miller, M. R., A. White, and M. Boots. 2006. The Evolution of Parasites in Response to Tolerance in Their Hosts: The Good, the Bad, and Apparent Commensalism. *Evolution* **60**:945–956. [1, 17]

Mills, S. A., and M. A. Marletta. 2005. Metal Binding Characteristics and Role of Iron Oxidation in the Ferric Uptake Regulator from *Escherichia coli*. *Biochemistry* **44**:13553–13559. [5]

Min, K.-S., H. Ueda, T. Kihara, and K. Tanaka. 2008. Increased Hepatic Accumulation of Ingested Cd Is Associated with Upregulation of Several Intestinal Transporters in Mice Fed Diets Deficient in Essential Metals. *Toxicol. Sci.* **106**:284–289. [6]

Mishra, D., and S. J. S. Flora. 2008. Differential Oxidative Stress and DNA Damage in Rat Brain Regions and Blood Following Chronic Arsenic Exposure. *Toxicol. Ind. Heath* **24**:247–256. [12]

Miyawaki, A., J. Llopis, R. Heim, et al. 1997. Fluorescent Indicators for $Ca^{2+}$ Based on Green Fluorescent Proteins and Calmodulin. *Nature* **388**:882–887. [20]

Moayeri, H., K. Bidad, S. Zadhoush, N. Gholami, and S. Anari. 2006. Increasing Prevalence of Iron Deficiency in Overweight and Obese Children and Adolescents (Tehran Adolescent Obesity Study). *Eur. J. Pediatr.* **165**:813–814. [12]

Mocchegiani, E., J. Romeo, M. Malavolta, et al. 2013. Zinc: Dietary Intake and Impact of Supplementation on Immune Function in Elderly. *Age* **35**:839–860. [8]

Modell, B., and M. Darlison. 2008. Global Epidemiology of Haemoglobin Disorders and Derived Service Indicators. *Bull. WHO* **86**:480–487. [6]

Modi, M., R. K. Kaul, G. M. Kannan, and S. J. S. Flora. 2006. Co-Administration of Zinc and N-Acetylcysteine Prevents Arsenic-Induced Tissue Oxidative Stress in Male Rats. *J. Trace Elem. Med. Biol.* **20**:197–204. [14]

Monachese, M., J. P. Burton, and G. Reid. 2012. Bioremediation and Tolerance of Humans to Heavy Metals through Microbial Processes: A Potential Role for Probiotics? *Appl. Environ. Microbiol.* **78**:6397–6404. [17]

Montefusco, S., R. Esposito, L. D'Andrea, et al. 2013. Copper Promotes TFF1-Mediated *Helicobacter pylori* Colonization. *PLoS One* **8**:e79455. [11]

Monteiro, C. A., E. C. Moura, W. L. Conde, and B. M. Popkin. 2004. Socioeconomic Status and Obesity in Adult Populations of Developing Countries: A Review. *Bull. WHO* **282**:940–946. [12]

Montenegro, M. F., F. Barbosa, Jr., V. C. Sandrim, R. F. Gerlach, and J. E. Tanus-Santos. 2006. A Polymorphism in the Delta-Aminolevulinic Acid Dehydratase Gene Modifies Plasma/Whole Blood Lead Ratio. *Arch. Toxicol.* **80**:394–398. [17]

Moon, S. S. 2013. Additive Effect of Heavy Metals on Metabolic Syndrome in the Korean Population: The Korea National Health and Nutrition Examination Survey (KNHANES) 2009–2010. *Endocrine* **46**:263–271. [17]

Moore, K. L., Y. Chen, A. M. L. van de Meene, et al. 2014. Combined NanoSIMS and Synchrotron X-Ray Fluorescence Reveal Distinct Cellular and Subcellular Distribution Patterns of Trace Elements in Rice Tissues. *New Phytol.* **201**:104–115. [20]

Moore, K. L., M. Schroder, E. Lombi, et al. 2010. NanoSIMS analysis of arsenic and selenium in cereal grain. *New Phytologist.* **185**:434–445. [20]

Moos, T. 1993. Simultaneous Application of Timm's Sulphide Silver Method and Immunofluorescence Histochemistry. *J. Neurosci. Meth.* **48**:149–156. [19]

Moreno, F., T. García-Barrera, and J. L. Gómez-Ariza. 2010. Simultaneous Analysis of Mercury and Selenium Species Including Chiral Forms of Selenomethionine in Human Urine and Serum by HPLC Column-Switching Coupled to ICP-MS. *Analyst* **135**:2700–2705. [14]

Moreno-Gordaliza, E., B. Canas, M. A. Palacios, and M. M. Gomez-Gomez. 2009. Top-Down Mass Spectrometric Approach for the Full Characterization of Insulin-Cisplatin Adducts. *Anal. Chem.* **81**:3507–3516. [20]

———. 2010. Novel Insights into the Bottom-up Mass Spectrometry Proteomics Approach for the Characterization of Pt-Binding Proteins: The Insulin-Cisplatin Case Study. *Analyst* **135**:1288–1298. [20]

Moreno-Gordaliza, E., C. Giesen, A. Lazaro, et al. 2011. Elemental Bioimaging in Kidney by LA-ICP-MS as a Tool to Study Nephrotoxicity and Renal Protective Strategies in Cisplatin Therapies. *Anal. Chem.* **83**:7933–7940. [20]

Morgan, O. W., A. Bramley, A. Fowlkes, et al. 2010. Morbid Obesity as a Risk Factor for Hospitalization and Death Due to 2009 Pandemic Influenza A(H1N1) Disease. *PLoS ONE* **5**:e9694. [12]

Morgenthau, A., A. Pogoutse, P. Adamiak, T. F. Moraes, and A. B. Schryvers. 2013. Bacterial Receptors for Host Transferrin and Lactoferrin: Molecular Mechanisms and Role in Host-Microbe Interactions. *Fut. Microbiol.* **8**:1575–1585. [2]

Mori, R., E. Ota, P. Middleton, et al. 2012. Zinc Supplementation for Improving Pregnancy and Infant Outcome. *Cochrane Database Syst. Rev.* **7**:CD000230. [8]

Morrens, B., L. Bruckers, E. D. Hond, et al. 2012. Social Distribution of Internal Exposure to Environmental Pollution in Flemish Adolescents. *Int. J. Hyg. Environ. Health* **215**:474–481. [11]

Moukarzel, A. 2009. Chromium in Parenteral Nutrition: Too Little or Too Much? *Gastroenterology* **137(Suppl 5)**:S18–S28. [8]

Mounicou, S., J. Szpunar, and R. Lobinski. 2009. Metallomics: The Concept and Methodology. *Chem. Soc. Rev.* **38**:1119–1138. [14, 18]

Moutafchiev, D., L. Sirakov, and P. Bontchev. 1998. The Competition between Transferrins Labeled with $^{59}$Fe, $^{65}$Zn, and $^{54}$Mn for the Binding Sites on Lactating Mouse Mammary Gland Cells. *Biol. Trace Elem. Res.* **61**:181–191. [3]

Mshvildadze, M., and J. Neu. 2010. The Infant Intestinal Microbiome: Friend or Foe? *Early Hum. Dev.* **86**:S67–S71. [17]

Mu, M., A. Wu, P. An, et al. 2014. Black Soyabean Seed Coat Extract Regulates Iron Metabolism by Inhibiting the Expression of Hepcidin. *Br. J. Nutr.* **111**:1181–1189. [6]

Muayed, M. E., M. R. Raja, X. Zhang, et al. 2012. Accumulation of Cadmium in Insulin-Producing Beta Cells. *Islets* **4**:405–416. [12]

Müller, M. J., H. Maier, and R. Mann. 2007. Nationaler Aktionsplan Gegen Das Übergewicht (a German National Action Plan against Obesity). Stuttgart: Georg Thieme Verlag. [8]

Munson, G. P., D. L. Lam, F. W. Outten, and T. V. O'Halloran. 2000. Identification of a Copper-Responsive Two-Component System on the Chromosome of *Escherichia coli* K-12. *J. Bacteriol.* **182**:5864–5871. [5]

Mustafa, A. K., M. M. Gadalla, and S. H. Snyder. 2009. Signaling by Gasotransmitters. *Sci. Signal.* **2**:re2. [13]

Nairz, M., U. Schleicher, A. Schroll, et al. 2013. Nitric Oxide-Mediated Regulation of Ferroportin-1 Controls Macrophage Iron Homeostasis and Immune Function in *Salmonella* Infection. *J. Exp. Med.* **210**:855–873. [9, 13]

Nairz, M., A. Schroll, T. Sonnweber, and G. Weiss. 2010. The Struggle for Iron: A Metal at the Host–Pathogen Interface. *Cell. Microbiol.* **12**:1691–1702. [3, 9, 13]

Nairz, M., I. Theurl, A. Schroll, et al. 2009. Absence of Functional Hfe Protects Mice from Invasive *Salmonella enterica* serovar *Typhimurium* Infection via Induction of Lipocalin-2. *Blood* **114**:3642–3651. [9, 13]

Naka, T., H. Kaneto, N. Katakami, and et al. 2013. Association of Serum Copper Levels and Glycemic Control in Patients with Type 2 Diabetes. *Endocrine J.* **60**:393–396. [12]

Nanamiya, H., G. Akanuma, Y. Natori, et al. 2004. Zinc Is a Key Factor in Controlling Alteration of Two Types of L31 Protein in the *Bacillus subtilis* Ribosome. *Mol. Microbiol.* **52**:273–283. [5, 7]

Nandal, A., C. C. Huggins, M. R. Woodhall, et al. 2010. Induction of the Ferritin Gene (*ftnA*) of *Escherichia coli* by $Fe^{(2+)}$-Fur Is Mediated by Reversal of H-NS Silencing and Is RyhB Independent. *Mol. Microbiol.* **75**:637–657. [5]

Naranuntarat, A., L. T. Jensen, S. Pazicni, J. E. Penner-Hahn, and V. C. Culotta. 2009. The Interaction of Mitochondrial Iron with Manganese Superoxide Dismutase. *J. Biol. Chem.* **284**:22633–22640. [4]

Nathan, C. F. 2008. Epidemic Inflammation: Pondering Obesity. *Mol. Med.* **14**:485–492. [12]

Natvig, D. O., K. Imlay, D. Touati, and R. A. Hallewell. 1987. Human Copper-Zinc Superoxide Dismutase Complements Superoxide Dismutase-Deficient *Escherichia coli* Mutants. *J. Biol. Chem.* **262**:14697–14701. [5]

Navarro, M. 2009. Gold Complexes as Potential Anti-Parasitic Agents. *Coord. Chem. Rev.* **253**:1619–1626. [10]

Navarro, M., W. Castro, and C. Biot. 2012. Bioorganometallic Compounds with Antimalarial Targets: Inhibiting Hemozoin Formation. *Organometallics* **31**:5715–5727. [10, 13]

Navarro, M., C. Gabbiani, L. Messori, and D. Gambino. 2010. Metal-Based Drugs for Malaria, Trypanosomiasis and Leishmaniasis: Recent Achivements and Perspectives. *Drug Discov. Today* **15**:1070–1078. [10, 13]

Navarro, M., G. Visbal, and E. Marchan. 2007. DNA Metallo-Intercalators with Leishmanicidal Activity. In: Programmed Cell Death in Protozoa, ed. J. M. P. Martin. New York: Landes Bioscience and Springer Science + Business Media. [10]

Navarro-Alarcon, M., and C. Cabrera-Vique. 2008. Selenium in Food and the Human Body: A Review. *Sci. Total Environ.* **400**:115–141. [11]

Nave, H., G. Beutel, and J. T. Kielstein. 2011. Obesity-Related Immunodeficiency in Patients with Pandemic Influenza H1N1. *Lancet Infect. Dis.* **11**:14–15. [12]

Nead, K. G., J. S. Halterman, J. M. Kaczorowski, P. Auinger, and M. Weitzman. 2004. Overweight Children and Adolescents: A Risk Group for Iron Deficiency. *Pediatrics* **114**:104–108. [12]

Nechay, B. R., L. B. Nanninga, and P. S. Nechay. 1986. Vanadyl (IV) and Vanadate (V) Binding to Selected Endogenous Phosphate, Carboxyl, and Amino Ligands: Calculations of Cellular Vanadium Species Distribution. *Arch. Biochem. Biophys.* **251**:128–138. [8]

Nelson, A. L., J. M. Barasch, R. M. Bunte, and J. N. Weiser. 2005. Bacterial Colonization of Nasal Mucosa Induces Expression of Siderocalin, an Iron-Sequestering Component of Innate Immunity. *Cell. Microbiol.* **7**:1404–1417. [3]

Nelson, A. L., A. J. Ratner, J. Barasch, and J. N. Weiser. 2007. Interleukin-8 Secretion in Response to Aferric Enterobactin Is Potentiated by Siderocalin. *Infect. Immun.* **75**:3160–3168. [3]

Neumann, M., and S. Leimkühler. 2011. The Role of System-Specific Molecular Chaperones in the Maturation of Molybdoenzymes in Bacteria. *Biochem. Res. Int.* **2011**:850924. [4]

Nevitt, T., and D. J. Thiele. 2011. Host Iron Withholding Demands Siderophore Utilization for *Candida Glabrata* to Survive Macrophage Killing. *PLoS Pathog.* 7:e1001322. [7]

Ngu, T. T., and M. J. Stillman. 2006. Arsenic Binding to Human Metallothionein. *J. Am. Chem. Soc.* **128**:12473–12483. [20]

Nicholson, J. K., J. C. Lindon, and E. Holmes. 1999. "Metabonomics": Understanding the Metabolic Responses of Living Systems to Pathophysiological Stimuli via Multivariate Statistical Analysis of Biological NMR Spectroscopic Data. *Xenobiotica* **29**:1181. [14]

Nieman, D. C., D. A. Henson, S. L. Nehlsen-Cannarella, et al. 1999. Influence of Obesity on Immune Function. *J. Am. Diet. Assoc.* **99**:294–299. [12]

Nies, D. H. 2003. Efflux-Mediated Heavy Metal Resistance in Prokaryotes. *FEMS Microbiol. Rev.* **27**:313–339. [4]

———. 2007. Bacterial Transition Metal Homeostasis. In: Molecular Microbiology of Heavy Metals, ed. D. H. Nies and S. Silver, pp. 117–142. Berlin: Springer-Verlag. [4]

Nies, D. H., A. Nies, L. Chu, and S. Silver. 1989. Expression and Nucleotide Sequence of a Plasmid-Determined Divalent Cation Efflux System from *Alcaligenes eutrophus*. *PNAS* **86**:7351–7355. [4]

NIH HMP Working Group. 2009. The NIH Human Microbiome Project. *Genome Res.* **19**:2317–2323. [7]

Nikonorova, A., M. G. Skalnaya, A. A. Tinkova, and A. V. Skalny. 2014. Mutual Interaction between Iron Homeostasis and Obesity Pathogenesis. *J. Trace Elem. Med. Biol.* May 24, pii: S0946–0672X(14)00071–76. [Epub ahead of print]. [12]

Niu, G., K. J. Krager, M. M. Graham, R. D. Hichwa, and F. E. Domann. 2005. Noninvasive Radiological Imaging of Pulmonary Gene Transfer and Expression Using the Human Sodium Iodide Symporter. *Eur. J. Nucl. Med. Mol. Imaging* **32**:534–540. [20]

Nizet, V., and R. S. Johnson. 2009. Interdependence of Hypoxic and Innate Immune Responses. *Nat. Rev. Immunol.* **9**:609–617. [17]

Nohynek, G. J., R. Fautz, F. Benech-Kieffer, and H. Toutain. 2004. Toxicity and Human Health Risk of Hair Dyes. *Food Chem. Toxicol.* **42**:517–543. [11]

Noinaj, N., M. Guillier, T. J. Barnard, and S. K. Buchanan. 2010. TonB-Dependent Transporters: Regulation, Structure, and Function. *Annu. Rev. Microbiol.* **64**:43–60. [2]

Nonaka, H., R. Hata, T. Doura, et al. 2013. A Platform for Designing Hyperpolarized Magnetic Resonance Chemical Probes. *Nat. Commun.* **4**:2411. [20]

Nordberg, M., and G. F. Nordberg. 2000. Toxicological Aspects of Metallothionein. *Cell. Mol. Biol.* **46**:451–463. [17]

Norowski, P. A., and J. D. Bumgardner. 2009. Biomaterial and Antibiotic Strategies for Peri-Implantitis. *J. Biomed. Mater. Res.* **88**:530–543. [16]

Norris, V., M. Chen, M. Goldberg, et al. 1991. Calcium in Bacteria: A Solution to Which Problem? *Mol. Microbiol.* **5**:775–778. [4]

Northrop-Clewes, C. A., and D. I. Thurnham. 2007. Monitoring Micronutrients in Cigarette Smokers. *Clin. Chim. Acta* **377**:14–38. [11]

Noyce, J. O., H. Michels, and C. W. Keevil. 2006. Potential Use of Copper Surfaces to Reduce Survival of Epidemic Meticillin-Resistant *Staphylococcus aureus* in the Healthcare Environment. *J. Hosp. Infect.* **63**:289–297. [11]

Nriagu, J. O., ed. 1984. Changing Metal Cycles and Human Health. Life Sciences Research Report 28. Berlin: Springer-Verlag. [17]

Nriagu, J. O., P. Bhattacharya, A. B. Mukherjee, et al. 2007. Arsenic in Soil and Groundwater: An Overview. In: Trace Metals and Other Contaminants in the Environment, ed. P. Bhattacharya et al., vol. 9, pp. 3–60 Amsterdam: Elsevier. [12]

Nriagu, J. O., and J. M. Pacyna. 1988. Quantitative Assessment of Worldwide Contamination of Air, Water and Soils by Trace Metals. *Nature* **333**:134–139. [15]

Nucifora, G., L. Chu, T. K. Misra, and S. Silver. 1989. Cadmium Resistance from *Staphylococcus aureus* Plasmid pl258 *cadA* Gene Results from a Cadmium-Efflux ATPase. *PNAS* **86**:3544–3548. [4]

Nyasae, L., R. Bustos, L. Braiterman, B. Eipper, and A. Hubbard. 2007. Dynamics of Endogenous ATP7A (Menkes Protein) in Intestinal Epithelial Cells: Copper-Dependent Redistribution between Two Intracellular Sites. *Am. J. Physiol Gastrointest. Liver Physiol.* **292**:G1181–G1194. [8]

Nyland, J. F., D. Fairweather, D. L. Shirley, et al. 2012. Low-Dose Inorganic Mercury Increases Severity and Frequency of Chronic Coxsackievirus-Induced Autoimmune Myocarditis in Mice. *Toxicol. Sci.* **125**:134–143. [17]

Ochi, A., E. Ishimura, Y. Tsujimoto, et al. 2011. Trace Elements in the Hair of Hemodialysis Patients. *Biol. Trace Elem. Res.* **143**:825–834. [11]

O'Donnell, R. T., G. L. DeNardo, D. L. Kukis, et al. 1999. A Clinical Trial of Radioimmunotherapy with [67]Cu-2IT-BAT-Lym-1 for Non-Hodgkin's Lymphoma. *J. Nucl. Med.* **40**:2014–2020. [20]

Offenbacher, E. G., H. Spencer, H. J. Dowling, and F. X. Pi-Sunyer. 1986. Metabolic Chromium Balances in Men. *Am. J. Clin. Nutr.* **44**:77–82. [8]

Ogra, Y., and Y. Annan. 2012. Selenometabolomics Explored by Speciation. *Biol. Pharm. Bull.* **35**:1863–1869. [14]

O'Halloran, T. V., and V. C. Culotta. 2000. Metallochaperones: An Intracellular Shuttle Service for Metal Ions. *J. Biol. Chem.* **275**:25057–25060. [14]

Okamoto, S., and L. D. Eltis. 2011. The Biological Occurrence and Trafficking of Cobalt. *Metallomics* **3**:963–970. [4]

Okazaki, Y., and E. Gotoh. 2013. Metal Ion Effects on Different Types of Cell Line, Metal Ion Incorporation into L929 and MC3T3-E1 Cells, and Activation of Macrophage-Like J774.1 Cells. *Mater. Sci. Eng. C Mater. Biol. Appl.* **33**:1993–2001. [16]

Olmedo, P., A. F. Hernandez, A. Pla, et al. 2013. Determination of Essential Elements (Copper, Manganese, Selenium and Zinc) in Fish and Shellfish Samples: Risk and Nutritional Assessment and Mercury-Selenium Balance. *Food Chem. Toxicol.* **62**:299–307. [11]

Olson, J. W., and R. J. Maier. 2002. Molecular Hydrogen as an Energy Source for *Helicobacter pylori*. *Science* **298**:1788–1790. [4]

Omara, F. O., and B. R. Blakley. 1994. The Effects of Iron Deficiency and Iron Overload on Cell-Mediated Immunity in the Mouse. *Br. J. Nutr.* **72**:899–909. [9, 13]

O'Neill, M. S., A. J. McMichael, J. Schwartz, and D. Wartenberg. 2007. Poverty, Environment, and Health: The Role of Environmental Epidemiology and Environmental Epidemiologists. *Epidemiology* **18**:664–668. [11]

Oppenheimer, S. J. 2001. Iron and Its Relation to Immunity and Infectious Disease. *J. Nutr.* **131**:616S–633S; discussion 633S–635S. [9, 13]

Ordway, D., M. Henao-Tamayo, E. Smith, et al. 2008. Animal Model of *Mycobacterium abscessus* Lung Infection. *J. Leukoc. Biol.* **83**:1502–1511. [12]

Orisakwe, O. E., O. J. Afonne, E. Nwobodo, L. Asomugha, and C. E. Dioka. 2001. Low-Dose Mercury Induces Testicular Damage Protected by Zinc in Mice. *Eur. J. Obstet. Gynecol. Reprod. Biol.* **95**:92–96. [14]

Ortega, R. 2009. Synchrotron Radiation for Direct Analysis of Metalloproteins on Electrophoresis Gels. *Metallomics* **1**:137–141. [18]

Osman, D., C. J. Patterson, K. Bailey, et al. 2013. The Copper Supply Pathway to a *Salmonella* Cu,Zn-Superoxide Dismutase (SodCII) Involves P(1b)-Type ATPase Copper Efflux and Periplasmic CueP. *Mol. Microbiol.* **87**:466–477. [5, 7]

Osman, D., K. J. Waldron, H. Denton, et al. 2010. Copper Homeostasis in *Salmonella* Is Atypical and Copper-CueP Is a Major Periplasmic Metal Complex. *J. Biol. Chem.* **285**:25259–25268. [7]

Ostrowski, K., C. Hermann, A. Bangash, et al. 1998. A Trauma-Like Elevation of Plasma Cytokines in Humans in Response to Treadmill Running. *J. Physiol.* **513(Pt 3)**:889–894. [11]

Oteiza, P. I. 2012. Zinc and the Modulation of Redox Homeostasis. *Free Radic. Biol. Med.* **53**:1748–1759. [12]

Outten, C. E., and T. V. O'Halloran. 2001. Femtomolar Sensitivity of Metalloregulatory Proteins Controlling Zinc Homeostasis. *Science* **292**:2488–2492. [4, 5]

Outten, F. W., O. Djaman, and G. Storz. 2004. A Suf Operon Requirement for Fe-S Cluster Assembly During Iron Starvation in *Escherichia coli. Mol. Microbiol.* **52**:861–872. [5]

Outten, F. W., C. E. Outten, J. Hale, and T. V. O'Halloran. 2000. Transcriptional Activation of an *Escherichia coli* Copper Efflux Regulon by the Chromosomal MerR Homologue, Cuer. *J. Biol. Chem.* **275**:31024–31029. [5]

Owen, G. A., B. Pascoe, D. Kallifidas, and M. S. Paget. 2007. Zinc-Responsive Regulation of Alternative Ribosomal Protein Genes in *Streptomyces coelicolor* Involves Zur and Sigma R. *J. Bacteriol.* **189**:4078–4086. [5]

Ozata, M., M. Mergen, C. Oktenli, et al. 2002. Increased Oxidative Stress and Hypozincemia in Male Obesity. *Clin. Biochem.* **35**:627–631. [12]

Paauw, A., M. A. Leverstein-van Hall, K. P. M. van Kessel, J. Verhoef, and A. C. Fluit. 2009. Yersiniabactin Reduces the Respiratory Oxidative Stress Response of Innate Immune Cells. *PLoS One* **4**:e8240. [3]

Pacyna, E. G., J. M. Pacyna, K. Sundseth, et al. 2010. Global Emission of Mercury to the Atmosphere from Anthropogenic Sources in 2005 and Projections to 2020. *Atmosph. Environ.* **44**:2487–2499. [17]

Pacyna, J. M., and E. G. Pacyna. 2001. Assessment of Global and Regional Emissions of Trace Metals to the Atmosphere from Anthropogenic Sources Worldwide. *Can. J. Environ. Rev.* **9**:269–298. [15, 17]

Padial-Molina, M., P. Galindo-Moreno, J. E. Fernández-Barbero, et al. 2011. Role of Wettability and Nanoroughness on Interactions between Osteoblast and Modified Silicon Surfaces. *Acta Biomater.* **7**:771–778. [16]

Padilla-Benavides, T., C. J. McCann, and J. M. Arguello. 2013. The Mechanism of $Cu^+$ Transport ATPases: Interaction with $Cu^+$ Chaperones And the Role of Transient Metal-Binding Sites. *J. Biol. Chem.* **288**:69–78. [5]

Palmer, A. E., Y. Qin, J. G. Park, and J. E. McCombs. 2011. Design and Application of Genetically Encoded Biosensors. *Trends Biotechnol.* **29**:144–152. [20]

Palmer, C., E. M. Bik, D. B. DiGiulio, D. A. Relman, and P. O. Brown. 2007. Development of the Human Infant Intestinal Microbiota. *PLoS Biol.* **5**:e177. [17]

Palmiter, R. D. 2004. Protection against Zinc Toxicity by Metallothionein and Zinc Transporter 1. *PNAS* **101**:4918–4923. [16]

Pamplona, A., A. Ferreira, J. Balla, et al. 2007. Heme Oxygenase-1 and Carbon Monoxide Suppress the Pathogenesis of Experimental Cerebral Malaria. *Nat. Med.* **13**:703–710. [13]

Panel on Dietary Antioxidants and Related Compounds. 2000. Dietary Reference Intakes for Vitamin C, Vitamin E, Selenium, and Carotenoids: Report of the Panel on Dietary Antioxidants and Related Compounds. Washington, D.C.: National Academy Press. [8]

Panel on Micronutrients. 2001. Dietary Reference Intakes for Vitamin a, Vitamin K, Arsenic, Boron, Chromium, Copper, Iodine, Iron, Manganese, Molybdenum, Nickel, Silicon, Vanadium, and Zinc Washington, D. C.: National Academy Press. [8]

Pantopoulos, K., S. K. Porwal, A. Tartakoff, and L. Devireddy. 2012. Mechanisms of Mammalian Iron Homeostasis. *Biochemistry* **51**:5705–5724. [9, 13]

Papp, J. F., E. L. Bray, D. L. Edelstein, et al. 2008. Factors That Influence the Price of Al, Cd, Co, Cu, Fe, Ni, Pb, Rare Earth Elements, and Zn. Open-File Report 2008–1356. Reston, VA: U.S. Geological Survey. [15]

Parizek, J., and I. Ostadalova. 1967. The Protective Effect of Small Amounts of Selenite in Sublimate Intoxication. *Experientia* **23**:142–143. [14]

Park, B., V. Nizet, and G. Y. Liu. 2008. Role of *Staphylococcus aureus* Catalase in Niche Competition against *Streptococcus pneumoniae*. *J. Bacteriol.* **190**:2275–2278. [3]

Park, S., J. Rich, F. Hanses, and J. C. Lee. 2009. Defects in Innate Immunity Predispose C57BL/6J-*Lepr*[db]/*Lepr*[db] Mice to Infection by *Staphylococcus aureus*. *Infect. Immun.* **77**:1008–1014. [12]

Park, S., X. You, and J. A. Imlay. 2005. Substantial DNA Damage from Submicromolar Intracellular Hydrogen Peroxide Detected in Hpx⁻ Mutants of *Escherichia coli*. *PNAS* **102**:9317–9322. [5]

Park, S. K., J. Schwartz, M. Weisskopf, et al. 2006. Low-Level Lead Exposure, Metabolic Syndrome, and Heart Rate Variability: The VA Normative Aging Study. *Environ. Health Perspect.* **114**:1718–1724. [12]

Park, Y. J., Y. H. Song, J. H. An, H. J. Song, and K. J. Anusavice. 2013. Cytocompatibility of Pure Metals and Experimental Binary Titanium Alloys for Implant Materials. *J. Dent.* **41**:1251–1258. [16]

Paternain, J. L., J. L. Domingo, M. Gomez, A. Ortega, and J. Corbella. 1990. Developmental Toxicity of Vanadium in Mice after Oral Administration. *J. Appl. Toxicol.* **10**:181–186. [8]

Patzer, S. I., and K. Hantke. 1998. The ZnuABC High-Affinity Zinc Uptake System and Its Regulator Zur in *Escherichia coli*. *Mol. Microbiol.* **28**:1199–1210. [5]

———. 2001. Dual Repression by $Fe^{(2+)}$-Fur and $Mn^{(2+)}$-MntR of the mntH Gene, Encoding an NRAMP-Like $Mn^{(2+)}$ Transporter in *Escherichia coli*. *J. Bacteriol.* **183**:4806–4813. [5]

Pauporte, T., D. Lincot, B. Viana, and F. Pelle. 2006. Toward Laser Emission of Epitaxial Nanorod Arrays of ZnO Grown by Electro-Deposition. *Appl. Phys. Lett.* **89**:233112. [15]

Paustenbach, D. J., D. A. Galbraith, and B. L. Finley. 2014. Interpreting Cobalt Blood Concentrations in Hip Implant Patients. *Clin. Toxicol.* **52**:98–112. [8]

Pecharsky, A. O., K. A. Gschneidner, and V. K. Pecharsky, Jr. 2003. The Giant Magnetocaloric Effect of Optimally Prepared Gd5Si2Ge2. *J. App. Physics* **93**:4722–4728. [15]

Pecher, K., D. McCubbery, E. Kneedler, et al. 2003. Quantitative Charge State Analysis of Manganese Biominerals in Aqueous Suspension Using Scanning Transmission X-Ray Microscopy (STXM). *Geochim. Cosmochim. Acta* **67**:1089–1098. [20]

Pechter, K. B., F. M. Meyer, A. W. Serio, J. Stulke, and A. L. Sonenshein. 2013. Two Roles for Aconitase in the Regulation of Tricarboxylic Acid Branch Gene Expression in *Bacillus subtilis*. *J. Bacteriol.* **195**:1525–1537. [5]

Pedrero, Z., L. Ouerdane, S. Mounicou, et al. 2012. Identification of Mercury and Other Metals Complexes with Metallothioneins in Dolphin Liver by Hydrophilic Interaction Liquid Chromatography with the Parallel Detection by ICP MS and Electrospray Hybrid Linear/Orbital Trap MS/MS. *Metallomics* **4**:473–479. [20]

Peeling, P. 2010. Exercise as a Mediator of Hepcidin Activity in Athletes. *Eur. J. Appl. Physiol.* **110**:877–883. [11]

Peeling, P., B. Dawson, C. Goodman, G. Landers, and D. Trinder. 2008. Athletic Induced Iron Deficiency: New Insights into the Role of Inflammation, Cytokines and Hormones. *Eur. J. Appl. Physiol.* **103**:381–391. [11]

Pena, A. C., N. Penacho, L. Mancio-Silva, et al. 2012. A Novel Carbon Monoxide-Releasing Molecule Fully Protects Mice from Severe Malaria. *Antimicrob. Agents Chemother.* **56**:1281–1290. [10]

Pena, M. M., J. Lee, and D. J. Thiele. 1999. A Delicate Balance: Homeostatic Control of Copper Uptake and Distribution. *J. Nutr.* **129**:1251–1260. [8]

Pericone, C. D., K. Overweg, P. W. Hermans, and J. N. Weiser. 2000. Inhibitory and Bactericidal Effects of Hydrogen Peroxide Production by *Streptococcus pneumoniae* on Other Inhabitants of the Upper Respiratory Tract. *Infect. Immun.* **68**:3990–3997. [3–5]

Pericone, C. D., S. Park, J. A. Imlay, and J. N. Weiser. 2003. Factors Contributing to Hydrogen Peroxide Resistance in *Streptococcus pneumoniae* Include Pyruvate Oxidase (SpxB) and Avoidance of the Toxic Effects of the Fenton Reaction. *J. Bacteriol.* **185**:6815–6825. [3, 20]

Perry, R. D., S. K. Craig, J. Abney, et al. 2012. Manganese Transporters Yfe and MntH Are Fur-Regulated and Important for the Virulence of *Yersinia pestis* in Bubonic Plague. *Microbiology* **158**:804–815. [7]

Perry, R. D., T. S. Lucier, D. J. Sikkema, and R. R. Brubaker. 1993. Storage Reservoirs of Hemin and Inorganic Iron in *Yersinia pestis*. *Infect. Immun.* **61**:32–39. [7]

Perry, R. D., I. Mier, Jr., and J. D. Fetherston. 2007. Roles of the Yfe and Feo Transporters of *Yersinia pestis* in Iron Uptake and Intracellular Growth. *Biometals* **20**:699–703. [7]

Peterson, J. I., S. R. Goldstein, R. V. Fitzgerald, and D. K. Buckhold. 1980. Fiber Optic pH Probe for Physiological Use. *Anal. Chem.* **52**:864–869. [20]

Peterson, V. M., J. F. Hansbrough, X. W. Wang, R. Zapata-Sirvent, and J. A. Boswick, Jr. 1985. Topical Cerium Nitrate Prevents Postburn Immunosuppression. *J. Trauma* **25**:1039–1044. [17]

Peyssonnaux, C., V. Datta, T. Cramer, et al. 2005. HIF-1α Expression Regulates the Bactericidal Capacity of Phagocytes. *J. Clin. Invest.* **115**:1806–1815. [3]

Picarelli, A., M. Di Tola, A. Vallecoccia, et al. 2011. Oral Mucosa Patch Test: A New Tool to Recognize and Study the Adverse Effects of Dietary Nickel Exposure. *Biol. Trace Elem. Res.* **139**:151–159. [11]

Pilones, K., A. Tatum, and J. Gavalchin. 2009. Gestational Exposure to Mercury Leads to Persistent Changes in T-Cell Phenotype and Function in Adult DBF1 Mice. *J. Immunotox.* **6**:161–170. [17]

Pinhas-Hamiel, O., R. S. Newfield, I. Koren, et al. 2003. Greater Prevalence of Iron Deficiency in Overweight and Obese Children and Adolescents. *Int. J. Obes. Relat. Metab. Disord.* **27**:416–418. [12]

Pirzadeh, A., M. M. Hazavei, M. H. Entezari, and A. Hasanzadeh. 2014 The Effect of Educational Intervention on Girl's Behavior Regarding Nutrition: Applying the Beliefs, Attitudes, Subjective Norms, and Enabling Factors. *J. Educ. Health Promot.* **3**:2277–9531. [8]

Pishchany, G., and E. P. Skaar. 2012. Taste for Blood: Hemoglobin as a Nutrient Source for Pathogens. *PLoS Pathog.* **8**:e1002535. [20]

Piwnica-Worms, D., D. P. Schuster, and J. R. Garbow. 2004. Molecular Imaging of Host-Pathogen Interactions in Intact Small Animals. *Cell. Microbiol.* **6**:319–331. [20]

Plenevaux, A., R. Cantineau, C. Brihaye, et al. 1990. Synthesis and Tissue Distribution of Four Se-Labeled Tertiary Amines, Potential Brain pH Imaging Agents. *Int. J. Rad. Appl. Instrum. B* **17**:601–607. [20]

Polacco, B. J., S. O. Purvine, E. M. Zink, et al. 2011. Discovering Mercury Protein Modifications in Whole Proteomes Using Natural Isotope Distributions Observed in Liquid Chromatography-Tandem Mass Spectrometry. *Mol. Cell. Proteomics* **10**:M110.004853. [17]

Porcheron, G., A. Garénaux, J. Proulx, M. Sabri, and C. M. Dozois. 2013. Iron, Copper, Zinc, and Manganese Transport and Regulation in Pathogenic Enterobacteria: Correlations between Strains, Site of Infection and the Relative Importance of the Different Metal Transport Systems for Virulence. *Front. Cell. Infect. Microbiol.* **3**:90. [13]

Portas, A. D. S., D. C. Miguel, J. K. U. Yokoyama-Yasunaka, S. R. Bortolin Uliana, and B. P. Espósito. 2012. Increasing the Activity of Copper(II) Complexes against Leishmania through Lipophilicity and Pro-Oxidant Ability. *J. Biol. Inorg. Chem.* **17**:107–112. [10]

Portugal, S., C. Carret, M. Recker, et al. 2011. Host-Mediated Regulation of Superinfection in Malaria. *Nat. Med.* **17**:732–737. [9, 13]

Posey, J. E., and F. C. Gherardini. 2000. Lack of a Role for Iron in the Lyme Disease Pathogen. *Science* **288**:1651–1653. [4, 5, 7]

Poskitt, E. M. 2014. Childhood Obesity in Low- and Middle-Income Countries. *Paediatr. Int. Child Health* **9**:2046905514Y0000000147. [Epub ahead of print]. [12]

Poss, K. D., and S. Tonegawa. 1997. Heme Oxygenase 1 Is Required for Mammalian Iron Reutilization. *PNAS* **94**:10919–10924. [13]

Prado, J. V., A. R. Vidal, and T. C. Duran. 2012. Application of Copper Bactericidal Properties in Medical Practice. *Rev. Med. Chile* **140**:1325–1332. [8]

Prasad, A. S. 2012. Discovery of Human Zinc Deficiency: 50 Years Later. *J. Trace Elem. Med. Biol.* **26**:66–69. [8]

———. 2013. Discovery of Human Zinc Deficiency: Its Impact on Human Health and Disease. *Adv. Nutr.* **4**:176–190. [7, 8]

Prentice, A. 1993. Does Mild Zinc Deficiency Contribute to Poor Growth Performance? *Nutr. Rev.* **5**:268–270. [12]

Prentice, A. M., H. Ghattas, C. Doherty, and S. E. Cox. 2007. Iron Metabolism and Malaria. *Food Nutr. Bull.* **28**:524S–539S. [6]

Pressler, U., H. Staudenmaier, L. Zimmermann, and V. Braun. 1988. Genetics of the Iron Dicitrate Transport System of *Escherichia coli*. *J. Bacteriol.* **170**:2716–2724. [5]

Price, J. S., A. F. Tencer, D. M. Arm, and G. A. Bohach. 1996. Controlled Release of Antibiotics from Coated Orthopedic Implants. *J. Biomed. Mater. Res.* **30**:281–286. [16]

Prodromou, C., P. J. Artymiuk, and J. R. Guest. 1992. The Aconitase of *Escherichia coli*. *Eur. J. Biochem.* **204**:599–609. [4]

Prohaska, J. R., and A. A. Gybina. 2004. Intracellular Copper Transport in Mammals. *J. Nutr.* **134**:1003–1006. [8]

Pruteanu, M., S. B. Neher, and T. A. Baker. 2007. Ligand-Controlled Proteolysis of the *Escherichia coli* Transcriptional Regulator ZntR. *J. Bacteriol.* **189**:3017–3025. [5]

Puckett, J., S. Westervelt, R. Gutierrez, and T. Takamiya. 2005. The Digital Dump. Exporting Re-Use and Abuse to Africa. Report from the Basel Action Network, Seattle. http://ban.org/library/TheDigitalDump.pdf (accessed Oct. 10, 2014). [15]

Puckett, S. P., E. Taylor, T. Raimondo, and T. J. Webster. 2010. The Relationship between the Nanostructure of Titanium Surfaces and Bacterial Attachment. *Biomaterials* **31**:706–713. [16]

Pugh, S. Y. R., J. L. DiGuiseppi, and I. Fridovich. 1984. Induction of Superoxide Dismutases in *Escherichia coli* by Manganese and Iron. *J. Bacteriol.* **160**:137–142. [5]

Puri, S., T. H. Hohle, and M. R. O'Brian. 2010. Control of Bacterial Iron Homeostasis by Manganese. *PNAS* **107**:10691–10695. [5]

Qaim, S. M. 2011. Development of Novel Positron Emitters for Medical Applications: Nuclear and Radiochemical Aspects. *Radiochim. Acta* **99**:611–625. [20]

———. 2012. The Present and Future of Medical Radionuclide Production. *Radiochim. Acta* **100**: [20]

———. 2013. New Trends in Nuclear Data Research for Medical Radionuclide Production. *Radiochim. Acta* **101**:473–480. [20]

Qin, Y., P. J. Dittmer, J. G. Park, K. B. Jansen, and A. E. Palmer. 2011. Measuring Steady-State and Dynamic Endoplasmic Reticulum and Golgi $Zn^{2+}$ with Genetically Encoded Sensors. *PNAS* **108**:7351–7356. [20]

Queiroz, D. M., P. R. Harris, I. R. Sanderson, et al. 2013. Iron Status and *Helicobacter pylori* Infection in Symptomatic Children: An International Multi-Centered Study. *PLoS One* **8**:e68833. [11]

Quigley, E. M. 2013. Gut Bacteria in Health and Disease. *Gastroenterol. Hepatol.* **9**:560–569. [17]

Quihui, L., G. G. Morales, R. O. Mendez, et al. 2010. Could Giardiasis Be a Risk Factor for Low Zinc Status in Schoolchildren from Northwestern Mexico? A Cross-Sectional Study with Longitudinal Follow-Up. *BMC Public Health* **10**:85. [11]

Raffatellu, M., M. D. George, Y. Akiyama, et al. 2009. Lipocalin-2 Resistance Confers an Advantage to *Salmonella enterica* Serotype Typhimurium for Growth and Survival in the Inflamed Intestine. *Cell Host Microbe* **5**:476–486. [7]

Rahman, A., M. Vahter, E. C. Ekstrom, and L. A. Persson. 2011. Arsenic Exposure in Pregnancy Increases the Risk of Lower Respiratory Tract Infection and Diarrhea During Infancy in Bangladesh. *Environ. Health Perspect.* **119**:719–724. [8]

Rajkumar, M., N. Ae, M. N. V. Prasad, and H. Freitas. 2010. Potential of Siderophore-Producing Bacteria for Improving Heavy Metal Phytoextraction. *Trends Biotechnol.* **28**:142–149. [17]

Rajkumar, M., M. N. V. Prasad, S. Swaminathan, and H. Freitas. 2013. Climate Change Driven Plant–Metal–Microbe Interactions. *Environ. Int.* **53**:74–86. [17]

Rakoff-Nahoum, S., J. Paglino, F. Eslami-Varzaneh, S. Edberg, and R. Medzhitov. 2004. Recognition of Commensal Microflora by Toll-Like Receptors Is Required for Intestinal Homeostasis. *Cell* **118**:229–241. [17]

Ramos, E., P. Ruchala, J. B. Goodnough, et al. 2012. Minihepcidins Prevent Iron Overload in a Hepcidin-Deficient Mouse Model of Severe Hemochromatosis. *Blood* **120**:3829–3836. [6]

Ramsey, K. A., R. E. Foong, P. D. Sly, A. N. Larcombe, and G. R. Zosky. 2013. Early Life Arsenic Exposure and Acute and Long-Term Responses to Influenza a Infection in Mice. *Environ. Health Perspect.* **121**:1187–1193. [11]

Rappaport, S. M., D. K. Barupal, D. Wishart, P. Vineis, and A. Scalbert. 2014. The Blood Exposome and Its Role in Discovering Causes of Disease. *Environ. Health Perspect.* **122**: 769–774. [17]

Rashed, M. N. 2011. The Role of Trace Elements on Hepatitis Virus Infection. *J. Trace Elem. Med. Biol.* **25**:181–187. [17]

Rauch, J. N., and J. M. Pacyna. 2009. Earth's Global Anthrobiogeochemical Ag, Al, Cr, Cu, Fe, Ni, Pb, and Zn Cycles. *Global Biogeochem. Cycles* **23**:GB2001. [15]

Rayman, M. P. 2000. The Importance of Selenium to Human Health. *Lancet* **356**:233–241. [2]

———. 2008. Food-Chain Selenium and Human Health: Emphasis on Intake. *Br. J. Nutr.* **100**:254–268. [11]

Rayman, M. P., and J. British. 2004. The Use of High-Selenium Yeast to Raise Selenium Status: How Does It Measure Up? *J. Nutr.* **92**:557–573. [14]

Razi, C. H., A. Z. Akelma, O. Akin, et al. 2012. Hair Zinc and Selenium Levels in Children with Recurrent Wheezing. *Pediatr. Pulmonol.* **47**:1185–1191. [11]

Razia, C. H., O. Akin, K. Harmancic, B. Akind, and R. Renda. 2011. Serum Heavy Metal and Antioxidant Element Levels of Children with Recurrent Wheezing. *Allergol. Immunopathol.* **39**:85–89. [17]

Recalcati, S., M. Locati, A. Marini, et al. 2010. Differential Regulation of Iron Homeostasis During Human Macrophage Polarized Activation. *Eur. J. Immunol.* **40**:824–835. [9, 13]

Rees, D. C., E. Johnson, and O. Lewinson. 2009. Abc Transporters: The Power to Change. *Nat. Rev. Mol. Cell Biol.* **10**:218–227. [2]

Rehder, D. 2012. The Potentiality of Vanadium in Medicinal Applications. *Fut. Med. Chem.* **4**:1823–1837. [13]

———. 2014. Vanadium: Its Role for Humans. In: Interrelations between Essential Metal Ions and Human Diseases, Vol. 13, Metal Ions in Life Sciences, ed. A. Sigel et al. Dordrecht: Springer Science + Business Media B.V. [13]

Reichard, J. F., and A. Puga. 2010. Effects of Arsenic Exposure on DNA Methylation and Epigenetic Gene Regulation. *Epigenomics* **2**:87–104. [17]

Reichmann, D., O. Rahat, M. Cohen, H. Neuvirth, and G. Schreiber. 2007. The Molecular Architecture of Protein-Protein Binding Sites. *Curr. Opin. Struct. Biol.* **17**:67–76. [4]

Reid, G. 2010. The Potential Role for Probiotic Yogurt for People Living with HIV/AIDS. *Gut Microbe* **1**:411–414. [17]

Reinke, C. M., J. Breitkreutz, and H. Leuenberger. 2003. Aluminium in over-the-Counter Drugs: Risks Outweigh Benefits? *Drug Saf.* **26**:1011–1025. [8]

Ren, X. Y., L. Xu, H. Meng, et al. 2009. Family-Based Association Analysis of S100A8 Genetic Polymorphisms with Aggressive Periodontitis. *J. Periodontal Res.* **44**:184–192. [20]

Reniere, M. L., and E. P. Skaar. 2008. *Staphylococcus aureus* Haem Oxygenases Are Differentially Regulated by Iron and Haem. *Mol. Microbiol.* **69**:1304–1315. [20]

Rensing, C., B. Fan, R. Sharma, B. Mitra, and B. P. Rosen. 2000. Copa: An *Escherichia coli* Cu(I)-Translocating P-Type ATPase. *PNAS* **97**:652–656. [5]

Rensing, C., and S. F. McDevitt. 2013. The Copper Metallome in Prokaryotic Cells. In: Metallomics and the Cell, ed. L. Banci, pp. 417–450. Dordrecht: Springer Science+Business Media. [4]

Rensing, C., B. Mitra, and B. P. Rosen. 1997. The *zntA* Gene of *Escherichia coli* Encodes a Zn(II)-Translocating P-Type ATPase. *PNAS* **94**:14326–14331. [5]

Restrepo, B. I. 2007. Convergence of the Tuberculosis and Diabetes Epidemics: Renewal of Old Acquaintances. *Clin. Infect. Dis.* **45**:436–438. [12]

Ridge, P. G., Y. Zhang, and V. N. Gladyshev. 2008. Comparative Genomic Analyses of Copper Transporters and Cuproproteomes Reveal Evolutionary Dynamics of Copper Utilization and Its Link to Oxygen. *PLoS One* **3**:e1378. [5]

Rink, L., ed. 2011. Zinc in Human Health. Amsterdam: IOS Press. [13]

Rink, L., and M. Maywald. 2014. Zinc Signals in Immunology. In: Zinc Signals in Cellular Functions and Disorders, ed. T. Fukada and T. Kambe, p. 197. New York: Springer. [13]

Riojas-Rodriguez, H., R. Solis-Vivanco, A. Schilmann, et al. 2010. Intellectual Function in Mexican Children Living in a Mining Area and Environmentally Exposed to Manganese. *Environ. Health Perspect.* **118**:1465–1470. [11]

Robbins, L. J., S. V. Lalonde, M. A. Saito, et al. 2013. Authigenic Iron Oxide Proxies for Marine Zinc over Geological Time and Implications for Eukaryotic Metallome Evolution. *Geobiology* **11**:295–306. [5]

Roberts, A. A., S. V. Sharma, A. W. Strankman, et al. 2013. Mechanistic Studies of Fosb: A Divalent-Metal-Dependent Bacillithiol-S-Transferase That Mediates Fosfomycin Resistance in *Staphylococcus aureus*. *Biochem. J.* **451**:69–79. [4]

Roberts, S. A., A. Weichsel, G. Grass, et al. 2002. Crystal Structure and Electron Transfer Kinetics of CueO, a Multicopper Oxidase Required for Copper Homeostasis in *Escherichia coli*. *PNAS* **99**:2766–2771. [4]

Robinson, B. H. 2009. E-Waste: An Assessment of Global Production and Environmental Impacts. *Sci. Total Environ.* **408**:183–191. [15]

Robinson, N. J., and D. R. Winge. 2010. Copper Metallochaperones. *Annu. Rev. Biochem.* **79**:537–562. [4, 7]

Rochford, E. T., R. G. Richards, and T. F. Moriarty. 2012. Influence of Material on the Development of Device-Associated Infection. *Clin. Microbiol. Infect.* **18**:1162–1167. [16]

Roelcke, U., K. L. Leenders, K. von Ammon, et al. 1996. Brain Tumor Iron Uptake Measured with Positron Emission Tomography and $^{52}$Fe-Citrate. *J. Neurooncol.* **29**:157–165. [20]

Rogalska, J., M. M. Brzóska, A. Roszczenko, and J. Moniuszko-Jakoniuk. 2009. Enhanced Zinc Consumption Prevents Cadmium-Induced Alterations in Lipid Metabolism in Male Rats. *Chem. Biol. Interactions* **177**:142–152. [14]

Rogalska, J., B. Pilat-Marcinkiewicz, and M. M. Brzóska. 2011. Protective Effect of Zinc against Cadmium Hepatotoxicity Depends on This Bioelement Intake and Level of Cadmium Exposure: A Study in a Rat Model. *Chem. Biol. Interactions* **193**:191–203. [14]

Roguska, A., A. Belcarz, T. Piersiak, et al. 2012. Evaluation of the Antibacterial Activity of Ag-Loaded TiO$_2$ Nanotubes. *Eur. J. Inorg. Chem.* **32**:5199–5206. [16]

Rohde, K. H., and D. W. Dyer. 2004. Analysis of Haptoglobin and Hemoglobin-Haptoglobin Interactions with the *Neisseria meningitidis* TonB-Dependent Receptor HpuAB by Flow Cytometry. *Infect. Immun.* **72**:2494–2506. [2]

Rolinski, O. J., and D. J. S. Birch. 1999. A Fluorescence Lifetime Sensor for Cu(I) Ions. *Meas. Sci. Technol.* **10**:127–136. [20]

Romach, E. H., C. Q. Zhao, L. M. Del Razo, M. E. Cebrián, and M. P. Waalkes. 2000. Studies on the Mechanisms of Arsenic-Induced Self Tolerance Developed in Liver Epithelial Cells through Continuous Low-Level Arsenite Exposure. *Toxicol. Sci.* **54**:500–508. [8]

Roman, M., P. Jitaru, and C. Barbante. 2014. Selenium Biochemistry and Its Role for Human Health. *Metallomics* **6**:25–54. [14]

Roome, A. J., S. J. Walsh, M. L. Cartter, and J. L. Hadler. 1993. Hepatitis B Vaccine Responsiveness in Connecticut Public Safety Personnel. *JAMA* **270**:2931–2934. [12]

Rosch, F., H. Herzog, C. Plag, et al. 1996. Radiation Doses of Yttrium-90 Citrate and Yttrium-90 EDTMP as Determined via Analogous Yttrium-86 Complexes and Positron Emission Tomography. *Eur. J. Nucl. Med.* **23**:958–966. [20]

Rosch, J. W., G. Gao, G. Ridout, Y. D. Wang, and E. I. Tuomanen. 2009. Role of Themanganese Efflux System *mntE* for Signalling and Pathogenesis in *Streptococcus pneuumoniae*. *Mol. Microbiol.* **72**:12–25. [5]

Rosen, B. P., A. A. Ajees, and T. R. McDermott. 2011. Life and Death with Arsenic. Arsenic Life: An Analysis of the Recent Report: "A Bacterium That Can Grow by Using Arsenic Instead of Phosphorus." *Bioessays* **33**:350–357. [14]

Rosen, G. M., S. Pou, C. L. Ramos, M. S. Cohen, and B. E. Britigan. 1995. Free Radicals and Phagocytic Cells. *FASEB J.* **9**:200–209. [9]

Rosenzweig, A. C. 2002. Metallochaperones: Bind and Deliver. *Chem. Biol.* **9**:673–677. [4]

Ross, A. C. 2012. Modern Nutrition in Health and Disease. Philadelphia: Wolters Kluwer Health/Lippincott Williams & Wilkins. [8]

Roth, J. A. 2006. Homeostatic and Toxic Mechanisms Regulating Manganese Uptake, Retention, and Elimination. *Biol. Res.* **39**:45–57. [13]

Rouault, T. A. 2013. Iron Metabolism in the CNS: Implications for Neurodegenerative Diseases. *Nat. Rev. Neurosci.* **14**:551–564. [11]

Rowland, J. L., and M. Niederweis. 2013. A Multicopper Oxidase Is Required for Copper Resistance in *Mycobacterium tuberculosis*. *J. Bacteriol.* **195**:3724–3733. [4, 13]

Ruiz-Nunez, B., L. Pruimboom, D. A. Janneke Dijck-Brouwera, and F. A. J. Muskiet. 2013. Lifestyle and Nutritional Imbalances Associated with Western Diseases: Causes and Consequences of Chronic Systemic Low-Grade Inflammation in an Evolutionary Context. *J. Nutr. Biochem.* **24**:1183–1201. [12]

Runyen-Janecky, L. J., S. A. Reeves, E. G. Gonzales, and S. M. Payne. 2003. Contribution of the *Shigella Flexneri* Sit, Iuc, and Feo Iron Acquisition Systems to Iron Acquisition *in Vitro* and in Cultured Cells. *Infect. Immun.* **71**:1919–1928. [7]

Russell, L. A. 2013. Osteoporosis and Orthopedic Surgery: Effect of Bone Health on Total Joint Arthroplasty Outcome. *Curr. Rheumatol. Rep.* **15**:371. [16]

Sabino, P., S. Stranges, and P. Strazzullo. 2013. Does Selenium Matter in Cardiometabolic Disorders? A Short Review of the Evidence. *J. Endocrinol. Invest.* **36**:21S–27S. [11]

Sadarangani, M., A. J. Pollard, and S. D. Gray-Owen. 2011. Opa Proteins and Ceacams: Pathways of Immune Engagement for Pathogenic *Neisseria*. *FEMS Microbiol Rev* **35**:498–514. [2]

Sakr, Y., K. Reinhart, F. Bloos, et al. 2007. Time Course and Relationship between Plasma Selenium Concentrations, Systemic Inflammatory Response, Sepsis, and Multiorgan Failure. *Br. J. Anaesth.* **98**:775–784. [13]

Sakurai, T., T. Ohta, N. Tomita, et al. 2004. Evaluation of Immunotoxic and Immunodisruptive Effects of Inorganic Arsenite on Human Monocytes/ Macrophages. *Int. Immunopharmacol.* **4**:1661–1673. [8]

Salas, P. F., C. Herrmann, and C. Orvig. 2013. Metalloantimalarials. *Chem. Rev.* **113**:3450–3492. [10, 13]

Salas, S. D., J. E. Bennett, K. J. Kwon-Chung, J. R. Perfect, and P. R. Williamson. 1996. Effect of the Laccase Gene CNLAC1, on Virulence of *Cryptococcus neoformans*. *J. Exp. Med.* **184**:377–386. [7]

Saliba, W., R. El Fakih, and W. Shaheen. 2010. Heart Failure Secondary to Selenium Deficiency, Reversible after Supplementation. *Int. J. Cardiol.* **141**:e26–e27. [8]

Salnikow, K., and A. Zhitkovich. 2008. Genetic and Epigenetic Mechanisms in Metal Carcinogenesis and Cocarcinogenesis: Nickel, Arsenic, and Chromium. *Chem. Res. Toxicol.* **21**:28–44. [17]

Samanovic, M. I., C. Ding, D. J. Thiele, and K. H. Darwin. 2012. Copper in Microbial Pathogenesis: Meddling with the Metal. *Cell Host Microbe* **11**:106–115. [9]

Samman, S., B. Sandstrom, M. B. Toft, et al. 2001. Green Tea or Rosemary Extract Added to Foods Reduces Nonheme-Iron Absorption. *Am. J. Clin. Nutr.* **73**:607–612. [8]

Sánchez-Delgado, R. A., and A. Anzellotti. 2004. Metal Complexes as Chemotherapeutic Agents against Tropical Diseases: Trypanosomiais, Malaria and Leishmaniasis. *Mini Rev. Med. Chem.* **4**:23–30. [10]

Sánchez-Gárces, M. A., and C. Gay-Escoda. 2004. Periimplantitis. *Med. Oral Patol. Oral Cir. Bucal.* **9**:69–74. [16]

Sander, L. E., S. D. Sackett, U. Dierssen, et al. 2010. Hepatic Acute-Phase Proteins Control Innate Immune Responses During Infection by Promoting Myeloid-Derived Suppressor Cell Function. *J. Exp. Med.* **207**:1453–1464. [12]

Sandstrom, B., and A. Cederblad. 1980. Zinc Absorption from Composite Meals: II. Influence of the Main Protein Source. *Am. J. Clin. Nutr.* **33**:1778–1783. [11]

Santamaria, A. B., and S. I. Sulsky. 2010. Risk Assessment of an Essential Element: Manganese. *J. Toxicol. Environ. Health* **73**:128–155. [13]

Sardans, J., J. Penuelas, and M. Estiarte. 2008. Warming and Drought Change Trace Element Bioaccumulation Patterns in a Mediterranean Shrubland. *Chemosphere* **70**:874–885. [17]

Sathekge, M., J. Wagener, S. V. Smith, et al. 2013. Biodistribution and Dosimetry of 195mPt-Cisplatin in Normal Volunteers. Imaging Agent for Single Photon Emission Computed Tomography. *Nuklearmedizin* **52**:222–227. [20]

Sauni, R., A. Linna, P. Oksa, et al. 2010. Cobalt Asthma: A Case Series from a Cobalt Plant. *Occup. Med.* **60**:301–306. [8]

Saurat, M., and S. Bringezu. 2008. Platinum Group Metal Flows of Europe, Part 1. *J. Indus. Ecol.* **12**:754–767. [15]

Sayadi, A., A. T. Nguyen, F. A. Bard, and E. A. Bard-Chapeau. 2013. Zip14 Expression Induced by Lipopolysaccharides in Macrophages Attenuates Inflammatory Response. *Inflamm. Res.* **62**:133–143. [13]

Sayato, Y., T. Hasegawa, S. Taniguchi, et al. 1993. Acute and Subacute Oral Toxicity of Selenocysteine in Mice. *Eisei Kagaku* **39**:289–296. [14]

Sazawal, S., R. E. Black, M. K. Bhan, et al. 1995. Zinc Supplementation in Young Children with Acute Diarrhea in India. *N. Engl. J. Med.* **333**:839–844. [13]

Sazawal, S., R. E. Black, M. Ramsan, et al. 2006. Effects of Routine Prophylactic Supplementation with Iron and Folic Acid on Admission to Hospital and Mortality in Preschool Children in a High Malaria Transmission Setting: Community-Based, Randomised, Placebo-Controlled Trial. *Lancet* **367**:133–143. [6, 9, 13]

Sazawal, S., R. E. Black, M. Ramsan, et al. 2007. Effect of Zinc Supplementation on Mortality in Children Aged 1–48 Months: A Community-Based Randomised Placebo-Controlled Trial. *Lancet* **369**:927–934. [13]

Schalk, I. J., M. Hannauer, and A. Braud. 2011. New Roles for Bacterial Siderophores in Metal Transport and Tolerance. *Environ. Microbiol.* **13**:2844–2854. [4]

Schaumlöffel, D., P. Giusti, M. V. Zoriy, et al. 2005. Ultratrace Determination of Uranium and Plutonium by Nano-Volume Flow Injection Double-Focusing Sector Field Inductively Coupled Plasma Mass Spectrometry (nFI-ICP-SFMS). *Int. J. Mass Spectrom.* **242**:217–223. [14]

Schelert, J., V. Dixit, V. Hoang, et al. 2004. Occurrence and Characterization of Mercury Resistance in the Hyperthermophilic Archaeon *Sulfolobus solfataricus* by Use of Gene Disruption. *J. Bacteriol.* **186**:427–437. [4]

Scheuhammer, A. M., S. Onosaka, K. Rodgers, and M. G. Cherian. 1985. The Interaction of Zinc and Cadmium in the Synthesis of Hepatic Metallothionein in Rats. *Toxicology* **36**:101–108. [14]

Schiering, N., W. Kabsch, M. J. Moore, et al. 1991. Structure of the Detoxification Catalyst Mercuric Ion Reductase from *Bacillus* sp. Strain RC607. *Nature* **352**:168–172. [4]

Schmidt, A., M. Beck, J. Malmström, et al. 2011. Absolute Quantification of Microbial Proteomes at Different States by Directed Mass Spectrometry. *Mol. Syst. Biol.* **7**:510. [18]

Schmidt, P. J., C. Kunst, and V. C. Culotta. 2000. Copper Activation of Superoxide Dismtase 1 (SOD1) *in Vivo*: Role for Protein-Protein Interactions with the Copper Chaperone for SOD1. *J. Biol. Chem.* **275**:33771–33776. [5]

Schmitt, J., I. Joost, E. P. Skaar, M. Herrmann, and M. Bischoff. 2012. Haemin Represses the Haemolytic Activity of *Staphylococcus aureus* in an Sae-Dependent Manner. *Microbiology* **158**:2619–2631. [7]

Schneider, D. S., and J. S. Ayres. 2008. Two Ways to Survive Infection: What Resistance and Tolerance Can Teach Us About Treating Infectious Diseases. *Nat. Rev. Immunol.* **8**:889–895. [1, 17]

Schomburg, I., A. Chang, S. Placzek, et al. 2013. Brenda in 2013: Integrated Reactions, Kinetic Data, Enzyme Function Data, Improved Disease Classification: New Options and Contents in Brenda. *Nucl. Acids Res.* **41**:D764–D772. [4]

Schröder, J. M., and J. Harder. 2006. Antimicrobial Skin Peptides and Proteins. *Cell Mol. Life Sci.* **63**:469–486. [13]

Schroeder, H. A. 1971. Losses of Vitamins and Trace Minerals Resulting from Processing and Preservation of Foods. *Am. J. Clin. Nutr.* **24**:562–573. [17]

Schulz, H., H. Hennecke, and L. Thöny-Meyer. 1998. Prototype of a Heme Chaperone Essential for Cytochrome C Maturation. *Science* **281**:1197–1200. [4, 11]

Schwartz, C. J., J. L. Giel, T. Patschkowski, et al. 2001a. IscR, an Fe-S Cluster-Containing Transcription Factor, Represses Expression of *Escherichia coli* Genes Encoding Fe-S Cluster Assembly Proteins. *PNAS* **98**:14895–14900. [5]

Schwartz, J. A., E. K. Lium, and S. J. Silverstein. 2001b. Herpes Simplex Virus Type 1 Entry Is Inhibited by the Cobalt Chelate Complex CTC-96. *J. Virol.* **75**:4117–4128. [8]

Schwarz, G., R. R. Mendel, and M. W. Ribbe. 2009. Molybdenum Cofactors, Enzymes and Pathways. *Nature* **460**:839–847. [2]

Schwarze, S. R., A. Ho, A. Vocero-Akbani, and S. F. Dowdy. 1999. *In Vivo* Protein Transduction: Delivery of a Biologically Active Protein into the Mouse. *Science* **285**:1569–1572. [20]

Scott, B. J., and A. R. Bradwell. 1983. Identification of the Serum Binding Proteins for Iron, Zinc, Cadmium, Nickel, and Calcium. *Clin. Chem.* **29**:629–633. [8]

Scott, R. A., J. E. Shokes, N. J. Cosper, F. E. Jenney, and M. W. W. Adams. 2005. Bottlenecks and Roadblocks in High-Throughput XAS for Structural Genomics. *J. Synchrotron Rad.* **12**:19–22. [18]

Seixas, E., R. Gozzelino, A. Chora, A. Ferreira, and G. Silva. 2009. Heme Oxygenase-1 Affords Protection against Noncerebral Forms of Severe Malaria. *PNAS* **106**:15837–15842. [17]

Sela, H., Z. Karpas, H. Cohen, A. Tal, and Y. Zeiri. 2013. Trace Element Concentration in Hair Samples as an Indicator of Exposure of Population in the Negev, Israel. *Biol. Trace Elem. Res.* **155**:209–220. [11]

Seligman, P. A., J. Kovar, and E. W. Gelfand. 1992. Lymphocyte Proliferation Is Controlled by Both Iron Availability and Regulation of Iron Uptake Pathways. *Pathobiology* **60**:19–26. [9]

Seltzer, C. C., and J. Mayer. 1963. Serum Iron and Iron-Binding Capacity in Adolescents. II. Comparison of Obese and Nonobese Subjects. *Am. J. Clin. Nutr.* **13**:354–361. [12]

Setyawati, I. A., K. H. Thompson, V. G. Yuen, et al. 1998. Kinetic Analysis and Comparison of Uptake, Distribution, and Excretion of 48V-Labeled Compounds in Rats. *J. Appl. Physiol.* **84**:569–575. [20]

Sevcenco, A. M., L. E. Bevers, G. C. Krijger, et al. 2010. Molybdenum Incorporation in Tungsten Aldehyde Oxidoreductase Enzymes from *Pyrococcus furiosus*. *J. Bacteriol.* **192**:4143–4152. [18]

Sevcenco, A. M., W. R. Hagen, and P. L. Hagedoorn. 2012. Microbial Metalloproteomes Explored Using MIRAGE. *Chem. Biodivers.* **9**:1967–1980. [18]

Sevcenco, A. M., G. C. Krijger, M. W. Pinkse, et al. 2009a. Development of a Generic Approach to Native Metalloproteomics: Application to the Quantitative Identification of Soluble Copper Proteins in *Escherichia coli*. *J. Biol. Inorg. Chem.* **14**:631–640. [18]

Sevcenco, A. M., M. W. Pinkse, E. Bol, et al. 2009b. The Tungsten Metallome of *Pyrococcus furiosus*. *Metallomics* **1**:395–402. [18]

Sevcenco, A. M., M. W. H. Pinkse, H. T. Wolterbeek, et al. 2011. Exploring the Microbial Metalloproteome Using MIRAGE. *Metallomics* **3**:1324–1330. [5, 18, 20]

Shahar, A., K. V. Patel, R. D. Semba, et al. 2010. Plasma Selenium Is Positively Related to Performance in Neurological Tasks Assessing Coordination and Motor Speed. *Mov. Disord.* **25**:1909–1915. [8]

Shanbhag, A. S., C. T. Hasselman, J. J. Jacobs, and et al. 1998. Biological Response to Wear Debris. In: The Adult Hip, pp. 279–288. Philadelphia: Lippincott-Raven Publ. [16]

Shanbhag, A. S., J. J. Jacobs, J. Black, J. O. Galante, and T. T. Glant. 1995. Human Monocyte Response to Particulate Biomaterials Generated *in Vivo* and *in Vitro*. *J. Orthop. Res.* **13**:792–801. [16]

Sharma, A. 2007. Relationship between Nickel Allergy and Diet. *Indian J. Dermatol. Venereol. Leprol.* **73**:307–312. [11]

Sharma, A., E. K. Gaidamakova, V. Y. Matrosova, et al. 2013. Responses of $Mn^{2+}$ Speciation in *Deinococcus radiodurans* and *Escherichia coli* to Gamma-Radiation by Advanced Paramagnetic Resonance Methods. *PNAS* **110**:5945–5950. [20]

Sheline, C. T., M. M. Behrens, and D. M. Choi. 2000. Zinc-Induced Cortical Neuronal Death: Contribution of Energy Failure Attributable to Loss of $NAD^+$ and Inhibition of Glycolysis. *J. Neurosci.* **20**:3139–3146. [16]

Shen, Z., T. Luangtongkum, Z. Qiang, et al. 2014. Identification of a Novel Membrane Transporter Mediating Resistance to Organic Arsenic in *Campylobacter Jejuni*. *Antimicrob. Agents Chemother.* **58**:2021–2029. [4]

Sheng, Y., E. Butler Gralla, M. Schumacher, et al. 2012. Six-Coordinate Manganese(3+) in Catalysis by Yeast Manganese Superoxide Dismutase. *PNAS* **109**:14314–14319. [2]

Shi, J., W. P. Lindsay, J. W. Huckle, A. P. Morby, and N. J. Robinson. 1992. Cyanobacterial Metallothionein Gene Expressed in *Escherichia coli*: Metal-Binding Properties of the Expressed Protein. *FEBS Lett.* **303**:159–163. [4]

Shi, W., and M. R. Chance. 2011. Metalloproteomics: Forward and Reverse Approaches in Metalloprotein Structural and Functional Characterization. *Curr. Opin. Chem. Biol.* **15**:144–148. [18]

Shi, W., C. Zhan, A. Ignatov, et al. 2005. Metalloproteomics: High-Throuput Structural and Functional Annotation of Proteins in Structural Genomics. *Structure* **13**:1473–1486. [18]

Shi, X., R. A. Festa, T. R. Ioerger, et al. 2014. The Copper-Responsive RicR Regulon Contributes to *Mycobacterium tuberculosis* Virulence. *MBio* **5**:e00876–00813. [7, 13]

Shim, H., and Z. L. Harris. 2003. Genetic Defects in Copper Metabolism. *J. Nutr.* **133**:1527S–1531S. [8]

Shin, J. H., S. Y. Oh, S. J. Kim, and J. H. Roe. 2007. The Zinc-Responsive Regulator Zur Controls a Zinc Uptake System and Some Ribosomal Proteins in *Streptomyces coelicolor* A3(2). *J. Bacteriol.* **189**:4070–4077. [5]

Shultis, D. D., M. D. Purdy, C. N. Banchs, and M. C. Wiener. 2006. Outer Membrane Active Transport: Structure of the BtuB:TonB Complex. *Science* **312**:1396–1399. [2]

Si, J., X. Wu, C. Wan, et al. 2011. Peripubertal Exposure to Low Doses of Tributyltin Chloride Affects the Homeostasis of Serum T, E2, LH, and Body Weight of Male Mice. *Environ. Toxicol.* **26**:307–314. [12]

Sidoryk-Wegrzynowicz, M., E. Lee, J. Albrecht, and M. Aschner. 2009. Manganese Disrupts Astrocyte Glutamine Transporter Expression and Function. *J. Neurochem.* **110**:822–830. [8]

Sigrist, C. J. A., E. de Castro, L. Cerutti, et al. 2012. New and Continuing Developments at Prosite. *Nucl. Acids Res.* **41**:D344–D347. [18]

Silbergeld, E. K., and D. L. Davis. 1994. Role of Biomarkers in Identifying and Understanding Environmentally Induced Disease. *Clin. Chem.* **40**:1363–1367. [17]

Silbergeld, E. K., I. A. Silva, and J. F. Nyland. 2005. Mercury and Autoimmunity: Implications for Occupational and Environmental Health. *Toxicol. Appl. Pharmacol.* **207**:282–292. [17]

Sillanpää, M. 1982. Micronutrients and the Nutrient Status of Soils: A Global Study. FAO Soils Bulletin 48. Rome: Food and Agriculture Organization of the United Nations. [17]

Silva, G., V. Jeney, A. Chora, et al. 2009. Oxidized Hemoglobin Is an Endogenous Proinflammatory Agonist That Targets Vascular Endothelial Cells. *J. Biol. Chem.* **284**:29582–29595. [13]

Silva, I. A., M. El Nabawi, D. Hoover, and E. K. Silbergeld. 2005. Prenatal HgCl$_2$ Exposure in BALB/c Mice: Gender Specific Effects on the Ontogeny of the Immune System. *Dev. Comp. Immunol.* **29**:171–183. [17]

Silva, I. A., J. F. Nyland, A. Gorman, et al. 2004. Mercury Exposure, Malaria, and Serum Antinuclear/Antinucleolar Antibodies in Amazon Populations in Brazil: A Cross-Sectional Study. *Environ. Health* **3**:11. [17]

Silva-Gomes, S., R. Appelberg, R. Larsen, M. P. Soares, and M. S. Gomes. 2013. Heme Catabolism by Heme Oxygenase-1 Confers Host Resistance to *Mycobacterium* Infection. *Infect. Immun.* **81**:2536–2545. [13]

Silver, S., and L. T. Phung. 2005. A Bacterial View of the Periodic Table: Genes and Proteins for Toxic Inorganic Ions. *J. Ind. Microbiol. Biotechnol.* **32**:587–605. [4]

Simo-Minana, J., M. Gaztambide Ganuza, P. Fernandez-Millan, and M. Pena-Fernandez. 1996. Hepatitis B Vaccine Immunoresponsiveness in Adolescents: A Revaccination Proposal after Primary Vaccination. *Vaccine* **4**:103–106. [12]

Simonet, M., M. Berche, J. L. Fauchere, and Veron. 1984. Impaired Resistance to Listeria monocytogenes in Mice Chronically Exposed to Cadmium. *Immunology* **53**:155–163. [17]

Simonsen, L. O., H. Harbak, and P. Bennekou. 2012. Cobalt Metabolism and Toxicology: A Brief Update. *Sci. Total Environ.* **432**:210–215. [8]

Sinclair, D., B. Zani, S. Donegan, P. Olliaro, and G. P. 2009. Artemisinin-Based Combination Therapy for Treating Uncomplicated Malaria. *Cochrane Database Syst. Rev.* **8**:CD007483. [10]

Singh, M. V. 2008. Micronutrient Deficiencies in Crops and Soils in India. *Micronut. Def. Global Crop Prod.*93–125. [17]

Singh, R. B., R. Beegom, S. S. Rastogi, Z. Gaoli, and Z. Shoumin. 1998. Association of Low Plasma Concentrations of Antioxidant Vitamins, Magnesium and Zinc with High Body Fat Per Cent Measured by Bioelectrical Impedance Analysis in Indian Men. *Magnes. Res.* **11**:3–10. [12]

Singh, S. K., G. Grass, C. Rensing, and W. R. Montfort. 2004. Cuprous Oxidase Activity of CueO from *Escherichia coli*. *J. Bacteriol.* **186**:7815–7817. [5]

Singh, V., V. Arora, M. J. Alam, and K. W. Garey. 2012. Inhibition of Biofilm Formation by Esomeprazole in *Pseudomonas aeruginosa* and *Staphylococcus aureus*. *Antimicrob. Agents Chemother.* **56**:4360–4364. [16]

Sitte, J., K. Pollok, F. Langenhorst, and K. Küsel. 2012. Nanocrystalline Nickel and Cobalt Sulfides Formed by a Heavy Metal-Tolerant, Sulfate-Reducing Enrichment Culture. *Geomicrobiol. J.* **30**:36–47. [4]

Smeester, L., J. E. Rager, K. A. Bailey, et al. 2011. Epigenetic Changes in Individuals with Arsenicosis. *Chem. Res. Toxicol.* **24**:165–167. [12]

Smith, A. D., S. Botero, T. Shea-Donohue, and J. F. Urban, Jr. 2011. The Pathogenicity of an Enteric *Citrobacter Rodentium* Infection Is Enhanced by Deficiencies in the Antioxidants Selenium and Vitamin E. *Infect. Immun.* **79**:1471–1478. [13]

Smith, A. D., L. Cheung, E. Beshah, T. Shea-Donohue, and J. F. Urban, Jr. 2013. Selenium Status Alters the Immune Response and Expulsion of Adult *Heligmosomoides bakeri* Worms in Mice. *Infect. Immun.* **81**:2546–2553. [13]

Smith, A. G., P. A. Sheridan, J. B. Harp, and M.A. Beck. 2007. Diet-Induced Obese Mice Have Increased Mortality and Altered Immune Responses When Infected with Influenza Virus. *J. Nutr.* **137**:1236–1243. [12]

So, P. K., B. Hu, and Z. P. Yao. 2013. Mass Spectrometry: Towards *in Vivo* Analysis of Biological Systems. *Mol. Biosyst.* **9**:915–929. [7]

Soares, M. P., I. Marguti, A. Cunha, and R. Larsen. 2009. Immunoregulatory Effects of HO-1: How Does It Work? *Curr. Opin. Chem. Biol.* **9**:482–489. [13]

Sobota, J. M., M. Gu, and J. A. Imlay. 2014. Intracellular Hydrogen Peroxide and Superoxide Poison 3-deoxy-D-arabinoheptulosonate 7-Phosphate Synthase, the First Committed Enzyme in the Aromatic Biosynthetic Pathway of *Escherichia coli*. *J. Bacteriol.* **196**:1980–1991. [5]

Sobota, J. M., and J. A. Imlay. 2011. Iron Enzyme Ribulose-5-Phosphate 3-Epimerase in *Escherichia coli* Is Rapidly Damaged by Hydrogen Peroxide but Can Be Protected by Manganese. *PNAS* **108**:5402–5407. [3, 5]

Solioz, M., and J. V. Stoyanov. 2003. Copper Homeostasis in *Enterococcus hirae*. *FEMS Microbiol. Rev.* **27**:183–195. [5]

Song, M. K., M. J. Rosenthal, A. M. K. Song, et al. 2009. Body Weight Reduction in Rats by Oral Treatment with Zinc Plus Cyclo-(His-Pro). *Br. J. Pharmacol.* **158**:442–445. [12]

Sonkaria, S., S. H. Ahn, and V. Khare. 2012. Nanotechnology and Its Impact on Food and Nutrition: A Review. *Recent Pat. Food Nutr. Agric.* **4**:8–18. [17]

Soofi, S., S. Cousens, S. P. Iqbal, et al. 2013. Effect of Provision of Daily Zinc and Iron with Several Micronutrients on Growth and Morbidity among Young Children in Pakistan: A Cluster-Randomised Trial. *Lancet* **382**:29–40. [9]

Sprietsma, J. E. 1999. Modern Diets and Diseases: NO-Zinc Balance. Under Th1, Zinc and Nitrogen Monoxide (NO) Collectively Protect against Viruses, AIDS, Autoimmunity, Diabetes, Allergies, Asthma, Infectious Diseases, Atherosclerosis and Cancer. *Med. Hypotheses* **53**:6–16. [12]

Sreedhara, A., and J. A. Cowan. 2002. Structural and Catalytic Roles for Divalent Magnesium in Nucleic Acid Biochemistry. *Biometals* **15**:211–223. [4]

Stadlbauer, C., C. Reiter, B. Patzak, G. Stingeder, and T. Prohaska. 2007. History of individuals of the 18th/19th centuries stored in bones, teeth, and hair analyzed by LA-ICP-MS-a step in attempts to confirm the authenticity of Mozart's skull. *Anal. Bioanal. Chem.* **388**:593–602. [20]

Stalenhoef, J. E., B. Alisjahbana, E. J. Nelwan, et al. 2007. The Role of Interferon Gamma in the Increased Tuberculosis Risk in Type 2 Diabetes Mellitus. *Eur. J. Clin. Microbiol. Infect. Dis.* **27**:97–103. [12]

Stasenko, S., E. M. Bradford, M. Piasek, et al. 2010. Metals in Human Placenta: Focus on the Effects of Cadmium on Steroid Hormones and Leptin. *J. Appl. Toxicol.* **30**:242–253. [11]

Stathopoulou, M. G., S. Kanoni, G. Papanikolaou, et al. 2012. Mineral Intake. *Prog. Mol. Biol. Transl. Sci.* **108**:201–236. [11]

Stauff, D. L., and E. P. Skaar. 2009. *Bacillus anthracis* HssRS Signalling to HrtAB Regulates Haem Resistance During Infection. *Mol. Microbiol.* **72**:763–778. [20]

Steinbrenner, H., and H. Sies. 2013. Selenium Homeostasis and Antioxidant Selenoproteins in Brain: Implications for Disorders in the Central Nervous System. *Arch. Biochem. Biophys.* **536**:152–157. [8]

Stern, G. A., R. W. Macdonald, P. M. Outridge, et al. 2012. How Does Climate Change Influence Arctic Mercury? *Sci. Total Environ.* **414**:22–42. [17]

Sterritt, R. M., and J. N. Lester. 1980. Interactions of Heavy Metals with Bacteria. *Sci. Total Environ.* **14**:5–17. [8]

Stevenson, C. R., N. G. Forouhi, G. Roglic, et al. 2007. Diabetes and Tuberculosis: The Impact of the Diabetes Epidemic on Tuberculosis Incidence. *BMC Public Health* **7**:234. [12]

Stigter, M., J. Bezemer, K. Groot de, and P. Layrolle. 2004. Incorporation of Different Antibiotics into Carbonated Hydroxyapatite Coatings on Titanium Implants, Release and Antibiotic Efficacy. *J. Control Release* **99**:127–137. [16]

Stojanovic, D., D. Nikic, and K. Lazarevic. 2004. The Level of Nickel in Smoker's Blood and Urine. *Cent. Eur. J. Public Health* **12**:187–189. [8]

Stoltenberg, M., A. Bush, G. Bach, et al. 2007. Amyloid Plaques Arise from Zinc-Enriched Cortical Layers in APP/PS1 Transgenic Mice and Are Paradoxically Enlarged with Dietary Zinc Deficiency. *Neuroscience* **150**:357–369. [6]

Stone, C. K., B. T. Christian, R. J. Nickles, and S. B. Perlman. 1994. Technetium 94m-Labeled Methoxyisobutyl Isonitrile: Dosimetry and Resting Cardiac Imaging with Positron Emission Tomography. *J. Nucl. Cardiol.* **1**:425–433. [20]

Stone, S. F., D. Hancock, and R. Zeisler. 1987. Characterization of Biological Macromolecules by Electrophoresis and Neutron-Activation. *J. Radioan. Nucl. Ch. Ar.* **112**:95–108. [20]

Stork, M., M. P. Bos, I. Jongerius, et al. 2010. An Outer Membrane Receptor of *Neisseria meningitidis* Involved in Zinc Acquisition with Vaccine Potential. *PLoS Pathog.* **6**:e1000969. [2]

Stork, M., J. Grijpstra, M. P. Bos, et al. 2013. Zinc Piracy as a Mechanism of *Neisseria meningitides* for Evasion of Nutritional Immunity. *PLoS Pathog.* **9**:e1003733. [13]

Storrie, H., and S. I. Stupp. 2005. Cellular Response to Zinc-Containing Organoapatite: An *in Vitro* Study of Proliferation, Alkaline Phosphatase Activity and Biomineralization. *Biomaterials* **26**:5492–5499. [16]

Strandberg, L., M. Verdrengh, M. Enge, et al. 2009. Mice Chronically Fed High-Fat Diet Have Increased Mortality and Disturbed Immune Response in Sepsis. *PLoS One* **4**:e7605. [12]

Strange, H. R., T. A. Zola, and C. N. Cornelissen. 2011. The *fbpABC* Operon Is Required for Ton-Independent Utilization of Xenosiderophores by *Neisseria gonorrhoeae* Strain FA19. *Infect. Immun.* **79**:267–278. [3]

Su, H., G. M. van Dam, C. I. Buis, et al. 2006. Spatiotemporal Expression of Heme Oxygenase-1 Detected by *in Vivo* Bioluminescence after Hepatic Ischemia in HO-1/ Luc Mice. *Liver Transpl.* **12**:1634–1639. [20]

Sun, G., T. Van de Wiele, P. Alava, F. Tack, and G. Du Laing. 2012. Arsenic in Cooked Rice: Effect of Chemical, Enzymatic and Microbial Processes on Bioaccessibility and Speciation in the Human Gastrointestinal Tract. *Environ. Pollut.* **162**:241–246. [17]

Sun, H., G. Xu, H. Zhan, et al. 2010. Identification and Evaluation of the Role of the Manganese Efflux Protein in *Deinococcus radiodurans*. *BMC Microbiol.* **10**:319. [5]

Sun, X., H. Meng, D. Shi, et al. 2011. Analysis of Plasma Calprotectin and Polymorphisms of S100A8 in Patients with Aggressive Periodontitis. *J. Periodontal Res.* **46**:354–360. [20]

Sun, X., G. Yu, Q. Xu, et al. 2013. Putative Cobalt- and Nickel-Binding Proteins and Motifs in *Streptococcus pneumoniae*. *Metallomics* **5**:928–935. [18]

Sunda, W. G. 2012. Feedback Interactions between Trace Metal Nutrients and Phytoplankton in the Ocean. *Front. Microbiol.* **3**:204. [8]

Sundar, S., and V. K. Prajapati. 2012. Drug Targeting to Infectious Diseases by Nanoparticles Surface Functionalized with Special Biomolecules. *Curr. Med. Chem.* **19**:3196–3202. [17]

Sundseth, K., J. M. Pacyna, E. G. Pacyna, et al. 2009. Economic Benefits from Decreased Mercury Emissions: Projections for 2020. *J. Cleaner Prod.* **18**:386–394. [15]

Sussulini, A., A. Matusch, M. Klietz, et al. 2012. Quantitative Imaging of Cu, Fe, Mn, Zn in the L-Dopa Treated Unilateral 6-Hydroxydopamine Parkinson's Disease Mouse Model by LA-ICP-MS. *Biomed. Spect. Imag.* **1**:125–136. [20]

Sutherland, D. E., K. L. Summers, and M. J. Stillman. 2012. Noncooperative Metalation of Metallothionein 1a and Its Isolated Domains with Zinc. *Biochemistry* **51**:6690–6700. [20]

Suttle, N. F., and D. G. Jones. 1989. Recent Developments in Trace Element Metabolism and Function: Trace Elements, Disease Resistance and Immune Responsiveness in Ruminants. *J. Nutr.* **119**:1055–1061. [8]

Swem, D. L., L. R. Swem, A. Setterdahl, and C. E. Bauer. 2005. Involvement of SenC in Assembly of Cytochrome C Oxidase in *Rhodobacter capsulatus*. *J. Bacteriol.* **187**:8081–8087. [5]

Sword, C. P. 1966. Mechanisms of Pathogenesis in *Listeria monocytogenes* Infection. I. Influence of Iron. *J. Bacteriol.* **92**:536–542. [19]

Szmacinski, H., and J. R. Lakowicz. 1993. Optical Measurements of pH Using Fluorescence Lifetimes and Phase-Modulation Fluorometry. *Anal. Chem.* **65**:1668–1674. [20]

Szygula, R., A. Bunio, and S. Tubek. 2011. The Content of Elements in Rainwater and Its Relation to the Frequency of Hospitalization for Chronic Lymphocytic Leukemia and Chronic Myeloid Leukemia in Opole Voivodship, Poland, During 2000–2002. *Biol. Trace Elem. Res.* **141**:41–52. [11]

Tabuchi, H. 2010. Japan Recycles Minerals from Used Electronics. *New York Times.* Oct. 5, 2010. [15]

Tainer, A., V. A. Roberts, and E. D. Getzoff. 1991. Metal-Binding Sites in Proteins. *Curr. Opin. Biotechnol.* **2**:582–591. [14]

Taki, M., J. L. Wolford, and T. V. O'Halloran. 2004. Emission Ratiometric Imaging of Intracellular Zinc: Design of a Benzoxazole Fluorescent Sensor and Its Application in Two-Photon Microscopy. *J. Am. Chem. Soc.* **126**:712–713. [20]

Takiguchi, M., W. E. Achanzar, W. Qu, G. Li, and M. P. Waalkes. 2003. Effects of Cadmium on DNA-(Cytosine-5) Methyltransferase Activity and DNA Methylation Status During Cadmium-Induced Cellular Transformation. *Exp. Cell. Res.* **286**:355–365. [11]

Tan, S., J. M. Noto, J. Romero-Gallo, R. M. Peek, Jr., and M. R. Amieva. 2011. *Helicobacter pylori* Perturbs Iron Trafficking in the Epithelium to Grow on the Cell Surface. *PLoS Pathog.* **7**:e1002050. [2, 7]

Taneja, S. K., M. Jain, R. Mandal, and K. Megha. 2012. Excessive Zinc in Diet Induces Leptin Resistance in Wistar Rat through Increased Uptake of Nutrients at Intestinal Level. *J. Trace Elem. Med. Biol.* **26**:267–272. [12]

Taneja, S. K., M. Mahajan, and P. Arya. 1996. Excessive Bioavailability of Zn May Cause Obesity in Humans. *Experientia* **52**:31–33. [12]

Tang, Y., and J. R. Guest. 1999. Direct Evidence for mRNA Binding and Post-Transcriptional Regulation by *Escherichi coli* Aconitases. *Microbiology* **145**:3069–3079. [5]

Tanji, K., T. Imaizumi, T. Matsumiya, et al. 2001. Desferrioxamine, an Iron Chelator, Upregulates Cyclooxygenase-2 Expression and Prostaglandin Production in a Human Macrophage Cell Line. *Biochim. Biophys. Acta* **1530**:227–235. [3]

Taudte, N., and G. Grass. 2010. Point Mutations Change Specificity and Kinetics of Metal Uptake by Zupt from *Escherichia coli*. *Biometals* **23**:643–656. [5]

Taylor, E., and T. J. Webster. 2011. Reducing Infections through Nanotechnology and Nanoparticles. *Int. J. Nanomedicine* **6**:1463–1473. [16]

Templeton, D. M., F. Ariese, R. Cornelis, et al. 2000. Guidelines for Terms Related to Chemical Speciation and Fractionation of Elements: Definitions, Structural Aspects and Methodological Approaches. *Pure Appl. Chem.* **72**:1453–1470. [14]

Thiele, D. J., and J. D. Gitlin. 2008. Assembling the Pieces. *Nat. Chem. Biol.* **4**:145–147. [14]

Thierse, H. J., S. Helm, and P. Pankert. 2008. Metalloproteomics in the Molecular Study of Cell Physiology and Disease. In: 2D-Page: Sample Preparation and Fractionation, ed. A. Posch, pp. 139–147, Methods in Molecular Biology, vol. 2. Totowa, NJ: Humana Press. [18]

Thompson, B., and L. Amoroso. 2013. Combating Micronutrient Deficiencies: Food-Based Approaches. Nutrition and Consumer Protection Division, Rome: FAO and CAB Intl. http://www.fao.org/docrep/013/am027e/am027e00.pdf (accessed April 18, 2014). [17]

Thompson, K. H., and C. Orvig. 2003. Boon and Bane of Metal Ions in Medicine. *Science* **300**:936. [10]

Thompson, R. B., B. P. Maliwal, and H. H. Zeng. 2000. Zinc Biosensing with Multiphoton Excitation Using Carbonic Anhydrase and Improved Fluorophores. *J. Biomed. Optics* **5**:17–22. [20]

Thorson, J. A., K. M. Smith, F. Gomez, P. W. Naumann, and J. D. Kemp. 1991. Role of Iron in T Cell Activation: Th1 Clones Differ from Th2 Clones in Their Sensitivity to Inhibition of DNA Synthesis Caused by IgG Mabs against the Transferrin Receptor and the Iron Chelator Deferoxamine. *Cell. Immunol.* **134**:126–137. [9]

Thurman, R. B., C. P. Gerba, and G. Bitton. 1989. The Molecular Mechanisms of Copper and Silver Ion Disinfection of Bacteria and Viruses. *Crit. Rev. Environ. Control* **18**:295–315. [8]

Tiedemann, M. T., D. E. Heinrichs, and M. J. Stillman. 2012. Multiprotein Heme Shuttle Pathway in *Staphylococcus aureus*: Iron-Regulated Surface Determinant Cog-Wheel Kinetics. *J. Am. Chem. Soc.* **134**:16578–16585. [2]

Tielsch, J. M., S. K. Khatry, R. J. Stoltzfus, et al. 2007. Effect of Daily Zinc Supplementation on Child Mortality in Southern Nepal: A Community-Based, Cluster Randomised, Placebo-Controlled Trial. *Lancet* **370**:1230–1239. [13]

Tillander, J., K. Hagberg, L. Hagberg, and R. Branemark. 2010. Osseointegrated Titanium Implants for Limb Prostheses Attachments: Infectious Complications. *Clin. Orthop. Relat. Res.* **468**:2781–2788. [16]

Tjalve, H., S. Jasim, and A. Oskarsson. 1984. Nickel Mobilization by Sodium Diethyldithiocarbamate in Nickel-Carbonyl-Treated Mice. *IARC Sci. Publ.*311–320. [8]

Tocheva, E. I., J. Lopez-Garrido, H. V. Hughes, et al. 2013. Peptidoglycan Transformations During *Bacillus subtilis* Sporulation. *Mol. Microbiol.* **88**:673–686. [20]

Tokar, E. J., W. Qu, and M. P. Waalkes. 2011. Arsenic, Stem Cells, and the Developmental Basis of Adult Cancer. *Toxicol. Sci.* **120 (Suppl 1)**:S192–S203. [8]

Tombline, G., J. M. Schwingel, J. D. Lapek, Jr., et al. 2013. *Pseudomonas aeruginosa* PA1006 Is a Persulfide-Modified Protein That Is Critical for Molybdenum Homeostasis. *PLoS One* **8**:e55593. [20]

Topping, G. J., P. Schaffer, C. Hoehr, T. J. Ruth, and V. Sossi. 2013. Manganese-52 Positron Emission Tomography Tracer Characterization and Initial Results in Phantoms and *in Vivo*. *Med. Phys.* **40**:042502. [20]

Torjussen, W., H. Zachariasen, and I. Andersen. 2003. Cigarette Smoking and Nickel Exposure. *J. Environ. Monit.* **5**:198–201. [11]

Torres, A. G., and S. M. Payne. 1997. Haem Iron-Transport System in Enterohaemorrhagic *Escherichia coli* O157:H7. *Mol. Microbiol.* **23**:825–833. [5]

Torres, J., S. Danese, and J. F. Colombel. 2013. New Therapeutic Avenues in Ulcerative Colitis: Thinking out of the Box. *Gut* **62**:1642–1652. [17]

Torres, V. J., A. S. Attia, W. J. Mason, et al. 2010. *Staphylococcus aureus* Fur Regulates the Expression of Virulence Factors That Contribute to the Pathogenesis of Pneumonia. *Infect. Immun.* **78**:1618–1628. [4]

Tosco, A., B. Fontanella, R. Danise, et al. 2010a. Molecular Bases of Copper and Iron Deficiency-Associated Dyslipidemia: A Microarray Analysis of the Rat Intestinal Transcriptome. *Genes Nutr.* **5**:1–8. [11]

Tosco, A., M. C. Monti, B. Fontanella, et al. 2010b. Copper Binds the Carboxy-Terminus of Trefoil Protein 1 (TFF1), Favoring Its Homodimerization and Motogenic Activity. *Cell. Mol. Life Sci.* **67**:1943–1955. [11]

Tottey, S., D. R. Harvie, and N. J. Robinson. 2005. Understanding How Cells Allocate Metals Using Metal Sensors and Metallochaperones. *Acc. Chem. Res.* **38**:775–783. [4]

Tottey, S., K. J. Waldron, S. J. Firbank, et al. 2008. Protein-Folding Location Can Regulate Manganese-Binding versus Copper- or Zinc-Binding. *Nature* **455**:1138–1142. [18, 20]

Touati, D., M. Jacques, B. Tardat, L. Bouchard, and S. Despied. 1995. Lethal Oxidative Damage and Mutagenesis Are Generated by Iron in Delta *Fur* Mutants of *Escherichia coli*: Protective Role of Superoxide Dismutase. *J. Bacteriol.* **177**:2305–2314. [5]

Tran, P. L., A. A. Hammond, T. Mosley, et al. 2009. Organoselenium Coating on Cellulose Inhibits the Formation of Biofilms by *Pseudomonas aeruginosa* and *Staphylococcus aureus*. *Appl. Environ. Microbiol.* **75**:3586–3592. [13]

Treffry, A., E. R. Bauminger, D. Hechel, et al. 1993. Defining the Roles of the Threefold Channels in Iron Uptake, Iron Oxidation and Iron-Core Formation in Ferritin: A Study Aided by Site-Directed Mutagenesis. *Biochem. J.* **296**:721–728. [4]

Trejos, T., R. Koons, S. Becker, et al. 2013. Cross-Validation and Evaluation of the Performance of Methods for the Elemental Analysis of Forensic Glass by $\mu$-XRF, ICP-MS, and LA-ICP-MS. *Anal. Bioanal. Chem.* **405**:5393–5409. [20]

Trumbo, P., A. A. Yates, S. Schlicker, and M. Poos. 2001. Dietary Reference Intakes: Vitamin a, Vitamin K, Arsenic, Boron, Chromium, Copper, Iodine, Iron, Manganese, Molybdenum, Nickel, Silicon, Vanadium, and Zinc. *J. Am. Diet. Assoc.* **101**:294–301. [11]

Trunova, V., A. Sidorina, V. Zvereva, and B. Churin. 2013. Changes in the Elemental Content of Rat Heart as a Result of the Fixation in Formalin Analyzed by Synchrotron Radiation X-Ray Fluorescent Analysis. *J. Trace Elem. Med. Biol.* **27**:76–77. [19]

Tse, P.-K. 2011. China's Rare Earth Industry. Usgs Open File Report 2011–1042. Reston, VA: U.S. Geological Survey. [15]

Tseng, C. H. 2004. The Potential Biological Mechanisms of Arsenic-Induced Diabetes Mellitus. *Toxicol. Appl. Pharmacol.* **197**:67–83. [12]

Tu, W. Y., S. Pohl, J. Gray, et al. 2012. Cellular Iron Distribution in *Bacillus anthracis*. *J. Bacteriol.* **194**:932–940. [4]

Tubek, S., A. Bunio, R. Szygula, and G. Krasowski. 2011. The Content of Elements in Rainwater and Its Relation to the Frequency of Hospitalization for Gastric and Duodenal Peptic Ulcers in Opole Voivodship, Poland, During 2000–2002. *Biol. Trace Elem. Res.* **140**:253–261. [11]

Tuerk, M. J., and N. Fazel. 2009. Zinc Deficiency. *Curr. Opin. Gastroenterol.* **25**:136–143. [11]

Tungtrongchitr, R., P. Pongpaew, B. Phonrat, et al. 2003. Serum Copper, Zinc, Ceruloplasmin and Superoxide Dismutase in Thai Overweight and Obese. *J. Med. Assoc. Thai* **86**:543–551. [12]

Turnbaugh, P. J., R. E. Ley, M. Hamady, et al. 2007. The Human Microbiome Project. *Nature* **449**:804–810. [17]

Turski, M. L., and D. J. Thiele. 2009. New Roles for Copper Metabolism in Cell Proliferation, Signaling, and Disease. *J. Biol. Chem.* **284**:717–721. [2]

Uberos, J., A. Molina-Carballo, V. Fernández-Puentes, R. Rodriguez-Belmonte, and A. Munoz-Hoyos 2010. Overweight and Obesity as Risk Factors for the Asymptomatic Carrier State of Neisseria Meningitidis among a Paediatric Population. *Eur. J. Clin. Microbiol. Infect. Dis.* **29(3)**:333–334. [12]

UNEP. 2013. Environmental Challenges of Metals Cycles. UNEP Resource Panel. Geneva: United Nations Environment Programme. [15, 17]

Vacheethasanee, K., and R. E. Marchant. 2000. Mechanisms of Bacterial Adhesion and Pathogenesis of Implant and Tissue Infections. In: Handbook of Bacterial Adhesion: Principles, Methods, and Applications, ed. Y. H. An and R. J. Friedman, pp. 73–90. Totowa: Humana Press. [16]

Vahjen, W., R. Pieper, and J. Zentek. 2011. Increased Dietary Zinc Oxide Changes the Bacterial Core and Enterobacterial Composition in the Ileum of Piglets. *J. Anim. Sci.* **89**:2430–2439. [7]

Vahter, M., A. Akesson, C. Liden, S. Ceccatelli, and M. Berglund. 2007. Gender Differences in the Disposition and Toxicity of Metals. *Environ. Res.* **104**:85–95. [11]

Valderas, M. W., J. W. Gatson, N. Wreyford, and M. E. Hart. 2002. The Superoxide Dismutase Gene *sodM* Is Unique to *Staphylococcus aureus*: Absence of *sodM* in Coagulase-Negative Staphylococci. *J. Bacteriol.* **184**:2465–2472. [4]

Vallee, B. L., and K. H. Falchuk. 1993. The Biochemical Basis of Zinc Physiology. *Physiol. Rev.* **73**:79–118. [5]

Van der Voet, G. B., and F. A. de Wolff. 1996. Human Exposure to Lithium, Thallium, Antimony, Gold and Platinum. In: Toxicology of Metals, ed. L. W. Chang, vol. 1. Boca Raton: CRC Press. [15]

van Dongen, E. M. W. M., T. H. Evers, L. M. Dekkers, et al. 2007. Variation of Linker Length in Ratiometric Fluorescent Sensor Proteins Allows Rational Tuning of Zn(II) Affinity in the Picomolar to Femtomolar Range. *J. Am. Chem. Soc.* **129**:3494–3495. [20]

van Veen, H. W., T. Abee, G. J. Kortstee, W. N. Konings, and A. J. Zehnder. 1994. Translocation of Metal Phosphate via the Phosphate Inorganic Transport System of *Escherichia coli. Biochemistry* **33**:1766–1770. [5]

Varghese, S., Y. Tang, and J. A. Imlay. 2003. Contrasting Sensitivities of *Escherichia coli* Aconitases a and B to Oxidation and Iron Depletion. *J. Bacteriol.* **185**:221–230. [5]

Varghese, S., A. Wu, S. Park, K. R. C. Imlay, and J. A. Imlay. 2007. Submicromolar Hydrogen Peroxide Disrupts the Ability of Fur Protein to Control Free-Iron Levels in *Escherichia coli. Mol. Microbiol.* **64**:822–830. [5]

Vashchenko, G., and R. T. MacGillivray. 2013. Multi-Copper Oxidases and Human Iron Metabolism. *Nutrients* **5**:2289–2313. [2]

Vavere, A. L., and M. J. Welch. 2005. Preparation, Biodistribution, and Small Animal PET of [45]Ti-Transferrin. *J. Nucl. Med.* **46**:683–690. [20]

Vermes, C., R. Chandrasekaran, J. J. Jacobs, et al. 2001. The Effects of Particulate Wear Debris, Cytokines, and Growth Factors on the Functions of Mg-63 Osteoblasts. *J. Bone Joint Surg. Am.* **83-A**:201–211. [16]

Vickery, L. E., and J. R. Cupp-Vickery. 2007. Molecular Chaperones HscA/Ssq1 and HscB/Jac1 and Their Roles in Iron-Sulfur Protein Maturation. *Crit. Rev. Biochem. Mol. Biol.* **42**:95–111. [4]

Vieira, C., S. Morais, S. Ramos, C. Delerue-Matos, and M. B. Oliveira. 2011. Mercury, Cadmium, Lead and Arsenic Levels in Three Pelagic Fish Species from the Atlantic Ocean: Intra- and Inter-Specific Variability and Human Health Risks for Consumption. *Food Chem. Toxicol.* **49**:923–932. [8]

Vignesh, K. S., J. Landero-Figueroa, A. Porollo, J. A. Caruso, and G. S. Deepe. 2013a. Granulocyte Macrophage-Colony Stimulating Factor Induced Zn Sequestration Enhances Macrophage Superoxide and Limits Intracellular Pathogen Survival. *Immunity* **39**:697–710. [9, 20]

Vignesh, K. S., J. Landero-Figueroa, A. Porollo, J. A. Caruso, and G. S. Deepe. 2013b. Zinc Sequestration: Arming Phagocyte Defense against Fungal Attack. *PLoS Pathog.* **9**:e1003815. [20]

Viktorinova, A., E. Toserova, M. Krizko, and Z. Durackova. 2009. Altered Metabolism of Copper, Zinc, and Magnesium Is Associated with Increased Levels of Glycated Hemoglobin in Patients with Diabetes Mellitus. *Metabolism* **58**:1477–1482. [12]

Villalobos, M., C. Merino-Sánchez, C. Hall, et al. 2009. Lead (II) Detection and Contamination Routes in Environmental Sources, Cookware and Home-Prepared Foods from Zimatlán, Oaxaca, Mexico. *Sci. Total Environ.* **407**:2836–2844. [17]

Vincent, J. B. 2010. Chromium: Celebrating 50 Years as an Essential Element? *Dalton Trans.* **39**:3787–3794. [2, 8]

Vinson, J. A., and P. Bose. 1987. Comparison of the Toxicology of Inorganic and Natural Selenium. In: Selenium in Biology and Medicine (Part A), ed. G. F. Combs et al., pp. 513–515. New York: Van Nostrand Reinhold Co. [14]

Visbal, G., E. Marchán, A. Maldonado, Z. Simoni, and M. Navarro. 2008. Synthesis and Characterization of Platinum-Sterol Hydrazone Complexes with Biological Activity against Leishmania (L.) Mexicana. *J. Inorg. Biochem.* **102**:547–554. [10]

Vitale, S., C. Fauquant, D. Lascoux, et al. 2009. A $Zns_4$ Structural Zinc Site in the *Helicobacter pylori* Ferric Uptake Regulator. *Biochemistry* **48**:5582–5591. [4]

Volz, K. 2008. The Functional Duality of Iron Regulatory Protein 1. *Curr. Opin. Struct. Biol.* **18**:106–111. [5]

Vrijheid, M., R. Slama, O. Robinson, et al. 2014. The Human Early-Life Exposome (HELIX): Project Rationale and Design. *Environ. Health Perspect.* **122**:535–544. [17]

Wade, W. G. 2013. The Oral Microbiome in Health and Disease. *Pharmacol. Res.* **69**:137–143. [17]

Wagner, D., J. Maser, B. Lai, et al. 2005. Elemental Analysis of *Mycobacterium avium-*, *Mycobacterium tuberculosis-*, and *Mycobacterium smegmatis*-Containing Phagosomes Indicates Pathogen-Induced Microenvironments within the Host Cell's Endosomal System. *J. Immunol.* **174**:1491–1500. [9]

Waldron, K. J., and N. J. Robinson. 2009. How Do Bacterial Cells Ensure That Metalloproteins Get the Correct Metal? *Nat. Rev. Microbiol.* **7**:25–35. [14]

Walker, G., and K. Burningham. 2011. Flood Risk, Vulnerability and Environmental Justice: Evidence and Evaluation of Inequality in a UK Context. *Crit. Soc. Policy* **31**:216–240. [11]

Walser, T., F. Schwabe, L. Thoni, L. de Temmerman, and S. Hellweg. 2013. Nanosilver Emissions to the Atmosphere: A New Challenge? E3S Web of Conferences, 1, 14003. http://dx.doi.org/10.1051/e3sconf/20130114003 (accessed Oct. 19, 2014). [15]

Walter, R. M., Jr., J. Y. Uriu-Hare, K. L. Olin, et al. 1991. Copper, Zinc, Manganese, and Magnesium Status and Complications of Diabetes Mellitus. *Diabetes Care* **14**:1050–1056. [12]

Wandersman, C., and P. Delepelaire. 2004. Bacterial Iron Sources: From Siderophores to Hemophores. *Annu. Rev. Microbiol.* **58**:611–647. [2]

Wang, C., H. Wang, J. Luo, et al. 2009. Selenium Deficiency Impairs Host Innate Immune Response and Induces Susceptibility to *Listeria monocytogenes* Infection. *BMC Immunol.* **10**:55. [13]

Wang, D., and C. A. Fierke. 2013. The BaeSR Regulon Is Involved in Defense against Zinc Toxicity in *E. coli. Metallomics* **5**:372–383. [5]

Wang, D., O. Hosteen, and C. A. Fierke. 2012a. ZntR-Mediated Transcription of *zntA* Responds to Nanomolar Intracellular Free Zinc. *J. Inorg. Biochem.* **111**:173–181. [5, 7]

Wang, D., T. K. Hurst, R. B. Thompson, and C. A. Fierke. 2011a. Genetically Encoded Ratiometric Biosensors to Measure Intracellular Exchangeable Zinc in *Escherichia coli*. *J. Biomed. Opt.* **16**:087011. [4]

Wang, K., H. Cui, Y. Deng, et al. 2012b. Effect of Dietary Vanadium on Intestinal Microbiota in Broiler. *Biol. Trace Elem. Res.* **149**:212–218. [11]

Wang, L., and S. Busbey. 2005. Images in Clinical Medicine: Acquired *Acrodermatitis enteropathica*. *N. Engl. J. Med.* **352**:1121. [8]

Wang, L., J. E. Manson, and H. D. Sesso. 2012c. Calcium Intake and Risk of Cardiovascular Disease: A Review of Prospective Studies and Randomized Clinical Trials. *Am. J. Cardiovasc. Drugs* **12**:105–116. [16]

Wang, Q., and T. J. Webster. 2013. Short Communication: Inhibiting Biofilm Formation on Paper Towels through the Use of Selenium Nanoparticles Coatings. *Int. J. Nanomedicine* **8**:407–411. [16]

Wang, R. E., Y. Zhang, J. Cai, W. Cai, and T. Gao. 2011b. Aptamer-Based Fluorescent Biosensors. *Curr. Med. Chem.* **18**:4175–4184. [5, 20]

Wang, W., Z. Xie, Y. Lin, and D. F. Zhang. 2014. Association of Inorganic Arsenic Exposure with Type 2 Diabetes Mellitus: A Meta-Analysis. *J. Epidemiol. Comm. Health* **68**:176–184. [12]

Ward, S. K., B. Abomoelak, E. A. Hoye, H. Steinberg, and A. M. Talaat. 2010. CtpV: A Putative Copper Exporter Required for Full Virulence of *Mycobacterium tuberculosis*. *Mol. Microbiol.* **77**:1096–1110. [7]

Warnes, S. L., V. Caves, and C. W. Keevil. 2012. Mechanism of Copper Surface Toxicity in *Escherichia coli* O157:H7 and *Salmonella* Involves Immediate Membrane Depolarization Followed by Slower Rate of DNA Destruction Which Differs from That Observed for Gram-Positive Bacteria. *Environ. Microbiol.* **14**:1730–1743. [11]

Warszawska, J. M., R. Gawish, O. Sharif, et al. 2013. Lipocalin 2 Deactivates Macrophages and Worsens Pneumococcal Pneumonia Outcomes. *J. Clin. Invest.* **123**:3363–3372. [3, 9, 13]

Watanabe, T., and S. Hirano. 2013. Metabolism of Arsenic and Its Toxicological Relevance. *Arch. Toxicol.* **87**:969–979. [8]

Waters, L. S., M. Sandoval, and G. Storz. 2011. The *Escherichia coli* MntR Miniregulon Includes Genes Encoding a Small Protein and an Efflux Pump Required for Manganese Homeostasis. *J. Bacteriol.* **193**:5887–5897. [5]

Weaver, L., H. T. Michels, and C. W. Keevil. 2008. Survival of *Clostridium difficile* on Copper and Steel: Futuristic Options for Hospital Hygiene. *J. Hosp. Infect.* **68**:145–151. [11]

Weber, D. J., W. A. Rutala, G. P. Samsa, J. E. Santimaw, and S. M. Lemon. 1985. Obesity as a Predictor of Poor Antibody Response to Hepatitis B Plasma Vaccine. *JAMA* **254**:3187–3189. [12]

Wegner, S. V., H. Arslan, M. Sunbul, J. Yin, and C. He. 2010. Dynamic Copper(I) Imaging in Mammalian Cells with a Genetically Encoded Fluorescent Copper(I) Sensor. *J. Am. Chem. Soc.* **132**:2567–2569. [20]

Wehrens, A., T. Aebischer, T. F. Meyer, and A. K. Walduck. 2008. Leptin Receptor Signaling Is Required for Vaccine-Induced Protection against *Helicobacter pylori*. *Helicobacter* **13**:94–102. [12]

Wei, L., P. Liao, H. Wu, et al. 2008. Toxicological Effects of Cinnabar in Rats by NMR-Based Metabolic Profiling of Urine and Serum. *Toxicol. Appl. Pharmacol.* **227**:417–429. [14]

Weinberg, E. D. 1972. Infectious Diseases Influenced by Trace Element Enviroment. *Ann. NY Acad. Sci.* **199**:274–284. [3]

———. 1999. Iron Loading and Disease Surveillance. *Emerg. Infect. Dis.* **5**:346–352. [9, 13]

Weir, E., A. Lawlor, A. Whelan, and F. Regan. 2008. The Use of Nanoparticles in Antimicrobial Materials and Their Characterization. *Analyst* **133**:835–845. [17]

Weisinger, J. R., and E. Bellorin-Font. 1998. Magnesium and Phosphorus. *Lancet* **352**:391–396. [16]

Weiss, G. 2002. Iron and Immunity: A Double-Edged Sword. *Eur. J. Clin. Invest.* **32(Suppl 1)**:70–78. [9, 13]

Weiss, G., and G. Schett. 2013. Anaemia in Inflammatory Rheumatic Diseases. *Nat. Rev. Rheumatol.* **9**:205–215. [9]

Welch, R. M., G. F. Combs, Jr., and J. M. Duxbury. 1997. Toward a "Greener" Revolution. *Iss. Sci. Technol.* **14**:50–58. [17]

Welch, R. M., and R. D. Graham. 2005. Agriculture: The Real Nexus for Enhancing Bioavailable Micronutrients in Food Crops. *J. Trace Elem. Med. Biol.* **18**:299–307. [17]

———. 2012. Perspectives on Enhancing the Nutritional Quality of Food Crops with Trace Element. In: Fertilizing Crops to Improve Human Health: A Scientific Review, vol. 1, Food and Nutrition Security. Norcross, GA: International Plant Nutrition Institute. [17]

Wennerhold, J., A. Krug, and M. Bott. 2005. The Arac-Type Regulator RipA Represses Aconitase and Other Iron Proteins from *Corynebacterium* under Iron Limitation and Is Itself Repressed by DtxR. *J. Biol. Chem.* **280**:40500–40508. [5]

Wermuth, P. J., and S. A. Jimenez. 2012. Gadolinium Compounds Signaling through TLR4 and TLR7 in Normal Human Macrophages: Establishment of a Proinflammatory Phenotype and Implications for the Pathogenesis of Nephrogenic Systemic Fibrosis. *J. Immunol.* **189**:318–327. [17]

Wesch, H., H. Przuntek, and D. Feist. 1980. Wilson Disease: Rapid Diagnosis and Differentiation of Heterozygous and Homozygous Carriers with 64CuCl2 (Article in German). *Dtsch. Med. Wochenschr.* **105**:483–488. [20]

Wessells, K. R., and K. H. Brown. 2012. Estimating the Global Prevalence of Zinc Deficiency: Results Based on Zinc Availability in National Food Supplies and the Prevalence of Stunting. *PLoS One* **7**:e50568. [8]

Wessels, I., H. Haase, G. Engelhardt, L. Rink, and P. Uciechowski. 2013. Zinc Deficiency Induces Production of the Pro-Inflammatory Cytokines IL-1β and TNFα in Promyeloid Cells via Epigenetic and Redox-Dependent Mechanisms. *J. Nutr. Biochem.* **24**:289–297. [13, 17]

White, C., J. Lee, T. Kambe, K. Fritsche, and M. J. Petris. 2009. A Role for the ATP7A Copper-Transporting ATPase in Macrophage Bactericidal Activity. *J. Biol. Chem.* **284**:33949–33956. [7, 9]

Whittaker, J. W. 2003. The Irony of Manganese Superoxide Dismutase. *Biochem. Soc. Trans.* **31**:1318–1321. [5]

Whittaker, P. 1998. Iron and Zinc Interactions in Humans. *Am. J. Clin. Nutr.* **68(Suppl 2)**:442S–446S. [8]

WHO. 1987. Environmental Health Criteria 58: Selenium. Geneva: World Health Organization. [14]

———. 1993. Guidelines for Drinking-Water Quality, 2nd edition, vol. 1. Geneva: World Health Organization. [14]

———. 2002. Principles and Methods for the Assessment of Risk from Essential Trace Elements. Environmental Health Criteria 228. Geneva: World Health Organization. [17]

———. 2009. Infant and Young Child Feeding: Model Chapter for Textbooks for Medical Students and Allied Health Professionals. . Geneva: WHO. [17]

———. 2013a. Global Burden of Disease, 2000–2011, Global Summary Estimates. http://www.who.int/healthinfo/global_burden_disease/en/. (accessed April 15, 2013). [17]

———. 2013b. World Malaria Report 2013. Geneva: World Health Organization. [10]

WHO/FAO/IAEA. 1996. Trace Elements in Human Nutrition and Health. Geneva: World Health Organization. [14]

WHO/UNICEF. 2004. Clinical Management of Acute Diarrhoea: WHO/Unicef Joint Statement, Geneva: World Health Organization. http://www.unicef.org/publications/files/ENAcute_Diarrhoea_reprint.pdf (accessed Sept. 7, 2014). [6]

Wieland, C. W., S. Florquin, E. D. Chan, et al. 2005. Pulmonary *Mycobacterium tuberculosis* Infection in Leptin-Deficient ob/ob Mice. *Int. Immunol.* **17**:1399–1408. [12]

Wilber, C. G. 1980. Toxicology of Selenium: A Review. *Clin. Toxicol.* **17**:171–230. [14]

Wildman, R. E., and S. Mao. 2001. Tissue-Specific Alterations in Lipoprotein Lipase Activity in Copper-Deficient Rats. *Biol. Trace. Elem. Res.* **80**:221–229. [12]

Wilks, S. A., H. T. Michels, and C. W. Keevil. 2006. Survival of *Listeria monocytogenes* Scott A on Metal Surfaces: Implications for Cross-Contamination. *Int. J. Food Microbiol.* **111**:93–98. [11]

Williams, R. J. P. 2001. Chemical Selection of Elements by Cells. *Coord. Chem. Rev.* **216-217**:583–595. [14, 18]

Willis, M. S., S. A. Monaghan, M. L. Miller, et al. 2005. Zinc-Induced Copper Deficiency: A Report of Three Cases Initially Recognized on Bone Marrow Examination. *Am. J. Clin. Pathol.* **123**:125–131. [8]

Wilson, R. G. 1995. SIMS Quantification in Si, GaAs, and Diamond: An Update. *Int. J. Mass Spectrom.* **143**:43–49. [20]

Wimalawansa, S. J. 2013. Rational Food Fortification Programs to Alleviate Micronutrient Deficiencies. *J. Food Process. Technol.* **4**:8. [17]

Winans, B., M. C. Humble, and B. P. Lawrence. 2011. Environmental Toxicants and the Developing Immune System: A Missing Link in the Global Battle against Infectious Disease? *Reprod. Toxicol.* **31**:327–336. [1, 17]

Winter, S. E., M. G. Winter, M. N. Xavier, et al. 2013. Host-Derived Nitrate Boosts Growth of *E. coli* in the Inflamed Gut. *Science* **339**:708–711. [11]

Wintergerst, E. S., S. Maggini, and D. H. Hornig. 2007. Contribution of Selected Vitamins and Trace Elements to Immune Function. *Annu. Nutr. Metab.* **51**:301–323. [8]

Wolfbeis, O. S. 1985. The Fluorescence of Organic Natural Products. In: Molecular Luminescence Spectroscopy Methods and Applications: Part I, ed. S. G. Schulman, pp. 167–370, Chemical Analysis: A Series of Monographs on Analytical Chemistry and Its Applications, P. J. Elving and J. Winefordner, series ed. New York: Wiley-Interscience. [20]

Wood, R. C., K. L. MacDonald, K. E. White, et al. 1993. Risk Factors for Lack of Detectable Antibody Following Hepatitis B Vaccination of Minnesota Health Care Workers. *JAMA* **270**:2935–2939. [12]

Wood, R. J. 2009. Manganese and Birth Outcome. *Nutr. Rev.* **67**:416–420. [8]

Wright, R. O., C. Amarasiriwardena, A. D. Woolf, R. Jim, and D. C. Bellinger. 2006. Neuropsychological Correlates of Hair Arsenic, Manganese, and Cadmium Levels in School-Age Children Residing near a Hazardous Waste Site. *Neurotoxicology* 27:210–216. [11]

Wu, J., L. Wang, J. He, and C. Zhu. 2012. *In Vitro* Cytotoxicity of $Cu^{2+}$, $Zn^{2+}$, $Ag^+$ and Their Mixtures on Primary Human Endometrial Epithelial Cells. *Contraception* 85:509–518. [16]

Wu, M.-L., W.-J. Tsai, J. Ger, et al. 2001. Cholestatic Hepatitis Caused by Acute Gold Potassium Cyanide Poisoning. *Clin. Toxicol.* 39:739–743. [15]

Xia, T., M. Kovochich, M. Liong, et al. 2008. Comparison of the Mechanism of Toxicityof Zinc Oxide and Cerium Oxide Nanoparticles Based on Dissolution and Oxidative Stress Properties. *ACS Nano.* 2:2121–2134. [16]

Xie, H., J. Mire, Y. Kong, et al. 2012. Rapid Point-of-Care Detection of the Tuberculosis Pathogen Using a BlaC-Specific Fluorogenic Probe. *Nat. Chem.* 4:802–809. [20]

Xu, F. F., and J. A. Imlay. 2012. Silver(I), Mercury(II), Cadmium(II), and Zinc(II) Target Exposed Enzymic Iron-Sulfur Clsuters When the Toxify *Escherichia coli.* *Appl. Environ. Microbiol.* 78:3614–3621. [5]

Xu, J., G. Ding, J. Li, et al. 2010. Zinc-Ion Implanted and Deposited Titanium Surfaces Reduce Adhesion of *Streptococcccus Mutans.* *Appl. Surf. Sci.* 256:7540–7544. [16]

Xu, J., Z. Jia, M. D. Knutson, and C. Leeuwenburgh. 2012. Impaired Iron Status in Aging Research. *Int. J. Mol. Sci.* 13:2368–2386. [8]

Xu, X., H. Hui, A. B. Dailey, et al. 2013. Potential Health Impacts of Heavy Metals on HIV-Infected Population in USA. *PLoS One* 8:e74288. [11, 17]

Xue, Y., A. V. Davis, G. Balakrishnan, et al. 2008. Cu(I) Recognition via Cation-Π and Methionine Interactions in Cusf. *Nat. Chem. Biol.* 4:107–109. [4]

Yachie, A., Y. Niida, T. Wada, et al. 1999. Oxidative Stress Causes Enhanced Endothelial Cell Injury in Human Heme Oxygenase-1 Deficiency. *J. Clin. Invest.* 103:129–135. [13]

Yakinci, C., A. Pac, F. Z. Kucukbay, M. Tayfun, and A. Gul. 1997. Serum Zinc, Copper, and Magnesium Levels in Obese Children. *Acta Pediatr. Jpn.* 39:339–341. [12]

Yamamoto, S., T. Tsukamoto, A. Terai, et al. 1997. Genetic Evidence Supporting the Fecal-Perineal-Urethral Hypothesis in Cystitis Caused by *Escherichia coli. J. Urol.* 157:1127–1129. [4]

Yamasaki, S., K. Sakata-Sogawa, A. Hasegawa, et al. 2007. Zinc Is a Novel Intracellular Second Messenger. *J. Cell Biol.* 177:637–645. [2]

Yan, Y., J. G. Waite-Cusic, P. Kuppusamy, and A. E. Yousef. 2013. Intracellular Free Iron and Its Potential Role in Ultrahigh-Pressure-Induced Inactivation of *Escherichia coli. Appl. Environ. Microbiol.* 79:722–724. [4]

Yang, J., I. Sangwan, A. Lindemann, et al. 2006. *Bradyrhizobium japonicum* Senses Iron through the Status of Haem to Regulate Iron Homeostasis and Metabolism. *Mol. Microbiol.* 60:427–437. [5]

Yang, L., W. Wang, S. Hou, P. J. Peterson, and W. P. Williams. 2002. Effects of Selenium Supplementation on Arsenism: An Intervention Trial in Inner Mongolia. *Environ. Geochem. Health* 24:359–374. [14]

Yankovskaya, V., R. Horsefield, S. Tornroth, et al. 2003. Architecture of Succinate Dehydrogenase and Reactive Oxygen Species Generation. *Science* 299:700–704. [4]

Yanoff, L. B., C. M. Menzie, B. Denkinger, et al. 2007. Inflammation and Iron Deficiency in the Hypoferremia of Obesity. *Int. J. Obes.* 31:1412–1419. [12]

Yasmin, S., S. C. Andrews, G. R. Moore, and N. E. Le Brun. 2011. A New Role for Heme, Facilitating Release of Iron from the Bacterioferritin Iron Biomineral. *J. Biol. Chem.* **286**:3473–3483. [4]

Yasuda, H., K. Yoshida, Y. Yasuda, and T. Tsutsui. 2012. Two Age-Related Accumulation Profiles of Toxic Metals. *Curr. Aging Sci.* **5**:105–111. [8]

Yeo, W. S., J. H. Lee, K. C. Lee, and J. H. Roe. 2006. IscR Acts as an Activator in Response to Oxidative Stress for the *Suf* Operon Encoding Fe-S Assembly Proteins. *Mol. Microbiol.* **61**:206–218. [5]

Ylostalo, P., L. Suominen-Taipale, A. Reunanen, and M. Knuuttila. 2008. Association between Body Weight and Periodontal Infection. *J. Clin. Periodontol.* **35**:297–304. [12]

Yoon, M., J. D. Schroeter, A. Nong, et al. 2011. Physiologically Based Pharmacokinetic Modeling of Fetal and Neonatal Manganese Exposure in Humans: Describing Manganese Homeostasis During Development. *Toxicol. Sci.* **122**:297–316. [8]

Yorifuji, T., T. Tsuda, S. Inoue, et al. 2013. Critical Appraisal of the 1977 Diagnostic Criteria for Minamata Disease. *Arch. Environ. Occup. Health* **68**:22–29. [6]

Young, M., W. M. I. Gooch, A. J. Zuckerman, et al. 2001. Comparison of a Triple Antigen and a Single Antigen Recombinant Vaccine for Adult Hepatitis B Vaccination. *J. Med. Virol.* **64**:290–298. [12]

Yuan, X., M. D. Fleming, and I. Hamza. 2013. Heme Transport and Erythropoiesis. *Curr. Opin. Chem. Biol.* **17**:204–211. [13]

Zargar, A. H., N. A. Shah, S. R. Masoodi, et al. 1998. Copper, Zinc, and Magnesium Levels in Non-Insulin Dependent Diabetes Mellitus. *Postgrad. Med. J.* **74**:665–668. [12]

Zawadzka, A. M., R. L. Crawford, and A. J. Paszczynski. 2007. Pyridine-2,6-Bis(Thiocarboxylic Acid) Produced by *Pseudomonas stutzeri* KC Reduces Chromium(VI) and Precipitates Mercury, Cadmium, Lead and Arsenic. *Biometals* **20**:145–158. [4]

Zeng, H., R. Bozym, R. E. Rosenthal, et al. 2005. *In Situ* Measurement of Free Zinc in an Ischemia Model and Cell Culture Using a Ratiometric Fluorescence-Based Biosensor. SPIE Conf. on Advanced Biomedical and Clinical Diagnostic Systems III, ed. T. Vo-Dinh et al., pp. 51–59. San Jose: SPIE. [20]

Zeng, H., M. I. Jackson, W. H. Cheng, and G. F. Combs, Jr. 2011. Chemical Form of Selenium Affects Its Uptake, Transport, and Glutathione Peroxidase Activity in the Human Intestinal Caco-2 Cell Model. *Biol. Trace Elem. Res.* **143**:1209–1218. [2]

Zeng, H., R. B. Thompson, B. P. Maliwal, et al. 2003. Real-Time Determination of Picomolar Free Cu(II) in Seawater Using a Fluorescence-Based Fiber Optic Biosensor. *Anal. Chem.* **75**:6807–6812. [20]

Zeng, L., and L. Zhang. 2011. Efficacy and Safety of Zinc Supplementation for Adults, Children and Pregnant Women with HIV Infection: Systematic Review. *Trop. Med. Int. Health* **16**:1474–1482. [8]

Zeth, K. 2012. Dps Biomineralizing Proteins: Multifunctional Architects of Nature. *Biochem. J.* **445**:297–311. [4]

Zhang, A. S., and C. A. Enns. 2009. Iron Homeostasis: Recently Identified Proteins Provide Insight into Novel Control Mechanisms. *J. Biol. Chem.* **284**:711–715. [2]

Zhang, J., X. D. Wang, B. H. Zhao, and C. X. Li. 2006a. Facile Synthesis of Narrowly Dispersed Silver Nanoparticles in Hydrogel. *Chem. Lett.* **35**:40–41. [15]

Zhang, L., and T. J. Webster. 2012a. Decreased Lung Carcinoma Cell Functions on Select Polymer Nanometer Surface Features. *J. Biomed. Mater. Res.* **100**:94–102. [16]

———. 2012b. Poly-Lactic-Glycolic-Acid Surface Nanotopographies Selectively Decrease Breast Adenocarcinoma Cell Functions. *Nanotechnology* **23**:155101. [16]

Zhang, L., and T. J. Webster. 2013. Effects of Chemically Modified Nanostructured Plga on Functioning of Lung and Breast Cancer Cells. *Int. J. Nanomedicine* **8**:1907–1919. [16]

Zhang, L., and M. H. Wong. 2007. Environmental Mercury Contamination in China: Sources and Impacts. *Environ. Int.* **33**:108–121. [8]

Zhang, P., W. D. Yang, J. S. Liu, and X. L. Zhang. 2006b. Effect of Long-Term Intake of $Y^{3+}$ in Drinking Water on Immune Function of Rats (Article in Chinese). *Wei Sheng Yan Jiu* **35**:279–281. [17]

Zhang, W., P. R. Contag, J. Hardy, et al. 2002. Selection of Potential Therapeutics Based on *in Vivo* Spatiotemporal Transcription Patterns of Heme Oxygenase-1. *J. Molec. Med.* **80**:655–664. [20]

Zhang, W., J. Q. Feng, S. E. Harris, et al. 2001. Rapid *in Vivo* Functional Analysis of Transgenes in Mice Using Whole Body Imaging of Luciferase Expression. *Transgenic Res.* **10**:423–434. [20]

Zhang, Y., and V. N. Gladyshev. 2009. Comparative Genomics of Trace Elements: Emerging Dynamic View of Trace Element Utilization and Function. *Chem. Rev.* **109**:4828–4861. [18]

Zhao, H., A. Konishi, Y. Fujita, et al. 2012. Lipocalin 2 Bolsters Innate and Adaptive Immune Responses to Blood-Stage Malaria Infection by Reinforcing Host Iron Metabolism. *Cell Host Microbe* **12**:705–716. [9, 13]

Zhao, H., R. J. Wong, T. C. Doyle, et al. 2008. Regulation of Maternal and Fetal Hemodynamics by Heme Oxygenase in Mice. *Biol. Reprod.* **78**:744–751. [20]

Zhao, L., P. K. Chu, Y. Zhang, and Z. Wu. 2009. Antibacterial Coatings on Titanium Implants. *J. Biomed. Mater. Res.* **91**:470–480. [16]

Zhao, L., H. Wang, K. Huo, et al. 2011. Antibacterial Nano-Structured Titania Coating Incorporated with Silver Nanoparticles. *Biomaterials* **32**:5706–5716. [16]

Zheng, M., B. Doan, T. D. Schneider, and G. Storz. 1999. OxyR and Soxrs Regulation of *Fur. J. Bacteriol.* **181**:4639–4643. [5]

Zheng, W. 1996. Choroid Plexus and Metal Toxicity. In: *Toxicology of Metals*, ed. L. W. Chang, vol. 1. Boca Raton: CRC Press. [15]

Zimmermann, M. B., and R. F. Hurrell. 2007. Nutritional Iron Deficiency. *Lancet* **370**:511–520. [11]

Zimmermann, M. B., C. Zeder, S. Muthayya, et al. 2008. Adiposity in Women and Children from Transition Countries Predicts Decreased Iron Absorption, Iron Deficiency and a Reduced Response to Iron Fortification. *Int. J. Obes.* **32**:1098–1104. [12]

Zuo, Z., S. Chen, T. Wu, et al. 2011. Tributyltin Causes Obesity and Hepatic Steatosis in Male Mice. *Environ. Toxicol.* **26**:79–85. [12]

# Subject Index